AF616422

Placental Bed Disorders

Placental Bed Disorders

Basic Science and its Translation to Obstetrics

Edited by

Robert Pijnenborg
Katholieke Universiteit Leuven, Department Woman & Child, University Hospital Leuven, Belgium

Ivo Brosens
Leuven Institute for Fertility and Embryology, Leuven, Belgium

Roberto Romero
National Institute of Child Health and Human Development, Perinatology Research Branch, Detroit, USA

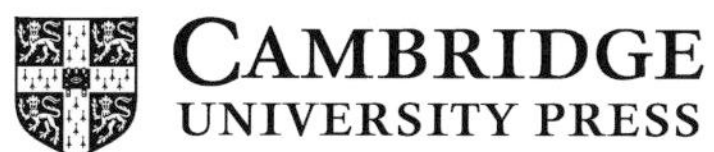

CAMBRIDGE UNIVERSITY PRESS
Cambridge, New York, Melbourne, Madrid, Cape Town, Singapore, São Paulo, Delhi, Dubai, Tokyo

Cambridge University Press
The Edinburgh Building, Cambridge CB2 8RU, UK

Published in the United States of America by Cambridge University Press, New York

www.cambridge.org
Information on this title: www.cambridge.org/9780521517850

First published 2010

Printed in the United Kingdom at the University Press, Cambridge

A catalog record for this publication is available from the British Library

Library of Congress Cataloging in Publication data
Placental bed disorders: basic science and its translation to obstetrics / edited by Robert Pijnenborg, Ivo Brosens, Roberto Romero.
p. ; cm.
Includes bibliographical references and index.
Summary: "The role of the placental bed in normal pregnancy and its complications has been intensively investigated for 50 years, following the introduction of a technique for placental bed biopsy. It is now recognized that disorders of the maternal–fetal interface in humans have been implicated in a broad range of pathologic conditions, including spontaneous abortion, preterm labor, preterm premature rupture of membranes, preeclampsia, intrauterine growth restriction, abruptio placentae and fetal death." – Provided by publisher.
ISBN 978-0-521-51785-0 (hardback : alk. paper)
1. Placenta – Diseases. 2. Placenta. I. Pijnenborg, Robert, 1945– II. Brosens, I. A. III. Romero, Roberto. IV. Title.
[DNLM: 1. Placenta Diseases. 2. Maternal–Fetal Exchange. 3. Placentation. WQ 212 P6979 2010]
RG591.P63 2010
618.3′4–dc22

2009052766

ISBN 978-0-521-51785-0 Hardback

We would like to dedicate this book 'Placental Bed Disorders' to the late William B. Robertson (1923–2008), who was one of the 'founding fathers' of placental bed research.

William (Bill) Robertson began to conduct collaborative research with Geoffrey Dixon, who had been at the Hammersmith Hospital (London, UK) when they both joined efforts at the University of the West Indies in Jamaica (1956–1964). Hypertension in pregnancy and its complications was a common and important problem in Jamaica.

William Robertson and Geoffrey Dixon introduced a new technique in which uterine tissue beneath the placenta was obtained during a cesarean delivery for histological studies. They coined the term 'placental bed biopsy' for this procedure, which led not only to a greater appreciation of the normal development of the maternal blood supply to the placenta, but also demonstrated the vascular changes occurring during hypertensive pregnancies.

This work continued when both Professors Dixon and Robertson returned to London. Further developments occurred in conjunction with Professor Marcel Renaer at the Department of Obstetrics and Gynaecology at the University of Leuven, Belgium, and in particular, with Professor Ivo Brosens, whom Bill had met when he was a Research Fellow with Professor Dixon at the Hammersmith Hospital.

In 1972, Bill Robertson spent a sabbatical year at the Catholic University in Leuven. This was an exciting time for all involved and led to the creation of a new research unit at the Catholic University, which was devoted to improving the understanding of the cellular and molecular biology of the placental bed. This unit expanded with the appointment of Professor Robert Pijnenborg, who joined the unit as Principal Investigator and scientific leader of the unit.

It was fitting that Bill Robertson was invited to open the International Symposium on the Placental Bed held in Leuven in 2007. Unfortunately, he was unable to join us at the meeting. However, committed to the milestone of 50 years of placental bed research, he sent a message to be shared with scientists and clinicians gathered in Belgium. In his message, Bill expressed how as Visiting Professor in the Department of Obstetrics and Gynaecology at the Catholic University he enjoyed some of the most stimulating, productive, and happiest times in his career and life.

We honor Bill Robertson for his contributions, teachings, and inspiring example.

The Editors

Robert Pijnenborg

Ivo Brosens

Roberto Romero

Contents

The color plates will be found between pages 242 and 243.

Contributors

Sayeda Abu-Amero
Clinical and Molecular Genetics
Institute of Child Health
University College London
London, UK

Ivo Brosens
Leuven Institute for Fertility and Embryology
Leuven, Belgium

Jan Brosens
Institute of Reproductive and Developmental Biology
Imperial College School of Hammersmith Hospital
London, UK

Graham J. Burton
Centre for Trophoblast Research
University of Cambridge
Cambridge, UK

Anthony M. Carter
Department of Cardiovascular and Renal Research
University of Southern Denmark
Odense, Denmark

Judith E. Cartwright
Division of Basic Medical Sciences
St George's, University of London
London, UK

Brianna Cloke
Institute of Reproductive and Developmental Biology
Imperial College School of Hammersmith Hospital
London, UK

Christophe L. Depoix
Laboratoire d'Obstétrique
Université Catholique de Louvain
Brussels, Belgium

Sascha Drewlo
Samuel Lunenfeld Research Institute
Mount Sinai Hospital
Toronto, Ontario, Canada

Caroline Dunk
Samuel Lunenfeld Research Institute
Mount Sinai Hospital
Toronto, Ontario, Canada

Qi Fu
Department of Pediatrics
University of Utah School of Medicine
Salt Lake City, USA

Luca Fusi
Institute of Reproductive and Developmental Biology
Imperial College School of Hammersmith Hospital
London, UK

David Haig
Department of Organismic and Evolutionary Biology
Harvard University
Cambridge, USA

Myriam C. Hanssens
Department of Obstetrics and Gynecology
University Hospital Gasthuisberg
Leuven, Belgium

Frans M. Helmerhorst
Department of Gynaecology and Reproductive Medicine and Department of Clinical Epidemiology
Leiden University Medical Center
Leiden, the Netherlands

Pak Chung Ho
Department of Obstetrics and Gynaecology
The University of Hong Kong Queen Mary Hospital
Pokfulam, Hong Kong

Eric Jauniaux
Academic Department of Obstetrics and Gynaecology
UCL EGA Institute for Women's Health
Royal Free and University College Hospitals
London, UK

S. Ananth Karumanchi
Department of Medicine, Obstetrics and Gynecology
Beth Israel Deaconess Medical Center and Harvard Medical School
Boston, MA, USA

Marc J. N. C. Keirse
Department of Obstetrics and Reproductive Medicine
Flinders University
Adelaide, Australia

Eliyahu V. Khankin
Division of Molecular and Vascular Medicine
Beth Israel Deaconess Medical Center
Boston, MA, USA

T. Yee Khong
Department of Histopathology
Women's and Children's Hospital
North Adelaide, Australia

Stephen R. Killick
Department of Obstetrics and Gynaecology
Women and Children's Hospital
Hull, UK

Chong Jai Kim
Perinatology Research Branch
NICHD/NIH/DHHS
Bethesda, Maryland and
Department of Pathology
Wayne State University School of Medicine
Detroit, USA

John C. P. Kingdom
Department of Obstetrics and Gynecology
Mount Sinai Hospital
Toronto, Ontario, Canada

Juan Pedro Kusanovic
Perinatology Research Branch
NICHD/NIH/DHHS
Bethesda, Maryland and
Department of Pathology
Wayne State University School of Medicine
Detroit, USA

Robert H. Lane
Department of Pediatrics
University of Utah School of Medicine
Salt Lake City, USA

Piotr Lesny
Department of Obstetrics and Gynaecology
Women and Children's Hospital
Hull, UK

Robert D. Martin
The Field Museum
Department of Anthropology
Chicago, USA

Robert A. McKnight
Department of Pediatrics
University of Utah School of Medicine
Salt Lake City, USA

Kari K. Melve
Medical Birth Registry of Norway
University of Bergen
Bergen, Norway

Ashley Moffett
Department of Pathology
University of Cambridge
Cambridge, UK

Gudrun E. Moore
Clinical and Molecular Genetics
Institute of Child Health
University College London
London, UK

Linda Morgan
Division of Clinical Chemistry
University Hospital
Queen's Medical Centre
Nottingham, UK

Ernest Hung Yu Ng
Department of Obstetrics and Gynaecology
The University of Hong Kong
Queen Mary Hospital
Pokfulam, Hong Kong

Robert Pijnenborg
Katholieke Universiteit Leuven
Department Woman & Child
University Hospital Leuven
Leuven, Belgium

Leslie Proctor
Department of Obstetrics and Gynecology
Mount Sinai Hospital
Toronto, Ontario, Canada

Sarosh Rana
Obstetrics and Gynecology
Maternal Fetal Medicine Division
Beth Israel Deaconess Medical Center
Boston, MA, USA

Roberto Romero
National Institute of Child Health and Human Development
Perinatology Research Branch
Detroit, USA

Rolv Skjaerven
Medical Birth Registry of Norway
University of Bergen
Bergen, Norway

Gordon C. S. Smith
University Department of Obstetrics and Gynecology
Rosie Maternity Hospital
Cambridge, UK

Robert N. Taylor
Department of Gynecology and Obstetrics
Emory University School of Medicine
Atlanta, USA

May Lee Tjoa
Division of Molecular and Vascular Medicine
Beth Israel Deaconess Medical Centre
Boston, USA

Lars J. Vatten
Department of Public Health
Norwegian University of Science and Technology
Trondheim, Norway

Lisbeth Vercruysse
Department of Obstetrics and Gynecology
University Hospital Gasthuisberg
Leuven, Belgium

Guy St. J. Whitley
Division of Basic Medical Sciences
St George's, University of London
London, UK

Preface

The role of the placental bed in normal pregnancy and its complications has been intensively investigated for 50 years, following the introduction of a technique for placental bed biopsy. It is now recognized that disorders of the maternal–fetal interface in humans have been implicated in a broad range of pathological conditions, including spontaneous abortion, preterm labor, preterm premature rupture of membranes, preeclampsia, intrauterine growth restriction, abruptio placentae, and fetal death.

These clinical disorders (referred to as 'obstetrical syndromes') are the major complications of pregnancy and leading causes of perinatal and maternal morbidity and mortality. Moreover, recent evidence indicates that these disorders have the potential to reprogram the endocrine, metabolic, vascular, and immune responses of the human fetus, and predispose to adult diseases. Thus, premature death from cardiovascular disease (myocardial infarction or stroke), diabetes mellitus, obesity, and hypertension may have their origins in abnormal placental development.

This is the first book devoted exclusively to the anatomy, physiology, immunology, and pathology of the placental bed. Experts in clinical and basic sciences have made important contributions to bring, in a single volume, a large body of literature on the normal and abnormal placental bed. Thus, readers will find informative, well-illustrated, and scholarly contributions in the cell biology of the placental bed, immunology, endocrinology, pathology, genetics, and imaging.

The aim of the book is to inform the reader about the exciting developments in the study of the placental bed as well as the novel approaches to the assessment of this unique tissue interface and its implications for the diagnosis and treatment of complications of pregnancy. It is believed that this book will be essential reading for those interested in clinical obstetrics, maternal–fetal medicine, perinatal pathology, neonatology, and reproductive medicine. Those interested in imaging of the maternal–fetal circulation or its interrogation with Doppler would also benefit from reading this book.

Section 1 Chapter 1

Introducing the placental bed

The placental bed in a historical perspective

Robert Pijnenborg

Katholieke Universiteit Leuven, Department Woman & Child, University Hospital Leuven, Leuven, Belgium

The discovery of the placental bed vasculature

Placental vasculature, in particular the relationship between maternal and fetal blood circulations, has been a contentious issue for a long time. It was indeed a matter of dispute whether or not the fetal blood circulation was separate from or continuous with the circulation of the mother as stated by the Roman physician Galen (129–200). The Renaissance anatomist Julius Caesar Arantius (1530–1589) is usually quoted for being the first who explicitly denied the existence of any vascular connection between the mother and the fetus *in utero* [1,2]. Although this opinion was seemingly based on careful dissections of human placentas *in situ*, he obviously did not have the tools to trace small blood vessels in sufficient detail to provide full support for this idea. Moreover, before William Harvey (1578–1657) anatomists did not understand the relationship between arteries and veins, and thus their knowledge about the uteroplacental blood flow in the placenta must have been rather confused.

The brothers William (1718–1783) and John Hunter (1728–1793) are credited for having demonstrated the separation of maternal and fetal circulations by using colored wax injections of human placentas *in utero*. It was probably the younger brother John who did all the work, and he claimed afterwards most of the credit for this finding [3]. In his magnificent *Anatomy of the human gravid uterus* (1774) William Hunter included the first drawing of spiral arteries ('convoluted arteries'), in what must have been the very first illustration of a human placental bed (Fig. 1.1) [4]. These 'convoluted arteries' are embedded in the decidualized uterine mucosa, the term 'decidua' being used for the first time by William Hunter to describe the 'membrane' enveloping the conceptus, which is discarded at parturition (Latin *decidere*, to fall off). This obviously referred to the decidua capsularis, typical for humans and anthropoid apes, which is formed as a result of the deep interstitial implantation of the blastocyst in these species. John Hunter, however, pointed out that there is also a 'decidua basalis' underneath the placenta. In a tubal pregnancy case he noticed that a similar tissue had developed within the uterus, and he therefore concluded that the decidua originates from the uterine mucosa [5].

Early ideas about placental function

Hunter's demonstration of separate vascular systems coincided with Lavoisier's discovery of oxygen and its role in respiration. It was found that the uptake of oxygen by the blood is associated with a shift in color from a dark to a light red. This color-shift was observed in lungs as well as in the gills of fish, and it was Erasmus Darwin (1731–1802), grandfather of Charles Darwin, who pointed out that exactly the same happens in the placenta [6]. Furthermore, Erasmus Darwin tried to understand how the oxygenated maternal blood is delivered to the fetus. He had noticed that after separation of the placenta, uterine blood vessels start bleeding, while the placental vessels do not. For him this was an indication that the terminations of the placental vessels must be inserted into the uterine vasculature while remaining closed off from the maternal circulation. He thought that structures, referred to as 'lacunae of the placentae' by John Hunter, might represent 'cells' filled with maternal blood from the uterine arteries. It is obvious that these 'cells' referred to compartments of the intervillous space. Erasmus Darwin went as far as to equate these 'lacunae of the placentae' to the 'air-cells' (alveoli) of the lungs. Also interesting is the comparison he made with cotyledonary placentas of cows, which after separation do not result in bleeding of uterine blood vessels. Of course he was unaware of structural differences between the human hemochorial

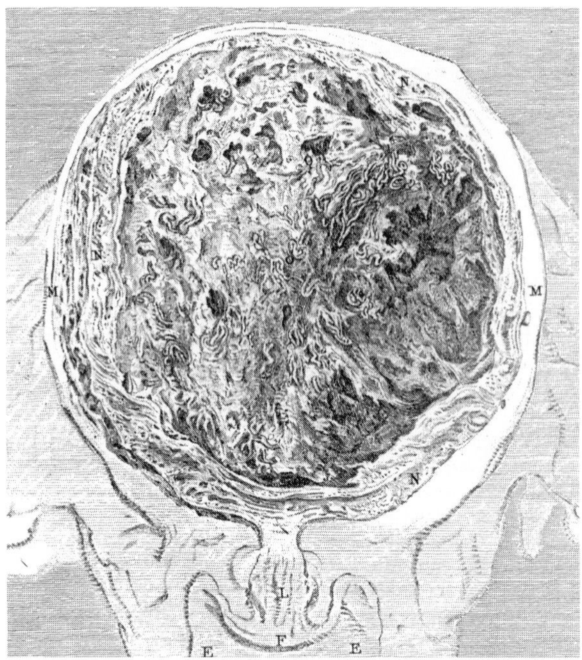

Fig. 1.1 View of the placental bed after removal of the placenta, showing stretches of spiral arteries. Illustration from William Hunter's *Anatomy of the human gravid uterus* (1774).

and the cow's epitheliochorial placenta. His speculation on a 'greater power of contractions' of uterine arteries in cows almost suggests an intuitive grasp about differences in uteroplacental blood supply between humans and cows [7], foreshadowing the later concept of 'physiologically changed' spiral arteries in the human [8].

While the ideas of eighteenth century investigators about the respiratory function of the placenta were essentially correct, opinions about a possible nutritive function of the placenta were very confused. The Scottish anatomist Alexander Monro (1697–1767) thought that, analogous to nutrient uptake in the intestines, a 'succulent' substance appeared between the uterine muscle and the placenta (i.e. the decidual region), which he thought would be absorbed by 'lacteal vessels' of the placenta [2]. In his opinion these placental vessels had to be open-tipped and had to cross the placental–uterine border for absorbing the uterine nutritious material. This idea was of course refuted by Hunter's injection experiments, which clearly showed that fetal vessels never end up in the uterine wall. Transmembrane transport mechanisms for glucose, lipid and amino acid transfer were obviously unknown at that time, and investigators like Erasmus Darwin therefore tended to minimize the idea of a possible nutritive function of the placenta. Instead he favored the view that the amniotic fluid was the main source of fetal nutrition, an idea that he had borrowed from William Harvey, but which became overruled by later findings.

The discovery of trophoblast invasion

A major technological advance in the nineteenth century was the perfection of the microscope together with the development of histological techniques for tissue sectioning and staining. The first microscopic images of the human placenta were obtained in 1832 by Ernst Heinrich Weber, revealing the organization of fetal blood vessels within villi, which are lined by a 'membrane' separating the fetal from the maternal blood. For several decades there was uncertainty about the nature of this outer villous 'membrane', and it was originally thought that this layer represented the maternal lining (endothelium) of the extremely dilated uterine vasculature [9]. The origin of this tissue layer and the real nature of the intervillous space could only be clarified by histological investigations from early implantation stages onwards. An early pioneer was the Dutch embryologist Ambrosius Hubrecht (1853–1915), who undertook the study of implantation in what he considered to be representative species of primitive mammals, hedgehogs and shrews. The idea behind this work was that the implantation events in primitive mammals might offer clues about the evolution of viviparity. His famous hedgehog study revealed early appearance of maternal blood lacunae engulfed by the outer layer of extraembryonic cells. He considered the latter as feeding cells and hence introduced the term 'trophoblast' [10].

Slowly investigators began to realize the invasive potential of this trophoblast. The French anatomist Mathias Duval (1844–1907) was probably the first to recognize the invasion of trophoblast (placenta-derived 'endovascular plasmodium' in his terminology) into endometrial arteries, in this case in the rat [11]. He published his findings in 1892, but he was not the first to have seen endovascular cells in maternal vessels. Twenty years before, in 1870, Carl Friedländer had reported the presence of endovascular cells in 'uterine sinuses' of a human uterus of 8 months' pregnancy [12]. He notified the rare occurrence of arteries in this specimen, obviously not realizing that these might have been transformed by endovascular cell invasion. He was unable to decide whether these cells

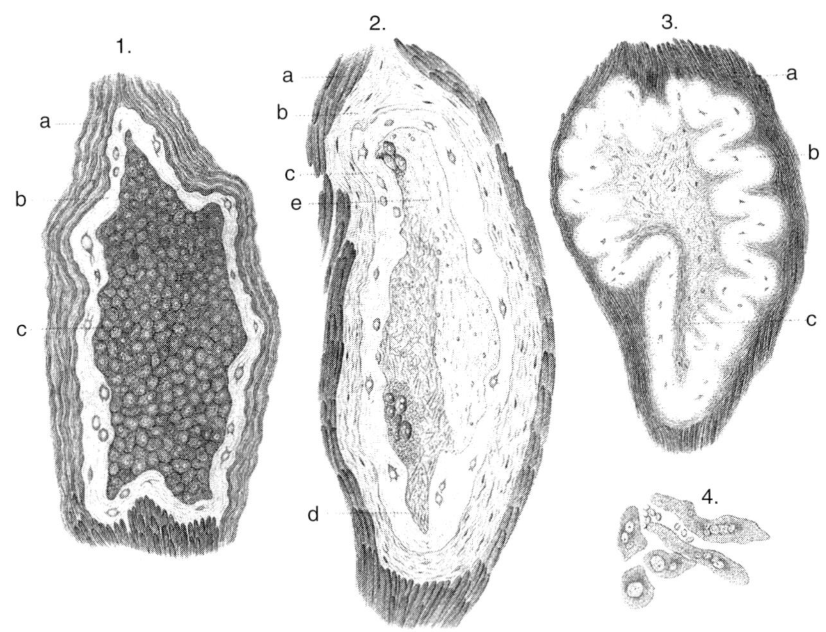

Fig. 1.2 'Uterine sinus' showing a plug of endovascular cells (1) and a similar vessel with embedded cells (2) in an 8 months' pregnant uterus. (3) shows a similar vessel in a postpartum uterus. Details of so-called multinuclear endovascular cells are shown in (4). Reproduced from Friedländer (1870).

were derived from the placenta or the surrounding maternal tissue, but he reported their presence as deep as the inner myometrium. His illustrations show two vessels of his 8 months specimen, one completely plugged, the other containing only a few intraluminal cells (Fig. 1.2). In the latter he noted the presence of a thickened homogeneous 'membrane' containing dispersed cells in the vessel wall (Fig. 1.2, parts 1b and 2c, recognizable as the fibrinoid layer with embedded trophoblast), and also an organized thrombus with young connective tissue (Fig 1.2, part 2e, recognizable as a thickened intima overlying the fibrinoid layer). He also obtained a postpartum uterus in which he thought he could recognize similar 'sinuses' (Fig 1.2, part 3). Surprisingly, Friedländer thought that most intravascular cells were multinuclear (Fig 1.2, part 4). He reasoned that the presence of endovascular cells must considerably slow down and even interrupt the maternal blood supply to the placenta, and considered that failed vascular plugging might result in intrauterine bleeding and maternal death. Friedländer's contemporaries favored the idea that the intravascular cells must have been sloughed off from the maternal vascular wall. It wasn't until the early twentieth century that investigators such as Otto Grosser [13] began to consider these cells as trophoblastic.

The actual depth of invasion was underrated for a long time, partly because of the increasing popularity of the decidual barrier concept. This idea originated in 1887 from Raissa Nitabuch's description of a fibrinoid layer which was thought to form a continuous separation zone between the anchoring 'chorionic' cells in the basal plate and the underlying decidua [14]. It is interesting that she also described cross-sections of decidual spiral arteries close to the intervillous space, mentioning (but not illustrating) a breaching of the endothelium by cells which were morphologically similar to those occurring on the inside of the fibrinoid layer. She did not further comment upon the nature of these cells, and neither did she quote Friedländer's 1870 publication. Unfortunately, the alleged barrier function of Nitabuch's layer was overemphasized in later years, and was also thought to act in the opposite sense by warding off a maternal immune attack on the semi-allogeneic trophoblastic cells [15]. These early concepts had to be considerably modified in later years, when it became clear that deep trophoblast invasion and associated spiral artery remodeling are essential for a healthy pregnancy. Indeed, this research received a considerable boost within the clinical context of preeclampsia and fetal growth restriction, as will be described in Chapters 2 and 3.

Conclusion

The phenomenon of trophoblast invasion – for a long time considered as merely playing a role in anchoring the placenta – has to be understood in the context of growing insights into placental function, notably fetal respiration and nutrition. The elucidation of the anatomical relationship between fetal and maternal circulations was therefore of fundamental importance. Early observations of trophoblast invasion into the spiral arteries set the stage for understanding the maternal blood supply to the placenta via the spiral arteries of the placental bed. This historical context provides an appropriate starting point for understanding the development of the present research directions, which are closely linked to the clinical problems of preeclampsia and fetal growth restriction.

References

1. Needham J. *A history of embryology*. Cambridge: Cambridge University Press; 1934: pp. 86–7.
2. Boyd J D, Hamilton W J. Historical survey. In: *The human placenta*. Cambridge: W Heffer & Sons; 1970: pp. 1–9.
3. Hunter J. On the structure of the placenta. In: *Observations on certain parts of the animal oeconomy*. Philadelphia: Haswell, Barrington & Haswell; 1840: pp. 93–103 [reprint of the original 1786 edition, with notes by Richard Owen].
4. Hunter W. *Anatomia uterina humani gravidi tabulis illustrata (The anatomy of the human gravid uterus exhibited in figures)*. Birmingham, Alabama: Gryphon Editions; 1980 [facsimile edition of the original edition by John Baskerville, Birmingham; 1774].
5. De Wit F. A historical study on theories of the placenta to 1900. *J Hist Med Allied Sci* 1959; **14**: 360–74.
6. Darwin E. Of the oxygenation of the blood in the lungs, and in the placenta. In: *Zoonomia; or the laws of organic life*, 3rd ed. London: J. Johnson; 1801: ch 38.
7. Pijnenborg R, Vercruysse L. Erasmus Darwin's enlightened views on placental function. *Placenta* 2007; **28**: 775–8.
8. Brosens I, Robertson W B, Dixon H G. The physiological response of the vessels of the placental bed to normal pregnancy. *J Pathol Bacteriol* 1967; **93**: 569–79.
9. Pijnenborg R, Vercruysse L. Shifting concepts of the fetal-maternal interface: a historical perspective. Placenta 2008; **29** Suppl: A S20–S25.
10. Hubrecht A A W. Studies in mammalian embryology. I. The placentation of *Erinaceus europaeus*, with remarks on the phylogeny of the placenta. *Q J Microsc Sci* 1889; **30**: 283–404.
11. Duval M. *Le placenta des rongeurs*. Paris: Felix Alcan; 1892.
12. Friedländer C. *Physiologisch-anatomische Untersuchungen über den Uterus*. Leipzig: Simmel; 1870: pp. 31–6.
13. Grosser O. *Frühentwicklung, Eihautbildung und Placentation des Mensch und der Säugetiere*. Munich: J.F. Bergmann; 1927.
14. Nitabuch R. *Beiträge zur Kenntniss der menschlichen Placenta*. Bern: Stämpfli'sche Buchdruckerei; 1887.
15. Bardawil W A, Toy B L. The natural history of choriocarcinoma: problems of immunity and spontaneous regression. *Ann N Y Acad Sci* 1959; **80**: 197–261.

Chapter 2

Unraveling the anatomy

Ivo Brosens

Leuven Institute for Fertility and Embryology Leuven, Belgium

Introduction

Although the gross anatomy of the maternal blood supply to and drainage from the intervillous space was well documented by William Hunter [1] in 1774 a considerable degree of confusion persisted, and in particular the understanding of the anatomical structure of the 'curling' arteries remained incomplete and often not based on data. Therefore as an introduction to the chapters on placental bed vascular disorders the early literature on the maternal blood supply to the placenta is briefly reviewed.

The term 'placental bed' was introduced 50 years ago by Dixon and Robertson [2] and can be grossly described as that part of the decidua and adjoining myometrium which underlies the placenta and whose primary function is the maintenance of an adequate blood supply to the intervillous space of the placenta. Certainly, there is no sharp anatomical demarcation line between the placental bed and the surrounding structures, but, as this part of the uterine wall has its own particular functional and pathological aspects, it has proven to be a most useful term for describing the maternal part of the placenta in contrast to the fetal portion.

The uteroplacental arteries

Anatomically the uteroplacental arteries can be defined as the radial and spiral arteries which link the arcuate arteries in the outer third of the myometrium to the intervillous space of the placenta. Before reaching the myometrio-decidual junction, the radial arteries usually split into two or three spiral arteries. When they enter the endometrium the spiral arteries are separated from each other by a 1–6 mm gap [3]. Small arteries, the so-called basal arterioles, branch off from the proximal part of the spiral arteries and vascularize the myometrio-decidual junction and the basal layer of the decidua. They are considered to be less responsive, if at all, to cyclic maternal hormones [4].

Two comments are appropriate here. First, some confusion existed as to whether the spiral arteries of the placental bed should be called 'arteries', which was commonly used in German literature, or 'arterioles', which was more common in the English literature. In view of the size of the spiral vessels, which communicate with the intervillous space, the terminology of 'spiral arteries' was adopted for these vessels in order to distinguish them from the 'spiral arterioles' of the decidua vera. A second comment relates to the spiral course as described by Kölliker [5]. Because during pregnancy these arteries increase in length as well as in size, Bloch [6] suggested that in the human the terminal part of the spiral artery is no longer spiral or cork-screw, but has a more undulating course as was demonstrated in the Rhesus monkey (*Macaca mulatta*) by Ramsey [7].

The origin of placental septa and the orifices of spiral arteries have been the subject of great controversy. Bumm [8,9] pointed out that the arteries are mainly lying in the decidual projections and septa, and eject their blood from the side of the cotyledon into the intervillous space (Fig. 2.1). Bumm's statement has been quoted as implying that the arteries open in the intervillous space near the chorionic plate, while Bumm obviously regarded the subchorionic blood as somewhat venous in nature. Wieloch [10] and Stieve [11] have corrected Bumm's observation in that they specified that the spiral arteries mainly open at the base of the septa. Boyd and Hamilton [4] confirmed that the septa are of dual maternal and trophoblastic origin and that arterial orifices are scattered more or less at random over the basal plate. The orifices of several arteries may be grouped closely together and, in individual vessels, are usually at their terminal portions. Spiral arteries may have initially multiple openings. Such multiple openings can later become separated by the straightening out and dilatation of the artery and the unwinding of the coils during placental growth. When multiple openings are present the segment of the artery between successive ones may show obliteration of the lumen.

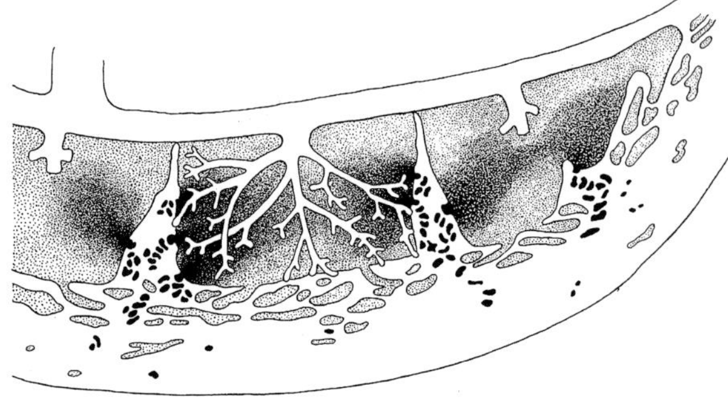

Fig. 2.1 Diagrammatic representation of the course of the maternal circulation through the intervillous space of the placenta. After Bumm [9].

Attempts to count the number of spiral arteries communicating with the intervillous space have been made by several investigators. Klein [12] counted in one separated placenta 15 maternal cotyledons with 87 arteries and 39 veins and in a second 10 cotyledons with 45 arteries and 27 veins. Spanner [13] working with a corrosion preparation of about 6 months' gestation found 94 arteries communicating with the intervillous space. Boyd [3] made calculations of total numbers based on sample counts of openings of the spiral arteries in the basal plate in three placentae of the third and fourth months of pregnancy. The calculations for full-term placentae varied between 180 and 320 openings but all three counts can only be considered as first appreciations. On the other hand, Ramsey [7] showed by serial sections in the Rhesus monkey the uneven distribution of arterial communications with the intervillous space and suggested that partial counts may have introduced errors in the calculations. In an anatomical reconstruction of two-fifths of the maternal side of a placenta *in situ* at term Brosens and Dixon [14] confirmed the irregular arrangement of septa and arterial and venous openings. All arteries opened into the intervillous space by a solitary orifice. They found in a normal placenta 45 openings for a surface area of 32 cm^2 [15] and in a uterus with placenta *in situ* from a woman with severe preeclampsia 10 spiral arteries for a surface area of 7 cm^2 [16], which in both cases amounts to one spiral artery for every 0.7 cm^2 of placental bed.

A bird's-eye view of the three-dimensional basal plate shows septa of various sizes with the majority of arterial orifices at the base of a septum. Septa are likely to represent uplifted basal plate reflecting differences in depth of decidual trophoblast invasion and resulting in a conchiform base for the anchoring of a fetal cotyledon. Arterioles high up in the septa and without an orifice into the intervillous space are likely to be basal arterioles.

The anatomy of the venous drainage has also been the subject of much discussion. Kölliker [5] stressed in 1879 the role of the marginal sinus, partly lying in the placenta and partly in the decidua vera. Spanner [13] revived this theory in 1935, however without quoting Kölliker. The anatomical work by many authors has subsequently shown that venous drainage occurs all over the basal plate. The veins fuse beneath the basal plate to form the so-called 'venous lakes' [7]. The term 'sinusoid' has been applied to these vessels, but has caused much confusion in the literature as the term has been used for the intervillous space and the spiral arteries.

The question of arteriovenous anastomoses in the decidua arose when Hertig and Rock [17] described extensive anastomoses in the decidua. Bartelmez [18], however, after re-examination of the original histological sections of Hertig and Rock [17] cast doubt on the drawings published by these authors in 1941 and the existence of such shunts was later disproved. Recently, Schaaps and collaborators [19] used three-dimensional sonography and anatomical reconstruction to investigate the placental bed vasculature and demonstrated an extensive vascular anastomotic network in the myometrium underlying the placenta. No such network was seen outside the placental bed. It can be speculated that the subendometrial network is formed by the hypertrophied basal arterioles and veins in the placental bed.

Pregnancy changes, intraluminal cells and giant cells

The morphological changes of the uteroplacental arteries were extensively studied, mainly by German investigators, around the turn of the last century and particularly in the context of the mechanism preventing the uterus from bleeding during the postpartum period.

Almost all authors before 1925 agreed that thickening of the intima occurs in myometrial arteries of the uterus as a result of gestation. Wermbter [20] in an extensive study showed that this change is not specific for pregnancy, but is also related to some degree with parity. The importance attached by these authors to intimal thickening was that under the influence of contractions the vessel becomes occluded and that the projections caused by the intimal proliferation could act as supports for the formation of thrombi causing primary occlusion of the vessel in the post-partum period. The large myometrial arteries of the multigravida are characterized by an abundance of elastic and collagenous tissue in the adventitia, although the amount of increase in elastic tissue does not necessarily correlate with the number of gestations.

While most authors seemed to be agreed on the changes in the myometrial arteries much confusion and discussion existed with respect to vessel changes in the placental bed. Friedländer [21] described in 1870 an outstanding vessel change in the placental bed, which was wrongly described by Leopold [22] as 'die Spontane Venenthrombose'. Friedänder's description is as follows:

> *One finds .... that many of these blood spaces are surrounded by a moderately thick coat e.g. for a sinus of 0.5 mm diameter a coat as thick as 0.04 mm, which contains many apparently large cells with prominent nuclei and a clear, nearly homogeneous ground substance staining intensively with Carmin stain .... The next remarkable phenomenon is that the content of the sinus is no longer made up of red and white blood cells, but contains, in a more or less great number very dark, large and granulated cells .... These cells are sometimes lying singly in the centre of the sinus, sometimes adherent to and lining, as a continuous epithelium, a part of the wall, and, at last, can become so numerous that they completely block the sinus only leaving here and there gaps for an occasional red blood cell.*

In 1904 Schickele [23] drew attention to the fact that the vessel changes described by Friedländer [21] and Leopold [22] occurred mainly in arteries and only occasionally in veins. However, they were incorrect in thinking that the cells in the arterial lumen were most marked in late pregnancy as their description included two different changes which, although related to each other, appear in the spiral arteries at a different time during the course of pregnancy. A confusing terminology has been used to describe the changes which occur in the wall of the spiral arteries communicating with the intervillous space, such as 'physiologische regressive Metamorphose', 'hyalin Rohr mit grössen Zellen', fibrinoid and hyaline structures of bizarre outline in collapsed vessels, and diffuse thickening of the entire wall.

The intrusive cells in the lumen as described by Friedländer [21] were intensively studied by Boyd and Hamilton [24] and Hamilton and Boyd [25,26] using their large collection of uterine specimens with the placenta *in situ*. They demonstrated the continuity of these cells with the cytotrophoblastic cells of the basal plate of the placenta. The intraluminal cells first appear in the arteries when the latter are being tapped by the invading trophoblast; the maternal blood then reaches the intervillous space by percolating through the gaps between the intraluminal cells. They decided that the most acceptable explanation was that these cells were derived from the cytotrophoblastic shell and migrated antidromically along the vessel lumen. The intraluminal cells can pass several centimeters along a spiral artery and, indeed, may be found in its myometrial segment. Such plugging by intraluminal cells was illustrated in a myometrial artery from a pregnant uterus with a fetus of 118 mm CR length [4]. The plugs were present in all the spiral arteries of the basal plate during the middle 3 months of pregnancy, although their numbers varied, and they disappeared altogether in the last months. They were never observed in the veins. Boyd and Hamilton [4] speculated that the intravascular plugs damped down the arterial pressure in arteries that had already lost their contractility.

Kölliker [5] was the first to describe in 1879 the giant cells ('Riesenzellen') in the placental bed and indicated that these cells are restricted to the decidua basalis. Opinions diverged on the origin of these cells. The fetal origin was demonstrated by Hamilton and Boyd [26] when they examined uteri with placenta *in situ* at closely related time intervals during pregnancy and observed continuity in the outgrowth of fetal syncytial elements into the maternal tissue. Suggested functions of the giant cells were the production of enzymes, possibly to 'soften up' the maternal tissue, and the elaboration of hormones. Hamilton and Boyd had the impression that there was no marked effect, cytolytic or otherwise, of the giant cells on the maternal tissue. These cells seemed to push aside the maternal cells and to dissolve the surrounding reticulin and collagen, but there was no apparent destructive effect on the adjacent maternal cells. The possibility of hormone production by giant cells was suggested by their histological and histochemical appearance.

Functional aspects

In the early 1950s the hemodynamic aspects of the maternal circulation of the placenta were investigated using different new functional techniques such as the determination of the ^{24}Na clearance time in the intervillous space [27], cineradiographic visualization of the uteroplacental circulation in the monkey [28,29], and determination of the pressure in the intervillous space [30].

Measurements of the amount of maternal blood flowing through the uterus and the intervillous space made by Browne and Veall [27] and Assali and coworkers [31] showed that maternal blood flows through the uterus during the third trimester at a rate of approximately 750 ml/min, and 600 ml/min through the placenta. Browne and Veall [27] found a slight but progressive slowing of the flow in late pregnancy up to term. However, in the presence of maternal hypertension a considerable decrease of flow was found and the extent of change appeared to be related to the severity of maternal hypertension.

Pathology of uteroplacental arteries

Vascular lesions of the uteroplacental arteries have been described since the beginning of the last century. Seitz [32] described in 1903 the intact uteri with placentae from two eclamptic patients with abruptio placentae and noted a proliferative and degenerative lesion in the spiral arteries, with narrowing and even occlusion of the vascular lumen. He found occluded arteries underlying an infarcted area of the *in situ* placenta, and related the vascular and decidual degeneration to the toxemic state. In later literature this excellent report on the uteroplacental pathology in eclampsia has been completely ignored, probably because at that time most authors were mainly interested in the presence of inflammatory cells in the decidua as a possible cause of eclampsia.

The delivered placenta and fetal membranes were for many years the commonest method of obtaining material for the study of spiral artery pathology, and there were large discrepancies between the findings in this material. In preeclampsia lesions such as acute degenerative arteriolitis [33], acute atherosis [34], and arteriosclerosis [35] were described.

Dixon and Robertson [2] introduced 50 years ago at the University of Jamaica the technique of placental bed biopsy at the time of cesarean section, while the Leuven group [36,37] obtained biopsies after vaginal delivery using sharpened ovum forceps. Both groups described hypertensive changes that showed the characteristic features of vessels exposed to systemic hypertension, i.e. hyalinization of true arterioles and intimal hyperplasia with medial degeneration and proliferative fibrosis of small arteries.

Physiological changes of placental bed spiral arteries

The method of placental bed biopsy produced useful material, but nevertheless was criticized by Hamilton and Boyd (personal communication). They strongly recommended the examination of intact uteri with the placenta *in situ* for the simple reason that the placental bed is such a battlefield that fetal and maternal tissues are hard to distinguish on biopsy material and maternal vessels are disrupted after placental separation. In 1958, independent from the British group in Jamaica, the Department of Obstetrics and Gynaecology of the Catholic University of Leuven had also started to collect placental bed biopsies, and in 1963 they began to collect uteri with the placenta *in situ* [37,38]. The hysterectomy specimens were obtained from women under normal and abnormal conditions whereas today tubal sterilization would have been performed at the time of cesarean section. The technique for keeping the placenta *in situ* at the time of cesarean hysterectomy was rather heroic. Immediately after delivery of the baby the uterine cavity was tightly packed with towels in order to reduce uterine retraction and prevent the placenta from separating from the wall. The large uterine specimens with placenta *in situ* were examined by semiserial sections to trace the course of spiral arteries from the basal plate to deep into the myometrium. As a result Brosens, Robertson and Dixon [39] described in 1967 the structural alterations in the uteroplacental arteries as part of the physiological response to the pregnancy and introduced for these vascular adaptations the term 'physiological changes' (Fig. 2.2). In 1972 the same authors [40] published the observation that preeclampsia is associated with defective physiological changes of the uteroplacental arteries in the junctional zone myometrium.

In subsequent studies the remodeling of the spiral arteries was investigated during the early stages of pregnancy. While abortion for medical reasons was allowed in the UK, it was not uncommon for older women to have a hysterectomy. When Geoffrey Dixon moved to the Academic Department of Obstetrics and Gynaecology of the University of Bristol in the 1970s he started to collect uteri with the fetus and placenta *in situ* from terminations of pregnancy by hysterectomy. The Bristol collection of uteri with placenta *in situ* was the starting point for the study of the development of uteroplacental arteries by Pijnenborg and colleagues [41].

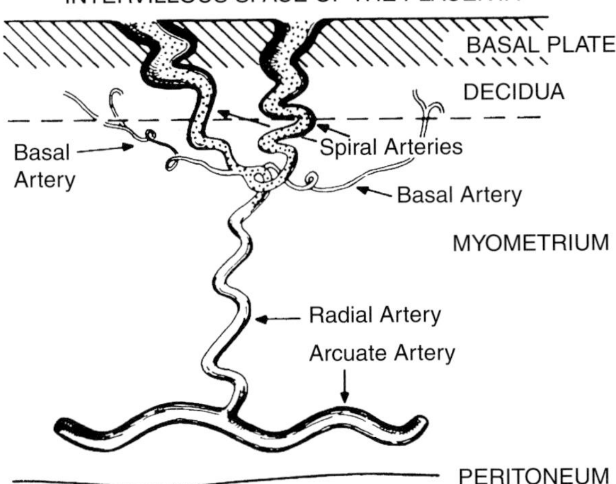

Fig. 2.2 Diagram of the maternal blood supply to the placental bed and intervillous space of the placenta showing physiological changes of the spiral arteries in the basal plate, decidua and junctional zone myometrium. After Brosens *et al.* [39].

Conclusions

The history outlined above illustrates the vascular complexity of deep placentation in humans. The spiral artery anatomy as well as the vascular pathology were only revealed after studying uteri with *in situ* placentae. There is no doubt that the main issue has been the recognition of the structural adaptation of the spiral arteries in the placental bed and the association of defective deep placentation with clinical conditions such as preeclampsia.

The main challenge today is to understand the mechanisms of the vascular adaptations and the role of the trophoblast and the maternal tissues in the interactions that can lead to a spectrum of obstetrical disorders.

References

1. Hunter W. *An anatomic description of the human gravid uterus.* London: Baskerville; 1774.
2. Dixon H G, Robertson W B. A study of vessels of the placental bed in normotensive and hypertensive women. *J Obstet Gynaecol Br Emp* 1958; **65**: 803–9.
3. Boyd J D. Morphology and physiology of the uteroplacental circulation: In: Villee C A, ed. *Gestation, transactions of the second conference the Josiah Macy Foundation.* New York: Macy Found; 1955: pp. 132–94.
4. Boyd J D, Hamilton W J. *The human placenta.* Cambridge: W. Heffer & Sons; 1970.
5. Kölliker A. *Entwicklungsgeschichte des Menschen und der höheren Tiere*, 2nd ed. Leipzig: Engelmann; 1879.
6. Bloch L. Ueber den Bau der menschlichen Placenta. *Beitr Path Anat* 1889; **4**: 557–92.
7. Ramsey E M. Circulation in the maternal placenta of primates. *Am J Obstet Gynec* 1954; **87**: 1–14.
8. Bumm E. Zur Kenntniss der Uteroplacentargefässe. *Arch Gynäk* 1980; **37**: 1–15.
9. Bumm E. Ueber die Entwicklung der mütterlichen Bluttlaufes in der menschlichen Placenta. *Arch Gynäk* 1893; **43**: 181–95.
10. Wieloch J. Beitrag zur Kenntnis des Baues der Placenta. *Arch Gynäk* 1923; **118**: 112–9.
11. Stieve H. Die Entwicklung und der Bau der mensclichen Placenta. 2. Zotten, Zottenraumglitter und Gefässe in der zweiten Hälfte der Schwangerschaft. *Z Mikr-anat Forsch* 1941; **50**: 1–120.
12. Klein G. Makroskopische Verhälten der Utero-Placentargefässe. In: Hofmeier, ed. *Die menschliche Placenta.* Leipzig: Wiesbaden; 1890: pp. 72–87.
13. Spanner R. Mütterlicher und kindlicher Kreislauf der menschlichen Placenta und seine Strombahnen. *Z Anat Entw* 1935; **105**: 163–242.
14. Brosens I, Dixon H G. The anatomy of the maternal side of the placenta. *J Obstet Gynaec Br Cwth* 1966; **73**: 357–63.
15. Brosens I A. The utero-placental vessels at term: the distribution and extent of physiological changes. *Trophoblast Res* 1988; **3**: 61–7.
16. Brosens I, Renaer M. On the pathogenesis of placental infarcts in pre-eclampsia. *J Obstet Gynaec Br Cwth* 1972; **79**: 794–9.
17. Hertig A T, Rock J. Two human ova of the pre-villous stage having an ovulation age of about eleven and twelve days respectively. *Contrib Embryol Carneg Inst* 1941; **29**: 127–56.
18. Bartelmez G W. Premenstrual and menstrual ischemia and the myth of endometrial arteriovenous anastomoses. *Am J Anat* 1956; **98**: 69–95.
19. Schaaps J-P, Tsatsaris V, Goffin F *et al.* Shunting the intervillous space: new concepts in human uteroplacental vascularization. *Am J Obstet Gynec* 2005; **192**: 323–32.
20. Wermbter F. Über den Umbau der Uterusgefäße in verschiedenen Monaten der Schwangerschaft erst- und mehrgebärender Frauen unter Berücksichtigung des Verhaltens der Zwischensubstanz der Arterienwände. *Virchow's Arch Path Anat* 1925; **257**: 249–83.
21. Friedländer C. *Physiologisch-anatomische Untersuchungen über den Uterus.* Leipzig: Simmel; 1870.

22. Leopold G. Die spontane Thrombose zahlreicher Uterinvenen in den letsten Monaten der Schwangerschaft. *Zblt Gynäk* 1877; **1**: 49.

23. Schickele G. Die vorzeitige Lösung der normal sitzenden Placenta. *Beitr Geburtsh Gynäk* 1904; **8**: 337.

24. Boyd J D, Hamilton W J. Cells in the spiral arteries of the pregnant uterus. *J Anat* 1956; **90**: 595.

25. Hamilton W J, Boyd J D. Development of the human placenta in the first three months of gestation. *J Anat* 1960; **94**: 297–328.

26. Hamilton W J, Boyd J D. Trophoblast in human utero-placental arteries. *Nature* 1966; **212**: 906–8.

27. Browne J C M, Veall N. The maternal placental blood flow in normotensive and hypertensive women. *J Obstet Gynaecol Br Emp* 1953; **60**: 141–7.

28. Ramsey E M. Circulation in the intervillous space of the primate placenta. *Am J Obstet Gynecol* 1962; **84**: 1649–63.

29. Martin Jr C B, McGaughey Jr H S, Kaiser I H, Donner M W, Ramsey E M. Intermittent functioning of the uteroplacental arteries. *Am J Obstet Gynecol* 1964; **90**: 819–23.

30. Alvarez H, Caldeyro-Barcia R. Contractility of the human uterus recorded by new methods. *Surg Gynec Obstet* 1950; **91**: 1–13.

31. Assali N S, Douglass Jr R A, Baird W W, Nicholson D B, Suyemoto R. Measurement of uterine blood flow and uterine metabolism. II. The techniques of catheterization and cannulation of the uterine veins and sampling of arterial and venous blood in pregnant women. *Am J Obstet Gynecol* 1953; **66**: 11–17.

32. Seitz L. Zwei sub partu verstorbene Fälle van Eklampsie mit vorzeitiger Lösung der normal sitzenden Placenta: mikroskopische Befunde an Placenta und Eihäuten. *Arch Gynäk* 1903; **69**: 71.

33. Hertig A T. Vascular pathology in the hypertensive albuminuric toxemias of pregnancy. *Clinics* 1945; **4**: 602–14.

34. Zeek P M, Assali N S. Vascular changes in the decidua associated with eclamptogenic toxemia of pregnancy. *Am J Clin Pathol* 1950; **20**: 1099–109.

35. Marais W D. Human decidual spiral arterial studies. Part III. Histological patterns and some clinical implications of decidual spiral arteriolosclerosis. *J Obstet Gynaecol Br Cwth* 1962; **69**: 225–33.

36. Brosens I. A study of the spiral arteries in the decidua basalis in normotensive and hypertensive pregnancies. *J Obstet Gynaec Br Cwth* 1964; **71**: 222–30.

37. Renaer M, Brosens I. Spiral arterioles in the decidua basalis in hypertensive complications of pregnancy. *Ned Tijdschr Verlosk Gynaecol* 1963; **63**: 103–318.

38. Brosens I. *The challenge of reproductive medicine at Catholic universities*. Leuven: Peeters-Dudley Publications; 2006.

39. Brosens I, Robertson W B, Dixon H G. The physiological response of the vessels of the placental bed to normal pregnancy. *J Pathol Bacteriol* 1967; **93**: 569–79.

40. Brosens I A, Robertson W B, Dixon H G. The role of the spiral arteries in the pathogenesis of preeclampsia. *Obstet Gynecol Ann* 1972; **1**: 177–91.

41. Pijnenborg R, Dixon G, Robertson W B, Brosens I. Trophoblastic invasion of human decidua from 8 to 18 weeks of pregnancy. *Placenta* 1980; **1**: 3–19.

Section 2 Chapter 3

Placental bed vascular disorders

Defective spiral artery remodeling

Ivo Brosens[1] and T. Yee Khong[2]

[1]Leuven Institute for Fertility and Embryology, Leuven, Belgium
[2]SA Pathology, Women's and Children's Hospital, North Adelaide, Australia

Introduction

Growth and decidualization are basic features of the response of uterine spiral arteries prior to pregnancy. In pregnancy unique structural changes occur first in endometrial and subsequently in myometrial segments in response to trophoblast invasion. Ultimately physiological changes are achieved that allow blood flow of some 600 ml/min into the intervillous space. The term 'placental bed' was deliberately chosen to emphasize that it includes 'not only basal decidua but also underlying myometrium containing the origins of the uteroplacental (spiral) arteries' [1].

In the initial studies of placental bed uteroplacental arteries in preeclampsia Dixon and Robertson [2] and Brosens [3] assumed that the response of the arteries to placentation was similar to that in normal pregnancy and the investigators were looking for typical hypertensive vascular lesions. However, after the identification of the physiological changes in the placental bed spiral arteries [4] (Fig. 3.1A), difficulty was experienced in identifying remodeled spiral arteries in the myometrium in cesarean hysterectomy specimens from women with hypertensive disease, and the question was raised whether physiological changes were defective in the myometrial segment. The study of two cesarean hysterectomy specimens with placenta *in situ* from women with severe preeclampsia showed that physiological changes were severely defective in the subendometrial myometrium [5].

In this chapter the features of defective physiological changes of the spiral arteries in the placental bed in association with preeclampsia and fetal growth restriction and the methodology of placental bed vascular studies are reviewed.

Defective spiral artery remodeling

Defective myometrial spiral artery remodeling in preeclampsia

Research on the presence and extent of physiological changes in the spiral arteries in the subendometrial myometrium was based on 15 hysterectomy specimens and over 300 placental bed biopsies [5]. The clinical groups included normotensive women, women with preeclampsia only, and women with preeclampsia complicating essential hypertension.

The study led to the following conclusions:

- In the third trimester of a *normal pregnancy* the physiological changes involve the myometrial segment of the spiral arteries except at the periphery of the placental bed. The mean external diameter of the myometrial spiral artery in the placental bed is approximately 500 μm. Acute atherosis was not observed in myometrial spiral arteries in or outside the placental bed.
- In *preeclampsia* physiological changes are almost completely restricted to the decidual segments of the spiral arteries (Fig. 3.2). The myometrial segment appears to have an essentially normal morphological structure including the retention of the internal elastic membrane. The mean external diameter is approximately 200 μm. Lesions of acute atherosis with intramural foam cell infiltrates occasionally occur.
- In *severe preeclampsia complicating essential hypertension*, physiological changes are present in the decidual segment of the spiral arteries, as is the case in preeclampsia, but seldom extend beyond the deciduo-myometrial junction except in the

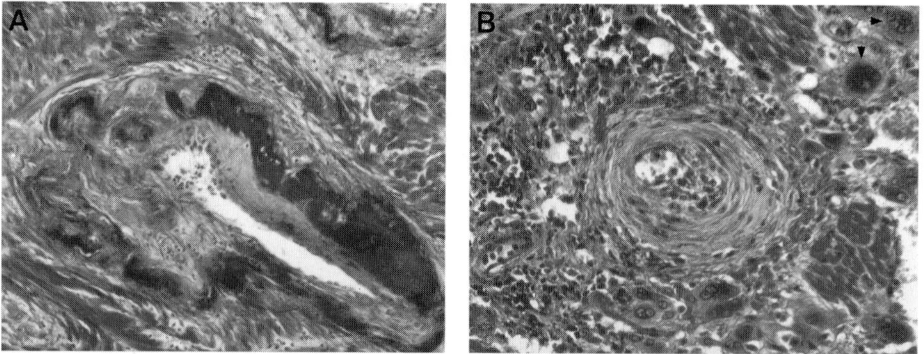

Fig. 3.1 (A) Uteroplacental artery showing marked distension and replacement of the muscular and elastic tissue in the wall by fibrinoid and invaded trophoblast. (B) A spiral artery in the junctional zone myometrium in severe preeclampsia showing absence of physiological changes and surrounded by interstitial trophoblast (Masson trichrome). See plate section for color version.

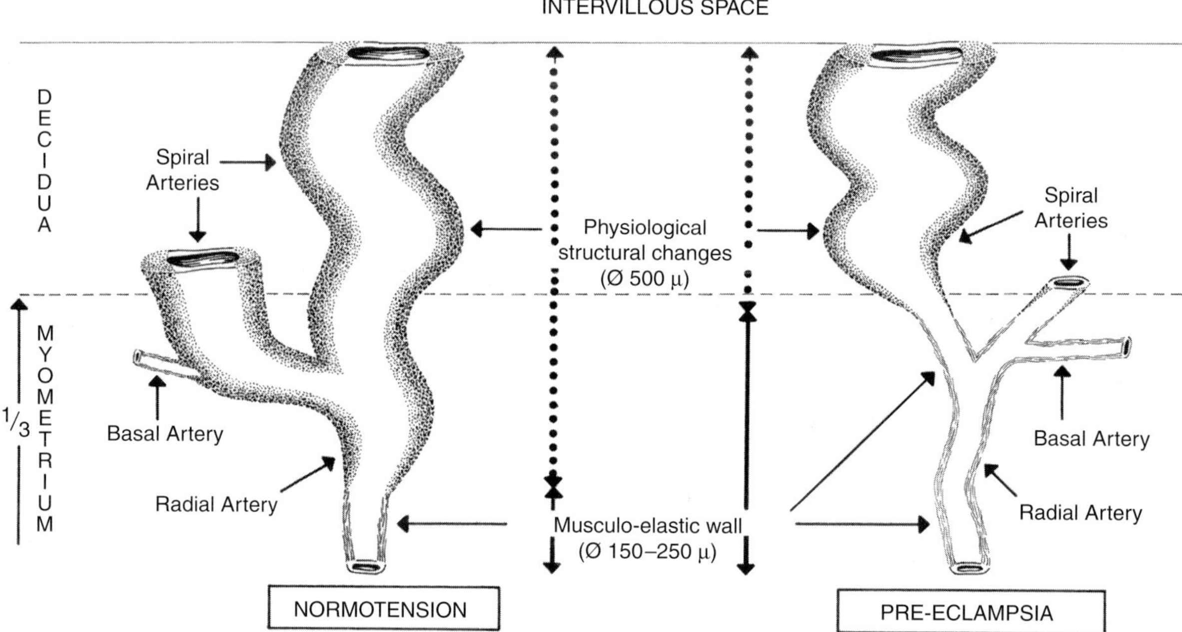

Fig. 3.2 Diagram of the extent of physiological changes in the placental bed in normal pregnancy and preeclampsia.

center of the placenta [6]. The mean external diameter of the myometrial spiral artery is similar to that in uncomplicated preeclampsia. However, the internal elastic lamina is frequently split or reduplicated and can be demonstrated in the hyperplastic intimal layer (Fig. 3.1B). In addition, atherosis is found in a vessel that is already hyperplastic. In fact, the combination of essential hypertension and preeclampsia produces severe obstructive lesions in the myometrial segment of uteroplacental bed arteries. The effect of the obstructive vascular lesions was reflected by a birth weight below the 10th percentile occurring in 27% of the infants born to women in the preeclampsia alone group and in 67% of the preeclampsia complicating essential hypertension group.

These results have been **consistently** confirmed by other studies (Table 3.1). The data do not imply that the inadequate response of the myometrial segments in placental bed spiral arteries is a causal factor in preeclampsia and that preeclampsia is the only condition in which poor vascular response is found. Although these clinical conditions are likely to be multifactorial

Table 3.1. Defective physiological changes in myometrial spiral arteries from women with preeclampsia

Author	Control n (%)	Preeclampsia n (%)
Placental bed biopsy (n: biopsies)		
Gerretsen [40]	1/23 (4%)	29/30 (97%)
Khong [7]	0/18 (0%)	Without FGR: 11/14 (79%) With FGR: 31/34 (91%)
Frusca [57]	1/14 (7%)	24/24 (100%)
Meekins [8][a]	5/21 (24%)	Severe PE 19/24 (82%)
Hanssens [10][b]	6/18 (33%)	Without FGR 16/23 (70%) With FGR 7/8 (88%)
Sagol [52][a]	4/20 (20%)	10/14 (71%)
Kim [58]	4/59 (7%)	12/23 (52%)
Kim [11]	4/103 (4%)	34/43 (81%)
Guzin [12]	4/20 (20%)	Mild: 6/12 (50%) Severe: 15/20 (75%)
Hysterectomy with placenta *in situ* (n: spiral arteries)		
Brosens [44]	45 (4%)	1(90%)

[a] Trophoblast invasion in spiral arteries.
[b] Based on number of spiral arteries.
FGR, fetal growth retardation; PE, preeclampsia.

disorders, there is strong clinical and morphological evidence to suggest that the degree of vascular resistance in the placental bed is a major factor in determining the fetal and neonatal outcome in these conditions.

Defective decidual spiral artery remodeling

In addition to the defect in remodeling the intramyometrial segment of the spiral artery in pregnancies complicated by preeclampsia and intrauterine growth restriction, it is now clear that the failure of trophoblastic invasion into the spiral arteries is not confined to the intramyometrial segments only.

In preeclampsia, a third to a half of the spiral arteries *in the decidual segment of the placental bed* lack the physiological changes [7] (Fig. 3.3). The absence of remodeling of the spiral artery at the level of the decidual segments is also seen in intrauterine growth restriction [7]. Although not described in

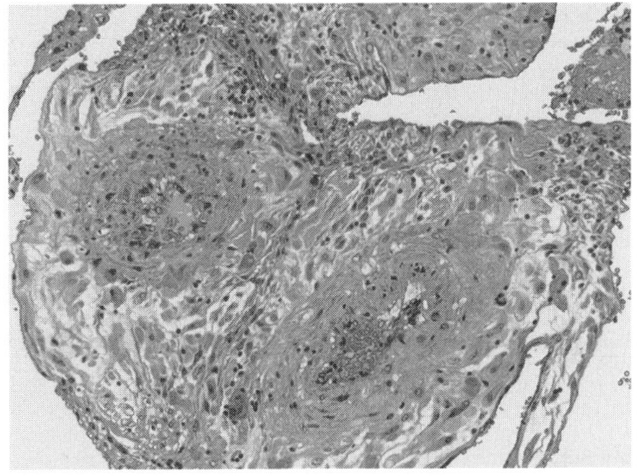

Fig. 3.3 An unconverted spiral artery in the decidual segment in preeclampsia. (From Keeling JW, Khong TY. *Fetal and neonatal pathology*. London: Springer.)

detail, Khong *et al.* also indicated in their publication that the lack of physiological change may also be confined to part of the circumference of the vessel with the remaining portion of the circumference showing physiological change [7]. These observations have since been confirmed by others [8,9].

Several authors have noted that the incidence of absence of physiological changes in preeclampsia with or without fetal growth restriction is higher in the myometrial than in the decidual segments (Table 3.2) [10,11,12]. The observations may suggest that there are differences in the extent of decidual defective physiological changes between different clinical conditions.

Defective spiral artery remodeling in fetal growth restriction

In the absence of hypertension, fetal growth restriction may have multiple causes. Failure of physiological transformation is thought to increase the vascular resistance in the placental bed and to reduce the blood flow to the intervillous space. The question whether fetal growth restriction in normotensive women is associated with defective physiological changes of the placental bed spiral arteries has been a subject of much controversy (Table 3.3). Sheppard and Bonnar found that in normotensive pregnancies complicated by fetal growth restriction, the physiological changes did not extend beyond the decidual segments of the utero-placental arteries [13]. However, Brosens *et al.* found absence of physiological changes in the myometrial segment in 10 (55%) out of 18 cases of fetal growth restriction in normotensive women versus 20% in a

Table 3.2. Absence of physiological changes in decidual and myometrial segments of spiral arteries in preeclampsia

	Placental bed	
	Decidua	Myometrium
Kim [11]		
Preeclampsia	14/43 (33%)	34/43 (80%)
Guzin [12]		
Mild preeclampsia	3/12 (25%)	6/12 (50%)
Severe preeclampsia	9/20 (45%)	15/20 (75%)

Table 3.3. Defective physiological changes and atherosis in myometrial spiral arteries in placental bed biopsies from normotensive women with fetal growth restriction

	Lesions	
Author	Defective	Atherosis
Brosens [14]	10/18 (55%)	Absent
Gerretsen [40]	8/16 (50%)	Not assessed
Hustin [24]	15/25 (60%)	Absent
Khong [7]	16/24 (67%)	Absent
Hanssens[a] [10]	3/6 (50%)	Absent

[a] number of spiral.

control group of normal weight fetuses [14]. De Wolf *et al.* described in five cases with borderline hypertension the defective physiological and hypertensive lesions changes and suggested that recurrent fetal growth restriction may be the first clinical manifestation of underlying vascular disease [15]. Khong *et al.* reported in 24 cases of fetal growth restriction without hypertension the absence of physiological changes in the myometrial segment in 67% of the cases [7].

A note of caution is that the number of cases is small and the topography of the defective lesions has not been confirmed on hysterectomy specimens with the placenta *in situ*. However, it is likely that defective physiological changes of the spiral arteries are a cause of fetal growth restriction in a group of small-for-age newborns. It is important to note that the lesions were not restricted to defective myometrial and decidual transformation, but also included vascular hypertensive lesions.

It can be concluded that in preeclampsia, whether or not it is a complication of essential hypertension, the failure of the spiral arteries to respond adequately to placentation must result in their suboptimal distension. The fetus is then subjected to poor intervillous blood flow from early gestation and not only during the period when preeclampsia is clinically manifest. In these circumstances low birth weight and liability to hypoxia of the infant of a woman who has shown the clinical features of preeclampsia for a few days should occasion no surprise. When preeclampsia complicates essential hypertension the high perinatal mortality and morbidity can be explained by the fact that associated hyperplastic changes cause a critically low level of intervillous space flow to be reached earlier than in preeclampsia alone.

Atherosis and other vascular lesions

A distinctive arteriopathy, subsequently called acute atherosis [16], was first described in the uterus in 'hypertensive albuminuric toxemia' of pregnancy [17]. The lesion is seen in preeclampsia, hypertensive disease not complicated by preeclampsia [3,18], normotensive intrauterine growth restriction [13,15,19,20,21], and systemic lupus erythematosus [22,23]. The relationship of acute atherosis to diabetes mellitus is complex. While some did not find acute atherosis in patients with uncomplicated diabetes mellitus or gestational diabetes [21,24], others have described the lesion in diabetes mellitus [18,25,26]. Unfortunately, these cases are complicated by hypertensive disease or by intrauterine growth restriction and it is unclear if it occurs in uncomplicated diabetes.

The incidence of acute atherosis ranges from 41% to 48% in a series examining placental bed biopsies, placental basal plates, and amniochorial membranes [27]. Some workers have found an inverse relationship between the presence of acute atherosis and birth weight [28,29] but this is not supported by critical statistical analysis of the data. No significant relation was found between the lesion and fetal outcome, including birth weight, degree of proteinuria, and severity or duration of the hypertension [27].

The lesion is seen in vessels that have not undergone the physiological changes of pregnancy and, accordingly, can also be seen in the maternal vessels in the decidua parietalis as well as those in the placental bed [21]. In established cases, this lesion is characterized by fibrinoid necrosis of the arterial wall, a perivascular lymphocytic infiltrate and, at a later stage, the presence of lipid-laden macrophages within the lumen and the damaged vessel wall (Fig. 3.4A). A fibrinoid necrosis is sometimes seen without either the lipophages or the

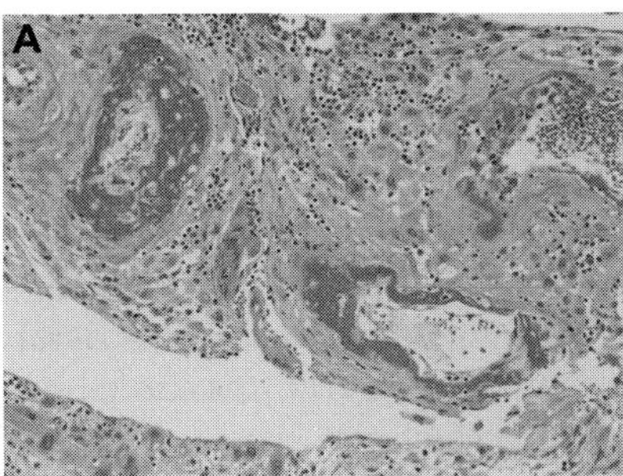

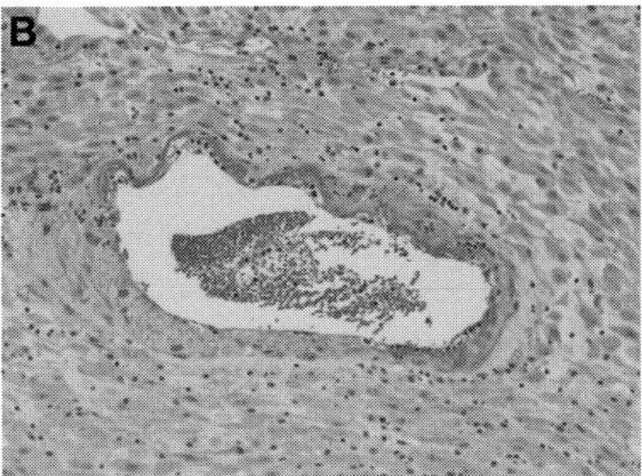

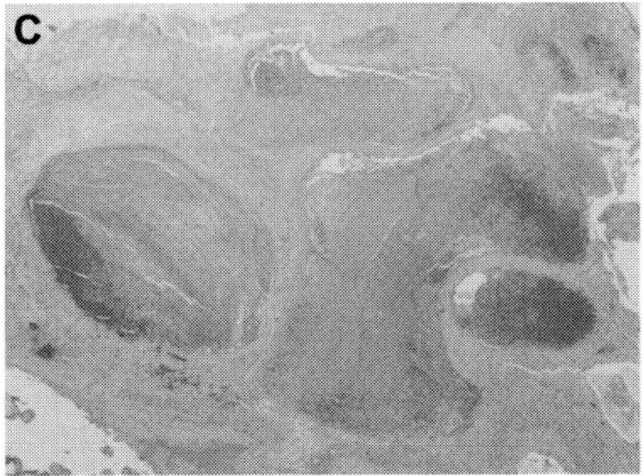

Fig. 3.4 (A) Established acute atherosis, with fibrinoid necrosis, lipid-laden macrophages, and a perivascular lymphocytic infiltrate. (B) Early acute atherosis with fibrinoid necrosis and a perivascular lymphocytic infiltrate; no lipophages are present at this stage. (C) Aneurysmal change in spiral arteries with thrombosis in vessel on the left.

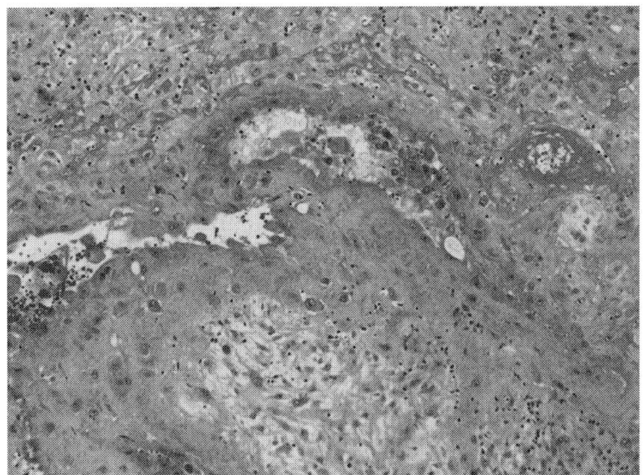

Fig. 3.5 Endovascular trophoblast is seen within the lumen of a uteroplacental artery in a third trimester preeclamptic pregnancy.

perivascular lymphocytic infiltrate suggesting that the earliest lesion that can be confidently identified as acute atherosis is fibrinoid necrosis [21] (Fig. 3.4B). This is consistent with ultrastructural studies examining the pathogenesis of the arteriopathy [30]. There is endothelial disruption and some vessels may show luminal obstruction by lipophages or thrombosis [31]. There is immunolabeling with lipoprotein (a), which is thrombogenic and atherogenic [32]. Aneurysmal formation associated with acute atherosis is sometimes seen and this may be the result of the weakened vessel wall as a result of the fibrinoid necrosis [31] (Fig. 3.4C).

Endovascular trophoblast is seen within the lumina of the spiral arteries in the first and second trimester as part of the retrograde or antidromic invasion of those arteries as part of the physiological vascular response to pregnancy (see Chapter 11). Whereas that is physiological, intraluminal endovascular trophoblast in the third trimester is pathological and is seen in the context of preeclampsia or intrauterine growth restriction [7,33] (Fig. 3.5). This has been argued as a teleological response by the fetal trophoblast to the hypoxia in the intervillous space resulting from the untransformed vessels [34]. Intravascular plugging by endovascular trophoblast in the first trimester has the effect of diminishing blood flow into the intervillous space and reducing oxidative stress [35] and, although the blood flow through the uteroplacental arteries would be considerably greater than that in the first trimester, nevertheless, there is still a physical impediment to the blood flow by the physical presence of endovascular trophoblast in the lumen in the third trimester. Additionally, there is disruption to the vascular endothelium [36].

Material for placental bed vascular studies

Basal plate

The basal plate of a delivered placenta is highly insufficient for the study of spiral arteries as it does not even represent the whole thickness of the decidua. However, the pathologist can choose a representative biopsy, such as the center of the placenta, and the number of biopsies is unlimited. Although decidual fragments may contain invaded spiral arteries, it should be clear that such material has only limited value for evaluating the depth and extent of trophoblast invasion and physiological changes. Khong *et al.* showed that in preeclampsia, not only are physiological changes restricted to decidual segments of spiral arteries, but also fewer arteries are invaded [7]. In that case, estimating the percentage of decidual arteries without physiological changes may be relevant, and therefore he recommended '*en face*' sectioning of flatly embedded basal plates in order to maximize the number of decidual spiral arteries examined [37]. Atherotic lesions may be detected in such material but, even in normal pregnancy, the basal plate may undergo lipid deposition, especially near term. A major limitation of basal plate studies, however, is that the structure of basal plate is variable including maternal arterioles in septa and that in the absence of physiological changes spiral and basal arterioles may have similar appearances.

Placental bed biopsies

Comparison of results based on placental bed biopsy is hampered by variations in the technique of obtaining placental bed biopsies and the examination of the biopsy [1,38]. The biopsy can vary in size (5 mm, 5–10 mm, or more than 10 mm), origin (central, paracentral, periphery), and thickness (decidua, myometrium). Moreover, the technique of examination of the biopsy can vary greatly, such as orientation of the biopsy and serial sectioning. These features are frequently not specified and therefore comparison of results between studies should be interpreted with caution.

The British and Belgian groups originally used two different techniques to obtain placental bed biopsies. Dixon and Robertson in Jamaica used a punch biopsy forceps or a curved scissor at the time of cesarean section [2]. On the other hand, Renaer and Brosens obtained biopsies predominantly at the time of vaginal delivery and used an ovum forceps with its edges sharpened [39]. The cups of the ovum forceps have a length of more than 1 cm and were laterally pressed against the uterine wall to obtain the biopsy. This technique provided a large piece of decidua and underlying myometrium. With about one spiral artery for $0.7\ cm^2$ placental bed surface (see 'Chapter 2') a biopsy with a size of $1\ cm^2$ is likely to include a spiral artery and, moreover, to include parts of both the decidual and myometrial segment. Criteria to confirm the placental bed origin of the biopsy included the presence of interstitial, endovascular or intramural trophoblast and/or an artery with physiological changes or an artery larger than 120 μm. However, the absence of both criteria does not necessarily exclude placental bed origin.

Gerretsen *et al.* and Robson *et al.* suggested that a single large biopsy is a more successful way for sampling spiral arteries with myometrial and decidual segments in the same biopsy than multiple biopsies [40,41]. Robson *et al.* recently used 310 mm-long biopsy forceps with 5 mm-wide cutting jaws to obtain under ultrasound guidance three or four biopsies from the presumed placental bed in early pregnancy and in late pregnancy at the time of cesarean section as well as after vaginal delivery. With this technique they obtained in late pregnancy biopsies with at least one spiral artery in 55% of cases. In these cases a third had both a decidual and myometrial vessel and a third had more than one myometrial vessel and there was no difference between normal and preeclampsia/small for gestational age groups [41].

In the literature the success rate of a biopsy specimen containing trophoblast and both decidual and myometrial segments of a spiral artery varied between 70% [14] and 44% [41]. However, vascular lesions do not occur in every spiral artery and they can be focal or segmental and therefore absent in random sections and even in biopsies [8].

Recently, Harsem *et al.* described the decidual suction method for more successful collection of decidual tissue [42]. Tissue was harvested in 51 cesarean sections by vacuum suction of the placental bed. In 44 (86%) cases one random section demonstrated at least one spiral artery and in 19 (37%) six or more spiral arteries were present. The authors proposed that the method is complementary to the placental bed biopsy method, but its greatest limitation is the lack of topographical oriented tissue yield, as well as the relative lack of myometrial tissue.

It is likely that a single biopsy specimen from the center of the placental bed reveals a different picture of the physiological changes of spiral arteries than multiple small biopsies taken at random. Therefore caution should be exercised when comparing the results of studies using different techniques.

Hysterectomy specimen with placenta *in situ*

Hysterectomy specimens with placenta *in situ* provide the ideal material for the study of structure and pathology of the uteroplacental vessels. Unfortunately the specimens collected by Boyd and Hamilton included no clinical information as they were mainly obtained in collaboration with coroners at the time of accidental maternal death [43]. However, in the late 1950s Hamilton recommended that Ivo Brosens should obtain cesarean hysterectomy specimens with the placenta *in situ* for the study of spiral arteries in maternal hypertensive disease. At that time tubal sterilization was illegal in Belgium, but cesarean hysterectomy could be performed for a range of medical reasons. Marcel Renaer and Joseph Schockaert, both senior gynecologists in the Department of Obstetrics and Gynaecology at the Catholic University of Leuven, introduced a rather heroic cesarean section technique. Immediately following the delivery of the baby the uterine cavity was tightly packed with towels in order to avoid retraction and separation of the placenta. In addition, in some cases a bold incision was made in the outer myometrium overlying the placenta to decrease retraction. A series of 15 cesarean hysterectomy specimens with placenta *in situ* was collected from normal and abnormal pregnancies [4,6,44]. The specimens containing uterine wall and placenta were cut on a sledge microtome in 8 µm sections and examined at 250 µm intervals (Figs. 3.6 and 3.7). The histological examination of the uterine wall with placenta *in situ* was the basis of the demonstration in 1967 of the presence of physiological changes of the spiral arteries in normal pregnancy and the discovery in 1972 of the absence of physiological changes in the myometrial junctional zone in preeclampsia [4,5].

Comments

Defective area of deep placentation

The study of the hysterectomy specimen with placenta *in situ* from a normotensive woman and a woman with severe preeclampsia revealed a similar number of spiral artery openings per 0.7 cm^2. The total number of spiral artery openings in the placental bed for a normal pregnancy was estimated at 120 and for severe preeclampsia 72 [44]. It is therefore likely that in severe cases not only the depth of physiological changes, but also the total number of uteroplacental arteries may be deficient.

The data add to the view that defective deep placentation starts with the beginning of implantation

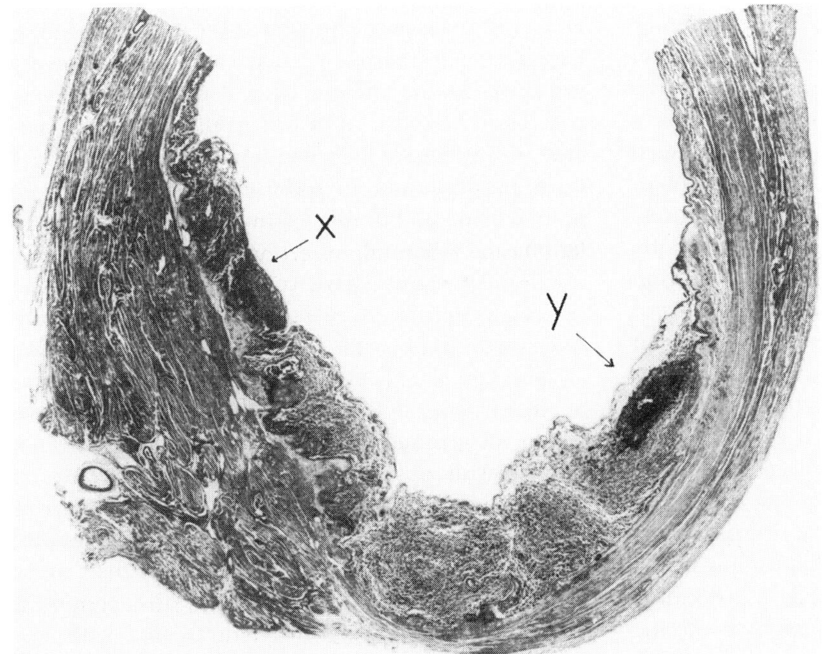

Fig. 3.6 Hysterectomy specimen from a patient with severe preeclampsia: the placenta *in situ* shows paracentral areas of placental infarction (X, Y).

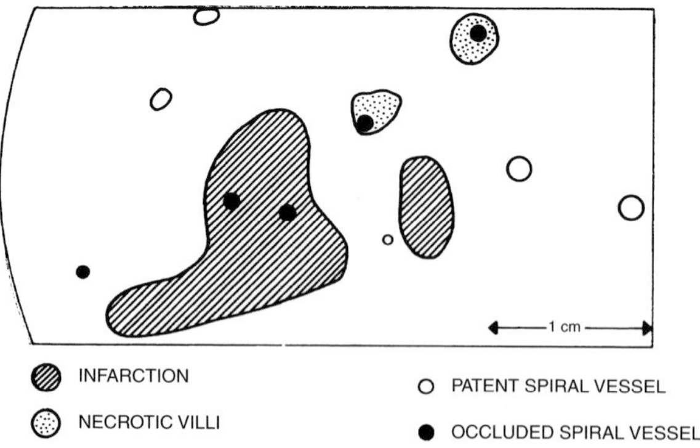

Fig. 3.7 Hysterectomy specimen from a patient with severe preeclampsia. Segment of maternal surface: the spiral artery in the central area is converted (○), while paracentral and peripheral spiral arteries are unconverted (•).

and that both defective deep placentation and a smaller number of uteroplacental arteries may result in a decreased central area of the placental bed with well-developed spiral arteries.

What causes failure of deep placentation?

Several observations point to different causes of defective deep placentation. Maternal hypertension has been a well-documented cause of deep placentation failure. Moreover, De Wolf *et al.* found that fetal growth restriction and severe lesions of placental bed spiral arteries can occur even in the absence of sustained hypertension [45]. Recently, Kim *et al.* showed that preterm premature rupture of the membranes or labour without rupture of the fetal membranes is also associated with defective deep placentation, although to a lesser degree, and with the absence of severe vascular lesions [11]. Ball and collaborators observed in late sporadic miscarriage that the disorganization of the spiral artery smooth muscle may not be entirely dependent on invaded trophoblast, as is currently assumed [46]. They referred to the work of Craven *et al.* who showed that disorganization of the media of spiral arteries is independent of trophoblast invasion and that progesterone effect may be a first step before typical physiological changes develop [47].

Recently, defective decidualization has been proposed as a cause of defective deep placentation [48] and maternal factors such as menstrual preconditioning may be a mechanism to prepare uterine tissues for deep placentation [49]. While decidualization in the endometrium refers to the stroma cells (i.e. decidual cells) it also involves immune cells such as uterine natural killer cells, macrophages, T cells, and growth factors and changes in the smooth muscle cells and spiral arteries in the myometrial junctional zone. Kim *et al.* suggested recently that in the absence of the decidual effect and dilatation the endovascular trophoblast cells may become arrested at the level of the myometrial junctional zone and fail to progress into myometrial spiral artery segments and that this could be the case in defective deep placentation, such as preterm premature rupture of the membranes or labor with intact membranes [11]. Interestingly, the percentage of nulliparous women is high in both groups of women with preeclampsia and preterm pregnancy complications. While the primary role of trophoblast in defective deep placentation remains controversial, defective preconditioning of the uterus and the presence of clinical or subclinical hypertensive vascular disease can be proposed as two independent maternal causes of defective deep placentation.

The future role of color Doppler ultrasound

The question arises as to whether Doppler findings throughout pregnancy can unravel the link between placental bed vascular development and the ultimate pregnancy outcome and shed more light on the clinical significance of defective deep placentation in different clinical conditions. Studies of the placental bed have in recent years shown that defective deep placentation is associated with a spectrum of clinical conditions. However, it has been shown that the extent of physiological changes and associated vascular lesions vary greatly between different clinical conditions. Severe preeclampsia and fetal growth restriction are associated with extensive failure of myometrial spiral artery transformation and, in addition, the arteries in both myometrium and decidua show hyperplastic vascular lesions and atherosis.

Doppler studies have consistently confirmed an increased uterine artery resistance in clinical conditions associated with defective deep placentation [12,50,51,52,53,54]. However, the question arises as to what extent the vascular resistance in the placental bed is determined by the decrease in number of arteries with physiological changes and the extent of defective physiological changes. In analogy with the findings of Matijevic *et al.* that impedance to blood flow in spiral arteries is lower in the central area of the placental bed than in the peripheral areas [55], the size of the central area with low impedance spiral arteries may be more important than the uterine artery resistance or the resistance in a few spiral arteries in the center of the placenta. Deurloo *et al.* recently performed measurements in the central region of the placenta, but failed to confirm previous findings of increased resistance in complicated pregnancies [56]. Indeed, examination of large hysterectomy specimens with placenta *in situ* has shown that in severe cases of preeclampsia a small, central part of the placenta may contain spiral arteries with fully developed physiological changes. This would suggest that comparison of the size of the central part with normal flow rather than the flow in a selected zone of the placenta may be a valuable method for estimating the severity of defective deep placentation.

References

1. Robertson W B, Khong T Y, Brosens I *et al.* The placental bed biopsy: review from three European centers. *Am J Obstet Gynecol* 1986; **155**: 401–12.
2. Dixon H G, Robertson W B. A study of the vessels of the placental bed in normotensive and hypertensive women. *J Obstet Gynaecol Br Emp* 1958; **65**: 803–9.
3. Brosens I. A study of the spiral arteries of the decidua basalis in normotensive and hypertensive pregnancies. *J Obstet Gynaecol Br Cwth* 1964; **71**: 222–30.
4. Brosens I, Robertson W B, Dixon H G. The physiological response of the vessels of the placental bed to normal pregnancy. *J Pathol Bacteriol* 1967; **93**: 569–79.
5. Brosens I A, Robertson W B, Dixon H G. The role of the spiral arteries in the pathogenesis of preeclampsia. *Obstet Gynecol Annu* 1972; **1**: 177–91.
6. Brosens I, Renaer M. On the pathogenesis of placental infarcts in pre-eclampsia. *J Obstet Gynaecol Br Commonw* 1972; **79**: 794–9.
7. Khong T Y, De Wolf F, Robertson W B, Brosens I. Inadequate maternal vascular response to placentation in pregnancies complicated by pre-eclampsia and by small-for-gestational age infants. *Br J Obstet Gynaecol* 1986; **93**: 1049–59.
8. Meekins J W, Pijnenborg R, Hanssens M, McFadyen I R, van Assche A. A study of placental bed spiral arteries and trophoblast invasion in normal and severe pre-eclamptic pregnancies. *Br J Obstet Gynaecol* 1994; **101**: 669–74.
9. Pijnenborg R, Anthony J, Davey D A *et al.* Placental bed spiral arteries in the hypertensive disorders of pregnancy. *Br J Obstet Gynaecol* 1991; **98**: 648–55.
10. Hanssens M, Pijnenborg R, Keirse M J *et al.* Renin-like immunoreactivity in uterus and placenta from normotensive and hypertensive pregnancies. *Eur J Obstet Gynecol Reprod Biol* 1998; **81**: 177–84.
11. Kim Y M, Bujold E, Chaiworapongsa T *et al.* Failure of physiologic transformation of the spiral arteries in patients with preterm labor and intact membranes. *Am J Obstet Gynecol* 2003; **189**: 1063–9.
12. Guzin K, Tomruk S, Tuncay Y A *et al.* The relation of increased uterine artery blood flow resistance and impaired trophoblast invasion in pre-eclamptic pregnancies. *Arch Gynecol Obstet* 2005; **272**: 283–8.
13. Sheppard B L, Bonnar J. The ultrastructure of the arterial supply of the human placenta in pregnancy complicated by fetal growth retardation. *Br J Obstet Gynaecol* 1976; **83**: 948–59.
14. Brosens I, Dixon H G, Robertson W B. Fetal growth retardation and the arteries of the placental bed. *Br J Obstet Gynaecol* 1977; **84**: 656–63.
15. De Wolf F, Brosens I, Renaer M. Fetal growth retardation and the maternal arterial supply of the human placenta in the absence of sustained hypertension. *Br J Obstet Gynaecol* 1980; **87**: 678–85.
16. Zeek P M, Assali N S. Vascular changes in the decidua associated with eclamptogenic toxemia of pregnancy. *Am J Clin Pathol* 1950; **20**: 1099–109.
17. Hertig A T. Vascular pathology in hypertensive albuminuric toxemias of pregnancy. *Clinics* 1945; **4**: 602–14.
18. Kitzmiller J L, Watt N, Driscoll S G. Decidual arteriopathy in hypertension and diabetes in pregnancy: immunofluorescent studies. *Am J Obstet Gynecol* 1981; **141**: 773–9.
19. Sheppard B L, Bonnar J. An ultrastructural study of utero-placental spiral arteries in hypertensive and normotensive pregnancy and fetal growth retardation. *Br J Obstet Gynaecol* 1981; **88**: 695–705.
20. Althabe O, Labarrere C, Telenta M. Maternal vascular lesions in placentae of small-for-gestational-age infants. *Placenta* 1985; **6**: 265–76.
21. Khong T Y. Acute atherosis in pregnancies complicated by hypertension, small-for-gestational-age infants, and diabetes mellitus. *Arch Pathol Lab Med* 1991; **115**: 722–5.
22. Abramowsky C R, Vegas M E, Swinehart G, Gyves M T. Decidual vasculopathy of the placenta in lupus erythematosus. *N Engl J Med* 1980; **303**: 668–72.
23. De Wolf F, Carreras L O, Moerman P *et al.* Decidual vasculopathy and extensive placental infarction in a patient with repeated thromboembolic accidents, recurrent fetal loss, and a lupus anticoagulant. *Am J Obstet Gynecol* 1982; **142**: 829–34.
24. Hustin J, Foidart J M, Lambotte R. Maternal vascular lesions in pre-eclampsia and intrauterine growth retardation: light microscopy and immunofluorescence. *Placenta* 1983; **4**: 489–98.

25. Emmrich P, Birke R, Gödel E. Morphology of myometrial and decidual arteries in normal pregnancy, in toxemia of pregnancy, and in maternal diabetes. *Pathol Microbiol (Basel)* 1975; **43**: 38–61.
26. Driscoll S G. The pathology of pregnancy complicated by diabetes mellitus. *Med Clin N Am* 1965; **49**: 1053–67.
27. Khong T Y, Pearce J M, Robertson W B. Acute atherosis in preeclampsia: maternal determinants and fetal outcome in the presence of the lesion. *Am J Obstet Gynecol* 1987; **157**: 360–3.
28. Maqueo M, Azuela J C, de la Vega M D. Placental pathology in eclampsia and preeclampsia. *Obstet Gynecol* 1964; **24**: 350–6.
29. McFadyen I R, Price A B, Geirsson R T. The relation of birthweight to histological appearances in vessels of the placental bed. *Br J Obstet Gynaecol* 1986; **93**: 476–81.
30. De Wolf F, Robertson W B, Brosens I. The ultrastructure of acute atherosis in hypertensive pregnancy. *Am J Obstet Gynecol* 1975; **123**: 164–74.
31. Khong T Y, Mott C. Immunohistologic demonstration of endothelial disruption in acute atherosis in pre-eclampsia. *Eur J Obstet Gynecol Reprod Biol* 1993; **51**: 193–7.
32. Meekins J W, Pijnenborg R, Hanssens M, Van Assche A, McFadyen I R. Immunohistochemical detection of lipoprotein(a) in the wall of placental bed spiral arteries in normal and severe preeclamptic pregnancies. *Placenta* 1994; **15**: 511–24.
33. Kos M, Czernobilsky B, Hlupic L, Kunjko K. Pathological changes in placentas from pregnancies with preeclampsia and eclampsia with emphasis on persistence of endovascular trophoblastic plugs. *Croat Med J* 2005; **46**: 404–9.
34. Khong T Y, Robertson W B. Spiral artery disease. In: Coulam C B, Faulk W P, McIntyre J A, eds. *Immunological obstetrics*. New York: W.W. Norton; 1992: pp. 492–501.
35. Jauniaux E, Hempstock J, Greenwold N, Burton G J. Trophoblastic oxidative stress in relation to temporal and regional differences in maternal placental blood flow in normal and abnormal early pregnancies. *Am J Pathol* 2003; **162**: 115–25.
36. Khong T Y, Sawyer I H, Heryet A R. An immunohistologic study of endothelialization of uteroplacental vessels in human pregnancy – evidence that endothelium is focally disrupted by trophoblast in preeclampsia. *Am J Obstet Gynecol* 1992; **167**: 751–6.
37. Khong T Y, Chambers H M. Alternative method of sampling placentas for the assessment of uteroplacental vasculature. *J Clin Pathol* 1992; **45**: 925–7.
38. Lyall F. The human placental bed revisited. *Placenta* 2002; **23**: 555–62.
39. Renaer M, Brosens I. [Spiral arterioles in the decidua basalis in hypertensive complications of pregnancy.] *Ned Tijdschr Verloskd Gynaecol* 1963; **63**: 103–18.
40. Gerretsen G, Huisjes H J, Elema J D. Morphological changes of the spiral arteries in the placental bed in relation to pre-eclampsia and fetal growth retardation. *Br J Obstet Gynaecol* 1981; **88**: 876–81.
41. Robson S C, Simpson H, Ball E, Lyall F, Bulmer J N. Punch biopsy of the human placental bed. *Am J Obstet Gynecol* 2002; **187**: 1349–55.
42. Harsem N K, Staff A C, He L, Roald B. The decidual suction method: a new way of collecting decidual tissue for functional and morphological studies. *Acta Obstet Gynecol Scand* 2004; **83**: **724**–30.
43. Boyd J D, Hamilton W J. *The human placenta*. Cambridge: Heffer and Sons; 1970.
44. Brosens I A. The utero-placental vessels at term: the distribution and extent of physiological changes. *Trophoblast Res* 1988; **3**: 61–7.
45. De Wolf F, De Wolf-Peeters C, Brosens I, Robertson W B. The human placental bed: electron microscopic study of trophoblastic invasion of spiral arteries. *Am J Obstet Gynecol* 1980; **137**: 58–70.
46. Ball E, Bulmer J N, Ayis S, Lyall F, Robson S C. Late sporadic miscarriage is associated with abnormalities in spiral artery transformation and trophoblast invasion. *J Pathol* 2006; **208**: 535–42.
47. Craven C M, Morgan T, Ward K. Decidual spiral artery remodelling begins before cellular interaction with cytotrophoblasts. *Placenta* 1998; **19**: 241–52.
48. Brosens J J, Pijnenborg R, Brosens I A. The myometrial junctional zone spiral arteries in normal and abnormal pregnancies: a review of the literature. *Am J Obstet Gynecol* 2002; **187**: 1416–23.
49. Brosens J J, Parker M, McIndoe A, Pijnenborg R, Brosens I A. A role for menstruation in preconditioning the uterus for successful pregnancy. *Am J Obstet Gynecol* 2009; **200**: 615.e1–615.e6.
50. Voigt H J, Becker V. Doppler flow measurements and histomorphology of the placental bed in uteroplacental insufficiency. *J Perinat Med* 1992; **20**: 139–47.
51. Lin S, Shimizu I, Suehara N, Nakayama M, Aono T. Uterine artery Doppler velocimetry in relation to trophoblast migration into the myometrium of the placental bed. *Obstet Gynecol* 1995; **85**: 760–5.
52. Sagol S, Özkinay E, Öztekin K, Özdemir N. The comparison of uterine artery Doppler velocimetry with the histopathology of the placental bed. *Aust N Z J Obstet Gynaecol* 1999; **39**: 324–9.
53. Aardema M W, Oosterhof H, Timmer A, van Rooy I, Aarnoudse J G. Uterine artery Doppler flow and

uteroplacental vascular pathology in normal pregnancies and pregnancies complicated by pre-eclampsia and small for gestational age fetuses. *Placenta* 2001; **22**: 405–11.

54. Madazli R, Somunkiran A, Calay Z, Ilvan S, Aksu M F. Histomorphology of the placenta and the placental bed of growth restricted foetuses and correlation with the Doppler velocimetries of the uterine and umbilical arteries. *Placenta* 2003; **24**: 510–6.

55. Matijevic R, Meekins J W, Walkinshaw S A, Neilson J P, McFadyen I R. Spiral artery blood flow in the central and peripheral areas of the placental bed in the second trimester. *Obstet Gynecol* 1995; **86**: 289–92.

56. Deurloo K L, Spreeuwenberg M D, Bolte A C, Van Vugt J M. Color Doppler ultrasound of spiral artery blood flow for prediction of hypertensive disorders and intra uterine growth restriction: a longitudinal study. *Prenat Diagn* 2007; **27**: 1011–6.

What is defective: decidua, trophoblast, or both?

Robert Pijnenborg and Myriam C. Hanssens

Katholieke Universiteit Leuven, Department Woman & Child, University Hospital Leuven, Leuven, Belgium

Introduction

It has been known for a long time that the occurrence of preeclampsia is somehow linked to the presence of a placenta [1]. During placentation the mother comes in close contact with semi-allogeneic fetal trophoblastic cells which play a key role in maternal–fetal physiological exchange. Because of the reduced number of layers separating the two circulations, the most intimate association between mother and fetus occurs in species with hemochorial placentation, in which fetal trophoblast is directly exposed to circulating maternal blood. In contrast to other placental types, hemochorial placentation is always associated with decidualization of the endometrium, which involves an 'epithelioid' transformation of the fibroblasts of the uterine mucosa [2], accompanied by extracellular matrix changes and infiltration by other cell types, notably uterine natural killer cells and macrophages. Multiple functions have been ascribed to the decidua, including the secretion of hormones and growth factors to allow embryo implantation and placental outgrowth in an orderly fashion, but at the same time also protecting the uterus against excessive damage [3]. Morphologically, various degrees of decidualization have been discerned in different species, notably in primates where a more elaborate decidua seems to be associated with deeper trophoblast invasion beyond the decidualized endometrium, as typically occurs in the human [4].

Decidualization not only involves the endometrial stroma, but also the spiral arteries which undergo a marked increase in length from the late luteal phase of the cycle onwards, leading to their spiral course [5]. After an early phase of 'plugging' by intraluminal trophoblast, spiral arteries undergo a retrograde ('antidromic') invasion by these cells, which are also largely responsible for the subsequent vascular remodeling (Chapter 11). Variations may occur in different species as to the involvement of endovascular and interstitial trophoblast, as well as to the depth of invasion which can either be restricted to the decidua or extended into the inner myometrium (Chapter 13). 'Physiologically changed' spiral arteries have undergone a loss of the vascular smooth muscle and the elastic lamina, resulting in a significant increase in vascular diameter to accommodate the increasing uteroplacental blood flow. Soon after the discovery of the characteristic spiral artery remodeling in the pregnant uterus, it was postulated that these changes resulted from a destructive action by invading trophoblast on the vessel wall [6] (see also Chapter 2). This initial emphasis on a primordial role of trophoblast in the process was subsequently toned down by the observation – in the human as well as in laboratory animals – that decidua-associated arterial changes, probably occurring under hormonal control, precede trophoblast invasion [7,8]. This seemed to imply that there exists an early preparatory phase which is essential for subsequent trophoblast-associated remodeling. Since in the human the trophoblast invades as deeply as the inner 'junctional zone' (JZ) myometrium, which is increasingly considered as a separate uterine compartment (see Chapter 9), the occurrence of a priming 'decidua-associated' vascular remodeling has to be considered also in this uterine compartment.

In 1972 Brosens and colleagues [9] showed for the first time that in preeclampsia the 'physiological changes' are restricted to the decidua. These observations were mainly based on studies of third trimester placental bed biopsies collected during cesarean sections, and since no data were available yet about an early 'decidualization' phase of vascular remodeling, it was logical to propose a failure of trophoblast invasion as a primary cause of the vascular defects. At that time little was known about the relationship between early invasive processes and vascular change during the first trimester. Although swelling of vascular smooth muscle in the decidual spiral arteries had already been described [10], an event obviously related to the development of perivascular decidual sheaths ('Streeter's columns'), nothing was known about the inner myometrium in early pregnancy, which was to be the site of the major vascular defects in preeclampsia. Subsequent histological studies of the junctional zone myometrial segments of spiral arteries in intact pregnant hysterectomy specimens of the first and early second trimester resulted in two major findings [11]. *First*, vascular changes including disorganization of the muscular wall are not exclusively due to the presence of trophoblast. Vascular smooth muscle becomes disorganized before the arrival of endovascular trophoblast and this process is enhanced in the presence of interstitial trophoblast. A *second* finding was the apparent occurrence of endovascular invasion in the inner myometrium as a second 'wave' occurring after a 4-week period of relative stability in the decidua. In later years this 'two waves concept' has been criticized, mainly following studies of large numbers of placental bed biopsies taken in early pregnancy [12,13]. Although the two waves concept is not definitely agreed upon, the point is relevant for considering possible mechanisms of failed invasion. Indeed, the occurrence of a distinct second wave might imply a specific mechanism for triggering deeper invasion, which might be disturbed in preeclampsia.

From the previous it follows that a failure of spiral artery remodeling might find its origin either in the fetal trophoblast or in the maternal environment (the decidualized endometrium and JZ myometrium, including the spiral arteries), or maybe even in both. In addition to these local uterine phenomena wider pathophysiological disturbances should also be considered, which may have an impact upon these local vascular defects.

Arguments for trophoblast defects

Focusing on spiral artery invasion, there is little direct evidence for the occurrence of intrinsic trophoblastic defects in early pregnancy. The only relevant observation so far might be the absence of endovascular trophoblast in myometrial spiral arteries in one out of seven post-15 weeks specimens in a study of early pregnant uteri [11]. While this finding is obviously very intriguing, it is of course pointless to guess whether or not preeclampsia would have occurred if the pregnancy had been allowed to continue.

Arguments for intrinsic defects in acquiring an 'invasive phenotype' during extravillous trophoblast differentiation were put forward during the high days of integrin research. A key observation was the discovery of a spatial gradient of shifting integrin expression within the cytotrophoblastic cell columns of anchoring villi, as revealed by immunohistochemistry on tissue samples of early abortions [14,15]. This integrin shift must result in an altered binding capacity to different extracellular matrix components, thought to be necessary for allowing trophoblast migration. This integrin shift could still be observed in late second trimester normal pregnancies, but was absent in preeclamptic women [16], thus indicating a possible cause for failed invasion. Although the idea was very attractive, no differences in integrin expression were observed in extravillous trophoblasts in the basal plate and associated decidua in third trimester placentae of normal and complicated pregnancies [17]. This observation does not refute the postulated role of a failed integrin shift in preeclampsia, however, since at this late stage of pregnancy all invasive activity may have stopped at the basal plate and associated decidua. Another problem with the defective integrin shift hypothesis is that mainly interstitial trophoblasts were evaluated in the quoted studies. While a defective endovascular invasion was implied by the restricted spiral artery remodeling, the question as to whether defective interstitial invasion might also be involved in preeclampsia has never been convincingly answered [18,19]. Although admittedly anecdotal, placental bed biopsies of even severe preeclamptic women may sometimes show intense interstitial invasion of the inner myometrium. This should not be surprising, since interstitial trophoblast numbers vary considerably throughout the whole extent of the placental bed, not only in preeclamptic women but also in normal pregnancies [18]. Recent evidence for defects in interstitial trophoblast in hypertensive pregnancies is the finding of an inadequate fusion of invading cytotrophoblast into multinuclear giant cells in both gestational hypertension and preeclampsia, associated with a maintenance of E-cadherin expression [20]. This finding is in agreement with a report of a failed down-regulation of E-cadherin in preeclampsia [16], but contradicts previous claims of increased fusion into multinuclear giant cells in this condition [21]. Whether alterations in E-cadherin expression may result from an intrinsic trophoblast defect, or rather are induced by maternal factors is not known.

Impaired trophoblast invasion in spiral arteries may not only be due to an intrinsic defect in invasive properties, but may also be induced by maternal cells. Inflammatory cells are inevitably present within invaded areas of the placental bed, and an aggravated maternal response might well lead to an 'overkill' of trophoblasts. Such events might be related to the concept that normal – and *a fortiori* preeclamptic – pregnancies represent a hyperinflammatory state [22]. Although not regularly seen in near-term placental bed biopsies, physiologically remodeled spiral arteries occasionally show extensive leukocytic infiltrations. It is possible, however, that invasion-related acute maternal inflammatory responses mainly occur in earlier stages of pregnancy when biopsies are not routinely taken, and this may account for the rarity of such observations.

Arguments for maternal defects

For a long time trophoblast invasion was thought to be controlled by a restrictive action of the decidua [3, 23]. One proposed mechanism, emerging from rodent studies, was the presence of a mechanical barrier, possibly effected by the tight intercellular junctions joining decidual stromal cells [2]. Such restriction would in the first place apply to interstitial trophoblasts which are directly in contact with the decidualized endometrial stroma. In the human, however, it is obvious that the decidua does not really act as a barrier but rather as a passage-way for trophoblasts to colonize the junctional zone myometrium, as witnessed by the tremendous numbers of interstitial trophoblasts appearing in this compartment during the first trimester [24]. Indeed, more recent evidence indicated that the human decidua may actually stimulate the invasive behavior of the trophoblasts by inducing their synthesis of matrix metalloproteinases (MMPs) [25]. This idea was already implicit in the comparative study by Ramsey and colleagues [4] who tried to find an explanation for the obviously higher degree of decidualization in the human as compared to other primate species with less deep trophoblast invasion. It is therefore conceivable that defective decidual function may be a possible reason for impaired trophoblast invasion in complicated pregnancies, although, as far as the interstitial invasion is concerned, the available (contradictory) evidence needs to be substantiated [18,19].

A stimulatory role of decidua for trophoblast invasion may also apply to the endovascular invasion of the spiral arteries. First, it is not inconceivable that the 'decidualized' vascular smooth muscle may also induce MMP production by the migrating endovascular trophoblasts and thus stimulate their invasion or incorporation into the vessel wall. Second, since the decidualization process of the spiral arteries implies a loss in the coherence of the vascular smooth muscle, this early vascular change might allow easier intramural penetration by the trophoblast. This loss in coherency of the smooth muscle must be related to alterations in the extracellular matrix, and such matrix changes have been reported for both the decidual stroma and the decidual segments of spiral arteries [26]. Decidua-associated vascular remodeling not only occurs in the decidua but also in the 'junctional zone' myometrial compartment [27]. Is there any evidence for a disturbed decidua-associated remodeling, either in the decidua or in the JZ myometrium, in complicated pregnancies? Unfortunately not, mainly because of the impossibility to routinely collect placental bed samples in the early stages of an ongoing pregnancy. There was certainly no morphological evidence of failed disorganization – i.e. maintenance of a tight vascular smooth muscle coherence – in myometrial spiral arteries of the one non-invaded post-15 weeks specimen in the previously quoted study [11].

Because of the disorganization of the vascular smooth muscle and subsequent vasodilatation, decidua-associated vascular remodeling may enhance blood flow to the implantation site. Doppler studies at the time of embryo replacement after IVF revealed an increased vascularity of the endometrium in conception cycles [28], which may result from angiogenic processes associated with early decidua-associated remodeling. It is not yet known to what degree defects in early endometrial and junctional zone vascularity are responsible for pregnancy complications. Disturbances in uterine arterial blood flow have been demonstrated as early as the twelfth week [29]. A marked increase in uteroplacental oxygenation has been observed after 12 weeks in normal pregnancies [30], i.e. before the onset of the alleged second wave of endovascular trophoblast invasion into the inner (junctional zone) myometrium. The question as to what comes first, increased blood flow or trophoblast invasion, has not yet been fully resolved. The most favored scenario still is that by their invasive action, trophoblasts open up the vessels, destroy the vascular smooth muscle, and transform the arteries into permanently dilated tubes, thus increasing maternal blood flow to the placenta. Taking a different point of view, one might envisage that, besides the invasion of the spiral arteries, the steroid-controlled rise in blood supply to the pregnant uterus also has to be taken into account [31]. Hemodynamics may indeed be a real, albeit imperfectly understood, factor directing trophoblast migration [32]. It is not unlikely that an inadequate rise in uteroplacental blood flow, which may result from various disturbances, is the real cause of failed trophoblast invasion and spiral artery remodeling in preeclampsia (Chapter 11).

Preeclampsia as a failure in the maternal–fetal dialogue

In the past the placental bed was frequently compared with a battle-field where invading trophoblasts are countered by a defense line of maternal decidua [33] (Chapter 16). This possible scenario appealed to many investigators who were looking for possible causes of the uniquely human disease preeclampsia, fueling the idea that the mother fights back against the threat of deeply invading trophoblast. It was silently assumed that deep trophoblast invasion was an exclusive feature of human pregnancy, and that there was no need to consider a maternal 'rejection' in other primate species which undergo only shallow invasion. However, a recent study of specimens from historical tissue collections revealed that deep invasion does occur in chimpanzees, and also in gorillas (Chapter 12). Interestingly, for both species case reports of suspected (pre-) eclampsia have been published [34,35,36]. Of course most pregnancies do not become preeclamptic, so that as a rule deep trophoblast invasion is well tolerated, without any ensuing 'battle'.

We have previously argued that a completely different concept of interaction may better reflect the reality, namely a concept of a mutual maternal–fetal support or 'dialogue' between uterus and trophoblast, as a result of an intricate coevolutionary process [37]. Although coevolution usually occurs at the level of interspecies interactions, the process is obviously also applicable to interactions between males and females, or between mothers and their offspring [38]. This could be considered as a 'Red Queen' scenario, in which both runners (mother and fetus) have to move as fast as possible in order to keep themselves 'at the same place'. Such stepwise coevolution between increasing trophoblast invasion and uterine adaptive (decidual) changes may have resulted in a progressively deeper invasion in the course of our evolution, thus setting a compromise in the inherent conflict between fetal nutrient requirements and maternal self-protection. Both partners then reap the benefit of optimizing their reproductive chances [39] (Chapter 16).

At this point we have to ask which benefits may be gained from the deeper trophoblast invasion and the associated deep vascular remodeling. At first sight there is no reason to consider the placenta of a baboon, which shows limited trophoblast invasion, to be less efficient than the human placenta. One possibility is that deep invasion may compensate for possible vascular disturbances due to our upright position [40]. Indeed, it has been reasoned that bipedalism may carry a risk of compressing the vena cava which may compromise uteroplacental blood flow. Since chimpanzees, which are basically knuckle-walkers, also show deep trophoblast invasion (Chapter 12), the upright position of the human has probably not been a major factor in the evolution of deep placentation. Another popular idea is that deep placentation provides a better support for a more extensive fetal brain development, and for that reason deep placentation used to be considered as being unique to humans. Also chimpanzee fetuses show considerable brain development [41] and this might also be related to their deep placentation. A possible link between fetal brain development, deep trophoblast invasion, and preeclampsia has been suggested [42]. Indeed, the extended reciprocal exposure of maternal and fetal cells must carry an increased risk for pregnancy complications such as preeclampsia due to the inevitable discordancies – genetic or other – between mother and fetus. It has even been proposed that accelerated fetal brain development in Neanderthalers, who had larger brains than the present *Homo sapiens*, must have been associated with more extensive trophoblast invasion and an associated higher risk of preeclampsia, contributing to their extinction [43]. More data are required, however, to support the proposed link between deep trophoblast invasion and increased fetal brain development, but also between deep invasion and placental efficiency. Following all these considerations, babies born after preeclamptic pregnancies must have been deprived of the benefits associated with deep placentation, and especially the long-term consequences of the disease should be a matter of concern.

Conclusion: defective remodeling as a disturbed partnership

This chapter provides a general overview of the two major components of pregnancy-associated spiral artery remodeling, the maternal (decidual) and the fetal (trophoblastic). A full understanding of the vascular remodeling process necessitates detailed knowledge of the fate of each arterial component. Based upon observations in early pregnancy specimens, we distinguished four major steps in arterial remodeling: (1) decidua-associated remodeling; (2) the intraluminal phase of trophoblast invasion; (3) intramural trophoblast incorporation (trophoblast-associated remodeling); and (4) a partial maternal repair [44].

Defects in each step may interfere with vascular remodeling and be associated with the whole spectrum of pregnancy complications. So far, most attention has been paid to the enigmatic disease preeclampsia, which is no longer considered as one specific disease, but rather as a syndrome which may have several underlying causes. The fact that different interfering steps may lead to failed spiral artery remodeling can be an additional reason for this multicausality. There is now general agreement that maternal constitutional factors play a role in the development of the preeclamptic syndrome [45]. Although such factors are usually considered in the light of the symptomatic 'second stage' of the disease, they might also have an impact on early remodeling steps in spiral arteries. It is known for instance that decidualization is impaired in diabetic rats [46] and diabetic NOD mice show underdevelopment of decidual spiral arteries [47]. It is not yet known whether in diabetic women the decidua-associated remodeling may be disturbed, but diabetes is a well-known risk factor for preeclampsia [48]. Other maternal physiological maladaptations to pregnancy such as a failure in plasma volume expansion or a failure in the redirection of maternal blood flow to the expanding uterus might have a direct negative effect on intraluminal trophoblast migration. Similar considerations may apply to other health issues, including fertility problems which may be due to a suboptimal uterine preparation for implantation and placental development, and which may contribute to poor pregnancy outcome after assisted reproduction (Chapter 20).

In order to unravel the possible causes of defective spiral artery remodeling it will be necessary to focus on early pregnancy, where the key of failed invasion and/or associated or preceding vascular defects has to be found. The big problem remains the impossibility of acquiring relevant study material of early placentation stages in ongoing pregnancies, and this problem is not likely to be solved in the foreseeable future.

References

1. Redman C W G. Pre-eclampsia and the placenta. *Placenta* 1991; **12**: 301–8.
2. Finn C A, Lawn A M. Specialized junctions between decidual cells in the uterus of the pregnant mouse. *J Ultrastr Res* 1967; **20**: 321–7.
3. Kirby D R S, Cowell T P. Trophoblast-host interactions. In: Fleischmajer R, Billingham R E, eds. *Epithelial-mesenchymal interactions*. Baltimore: Williams & Wilkins; 1968: pp. 64–77.
4. Ramsey E R, Houston M L, Harris J W S. Interactions of the trophoblast and maternal tissues in three closely related primate species. *Am J Obstet Gynecol* 1976; **124**: 647–52.
5. Ramsey E M, Donner M W. Vasculature of the nonpregnant uterus. In: *Placental Vasculature and Circulation*. Stuttgart: Georg Thieme Publishers; 1980: pp. 20–5.
6. Brosens I, Robertson W B, Dixon H G. The physiological response of the vessels of the placental bed to normal pregnancy. *J Path Bact* 1967; **93**: 569–79.
7. Brosens I A. Morphological changes in the utero-placental bed in pregnancy hypertension. *Clin Obstet Gynaecol* 1977; **4**: 573–93.
8. Pijnenborg R, Robertson W B, Brosens I. The arterial migration of trophoblast in the uterus of the golden hamster. *J Reprod Fert* 1974; **40**: 269–80.
9. Brosens I, Robertson W B, Dixon H G. The role of spiral arteries in the pathogenesis of preeclampsia. In: Wynn R M, ed. *Obstetrics and gynecology annual*. New York: Appleton-Century-Crofts; 1972: pp. 177–91.
10. Brettner A. Zum Verhalten der Sekundären Wand der Uteroplacentargefässe bei der Decidualen Reaktion. *Acta Anat* 1964; **57**: 367–76.
11. Pijnenborg R, Bland J M, Robertson W B, Brosens I. Uteroplacental arterial changes related to interstitial trophoblast migration in early human pregnancy. *Placenta* 1983; **4**: 397–414.
12. Robson S C, Ball E, Lyall F, *et al.* Endovascular trophoblast invasion and spiral artery transformation: the 'two wave' theory revisited. *Placenta* 2001; **22**: A.25.
13. Lyall F. The human placental bed revisited. *Placenta* 2002; **23**: 555–62.

14. Damsky C H, Fitzgerald M L, Fisher S J. Distribution patterns of extracellular matrix components and adhesion receptors are intricately modulated during first trimester cytotrophoblast differentiation along the invasive pathway, in vivo. *J Clin Invest* 1992; **89**: 210–22.
15. Aplin J D. Expression of integrin α6β4 in human trophoblast and its loss from extravillous cells. *Placenta* 1993; **14**: 203–15.
16. Zhou Y, Damsky C H, Chiu K, Roberts J M, Fisher S J. Preeclampsia is associated with abnormal expression of adhesion molecules by invasive cytotrophoblasts. *J Clin Invest* 1993; **91**: 950–60.
17. Divers M J, Bulmer J N, Miller D, Lilford R J. Beta 1 integrins in third trimester human placentae: no differential expression in pathological pregnancy. *Placenta* 1995; **16**: 245–60.
18. Pijnenborg R, Vercruysse L, Verbist L, Van Assche F A. Interaction of interstitial trophoblast with placental bed capillaires and venules of normotensive and pre-eclamptic pregnancies. *Placenta* 1998; **19**: 569–75.
19. Naicker T, Shedun S M, Moodley J, Pijnenborg R. Quantitative analysis of trophoblast invasion in preeclampsia. *Acta Obstet Gynecol Scand* 2003; **82**: 722–29.
20. Al-Nasiry S, Vercruysse L, Hanssens M, Luyten C, Pijnenborg R. Interstitial trophoblastic cell fusion and E-cadherin immunostaining in the placental bed of normal and hypertensive pregnancies. *Placenta* 2009; **30**: 719–725.
21. Gerretsen G, Huisjes H J, Hardonk M J, Elema J D. Trophoblast alterations in the placental bed in relation to physiological changes in spiral arteries. *Br J Obstet Gynaecol* 1983; **90**: 34–9.
22. Redman C W B, Sacks G P, Sargent I L. Preeclampsia: an excessive maternal inflammatory response to pregnancy. *Am J Obstet Gynecol* 1999; **180**: 499–506.
23. Billington W D. Biology of the trophoblast. *Adv Reprod Physiol* 1971; **5**: 27–66.
24. Pijnenborg R, Bland J M, Robertson W B, Dixon G, Brosens I. The pattern of interstitial trophoblast invasion of the myometrium in early human pregnancy. *Placenta* 1981; **2**: 303–16.
25. Jones R L, Findlay J K, Farnworth P G *et al.* Activin A and inhibin A differentially regulate human uterine matrix metalloproteinases: potential interactions during decidualization and trophoblast invasion. *Endocrinology* 2006; **147**: 724–32.
26. Aplin J D, Charlton A K, Ayad S. An immunohistochemical study of human endometrial extracellular matrix during the menstrual cycle and first trimester of pregnancy. *Cell Tissue Res* 1988; **253**: 231–40.
27. Brosens J J, Pijnenborg R, Brosens I. The myometrial junctional zone spiral arteries in normal and abnormal pregnancies. *Am J Obstet Gynecol* 2002; **187**: 1416–23.
28. Maugey-Laulom B, Commenges-Ducos M, Jullien V *et al.* Endometrial vascularity and ongoing pregnancy after IVF. *Eur J Obstet Gynecol Reprod Biol* 2002; **104**: 137–43.
29. Plasencia W, Maiz N, Bonino S, Kaihura C, Nicolaides K H. Uterine artery Doppler at 11+0 to 13+6 weeks in the prediction of pre-eclampsia. *Ultrasound Obstet Gynecol* 2007; **30**: 742–9.
30. Jauniaux E, Watson A L, Hempstock J *et al.* Onset of maternal arterial blood flow and placental oxidative stress. *Am J Pathol* 2000; **157**: 2111–22.
31. Chang K, Zhang L. Steroid hormones and uterine vascular adaptation to pregnancy. *Reprod Sci* 2008; **15**: 336–48.
32. Pijnenborg R. Uterine haemodynamics as a possible driving force for endovascular trophoblast migration in the placental bed. *Medical Hypoth* 2000; **55**: 114–18.
33. Labarrere C A, Faulk W P. Diabetic placentae: studies of the battlefield after the war. *Diabetes/Metabolism Rev* 1991; **7**: 253–63.
34. Baird J N Jr. Eclampsia in a lowland gorilla. *Am J Obstet Gynecol* 1981; **141**: 345–6.
35. Stout C, Lemmon W B. Glomerular capillary endothelial swelling in a pregnant chimpanzee. *Am J Obstet Gynecol* 1969; **105**: 212–5.
36. Thornton J G, Onwude J L. Convulsions in pregnancy in related gorillas. *Am J Obstet Gynecol* 1992; **167**: 240–1.
37. Pijnenborg R, Vercruysse L, Hanssens M. Fetal-maternal conflict, trophoblast invasion, pre-eclampsia and the Red Queen. *Hypertens Preg* 2008; **27**: 183–96.
38. Dawkins R, Krebs J R. Arms races between and within species. *Proc R Soc Lond B* 1979; **205**: 489–511.
39. Haig D. Genetic conflicts in human pregnancy. *Q Rev Biol* 1993; **68**: 495–532.
40. Rockwell L C, Vargas E, Moore L G. Human physiological adaptation to pregnancy: inter- and intraspecific perspectives. *Am J Hum Biol* 2003; **15**: 330–41.
41. DeSilva J, Lesnik J. Chimpanzee neonatal brain size: implications for brain growth in *Homo erectus*. *J Hum Evolution* 2006; **51**: 207–12.
42. Robillard P Y, Hulsey T C, Dekker G A, Chaouat G. Preeclampsia and human reproduction. An essay of a long term reflection. *J Reprod Immun* 2003; **59**: 93–100.
43. Chaline J. Increased cranial capacity in hominid evolution and preeclampsia. *J Reprod Immun* 2003; **59**: 137–52.

44. Pijnenborg R, Vercruysse L, Hanssens M. The uterine spiral arteries in human pregnancy: facts and controversies. *Placenta* 2006; **27**: 939–58.

45. Ness R B, Roberts J M. Heterogeneous causes constituting the single syndrome of preeclampsia: a hypothesis and its implications. *Am J Obstet Gynecol* 1996; **175**: 1365–79.

46. Garris D R. Effects of diabetes on uterine condition, decidualization, vascularization, and corpus luteum function in the pseudopregnant rat. *Endocrinology* 1988; **122**: 665–72.

47. Burke S D, Dong H, Hazan Q D, Croy B A. Aberrant endometrial features of pregnancy in diabetic NOD mice. *Diabetes* 2007; **56**: 2919–26.

48. Garner P R, D'Alton M E, Dudley D K, Huard P, Hardie M. Preeclampsia in diabetic pregnancies. *Am J Obstet Gynecol* 1990; **163**: 505–8.

Section 3 Chapter 5

Uterine vascular environment

Decidualization

Brianna Cloke, Luca Fusi, and Jan Brosens

Institute of Reproductive and Developmental Biology, Imperial College London, Hammersmith Hospital Campus, London, UK

Introduction

The maternal response to an implanting embryo is arguably the single most important factor in determining pregnancy outcome. This maternal response is termed decidualization, a process that occurs in all species where implantation involves breaching of the luminal endometrial epithelium [1]. Decidualization denotes pregnancy-associated remodeling of the endometrial stromal compartment, which is characterized by transient local edema, an abundance of macrophages and specialized uterine natural killer (uNK) cells, angiogenesis, and the extraordinary transformation of resident endometrial stromal fibroblasts into secretory, epithelioid decidual cells. From a functional perspective, the decidual process establishes maternal immunological tolerance to fetal antigens, protects the conceptus against environmental insults, and ensures tissue integrity and hemostasis during the process of trophoblast invasion and placenta formation [1]. Thus, perturbations in the decidual process inevitably result, depending on severity, in either implantation failure or impaired placental function.

Different evolutionary strategies have emerged to ensure reproductive success. For instance, many mammals display delayed implantation, also termed 'embryonic diapause', which is characterized by a temporary suspension of embryo development prior to implantation. Embryonic diapause can either be induced in response to environmental signals (facultative diapause) or occur in every gestation (obligate diapause) and is reversed when optimal environmental, metabolic, and hormonal conditions are achieved [2]. Activation of dormant blastocysts in the mouse uterus, for example, is dependent upon a rise in estrogen levels, which in turn synchronizes the multiple implantation events in this species [3]. Implantation in humans differs in several key aspects. First, there is no evidence of uncoupling of pre- and postimplantation development in human embryos. Second, human beings, unlike most species, must deal with a high incidence of embryonic aneuploidies. Finally, multiple implantations are relatively rare and the invasive potential of the human embryo is high. To deal with these 'unique' reproductive features, a number of adaptive responses must have evolved in human beings, one of which may well have been the emergence of 'spontaneous' cyclic decidualization of the endometrium. Once the decidual process is initiated, no additional implantation events can occur. In most mammals decidualization is triggered by signals from the implanting embryo(s) but in human beings this process is under maternal control and initiated around day 23 of each cycle (Fig. 5.1) [4]. Thus, 'spontaneous' decidualization of the human endometrium during the luteal phase of the cycle restricts the 'window of endometrial receptivity' during which an embryo can implant, which in turn may serve as an important selection mechanism that favors implantation of developmentally competent embryos and limits the likelihood of abnormal pregnancies. In support of this conjecture, Wilcox *et al.* demonstrated that late implantation beyond day 23 of a 28-day cycle, which presumably reflects impaired decidualization and a prolonged implantation window, is associated with an exponential increase in early pregnancy loss [5].

The process of endometrial decidualization is thus a key event with direct relevance to very early pregnancy as well as subsequent pregnancy outcome. Although decidualization encompasses all aspects of endometrial preparation for pregnancy, including the dramatic changes in local immune cells and vascular remodeling, this chapter first reviews our current understanding of the signals and pathways that control the morphological and biochemical differentiation of resident endometrial fibroblasts into secretory decidual cells, after which the functions of these cells at the feto-maternal interface are discussed.

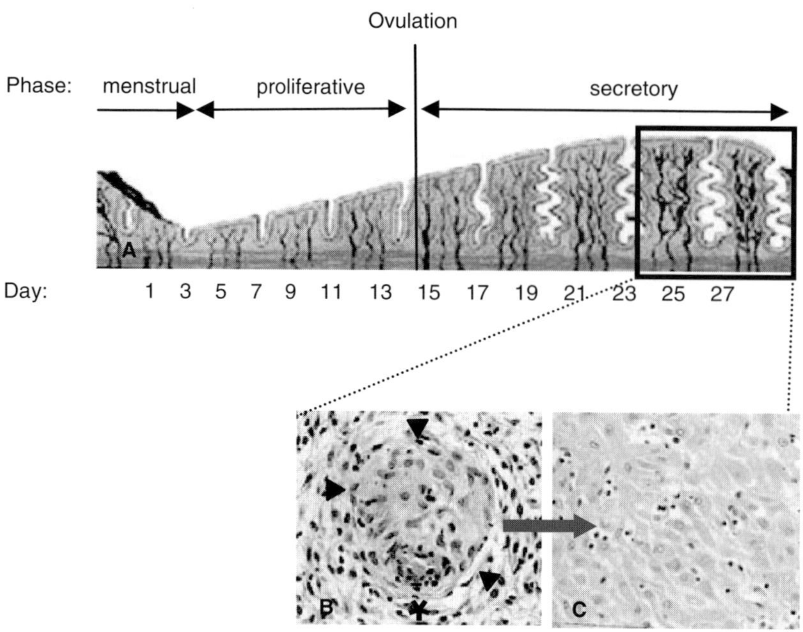

Fig. 5.1 Cyclic decidualization of the endometrial stromal compartment during the menstrual cycle. (A) The postovulatory rise in progesterone levels initiates endometrial differentiation in preparation for pregnancy. (B) As is the case in other menstruating species, the human endometrium exhibits spontaneous decidualization during the late secretory phase of the cycle, a process initiated around the terminal spiral arteries (*) and characterized by epithelioid transformation of stromal fibroblasts (arrowheads). (C) The decidual process continues to evolve and in pregnancy encompasses the entire stromal compartment. See plate section for color version.

Morphological and biochemical differentiation

Recent studies have shown that adult somatic cells can be reprogrammed to pluripotent stem cells by transduction of merely four factors: OCT3/4, SOX2, KLF4, and c-MYC [6]. Interestingly, manual mining of microarray data shows that differentiation of endometrial fibroblasts into decidualizing cells is associated with enhanced expression of three of these factors (Fig. 5.2) [7]. Not surprisingly, the decidual cell phenotype is not only complex but also dynamic. In their undifferentiated form, endometrial stromal cells have a spindle-shaped fibroblastic appearance. Progressive enlargement and rounding of the nucleus, cytoplasmic accumulation of glycogen and lipid droplets, and expansion of the Golgi complex and rough endoplasmic reticulum underpin the transformation of endometrial fibroblasts into decidual cells with a secretory, epithelioid-like phenotype [1]. Multiple projections appear on the cell surface, which extend into the extracellular matrix or indent adjacent cells. Decidualizing cells produce an abundance of extracellular matrix proteins, including laminin, type IV collagen, fibronectin, and heparan sulfate proteoglycan [8,9]. The abundantly secreted laminin and collagen IV are precipitated into a basement membrane-like pericellular material, which is not unlike 'real' basement

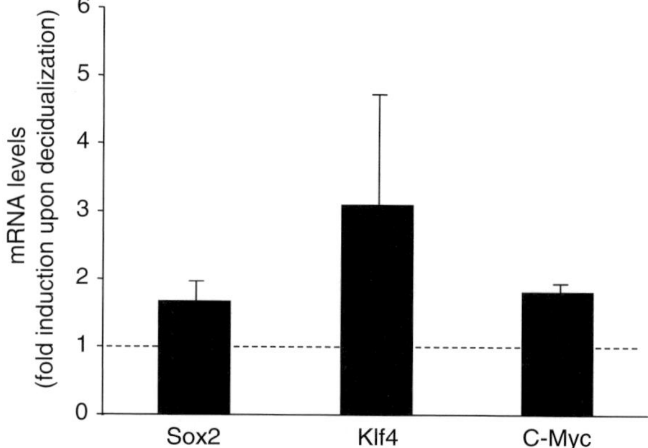

Fig. 5.2 Decidualization of human endometrial stromal cells is associated with induction of transcriptional mediators of cellular pluripotency. Primary human endometrial stromal cells were decidualized in culture for 3 days. Total mRNA was subjected to genome-wide expression profiling. Manual mining of the microarray data revealed that endometrial cells express higher levels of Oct3/4, Kfl4, and c-Myc transcripts upon differentiation into decidual cells. The data represent fold induction (± standard deviation) of normalized mRNA signal intensities, relative to expression levels in undifferentiated cells (dotted line), of three independent cultures.

membranes secreted by epithelia. Decidualization is also characterized by a dramatic increase in filamentous actin polymerization and stress fiber formation (Fig. 5.3) and loss of phosphorylation of the regulatory light chain of myosin 2 (MLC2), which in turn

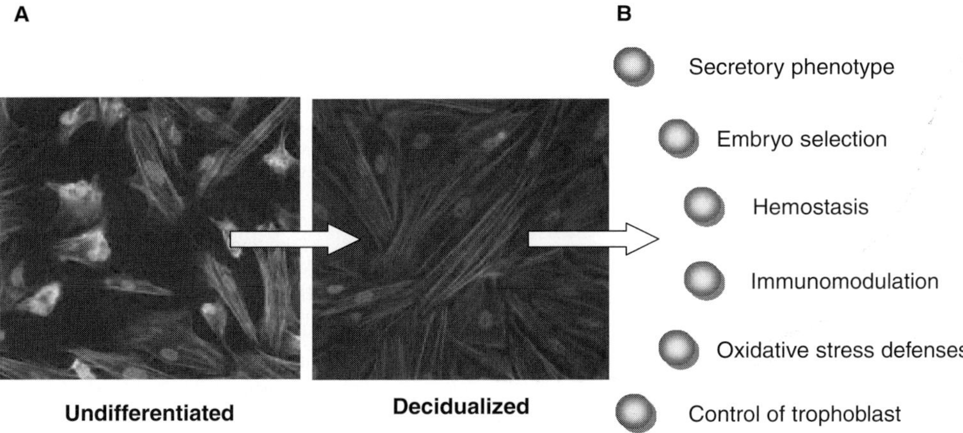

Fig. 5.3 Morphological changes and functional reprogramming upon decidualization. (A) Cytoskeletal organization and stress fiber formation. Phalloidin staining (red) of filamentous-actin in undifferentiated endometrial stromal cells (left panel) and cells decidualized in culture for 72 hours (right panel). (B) In concert, endometrial stromal cells acquire unique functions essential for pregnancy. See plate section for color version.

accounts for the marked reduction in cell motility [10]. In conjunction, expression of desmin, α-smooth muscle actin, and vimentin points towards the acquisition of a more contractile myofibroblastic phenotype [11].

Gene profiling studies have been instrumental in delineating the extent and magnitude of cellular reprogramming associated with decidualization. Using a genome-wide array approach, Takano *et al.* reported that treatment of primary endometrial stromal cell cultures with a decidualizing stimulus for only 3 days is sufficient to significantly alter the expression of 3307 genes [7]. In this study, more genes were downregulated (60%) than upregulated (40%) upon decidual transformation. Based on this and other gene profiling studies, decidualization can be described as a process of sequential reprogramming of functionally related families of genes involved in cell adhesion, signal transduction, stress responses, extracellular matrix reorganization, cytoskeletal organization, metabolism, cell cycle progression, apoptosis, and differentiation [7,10,12].

The acquisition of a secretory phenotype by endometrial stromal cells is associated with the expression of a myriad of genes (e.g. *SOD2*, *GADD45A*, *MAOB*, *SSP1*, *CLU*, and *FOXO1*) that are first either constitutively expressed in endometrial epithelial cells or induced in this cellular compartment upon ovulation [7]. Major secretory products of decidualized stromal cells, such as prolactin (PRL) and insulin-like growth factor binding protein-1 (IGFBP-1), have traditionally been used as markers of the differentiated cellular state [13,14]. Intriguingly, expression of PRL by differentiating endometrial cells, which requires transcriptional activation of an alternative promoter located 6 kilobases upstream of the pituitary transcription initiation site, has been shown to be a recent evolutionary innovation linked to the emergence of eutherian (placental) mammals that are capable of prolonged internal gestation [15]. Differentiating endometrial stromal cells also secrete a variety of factors, such as macrophage inflammatory protein-1β, interleukin (IL)-11, and IL-15, which are thought to provide chemotactic and activating signals for uNK cells [16,17]. Other major secretory products of decidual cells include Lefty-A, a novel member of the TGF-β superfamily originally identified as an endometrial bleeding-associated factor (Ebaf), Wnt4, and glutathione peroxidase 3, a secreted enzyme with potent extracellular antioxidant activity capable of reducing hydrogen peroxide and a broad range of fatty acid- and phospholipid-hydroperoxides [7,18,19].

Mechanism of decidualization

Decidual transformation of endometrial stromal cells can be faithfully recapitulated in culture and these *in vitro* studies have yielded invaluable insights into the signal pathways and downstream transcription factors that govern this differentiation process [7,9,12]. Contrary to what is often stated, progesterone is not the primary trigger of the decidual process. In vivo, decidual transformation is first apparent approximately 9 days after the postovulatory rise in circulating progesterone levels (see Fig. 5.1), further indicating that the expression of decidua-specific genes is not under direct transcriptional control of activated progesterone receptor (PR). It is now well established that initiation of the decidual process is dependent upon increased levels of the second messenger cyclic adenosine monophosphate (cAMP) and sustained activation of the protein kinase A (PKA) pathway [14]. Although exposure of primary cultures to progesterone, alone or in combination with estradiol, for 8–10 days will trigger expression of decidual markers, this response is mediated by a gradual increase in intracellular cAMP levels and abrogated in the presence of PKA inhibitor [20].

Cyclic AMP is a ubiquitous second messenger molecule that is generated from ATP by adenylate cyclase. This enzyme is activated upon binding of ligand to members of the family of G-protein-coupled receptors (GPCRs), which are coupled to a stimulatory heterotrimeric guanine nucleotide-binding protein (G-protein). Adenylate cyclase activity in the human endometrium increases during the menstrual cycle and the cAMP content in biopsies obtained from patients during the secretory phase is higher than that in the proliferative phase [21]. During the secretory phase of the cycle, local factors are produced capable of increasing cAMP levels in stromal cells, including relaxin, corticotropin-releasing hormone and prostaglandin E_2 [22,23,24]. The intracellular level of cAMP is determined not only by its production but also by its degradation. Members of the large family of phosphodiesterases (PDEs) convert cAMP to AMP, which no longer stimulates PKA activity. PDE4 and PDE8 are the principal PDE isoforms in endometrial stromal cells and inhibition of PDE4 is sufficient to induce expression of decidual markers [25]. Thus, sustained increase in cellular cAMP observed in decidualizing endometrium may, at least in part, be due to inhibition of PDE activity.

Although undifferentiated endometrial fibroblasts abundantly express PR, elevated cAMP levels are essential to sensitize these cells to progesterone. Convergence of cAMP and progesterone signaling is complex and appears to occur at multiple levels. First, cAMP activation of the PKA pathway has been shown to disrupt the interaction of PR with corepressors, such as nuclear receptor corepressor (NCoR) and silencing mediator for retinoid and thyroid hormone (SMRT), thereby facilitating recruitment of steroid receptor coactivators [26]. Second, cAMP induces the expression or activation of several transcription factors, including FOXO1, STAT5 (signal transducers and activators of transcription 5), and C/EBPβ CCAAT/enhancer-binding protein β, capable of interacting directly with PR [27,28]. This has led to the hypothesis that PR, and more specifically PR-A, may serve as a platform in endometrial cells for the formation of multimeric transcriptional complexes that regulate the expression of decidua-specific genes. Thus, by hijacking decidua-specific transcription factors, the liganded PR acquires transcriptional control over many more genes than would be predicted on the basis of consensus PR response elements in their promoter regions.

Another important mechanism whereby cAMP signaling sensitizes endometrial fibroblasts to progesterone involves downregulation of protein inhibitor of activated STAT 1 (PIAS1), the E3 SUMO ligase for PR [29]. SUMO (small ubiquitin-like modifier) proteins (SUMO-1, -2, -3, and -4) are posttranslational modifiers whose dynamic and reversible attachment to other proteins proceeds through a sequence of enzymatically directed steps. Sumoylation profoundly modulates the function of many diverse target proteins, by altering protein stability, protein–protein interactions, and cellular localization, and generally bestows repressive properties onto transcription factors [30]. In undifferentiated endometrial cells, PR is rapidly modified by covalent attachment of SUMO-1 upon hormone binding. Loss of PIAS1 expression upon decidualization greatly reduces this enzymatic modification of PR, resulting in much enhanced *trans*-activation potential of the receptor [29].

PIAS1 is also responsible for SUMO modification of other steroid receptors expressed in endometrial stromal cells, including the androgen receptor (AR) [10]. Consequently, decidualization is also characterized by increased cellular sensitivity to androgen signaling. In fact, there is an important but often overlooked role for androgens in establishing a functional decidua in early pregnancy. Serum androgen levels fluctuate throughout the menstrual cycle, with levels peaking around ovulation [31]. However, tissue androgen levels and conversion of androstenedione to testosterone are higher in secretory than proliferative endometrium [32]. Moreover, a rise in circulating androgen levels in the late luteal phase is associated with a conception cycle and levels continue to rise in early pregnancy [33]. By combining small interfering RNA technology with genome-wide expression profiling, we recently found that AR and PR regulate the expression of distinct decidual gene networks. Although the number of decidual genes under AR control was relatively small (~ 100), they were functionally indispensable for differentiation-dependent stress fiber formation, exocytosis, and cell cycle inhibition [10]. In comparison, PR depletion perturbed the expression of 10 times more genes, underscoring the importance of this nuclear receptor in regulating diverse cellular functions. However, several PR-dependent genes encode for signaling intermediates and knockdown of PR abolished activation of WNT/β-catenin, TGFβ/SMAD, and STAT pathways in decidualizing cells. Thus, PR regulates endometrial stromal cell differentiation, at least in part, by re-programming the cellular responses to growth factor and cytokine signal transduction.

At first glance decidualization may appear rather straightforward, requiring only enhanced cAMP signaling to sensitize endometrial fibroblasts to steroid hormones. It is in fact a constantly evolving differentiation process that entails activation and inhibition of a myriad of signal transduction pathways. Once initiated, decidualizing endometrial cells secrete various factors, including IL-11, IL-15, activin A, somatostatin, ghrelin, PRL, IGFBP-1, and sphingosine-1-phosphate, capable of amplifying and modifying the differentiated phenotype in an autocrine or paracrine fashion [16,34]. For example, decidual PRL is thought to be important in inhibiting 20α-hydroxysteroid dehydrogenase expression, an enzyme that catabolizes progesterone [35]. Another example is the ability of IGFBP-1 to enhance the decidual response, which is thought to involve binding of this protein to α5β1 integrin on the surface of endometrial stromal cells [36].

In vivo, numerous additional paracrine signals derived from local immune cells and interacting invading trophoblast will further modify decidual cell function in a dynamic fashion. The cellular tyrosine kinase c-Src has emerged as a possible focal point for the integration of various cytokine, growth factor, and steroid hormone signals in decidual cells. c-Src belongs to the Src family of protein tyrosine kinases (SFKs), which are probably best known for their roles downstream of integrin adhesion receptors. SFKs are necessary for the generation of 'outside-in signals' that regulate cytoskeletal organization, cell motility, and gene expression in response to cell adhesion. Decidualization is associated with strong c-Src activation, which in turn is an upstream regulator of several critical signal transduction cascades, including the mitogen-activated protein kinase (MAPK), phosphatidylinositol 3-kinase (PI3K), and STAT pathways [37]. Not surprisingly, the decidual response is greatly impaired in *c-Src* null mice [38].

Decidualization and vascular remodeling

Morphologically, decidualization is first apparent in stromal cells underlying the surface epithelium and surrounding the terminal spiral arteries during the mid to late luteal phase of the cycle [4]. At this stage, the spiral arteries are already being remodeled in preparation of pregnancy; a process characterized by endothelial swelling, vacuolation, and disorganization of the smooth muscle media. Decidual cells form a typical cuff around these vessels and ensure tissue hemostasis prior to and during endovascular trophoblast invasion through several mechanisms. For example, decidualizing endometrial stromal cells highly express tissue factor (TF), a membrane-anchored glycoprotein that serves as a receptor for coagulation factor VII/VIIa. TF triggers activation of the extrinsic coagulation pathway leading to the production of fibrin in a spatially and temporally controlled manner. The hemostatic functions of decidual cells are further enhanced by the concurrent induction of the fibrinolysis inhibitor plasminogen activator type 1 [39].

During the luteal phase, the endometrial stroma becomes dynamically populated with a wide variety of innate immune cells, including macrophages, uNK cells, and specialized uterine dendritic cells (uDCs) [40]. These immune cells are tolerogenic towards the invading semi-allogenic trophoblast, or allogenic in the case of recipients of donated oocytes, and have emerged as key regulators of angiogenesis in the decidua. Particularly, uNK cells, which reportedly make up 40% of cells in the decidua of pregnancy, are a rich source of angiogenic factors, endothelial cell mitogens, and various chemokines; key factors that coordinate trophoblast invasion with the vascular remodeling of the spiral arteries [41]. As mentioned, decidualizing stromal cells highly express IL-15 (Cloke, Fusi & Brosens, unpublished data), which is the primary trigger that converts inert endometrial NK cells into specialized tolerogenic cells capable of producing angiogenic growth factors. Moreover the expression levels of IL-15 transcripts, as well as the abundance of uNK cells, correlate with the subendometrial vascular flow during the luteal phase of the cycle [42].

A recent study has highlighted the critical role of uDCs in establishing a functional maternal–fetal interface [43]. In a transgenic mouse model, depletion of uDCs resulted in failure of decidualization, impaired implantation, and embryonic resorption. Interestingly, uDC ablation resulted in loss of both allogenic and syngenic pregnancies, indicating that the underlying mechanism did not involve an immunological response. Instead pregnancy loss was due to a delayed maternal angiogenic response, increased vascular permeability, and inhibited blood vessel maturation.

Decidualization and immunotolerance

Pregnancy involves complex immune regulation, necessary to prevent cytotoxic T cells from responding to fetal antigens, while simultaneously ensuring strong innate immunity at the maternal–fetal interface. Decidualizing stromal cells play an important role in local immunomodulation in more than one way. As mentioned, the postovulatory rise in progesterone levels induces expression of macrophage inflammatory protein-1β and interleukin-15 by differentiating endometrial stromal cells, which in turn provide the chemotactic and activating signals for uNK cells [44]. Gene expression studies of human uNK cells reported high expression of immunomodulatory molecules such as galectin-1 and glycodelin A [41]. Galectin-1 is known to inhibit T cell proliferation and survival and attenuates expression of proinflammatory cytokines by activated T cells [45]. Similarly, glycodelin A (also termed placental protein 14) potently inhibits T cell activation through its ability to interact with the tyrosine phosphatase receptor CD45 on the T cell surface [46]. The decidua, like syncytiotrophoblast, also expresses the tryptophan-catabolizing enzyme indoleamine 2,3-dioxygenase (IDO) [47]. Tryptophan is an essential amino acid required for cell proliferation. Studies in mice revealed an essential role for IDO in pregnancy [48]. Treatment of mothers with an IDO inhibitor, 1-methyl-tryptophan, induces extensive inflammation, massive complement deposition, and hemorrhagic necrosis at the feto-maternal interface, resulting in the resorption of semi-allogenic fetuses [49]. However, no inflammatory reaction is observed when syngenic mothers are given the IDO inhibitor and the pregnancy is not lost. These data strongly suggest that IDO activity protects the fetus by suppressing T cell-dependent inflammatory responses to fetal alloantigens.

Decidual cells display a variety of additional features that further suggest a key role for these cells in suppressing T cell-mediated cytotoxicity in pregnancy. For example, they highly express Fas ligand, a member of the tumor necrosis factor (TNF) superfamily that serves as a key death factor for activated T cells. However, decidual cells also express Fas, alternatively termed CD95 or APO-1, the cognate cell surface receptor for Fas ligand and a member of the TNF/nerve growth factor (NGF) receptor family [50]. Fas-induced cell death is, however, tightly controlled by various cytoplasmic regulators, amongst which is c-FLIP, a procaspase-8-like protease-deficient protein and potent inhibitor of death receptor-mediated apoptosis. In addition to Fas ligand and Fas, decidual cells abundantly express c-FLIP, which may serve to prevent autoactivation of the death receptor signaling pathway [51]. Another characteristic of endometrial stromal cell differentiation is the strong induction of *HSD11B1* expression (105-fold), which encodes for 11β-hydroxysteroid dehydrogenase type 1 (11β-HSD1) [7]. This enzyme operates predominantly as a reductase that converts inactive cortisone into active cortisol. In contrast, 11β-HSD2, which inactivates cortisol, localizes predominantly to placental syncytiotrophoblast [52]. The distinct expression pattern of these two isoenzymes suggests the presence of a cortisol gradient at the feto-maternal interface, which could constitute a major mechanism that protects the fetal allograft against a potential maternal immune response. Finally, like extravillous trophoblast, decidual stromal cells reportedly also express human leukocyte antigen G, an atypical non-polymorphic antigen suggested to reduce the potential cytotoxicity of maternal T lymphocytes and uNK cells [53].

Decidualization and cellular resistance

Decidualization is a rather paradoxical process. On the one hand, decidualizing stromal cells abundantly express various proapoptotic factors and are programmed to self-destruct upon falling progesterone levels, which plays an integral role in cyclic menstruation. On the other hand, this differentiation process is also characterized by strong resistance to cell death in response to oxidative or inflammatory insults [51]. Pregnancy has been described as a hyperinflammatory process and the ability of decidualizing endometrial cells to cope with proinflammatory and oxidative stress signals is key to safeguarding the integrity of the feto-maternal interface during the process of deep trophoblast invasion.

Major fluctuations in oxygen concentrations occur at the feto-maternal interface during normal pregnancy as a consequence of the profound vascular adaptations in the first trimester of pregnancy [54]. These changes in oxygen tension at the uteroplacental interface generate intracellular reactive oxygen species (ROS). In the absence of effective defense mechanisms, ROS, including superoxide anion, hydrogen peroxide, and hydroxyl radicals, cause indiscriminate damage to proteins, lipids, and nucleic acids. To counteract oxidative stress, cells constitutively express enzymes that neutralize ROS, which repair and replace the damage caused by ROS [55]. In addition, cells can also mount an 'adaptive response' to elevated levels of oxidative stress, such as increased expression of antioxidant enzymes, including glutathione S-transferases, peroxidases, and superoxide dismutases, and activation of protective and repair genes, such as heat shock proteins and GADD45α (growth arrest- and DNA damage-inducible protein α of 45 kDa), respectively [56]. Depending on the level of oxidative stress experienced, cells will either undergo transient cell cycle arrest and repair, senescence, apoptosis, or ultimately necrosis [57].

A variety of intracellular and extracellular free radical scavengers, such as superoxide dismutase 2, peroxiredoxin 2, thioredoxin, glutaredoxin and glutathione peroxidase 3, are induced upon decidualization [51,58]. In addition to increased scavenging capacity, other mechanisms are important for resistance to oxidative cell death upon decidualization. Exposure of undifferentiated endometrial cells to ROS triggers sustained activation of stress-dependent MAPK signaling pathways, more specifically the Jun N-terminal kinase (JNK) pathway, which in turn induces the expression and nuclear accumulation of FOXO3a, a member of the FOXO subfamily of Forkhead transcription factors [51]. Under conditions of cellular stress, FOXO3a activation in undifferentiated endometrial cells triggers the expression of pro-apoptotic target genes, such as *BIM*. In decidualizing cells, however, JNK activation in response to ROS is firmly silenced and FOXO3a is no longer induced, thereby disabling the apoptotic machinery responsible for oxidative cell death in undifferentiated endometrial stromal cells [51]. Decidualized cells also show a reduced activation of the p38 MAPK in response to proinflammatory cytokines, such as IL-1β [59].

The tumor suppressor protein p53 plays a fundamental role in protecting the genome from genotoxic insults. Wild-type p53 is massively upregulated upon cAMP-induced decidualization of endometrial stromal cells in culture [60]. Nuclear accumulation of p53 in the endometrial stromal cell compartment is also apparent *in vivo* during the secretory phase of the cycle. In most normal cells, it is present at very low levels because it is subject to rapid proteasomal degradation under physiological circumstances. In response to stress and DNA damage, the protein is stabilized and rapidly accumulates in the nucleus where it initiates events leading to cell cycle arrest and DNA repair or apoptosis, thus eliminating genotypically aberrant cells from the organism [61]. In addition to activating transcription of immediate target genes, p53 also exerts its functions by engaging in protein–protein interactions and suppression of transcription of a different set of target genes. Accumulation of p53 in the nuclei of decidualizing endometrial stromal cells is due to protein stabilization, as p53 mRNA levels remain unchanged. The presence of p53 is tightly linked to the decidualized status of the cells. Upon withdrawal of the decidualizing stimulus, stromal cells de-differentiate morphologically and lose expression of decidual PRL and IGFBP-1 along with the disappearance of p53 protein [60].

The role of p53 in the decidual process warrants further investigations. However, GADD45α, a putative p53 target gene, is also highly expressed in secretory phase endometrium [51]. GADD45 proteins are multifaceted factors implicated in the regulation of diverse stress responses, including cell cycle arrest at G2/M, chromatin remodeling, nucleotide excision repair, and apoptosis. They are presumed to serve as gatekeepers capable of killing cells unable to repair damaged DNA [62]. In addition to cytoprotection, another potential role of p53 and GADD45α in this system might be to halt proliferation and facilitate differentiation of the stromal compartment. Moreover, p53 and GADD45α could also play a role in safeguarding the genomic stability of endometrial cells during the cyclic process of rapid proliferation, differentiation, menstrual shedding, and regeneration.

Decidualization: clinical perspectives

The emergence in human beings of a cyclic decidual process has several major clinical implications; the most obvious of which is menstruation and its associated disorders. Menstruation, defined as shedding of the superficial endometrial layer in response to falling progesterone levels accompanied by overt bleeding, is a rare biological phenomenon found only in certain simian primates (Old World monkeys, apes, and humans), some bat species, such as wild fulvous fruit bats, and perhaps the elephant shrew. The unifying feature of the endometrium of menstruating species, including bats, is cyclic decidualization independent of pregnancy. All menstruating species also possess hemochorial placentae. Compared to most of our primate relatives, menstruation in humans is not only extraordinarily heavy but placentation is also exceptionally deep, with trophoblast invading not only the decidual endometrium but also the inner third of the myometrium, termed the uterine junctional zone, and its spiral arteries [63].

In addition to decidualizing stromal cells, all other cellular components in the superficial endometrial layer take part in menstrual shedding. Perhaps the first histological sign of impending endometrial breakdown is uNK cell apoptosis. As uNK cells do not express progesterone receptors (PR), cell death is likely a consequence of paracrine signals derived from PR-positive stromal cells [64]. Upon progesterone withdrawal, differentiated stromal cells also produce the chemokines and inflammatory mediators, such as IL-8, that trigger local infiltration of the endometrium by macrophages and other inflammatory cells. Approximately 2 days before the onset of menstruation, endometrial epithelial cells show a high degree of apoptosis, a low proliferative index, and loss of PR expression [65]. In contrast, stromal cell apoptosis is a later event, characterized by translocation of cytoplasmic FOXO1 to the nucleus, and induction and activation of proapoptotic BH3-only proteins, such as Bim [51]. Cell death in the endometrial stromal compartment is not pronounced but even limited apoptosis of decidualized cells surrounding the terminal spiral arteries may trigger focal interstitial hemorrhage. Ultimately, the shedding of endometrial tissue requires local and controlled degradation of the extracellular matrix, which in turn is dependent upon expression of matrix metalloproteinases (MMPs), secreted predominantly by differentiated stromal cells upon progesterone withdrawal [65].

Menstruation could be viewed as a rather unfortunate by-product of the process of extensive endometrial remodeling necessary to prepare uterine tissues for deep hemochorial placentation. However, the 'menstrual preconditioning hypothesis' recently challenged this view [66]. The term 'preconditioning' refers to the paradoxical yet ubiquitous biological phenomenon that a brief exposure to a harmful stimulus at a dose below the threshold for tissue injury provides robust protection against, or tolerance to, the injurious effects of a subsequent more severe insult. Analogously, the menstrual preconditioning hypothesis infers that modest cycle inflammation and oxidative stress associated with decidualization and menstruation may protect uterine tissues against the hyperinflammation associated with deep placentation. While speculative, this hypothesis fits well with the observation that disorders associated with impaired deep placentation, such as preeclampsia, are more prevalent and severe in very young women, especially in the first pregnancy [67].

In view of their specialized functions, it is rather surprising that few studies have addressed the role of decidual stromal cells in pathological pregnancy conditions. Moreover, as endometrial decidualization is cyclical, biochemical analysis of this differentiation process prior to conception may yield important cues for understanding subsequent pregnancy complications. Instead, several studies have focused on the uNK cell population during the putative window of implantation, especially in patients with a history of recurrent pregnancy loss [68,69]. These studies are fraught with difficulties. For example, timed endometrial samples of parous women are often used as a control reference but this approach does not take into account the possible effect of prior pregnancy on subsequent uNK cell counts. Moreover, analyses have been largely restricted to quantification of uNK cell numbers, which may not reflect or correlate with the function of these cells at the feto-maternal interface. Only two prospective studies, both very limited in size, have so far attempted to correlate uNK cell number in mid-secretory endometrial biopsy samples from recurrent miscarriage patients with subsequent pregnancy outcome [70,71]. The smallest study reported an association between increased uNK cell density and subsequent pregnancy loss but this was not confirmed in the subsequent larger study.

The role of decidual cells extends well beyond early pregnancy events. It is now also well established that common obstetrical disorders associated with impaired placentation, such as preeclampsia and fetal growth restriction, have their origins very early in pregnancy. For example, apoptotic responses are already enhanced in first trimester extravillous trophoblasts from pregnancies at risk of developing preeclampsia [72]. Consequently, there is considerable clinical interest in serum markers, such as placental protein 13 and circulating anti-angiogenic factors like soluble fms-like tyrosine kinase and endoglin, that may reflect impaired placental function during the first trimester of pregnancy [73,74]. However, there are as yet no circulating markers for the maternal decidual response. As the decidualization is characterized by secretory transformation of the endometrial stromal compartment, these markers are likely to exist. Moreover, identification of such serum markers raises the possibility of treatment of those women at risk of pregnancy complications prior to conception.

Acknowledgment

This work was supported by the Institute of Obstetrics and Gynaecology. We apologize to all those authors whose important contribution could not be referenced due to space restraints.

References

1. Gellersen B, Brosens I A, Brosens J J. Decidualization of the human endometrium: mechanisms, functions, and clinical perspectives. *Semin Reprod Med* 2007; **25**: 445–53.
2. Lopes F L, Desmarais J A, Murphy B D. Embryonic diapause and its regulation. *Reproduction* 2004; **128**: 669–78.
3. Hamatani T, Daikoku T, Wang H *et al.* Global gene expression analysis identifies molecular pathways distinguishing blastocyst dormancy and activation. *Proc Natl Acad Sci U S A* 2004; **101**: 10326–31.
4. de Ziegler D, Fanchin R, de Moustier B, Bulletti C. The hormonal control of endometrial receptivity: estrogen (E2) and progesterone. *J Reprod Immunol* 1998; **39**: 149–66.
5. Wilcox A J, Baird D D, Weinberg C R. Time of implantation of the conceptus and loss of pregnancy. *N Engl J Med* 1999; **340**: 1796–9.
6. Park I H, Zhao R, West J A *et al.* Reprogramming of human somatic cells to pluripotency with defined factors. *Nature* 2008; **451**: 141–6.
7. Takano M, Lu Z, Goto T *et al.* Transcriptional cross talk between the forkhead transcription factor forkhead box O1A and the progesterone receptor coordinates cell cycle regulation and differentiation in human endometrial stromal cells. *Mol Endocrinol* 2007; **21**: 2334–49.
8. Aplin J D, Charlton A K, Ayad S. An immunohistochemical study of human endometrial extracellular matrix during the menstrual cycle and first trimester of pregnancy. *Cell Tissue Res* 1988; **253**: 231–40.
9. Popovici R M, Betzler N K, Krause M S *et al.* Gene expression profiling of human endometrial-trophoblast interaction in a coculture model. *Endocrinology* 2006; **147**: 5662–75.
10. Cloke B, Huhtinen K, Fusi L *et al.* The androgen and progesterone receptors regulate distinct gene networks and cellular functions in decidualizing endometrium. *Endocrinology* 2008; **149**: 4462–74.
11. Oliver C, Montes M J, Galindo J A, Ruiz C, Olivares E G. Human decidual stromal cells express alpha-smooth muscle actin and show ultrastructural similarities with myofibroblasts. *Hum Reprod* 1999; **14**: 1599–605.
12. Brar A K, Handwerger S, Kessler C A, Aronow B J. Gene induction and categorical reprogramming during in vitro human endometrial fibroblast decidualization. *Physiol Genomics* 2001; **7**: 135–48.
13. Bell S C, Jackson J A, Ashmore J, Zhu H H, Tseng L. Regulation of insulin-like growth factor-binding protein-1 synthesis and secretion by progestin and relaxin in long term cultures of human endometrial stromal cells. *J Clin Endocrinol Metab* 1991; **72**: 1014–24.
14. Brosens J J, Hayashi N, White J O. Progesterone receptor regulates decidual prolactin expression in differentiating human endometrial stromal cells. *Endocrinology* 1999; **140**: 4809–20.
15. Lynch V J, Tanzer A, Wang Y *et al.* Adaptive changes in the transcription factor HoxA-11 are essential for the evolution of pregnancy in mammals. *Proc Natl Acad Sci U S A* 2008; **105**: 14928–33.
16. Dimitriadis E, White C A, Jones R L, Salamonsen L A. Cytokines, chemokines and growth factors in endometrium related to implantation. *Hum Reprod Update* 2005; **11**: 613–30.
17. Jones R L, Hannan N J, Kaitu'u T J, Zhang J, Salamonsen L A. Identification of chemokines important for leukocyte recruitment to the human endometrium at the times of embryo implantation and menstruation. *J Clin Endocrinol Metab* 2004; **89**: 6155–67.
18. Cornet P B, Picquet C, Lemoine P *et al.* Regulation and function of LEFTY-A/EBAF in the human endometrium: mRNA expression during the menstrual cycle, control by progesterone, and effect on matrix metalloprotineases. *J Biol Chem* 2002; **277**: 42496–504.
19. Riesewijk A, Martin J, van Os R *et al.* Gene expression profiling of human endometrial receptivity on days LH+2 versus LH+7 by microarray technology. *Mol Hum Reprod* 2003; **9**: 253–64.

20. Brar A K, Frank G R, Kessler C A, Cedars M I, Handwerger S. Progesterone-dependent decidualization of the human endometrium is mediated by cAMP. *Endocrine* 1997; **6**: 301–7.

21. Tanaka N, Miyazaki K, Tashiro H, Mizutani H, Okamura H. Changes in adenylyl cyclase activity in human endometrium during the menstrual cycle and in human decidua during pregnancy. *J Reprod Fertil* 1993; **98**: 33–9.

22. Milne S A, Perchick G B, Boddy S C, Jabbour H N. Expression, localization, and signaling of PGE(2) and EP2/EP4 receptors in human nonpregnant endometrium across the menstrual cycle. *J Clin Endocrinol Metab* 2001; **86**: 4453–9.

23. Palejwala S, Tseng L, Wojtczuk A, Weiss G, Goldsmith L T. Relaxin gene and protein expression and its regulation of procollagenase and vascular endothelial growth factor in human endometrial cells. *Biol Reprod* 2002; **66**: 1743–8.

24. Zoumakis E, Margioris A N, Stournaras C *et al.* Corticotrophin-releasing hormone (CRH) interacts with inflammatory prostaglandins and interleukins and affects the decidualization of human endometrial stroma. *Mol Hum Reprod* 2000; **6**: 344–51.

25. Bartsch O, Bartlick B, Ivell R. Phosphodiesterase 4 inhibition synergizes with relaxin signaling to promote decidualization of human endometrial stromal cells. *J Clin Endocrinol Metab* 2004; **89**: 324–34.

26. Rowan B G, Garrison N, Weigel N L, O'Malley B W. 8-Bromo-cyclic AMP induces phosphorylation of two sites in SRC-1 that facilitate ligand-independent activation of the chicken progesterone receptor and are critical for functional cooperation between SRC-1 and CREB binding protein. *Mol Cell Biol* 2000; **20**: 8720–30.

27. Mak I Y, Brosens J J, Christian M *et al.* Regulated expression of signal transducer and activator of transcription, Stat5, and its enhancement of PRL expression in human endometrial stromal cells in vitro. *J Clin Endocrinol Metab* 2002; **87**: 2581–8.

28. Christian M, Zhang X, Schneider-Merck T *et al.* Cyclic AMP-induced forkhead transcription factor, FKHR, cooperates with CCAAT/enhancer-binding protein beta in differentiating human endometrial stromal cells. *J Biol Chem* 2002; **277**: 20825–32.

29. Jones M C, Fusi L, Higham J H *et al.* Regulation of the SUMO pathway sensitizes differentiating human endometrial stromal cells to progesterone. *Proc Natl Acad Sci U S A* 2006; **103**: 16272–7.

30. Kerscher O, Felberbaum R, Hochstrasser M. Modification of proteins by ubiquitin and ubiquitin-like proteins. *Annu Rev Cell Dev Biol* 2006; **22**: 159–80.

31. Massafra C, De Felice C, Agnusdei D P, Gioia D, Bagnoli F. Androgens and osteocalcin during the menstrual cycle. *J Clin Endocrinol Metab* 1999; **84**: 971–4.

32. Bonney R C, Scanlon M J, Jones D L, Reed M J, James V H. Adrenal androgen concentrations in endometrium and plasma during the menstrual cycle. *J Endocrinol* 1984; **101**: 181–8.

33. Castracane V D, Stewart D R, Gimpel T, Overstreet J W, Lasley B L. Maternal serum androgens in human pregnancy: early increases within the cycle of conception. *Hum Reprod* 1998; **13**: 460–4.

34. Tanaka K, Minoura H, Isobe T *et al.* Ghrelin is involved in the decidualization of human endometrial stromal cells. *J Clin Endocrinol Metab* 2003; **88**: 2335–40.

35. Bao L, Tessier C, Prigent-Tessier A *et al.* Decidual prolactin silences the expression of genes detrimental to pregnancy. *Endocrinology* 2007; **148**: 2326–34.

36. Matsumoto H, Sakai K, Iwashita M. Insulin-like growth factor binding protein-1 induces decidualization of human endometrial stromal cells via alpha5beta1 integrin. *Mol Hum Reprod* 2008; **14**: 485–9.

37. Maruyama T, Yoshimura Y, Sabe H. Tyrosine phosphorylation and subcellular localization of focal adhesion proteins during in vitro decidualization of human endometrial stromal cells. *Endocrinology* 1999; **140**: 5982–90.

38. Kim H, Laing M, Muller W. c-Src-null mice exhibit defects in normal mammary gland development and ERalpha signaling. *Oncogene* 2005; **24**: 5629–36.

39. Lockwood C J, Krikun G, Schatz F. The decidua regulates hemostasis in human endometrium. *Semin Reprod Endocrinol* 1999; **17**: 45–51.

40. Dietl J, Honig A, Kammerer U, Rieger L. Natural killer cells and dendritic cells at the human feto-maternal interface: an effective cooperation? *Placenta* 2006; **27**: 341–7.

41. Koopman L A, Kopcow H D, Rybalov B *et al.* Human decidual natural killer cells are a unique NK cell subset with immunomodulatory potential. *J Exp Med* 2003; **198**: 1201–12.

42. Ledee N, Chaouat G, Serazin V *et al.* Endometrial vascularity by three-dimensional power Doppler ultrasound and cytokines: a complementary approach to assess uterine receptivity. *J Reprod Immunol* 2008; **77**: 57–62.

43. Plaks V, Birnberg T, Berkutzki T *et al.* Uterine DCs are crucial for decidua formation during embryo implantation in mice. *J Clin Invest* 2008; **118**: 3954–65.

44. Kitaya K, Yamaguchi T, Honjo H. Central role of interleukin-15 in postovulatory recruitment of

peripheral blood CD16(-) natural killer cells into human endometrium. *J Clin Endocrinol Metab* 2005; **90**: 2932–40.

45. Nguyen J T, Evans D P, Galvan M *et al.* CD45 modulates galectin-1-induced T cell death: regulation by expression of core 2 O-glycans. *J Immunol* 2001; **167**: 5697–707.
46. Rachmilewitz J, Borovsky Z, Riely G J, Miller R, Tykocinski M L. Negative regulation of T cell activation by placental protein 14 is mediated by the tyrosine phosphatase receptor CD45. *J Biol Chem* 2003; **278**: 14059–65.
47. Kudo Y, Hara T, Katsuki T *et al.* Mechanisms regulating the expression of indoleamine 2,3-dioxygenase during decidualization of human endometrium. *Hum Reprod* 2004; **19**: 1222–30.
48. Mellor A L, Chandler P, Lee G K *et al.* Indoleamine 2,3-dioxygenase, immunosuppression and pregnancy. *J Reprod Immunol* 2002; **57**: 143–50.
49. Munn D H, Zhou M, Attwood J T *et al.* Prevention of allogeneic fetal rejection by tryptophan catabolism. *Science* 1998; **281**: 1191–3.
50. Harirah H M, Donia S E, Parkash V, Jones D C, Hsu C D. Localization of the Fas-Fas ligand system in human fetal membranes. *J Reprod Med* 2002; **47**: 611–6.
51. Kajihara T, Jones M, Fusi L *et al.* Differential expression of FOXO1 and FOXO3a confers resistance to oxidative cell death upon endometrial decidualization. *Mol Endocrinol* 2006; **20**: 2444–55.
52. Driver P M, Kilby M D, Bujalska I *et al.* Expression of 11 beta-hydroxysteroid dehydrogenase isozymes and corticosteroid hormone receptors in primary cultures of human trophoblast and placental bed biopsies. *Mol Hum Reprod* 2001; **7**: 357–63.
53. Blanco O, Tirado I, Munoz-Fernandez R *et al.* Human decidual stromal cells express HLA-G: effects of cytokines and decidualization. *Hum Reprod* 2008; **23**: 144–52.
54. Jauniaux E, Watson A L, Hempstock J *et al.* Onset of maternal arterial blood flow and placental oxidative stress: a possible factor in human early pregnancy failure. *Am J Pathol* 2000; **157**: 2111–22.
55. Thannickal V J, Fanburg B L. Reactive oxygen species in cell signaling. *Am J Physiol Lung Cell Mol Physiol* 2000; **279**: L1005–28.
56. Tran H, Brunet A, Grenier J M *et al.* DNA repair pathway stimulated by the forkhead transcription factor FOXO3a through the Gadd45 protein. *Science* 2002; **296**: 530–4.
57. Davies K J. Oxidative stress, antioxidant defenses, and damage removal, repair, and replacement systems. *IUBMB Life* 2000; **50**: 279–89.
58. Borthwick J M, Charnock-Jones D S, Tom B D *et al.* Determination of the transcript profile of human endometrium. *Mol Hum Reprod* 2003; **9**: 19–33.
59. Strakova Z, Srisuparp S, Fazleabas A T. IL-1beta during in vitro decidualization in primate. *J Reprod Immunol* 2002; **55**: 35–47.
60. Pohnke Y, Schneider-Merck T, Fahnenstich J *et al.* Wild-type p53 protein is up-regulated upon cyclic adenosine monophosphate-induced differentiation of human endometrial stromal cells. *J Clin Endocrinol Metab* 2004; **89**: 5233–44.
61. Levine A J. p53, the cellular gatekeeper for growth and division. *Cell* 1997; **88**: 323–31.
62. Thyss R, Virolle V, Imbert V *et al.* NF-kappaB/Egr-1/Gadd45 are sequentially activated upon UVB irradiation to mediate epidermal cell death. *Embo J* 2005; **24**: 128–37.
63. Brosens I, Robertson W B, Dixon H G. The physiological response of the vessels of the placental bed to normal pregnancy. *J Pathol Bacteriol* 1967; **93**: 569–79.
64. King A. Uterine leukocytes and decidualization. *Hum Reprod Update* 2000; **6**: 28–36.
65. Brosens J J, Gellersen B. Death or survival – progesterone-dependent cell fate decisions in the human endometrial stroma. *J Mol Endocrinol* 2006; **36**: 389–98.
66. Brosens J J, Parker M G, McIndoe A, Pijnenborg R, Brosens I A. A role for menstruation in preconditioning the uterus for successful pregnancy. *Am J Obstet Gynecol* 2009; **200**: 615.e1–615.e6.
67. Saftlas A F, Olson D R, Franks A L, Atrash H K, Pokras R. Epidemiology of preeclampsia and eclampsia in the United States, 1979–1986. *Am J Obstet Gynecol* 1990; **163**: 460–5.
68. Hong Y, Wang X, Lu P, Song Y, Lin Q. Killer immunoglobulin-like receptor repertoire on uterine natural killer cell subsets in women with recurrent spontaneous abortions. *Eur J Obstet Gynecol Reprod Biol* 2008; **140**: 218–23.
69. Clifford K, Flanagan A M, Regan L. Endometrial CD56+ natural killer cells in women with recurrent miscarriage: a histomorphometric study. *Hum Reprod* 1999; **14**: 2727–30.
70. Tuckerman E, Laird S M, Prakash A, Li T C. Prognostic value of the measurement of uterine natural killer cells in the endometrium of women with recurrent miscarriage. *Hum Reprod* 2007; **22**: 2208–13.
71. Quenby S, Bates M, Doig T *et al.* Pre-implantation endometrial leukocytes in women with recurrent miscarriage. *Hum Reprod* 1999; **14**: 2386–91.

72. Whitley G S, Dash P R, Ayling L J *et al.* Increased apoptosis in first trimester extravillous trophoblasts from pregnancies at higher risk of developing preeclampsia. *Am J Pathol* 2007; **170**: 1903–9.

73. Huppertz B, Sammar M, Chefetz I *et al.* Longitudinal determination of serum placental protein 13 during development of preeclampsia. *Fetal Diagn Ther* 2008; **24**: 230–6.

74. Baumann M U, Bersinger N A, Mohaupt M G *et al.* First-trimester serum levels of soluble endoglin and soluble fms-like tyrosine kinase-1 as first-trimester markers for late-onset preeclampsia. *Am J Obstet Gynecol* 2008; **199**: 266 e1–6.

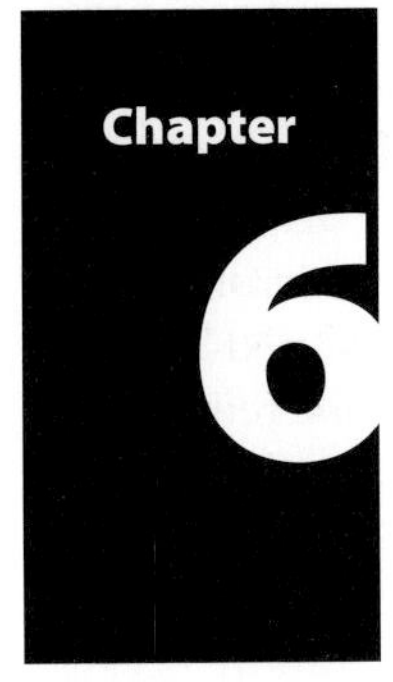

Immune cells in the placental bed

Ashley Moffett

Department of Pathology, University of Cambridge, Cambridge, UK

Introduction

At the site where the placenta implants there is intermingling of fetal trophoblast cells with maternal tissues [1,2]. This is therefore an important potential site of maternal–fetal allorecognition. The mucosal lining of the human uterus is transformed from endometrium in the non-pregnant state to the decidua of pregnancy [3]. Decidua has an unusual composition of leukocytes and lymphatics are also present [4]. Therefore, there must be mechanisms in place to avoid any type of immune 'rejection'. In addition to the avoidance of any damaging immune responses there is also the possibility that the decidual immune system might regulate placentation, in particular, the extent and depth of trophoblast invasion. It has long been known that trophoblast invasion proceeds quite differently when decidua is absent as seen when the placenta implants over scar tissue from a previous cesarean section as in an ectopic tubal pregnancy [5,2]. There is extensive destruction of the myometrium and this is never seen normally. Indeed, apart from the thin rim of Nitabuch's layer and the fibrinoid necrosis of the arterial media, there is remarkably little necrosis around the invading trophoblast cells in the decidua or myometrium. In addition, in the absence of decidua, such as when implantation occurs in the isthmus of the fallopian tube, individual interstitial trophoblast cells do not fuse to become placental bed giant cells (unpublished data). Although it is hard to infer functional capabilities from histological sections, these trophoblast giant cells are always seen at the deepest part of the implantation site and therefore have been considered static. The role of the decidua in controlling placentation does therefore seem clear [6]. Because such a conspicuous feature accompanying decidual change is the influx of large numbers of uterine natural killer (uNK) cells they have been proposed to provide the correct degree of trophoblast invasion [7]. Of course, it is not absolutely certain whether this controlling influence is exerted by the decidual tissue itself or specifically by the uNK cells within the decidua.

NK cells

The presence of mononuclear cells in the lining of the uterine mucosa has been well documented by histologists. Indeed, granulated cells were noted in the decidua long ago and were even then thought to be a type of lymphoid cell [8,9]: '*Quoi qu'il en soit, ce qui est indiscutable c'est que ce sont des cellules a type lymphoide propres a la decidua humain* (*Whatever, what is indisputable is that they are lymphoid-type cells specific to the human decidua*)'. These cells were subsequently also identified in the non-pregnant endometrium and were variously named as endometrial granulocytes, *Körnchenzellen*, or 'K' cells [10], globular leukocytes [11] and specific endometrial granular cells [12]. Several of the reports noted the apparent hormonal dependence of endometrial granulocytes and that they were particularly prominent in the secretory endometrium just before menstruation and persisted if decidualization occurred. Unless pregnancy intervenes, they show degenerative changes in the late secretory phase with mulberry-shaped nuclei. This appearance led to their name, endometrial granulocytes, because of the superficial resemblance to neutrophils. The distribution of the granulated cells is characteristic. There is a diffuse scattering of cells throughout the luteal phase stroma but also a tendency to aggregate around arteries and glands. In early decidua they amass in the decidua basalis at the implantation site but are mainly in the superficial decidual layer (decidua compacta) with only a few cells in the intervening stroma between the dilated glands of the deeper decidua spongiosa. Unlike in rodents, granulated cells are also present in decidua parietalis, which covers the uterine surface away from the site of placentation.

Outside the uterus, endometrial granulocytes have only been described in areas of ectopic decidualization, commonly in the fallopian tube and less often in the cervix or on the surface of the ovary [10]. Endometrial granulocytes are absent in the non-decidualized areas of the fallopian tube in an ectopic pregnancy, yet they are always present in the uterine decidua in such pregnancies even though no trophoblast is present in the uterus. They are also absent from any pathological conditions of the endometrium associated with excess estrogen such as endometrial hyperplasia and carcinoma. These observations all suggest that these cells are recruited under the hormonal influences of pregnancy and not as a response to invading trophoblast.

Once these cells were identified as CD56+ NK cells [13,14], it was possible to characterize their presence in the uterine mucosa more reliably. It was confirmed that the influx of NK cells into the uterine mucosa precedes decidualization in that the numbers of uNK cells already begin to increase in the mid-luteal phase of the non-pregnant endometrium, reaching a peak by the late secretory phase of the cycle and continuing until decidualization of pregnancy occurs [15,16]. This means that the accumulation of uNK cells in decidua is not related to the onset of pregnancy per se but is part of the cyclical changes occurring in the uterine mucosal lining. This temporal progression reinforced the view that the accumulation of uNK cells is likely to be under hormonal control, particularly progesterone, because their increase in numbers mirrors the rise in levels of this hormone. Interestingly, uNK cells do not express classical nuclear progesterone receptors so this hormone must exert its action indirectly, probably via other cells in the uterus [17,18]. IL-15 secreted by endometrial stromal cells is thought to have a major influence on uNK cell proliferation because stromal cells do express progesterone receptors and their production of IL-15 is increased by progesterone [19,20]. Another possible stromal cell product that could act on NK cells is prolactin whose progesterone dependence is well described [21].

Uterine NK cells are defined by the high expression of the surface marker CD56 so they are designated $CD56^{superbright}$ [22]. No other organs in the body possess such cells with their distinctive phenotypic profile (Table 6.1). There is a small population of $CD56^{bright}$ NK cells circulating in blood but these are not identical to those in the uterus in either morphology or phenotype [3,23]. The question has arisen as to how the $CD56^{bright}$ NK cells in blood and uterus are related. There could be CD34+ resident progenitors but it is difficult to rule out that these cells are

Table 6.1. A comparison of CD56+ NK subsets in peripheral blood and decidua

Marker	Decidua $CD56^{bright}$	Blood $CD56^{bright}$	Blood $CD56^{dim}$
CD9	+	–	–
CD16	–	–	+
CD69	+	–	–
CD151	++	–	+
CD160	–	–	+
L-selectin	–	++	+/–
α1 integrin	+	–	–
α6 integrin	–	+	+
KIR	+	–	+
NKG2A	+	+	+/–
CD94	++	++	+/–
NKG2D	+	+	+
NKp46	+	+	+
Perforin	+++	+	+++
Granzyme	+++	+	+++

contaminants from blood [24,25]. Another theory proposes that blood NK cells infiltrate the uterus where they proliferate and differentiate in the hormone-rich uterine mucosal environment. Many uNK cells do stain for the proliferation marker Ki-67 in the secretory phase as well as in early decidua [26]. Animal studies are in support of such a proposal. It has been shown that $CD56^{bright}$ NK cells from human peripheral blood selectively adhere to sections of mouse uterus in a Stamper-Woodruff assay and that splenic lymphocytes from pregnant mice can reconstitute uNK cells in NK cell-deficient mice [27]. The endometrium is also induced to express CXC chemokines by ovarian hormones [28]. These observations indicate that uNK cells might be constantly replenished by blood NK cells or by an NK cell progenitor from the blood.

The period between implantation and menstruation (LH 7–14) is critical for the endometrium to make the critical decision whether to continue the process of decidualization or to break down and be shed at menstruation [29,30]. The progesterone concentrations parallel this decision and either plummet or rapidly rise. If pregnancy does not occur, about 2 days before menstruation, nuclear changes appear in the uNK cells suggesting that they may be dying. The mechanism causing their death appears to be caspase-independent, which makes the process atypical of apoptosis [31,32]. These nuclear changes are present before any other features of impending menstrual breakdown such as neutrophil infiltration, clumping of stromal cells, and interstitial hemorrhage are seen. Death of uNK cells, therefore, appears to precede menstrual breakdown. Human endometrial NK cells produce a combination of cytokines that are influential in angiogenesis and vascular stability, such as vascular endothelial growth factor C (VEGF-C), placental growth factor (PlGF), and angiopoietin-2 (Ang-2) [33,34,35]. Indeed, they are preferentially located around the spiral arteries in early decidua and in late secretory endometrium. The withdrawal of these factors after the demise of the uNK cells would be expected to lead to menstrual breakdown where vascular collapse is known to be a critical event. In other mucosal sites in the body, populations of leukocytes do play a role in renewal and differentiation and recent reports have identified mucosal NK cells that secrete IL-22 to maintain mucosal integrity [36]. Uterine NK cells may well perform a similar function in endometrium and decidua.

NK cells and trophoblast invasion

When mammals evolved an invasive form of placentation where the uterine epithelium is breached, the mucosal NK cells could then have been co-opted from a mainly mucosal function to play a further additional role – that of regulating implantation by monitoring trophoblast invasion and ensuring that a balance between adequate fetal nutrition and maternal survival is achieved. In support of this view is the histological observation that NK cells are particularly abundant among the invading trophoblast cells in the decidua basalis. Trophoblast continues to penetrate the uterine wall as far as the inner myometrium where the cells fuse to become placental bed giant cells. NK cells are not a feature of the myometrium so the behavior of trophoblast in this deeper part of the uterus is independent of their influence. Unpublished observations from our laboratory do suggest though that if trophoblast has not first passaged through the NK-rich decidual environment before penetrating myometrium then giant cells do not form and there is deep invasion with destruction of the smooth muscle. This suggests that the role of decidua and its NK cells is to *modify* the trophoblast as it moves through so that the cells reaching the inner myometrium no longer have such invasive and destructive proclivities. In normal pregnancies, they do retain the ability to encircle and destroy the media of the spiral arteries with resulting fibrinoid necrosis and subsequent replacement of the endothelium by endovascular trophoblast. This is deficient in preeclampsia perhaps because of excess 'modification' by decidua and the NK cells?

How might uNK cells control trophoblast invasion? Several lines of evidence indicate that the local uterine immune system is involved. Trophoblast cells which invade into decidua during implantation express an unusual array of HLA molecules [2]. Instead of the usual combination of HLA-A, -B and -C of somatic cells, trophoblast expresses one classical (HLA-C) and two non-classical (HLA-E and HLA-G) [37,38,39] molecules. Of these molecules, only HLA-C is polymorphic whereas HLA-E and HLA-G are invariant. The functions of these trophoblast HLA molecules have been the focus of much research interest. Receptors for these HLA molecules are expressed by uNK cells thereby providing a potential molecular mechanism for maternal–fetal recognition.

A further potential site where maternal immune cells can interact with endovascular trophoblast is in the spiral arteries in the decidua basalis. Endovascular trophoblast expresses a similar array of HLA class I molecules to the interstitial trophoblast. At present nothing is known about how maternal peripheral blood NK cells, T cells, or monocytes might respond to the trophoblast ligands.

HLA-E

All uNK cells express high levels of the inhibitory receptor CD94/NKG2A whose ligand is HLA-E [40,37]. This interaction will, therefore, prevent lysis of trophoblast by uNK cells. The peptide that is bound to HLA-E is derived from the signal peptide of other MHC class I molecules expressed by the cell. The peptide bound to HLA-E that is derived from leader sequence of HLA-G has a particularly strong influence on the binding affinity of HLA-E to the CD94/NKG2 receptor [41]. In addition, demonstrable binding of HA-E to the homologous receptor, CD94/NKG2C (that is activating rather than the inhibitory CD94/NKG2A), is only seen when HLA-E has an HLA-G-derived bound peptide. This means that uNK cells could respond differently to trophoblast HLA-E compared to other surrounding cells in the vicinity which are also HLA-E positive but are binding peptides derived from leader sequences of maternal classical HLA-A, -B and -C.

HLA-G

HLA-G is a non-classical HLA class I molecule that was identified and found to be expressed by trophoblast cells nearly 20 years ago [42,43,44]. The HLA-G gene is located within the MHC at 6p21.3, one of the two most polymorphic regions of the human genome. In contrast to classical HLA class I genes HLA-G shows only minimal variation, with around 20 nucleotide alleles encoding less than 10 different protein sequences. This limited polymorphism is distributed between the α1, α2, and α3 domains, unlike the polymorphism in classical HLA class I molecules, where it is concentrated around the peptide binding groove. HLA-G is also unusual in having a stop codon in exon 7, resulting in a truncated cytoplasmic tail that affects HLA-G trafficking with retention in the ER until a high-affinity peptide is bound. Reduced endocytosis from the cell surface also occurs, meaning that HLA-G proteins have an extended surface half life. As predicted from the limited polymorphism and unusual cellular trafficking characteristics, HLA-G demonstrates a highly restricted peptide repertoire. These unique characteristics of HLA-G, limited polymorphism, restricted peptide repertoire and unusual cellular trafficking, suggest that a role in the presentation of intracellular peptide to T cells is unlikely [45,46]. Indeed, to date, HLA-G-restricted T cells have not been detected in humans.

HLA-G has been found in different conformations at the cell surface. Of most interest HLA-G can exist as a dimer of two conventional β_2m-associated HLA-G complexes. Dimers of HLA-G have been described with recombinant protein *in vitro*, on the surface of HLA-G transfectants and primary trophoblast cells [47,48,49]. The HLA-G homodimer is linked by a disulfide bond between extracellular cysteines at position 42 in the heavy chain α1 domain. Comparison of HLA class I sequences reveals that cysteine 42 is unique to HLA-G alleles implying that this homodimeric HLA class I complex is unique to HLA-G.

Genes orthologous to HLA-G can be identified in the closest evolutionary relatives of humans, chimpanzees and gorillas [50]. Interestingly because there is conservation of the cysteine 42 and limited MHC-G polymorphism a similar function is likely and this might be related to the deeply invasive placentation characteristic of these species [2] (see also Chapter 12). In contrast in the orangutans and Old and New World monkeys, cysteine 42 is substituted for a serine so dimerization of MHC-G will not occur and MHC-G is either a polymorphic classical MHC class I molecule or a pseudogene. Other MHC molecules have been suggested as functional homologues of HLA-G in Old World monkeys and rodents on the basis of limited polymorphism and expression in the placenta, but there is still a paucity of functional evidence for any of these 'trophoblast' MHC genes in any species.

There is still some controversy regarding the identity of the uNK cell receptors for HLA-G. This is surprising as HLA-G has held center stage in reproductive immunology research for some time. Only the invading trophoblast cells express HLA-G, implying that this molecule is likely to have a pivotal role to play in implantation, but what this role is remains unclear. The leukocyte receptor complex of chromosome 19 includes two polymorphic gene families, leukocyte immunoglobulin-like receptors (LILR), and killer cell immunoglobulin-like receptors (KIR) [51,52]. Members of both these families can bind HLA-G. The LILR family comprises 13 loci of which only the inhibitory LILRB1 and LILRB2 receptors recognize all

HLA class I molecules. LILRB1 and -2 are expressed by all peripheral macrophages and dendritic cells. LILRB1 is also expressed on undefined subsets of most B, some T, and NK cells. In the decidua, all HLA-DR$^+$ cells have been shown to express both LILRB1/2 and 20% of CD56$^+$ cells express LILRB1 [49].

LILRB1 and 2 have been shown to bind HLA-G by a range of experimental methods: LILRB1/2-Fc fusion proteins specifically bound to transfected cells expressing HLA class I molecules including HLA-G in the absence of HLA-E [53,51,54]. HLA-G tetramers bound cells transfected with LILRB1/2 and human PBMC; binding was blocked with anti-LILRB mAb [55]. Surface plasmon resonance (SPR) experiments with recombinant HLA-G molecules demonstrated that the affinity of LILRB1 and 2 binding to HLA-G is higher than other HLA class I molecules [56,57]. The co-crystal structure of LILRB1 binding to the α3 domain and β_2m molecule of HLA-A is now available and the HLA-G crystal structure is similar [58]. Importantly, given that formation of this dimer is unique to HLA-G, dimerization dramatically increases LILRB1 binding. A LILRB1-Fc fusion protein bound more strongly to wild type HLA-G transfectants than serine 42 mutants that do not dimerize [59]). SPR measurements of soluble monomeric and dimeric HLA-G complexes binding LILRB molecules confirmed this finding [60]. The increased binding avidity of the dimer translates into augmented signaling through LILRB1 because LILRB1-mediated inhibition of IgϵR-mediated serotonin release and inhibition of NK killing were both increased with cells expressing HLA-G that can form dimers, as opposed to a serine 42 mutant [59]. In addition, a LILRB1 chimera NFAT-GFP reporter cell assay showed that 100-fold lower concentrations of dimeric compared to monomeric HLA-G were necessary to induce a signal [60]. Most recently, LILRB1 has been shown to bind HLA-G expressed on trophoblast cells *in vivo*, and preferentially the homodimer was immunoprecipitated from the cell surface with a LILRB1-Fc fusion protein [49]. Overall the evidence is convincing that the HLA-G dimer binds LILRB1 and that this interaction is likely to be functional.

The KIR are another polygenic receptor family, some of which bind HLA-C molecules but one KIR, KIR2DL4, binds HLA-G. KIR2DL4 is a framework gene at the center of the KIR gene complex and is present in all KIR haplotypes. KIR2DL4 surface expression on peripheral and decidual NK cells *in vivo* has proved difficult to detect [61,62]). In addition, one allele of KIR2DL4 produces a transcript that lacks any transmembrane domain *in vitro* and is present in most populations at a frequency of around 50%. Presence of both a cytoplasmic ITIM motif and an argine residue in the transmembrane region indicates KIR2DL4 could be either a stimulating or inhibitory receptor. Like other aspects of this enigmatic molecule, whether KIR2DL4 can bind to HLA-G has been controversial. A KIR2DL4-Fc fusion protein bound HLA-G transfectants and this was blocked with anti-KIR2DL4 and anti-HLA-G mAb [61,62]) but others have disputed these findings [55]. A possible explanation for these contradictory findings is that KIR2DL4 binds to HLA-G in a low-affinity interaction that only takes place when the ligand is concentrated in endosomal compartments. KIR2DL4 was detected intracellularly in the early Rab 5$^+$ endosomes of peripheral NK cells using confocal microscopy [62]. When GFP-tagged KIR2DL4 transfected cells were incubated with soluble HLA-G molecules, intracellular co-localization of HLA-G and KIR2DL4 could be detected which was blocked with specific mAb. That NK cells might sense ligands via endosomal compartments is an interesting new area for research. What remains to be shown is conclusive evidence of KIR2DL4 protein expression *in vivo*, and in particular whether decidual NK cells also express KIR2DL4 in endosomes and how HLA-G can reach these compartments *in vivo*.

From the evidence available the most compelling is that relating to the HLA-G:LILRB1 interaction. The outcome of this interaction has been shown by many studies to result in deviating dendritic cells towards a tolerogenic rather than an immunogenic phenotype [63,64,65]. For a trophoblast molecule to direct the uterine dendritic cells towards becoming tolerogenic during early pregnancy and thus downregulate any possible allogenic responses is an attractive idea [49,46]. Decidual HLA-DR+ cells are abundant accounting for ~20% of decidual leukocytes [66]. In addition decidual NK cells may be stimulated by an HLA-G:KIR2DL4 interaction to produce a beneficial array of cytokines and chemokines that facilitate the vascular changes necessary in the placental bed. If both signaling pathways occur in parallel, HLA-G would be able to influence both decidual NK cells and HLA-DR$^+$ cells, accounting for ~90% of leukocytes at the placental implantation site. Thus, as the placental trophoblast cells infiltrate the uterine mucosa they could deliver a pregnancy-specific signal to most of the local maternal leukocytes and modify their function to accommodate the feto-placental unit.

HLA-C

The NK cell receptors for HLA-C are members of the Killer-cell Immunoglobulin-like Receptor (KIR) multigene family [67]. HLA-C has emerged as a dominant ligand for NK cells [68]). Individual KIR can distinguish between an epitope of all HLA-C allotypes that is based on a dimorphism at position 80 of the α1 domain. This divides HLA-C alleles into Group 1 (C1) or Group 2 (C2). There is great diversity of KIR haplotypes, with variations in the number of genes as well as polymorphism at individual loci. Some of the KIR genes encode an inhibitory receptor while others (with a similar extracellular domain) encode for a receptor that gives an activating signal. Broadly speaking, KIR haplotypes comprise two groups, A and B, that differ principally by having additional activating receptors in the B haplotype (Fig. 6.1). The distinction between these two haplotypes seems to indeed have a biological basis as there are many clinical correlations with KIR A or B haplotypes and infectious diseases (HIV, HCV, HSV) as well as autoimmune conditions [69,70]. In any pregnancy, the maternal KIR genotype can be AA (no activating KIR) or AB/BB (presence of between one and five activating KIRs).

That interaction between trophoblast HLA-C and uNK cell KIR plays a critical role in implantation is very persuasive. Recent studies have shown that the KIR repertoire in uNK cells is dynamic and changes dramatically during the early weeks of pregnancy [71,72]. Both the proportion of CD56+ cells expressing KIR specific for HLA-C and the levels of expression of these KIR are upregulated. The increased expression of HLA-C-specific KIR by uNK cells is a transient phenomenon, with high expression when samples first become available at around 6 weeks, which coincides with the time when trophoblast begins to migrate extensively into decidua to transform the spiral arteries. These changes in KIR expression by uNK cells contrast with peripheral blood NK cells where, in healthy individuals, both the frequency and expression levels of KIR are genetically determined and remain fixed for many years. Change in the KIR repertoire in uNK cells during pregnancy, therefore, is an unusual physiological phenomenon which is likely to be related to the role these receptors play in implantation. Of interest though is that in mice infected with MCMV there is transient expansion of NK subsets bearing receptors specific for the MCMV-encoded NK ligands [73]. The upregulation of uterine NK KIR is particular for those that bind to HLA-C because the HLA-B-specific KIR3DL1 do not increase significantly. This is relevant since invading trophoblast cells express HLA-C and not HLA-A or HLA-B. Both inhibitory and activating KIR for HLA-C are upregulated. The increase in level of KIR expression by uNK cells is also reflected in higher binding of HLA-C tetramers *in vitro*. This should be functionally important *in vivo* in relation to binding to trophoblast HLA-C [72]. The CD56^{bright} NK cell population in blood expresses no KIR at all. If blood CD56^{bright} NK cells are the source of CD56^{bright} uNK cells, then this observation indicates that KIR expression is indeed induced locally *in utero*. Products like IL-15 from decidual stromal cells could provide the necessary stimulus for this induction.

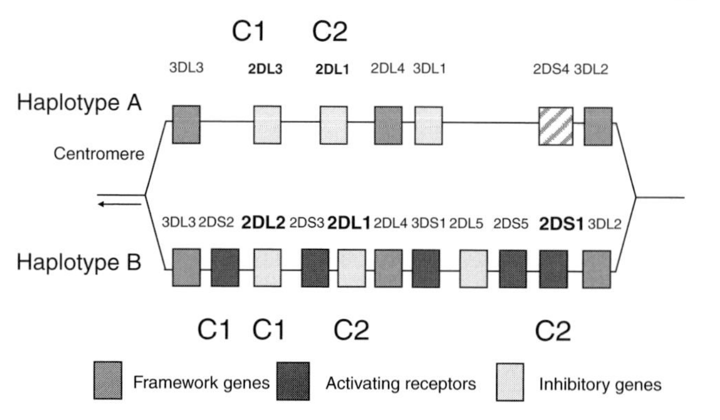

Fig. 6.1 Two representative KIR haplotypes of A and B type. See plate section for color version.

The conformation of HLA-C molecules on trophoblast is unusual in that it exists predominantly in the stable β_2m-associated form, with negligible levels of the unfolded HLA-C conformers that are seen on somatic cells [74]. There are several possible explanations for this including the increased availability of suitable high-affinity peptides in trophoblast cells compared to normal cells. It will be of interest to see if HLA-C is also more stable on virally infected cells allowing alteration in affinity for activating or inhibitory KIR. Possibly trophoblast is behaving like an infected cell? Certainly, tetramers of KIR2DL1 are observed to bind specifically to HLA-C molecules on trophoblast cells [72]. All these findings suggest that both KIR and HLA-C in the implantation site have features that are specially adapted for enhanced recognition of HLA-C on trophoblast by uNK cells.

Because both HLA-C and KIR genes are polymorphic it can be predicted that the interaction between maternal uNK cell KIR and paternal trophoblast HLA-C would have different outcomes in each pregnancy [75]. Some of these interactions could be disadvantageous for implantation and might contribute to the underlying pathogenesis of important diseases, such as preeclampsia. Initial histological studies over 50 years ago indicated that defective decidual arterial modification due to inadequate trophoblast invasion was frequently seen in the placental bed of women with preeclampsia (see Chapter 3). This has now been supported by Doppler ultrasound studies of maternal uterine blood flow. How the fine-tuning of trophoblast invasion to prevent under- or over-invasion is achieved is unknown. It has been reported that a KIR AA genotype (inhibitory KIR only) in the mother combined with the presence of an HLA-C2 group in the fetus increases the susceptibility to preeclampsia. However, the maternal KIR genotype appears to be unimportant when a homozygous C1/C1 is present in the fetus [76].

The obvious question that arises is what is the protective KIR gene or genes on the B haplotype that protects against preeclampsia when there is an HLA-C2 in the fetus? There is evidence that the KIR genes at the telomeric end of the haplotype might be important, in particular the activating receptor for HLA-C2 (KIR2DS1) (unpublished data). Women with preeclampsia, recurrent miscarriage, and fetal growth restriction all have reduced frequencies of KIR2DS1 compared to controls (unpublished data). Thus, it seems that the presence of HLA-C2 in the fetal trophoblast normally induces a strong inhibitory signal by binding to the inhibitory receptor KIR2DL1 that needs to be overcome by the presence of an activating KIR such as KIR2DS1 for pregnancy to be successful. Recent analyses have shown that this applies also to recurrent miscarriage and fetal growth restriction, two conditions that have a similar basic pathogenesis of failure of trophoblast to invade the spiral arteries correctly [77]. This reinforces the view that certain combinations of trophoblast HLA-C and maternal KIR interaction are responsible for many pathological pregnancies [78]. At present, it is unclear whether the HLA-C status of the mother or that of the invading fetal trophoblast can influence the KIR repertoire of the uNK cells. If the former, then the role of the self HLA-C ligands in setting the responsiveness of the mature maternal NK cells will also be important to consider [79]; if the latter, then the further question arises whether the uNK cell KIR repertoire will differ between the first and subsequent pregnancies. This would be an interesting mechanism for NK cell education. Recent studies in mice have demonstrated that NK cells do have 'memory' reminiscent of T cell memory [80]. If this NK 'memory' is confirmed in humans, there might perhaps be some persistence of the trophoblast-specific NK cells that are retained and more responsive in a subsequent pregnancy from the same father.

The exact mechanism by which uNK cells influence trophoblast invasion remains unclear. Despite its name of 'killer' cell, there is no good evidence that uNK cells can kill trophoblast. Instead, uNK cells are known to make a wide variety of cytokines and angiogenic factors including IFN-γ, IP-10, IL-8, VEGF-A, VEGF-C and Ang-2, all of which can influence either vascular function or trophoblast migration [81,35]. Secretion of several of these cytokines by uNK cells is altered following engagement of KIR by HLA-C ligands, so the cytokine milieu that the invading trophoblast cells are exposed to would be different in pregnancies with different KIR/HLA-C combinations, thereby modifying the extent of trophoblast invasion. Examination of the placental bed in mice genetically deficient in uNK cells shows that the transformation of decidual arteries typical of normal implantation does not occur [82]. This indicates that an important function of mouse uNK cells could be to directly modify decidual blood vessels by cytokines rather than indirectly via the control of trophoblast invasion as in humans.

Given the association of HLA-C2 and KIRAA genotypes with reproductive failure, it would seem logical to predict that these gene combinations would be selected against. Why are these KIR AA genotypes eventually not selected out given the deleterious effect for mothers with these genotypes? There are large differences in populations in the frequency of both KIRAA genotypes and HLA-C2 groups [67]. There must be balancing selective pressures, perhaps to provide defense against infections. Necessities for survival of human populations are to provide defense against infection as well as an ability to reproduce successfully [69]. The HLA-C locus has evolved relatively recently and is found only in humans, the African great apes and some (but not all) orangutans. Similarly, there are features of the KIR family of receptors which indicate that there has been rapid evolution of this gene family in primates. It is a fascinating speculation that selective pressures for reproductive success together with defense against infections could have contributed to the rapid change of HLA-C and KIR genes in primates. Possibly the expansion and diversification of KIR genes in great apes is related to the increasingly dangerous invasive proclivities of trophoblast compared with lower primates (see Chapter 12, [83]). However, even chimpanzees, which have comparable inhibitory KIR for their MHC-C allotypes, have minimal expansion of activating KIR and the large numbers of activating KIR seem to be specific to humans. The demands put on the human pelvis by walking upright as well as the increasing brain size may both have impacted on the placental blood supply [2].

The overall conclusion is that the local immunity in the human implantation site is an unusual one that is reflected in the cell types present. These are mainly immune effectors belonging to the innate rather than the adaptive immune system. The laws governing reproduction immunology, therefore, are not the same as those for transplantation immunology, in spite of superficial resemblance between the two allogeneic systems.

References

1. Loke Y W, King A. *Human implantation*. Cambridge: CUP; 1995.
2. Moffett A, Loke C. Immunology of placentation in eutherian mammals. *Nat Rev Immunol* 2006; **6**: 584–94.
3. Moffett-King A. Natural killer cells and pregnancy. *Nat Rev Immunol* 2002; **2**: 656–63.
4. Red-Horse K, Rivera J, Schanz A *et al.* Cytotrophoblast induction of arterial apoptosis and lymphangiogenesis in an in vivo model of human placentation. *J Clin Invest* 2006; **116**: 2643–52.
5. Kirby D R. Development of mouse eggs beneath the kidney capsule. *Nature* 1960; **187**: 707–8.
6. McLaren A. In: Park W W, ed. *The early conceptus, normal and abnormal*. Edinburgh: University of St Andrews Press; 1965: pp. 27–33.
7. Trundley A, Moffett A. Human uterine leukocytes and pregnancy. *Tissue Antigens* 2004; **63**: 1–12.
8. Marchand F. Ueber die sogenannten dezidualen Geschwülste im Anschluss an normale Geburt, Blasenmole und Extrauterinschwangerschaft. *Mschr Geburtsh Gynäk* 1895; **1**: 419.
9. Weill P. Etudes sur les leukocytes I. Les cellules granuleuses des muqueuses intestinales et utérines. *Arch Anat Microsc* 1921; **17**: 77–82.
10. Hamperl H, Hellweg G. Granular endometrial stroma cells. *Obstet Gynecol* 1958; **11**: 379–87.
11. Von Numers C. On the specific granular cells (globular leukocytes) of the human endometrium. *Acta Pathol Microbiol Scand* 1953; **33**: 250–6.
12. Kazzaz B A. Specific endometrial granular cells: a semiquantitative study. *Eur J Obstet Gynecol* 1972; **3**: 77–84.
13. Ritson A, Bulmer J N. Endometrial granulocytes in human decidua react with a natural killer (NK) cell marker NKH1. *Immunology* 1987; **62**: 329–31.
14. King A, Wellings V, Gardner L, Loke Y W. Immunocytochemical characterization of the unusual large granular lymphocytes in human endometrium throughout the menstrual cycle. *Hum Immunol* 1989; **24**(3):195–205.
15. King A. Uterine leukocytes and decidualization. *Hum Reprod Update* 2000; **6**: 28–36.
16. Bulmer J N, Lash G E. Human uterine natural killer cells: a reappraisal. *Mol Immunol* 2005; **42**:511–21 [Review].
17. King A, Gardner L, Loke Y W. Evaluation of oestrogen and progesterone receptor expression in uterine mucosal lymphocytes. *Hum Reprod* 1996; **11**: 1079–82.
18. Henderson T A, Saunders P T, Moffett-King A *et al.* Steroid receptor expression in uterine natural killer cells. *J Clin Endocrinol Metab* 2003; **88**: 440–9.
19. Verma S, Hiby S E, Loke Y W, King A *et al.* Human decidual natural killer cells express the receptor for and respond to the cytokine interleukin 15. *Biol Reprod* 2000; **62**: 959–68.
20. Kitaya K, Yamaguchi T, Honjo H. Central role of interleukin-15 in postovulatory recruitment of peripheral blood CD16(-) natural killer cells into human endometrium. *J Clin Endocrinol Metab* 2005; **90**: 2932–40.

21. Sun R, Li A L, Wei H M, Tian Z G. Expression of prolactin receptor and response to prolactin stimulation of human NK cell lines. *Cell Res* 2004; **14**: 67–73.

22. King A, Balendran N, Wooding P, Loke Y W *et al.* CD3-leukocytes present in the human uterus during early placentation: phenotypic and morphologic characterization of the CD56++ population. *Dev Immunol* 1991; **1**: 169–90.

23. Koopman L A, Kopcow H D, Rybalov B *et al.* Human decidual natural killer cells are a unique NK cell subset with immunomodulatory potential. *J Exp Med* 2003; **198**: 1201–12.

24. Lynch L, Golden-Mason L, Eogan M *et al.* Cells with haematopoietic stem cell phenotype in adult human endometrium: relevance to infertility? *Hum Reprod* 2007; **22**: 919–26.

25. Keskin D B, Allan D S, Rybalov B *et al.* TGFbeta promotes conversion of CD16+ peripheral blood NK cells into CD16- NK cells with similarities to decidual NK cells. *Proc Natl Acad Sci USA* 2007; **104**: 3378–83.

26. Pace D, Morrison L, Bulmer J N *et al.* Proliferative activity in endometrial stromal granulocytes throughout menstrual cycle and early pregnancy. *J Clin Pathol* 1989; **42**: 35–9.

27. Chantakru S, Miller C, Roach L E *et al.* Contributions from self-renewal and trafficking to the uterine NK cell population of early pregnancy. *J Immunol* 2002; **168**: 22–8.

28. Sentman C L, Meadows S K, Wira C R *et al.* Recruitment of uterine NK cells: induction of CXC chemokine ligands 10 and 11 in human endometrium by estradiol and progesterone. *J Immunol* 2004; **173**: 6760–6.

29. Critchley H O, Kelly R W, Brenner R M *et al.* The endocrinology of menstruation – a role for the immune system. *Clin Endocrinol* 2001; **55**: 701–10.

30. Jabbour H N, Kelly R W, Fraser H M *et al.* Endocrine regulation of menstruation. *Endocrin Rev* 2006; **27**: 17–46.

31. Pongcharoen S, Bulmer J N, Searle R F *et al.* No evidence for apoptosis of decidual leukocytes in normal and molar pregnancy: implications for immune privilege. *Clin Exp Immunol* 2004; **138**: 330–6.

32. Kroemer G, Martin S K. Caspase independent cell death. *Nat Med* 2005; **11**: 725–30.

33. Langer N, Beach D, Lindenbaum E S *et al.* Novel hyperactive mitogen to endothelial cells: human decidual NKG5. *Am J Reprod Immunol* 1999; **42**: 263–72.

34. Li X F, Charnock-Jones D S, Zhang E *et al.* Angiogenic growth factor messenger ribonucleic acids in uterine natural killer cells. *J Clin Endocrinol Metab* 2001; **86**: 1823–34.

35. Lash G E, Schiessl B, Kirkley M *et al.* Expression of angiogenic growth factors by uterine natural killer cells during early pregnancy. *J Leukoc Biol* 2006; **80**: 572–80.

36. Sanos S L, Bui V L, Mortha A *et al.* RORgammat and commensal microflora are required for the differentiation of mucosal interleukin 22-producing NKp46+ cells. *Nat Immunol* 2009; **10**: 11–2.

37. King A, Allan DS J, Bowen M J *et al.* HLA-E is expressed on trophoblast cells and interacts with CD94/NKG2A receptors on decidual NK cells. *Eur J Immunol* 2000; **30**: 1623–31.

38. King A, Burrows T D, Hiby S E *et al.* Surface expression of HLA-C antigen by human extravillous trophoblast. *Placenta* 2000; **21**: 376–87.

39. Apps R, Murphy S P, Fernando R *et al.* Human leukocyte antigen (HLA) expression by normal trophoblast cells and placental cell lines using a novel method to characterize allotype specificity of anti-HLA antibodies. *Immunology*, in press.

40. Lazetic S, Chang C, Houchins J P *et al.* Human natural killer cell receptors involved in MHC class I recognition are disulphide linked heterodimers of CD94 and NKG2 subunits. *J Immunol* 1996; **157**: 4741–5.

41. Llano M, Lee N, Navarro F *et al.* HLA-E-bound peptides influence recognition by inhibitory and triggering CD94/NKG2 receptors: preferential response to an HLA-G-derived nonamer. *Eur J Immunol* 1998; **28**: 2854–63.

42. Kovats S, Main E K, Librach C *et al.* A class I antigen, HLA-G, expressed in human trophoblasts. *Science* 1990; **248**: 220–3.

43. McMaster M T, Librach C L, Zhou Y *et al.* Human placental HLA-G expression is restricted to differentiated cytotrophoblasts. *J Immunol* 1995; **154**: 3771–8.

44. Loke Y W, King A, Burrows T *et al.* Evaluation of trophoblast HLA-G antigen with a specific monoclonal antibody. *Tissue Antigens* 1997; **50**: 135–46.

45. Bainbridge D, Ellis S, Le Bouteiller P, Sargent I. HLA-G remains a mystery. *Trends Immunol* 2001; **22**: 548–52.

46. Apps R, Gardner L, Moffett A *et al.* A critical look at HLA-G. *Trends Immunol* 2008; **29**: 313–21.

47. Boyson J E, Erskine R, Whitman M C *et al.* Disulfide bond-mediated dimerization of HLA-G on the cell surface. *Proc Natl Acad Sci USA* 2002; **99**: 16180–5.

48. Gonen-Gross T, Achdout H, Gazit R *et al.* Complexes of HLA-G protein on the cell surface are important for leukocyte Ig-like receptor-1 function. *J Immunol* 2003; **171**: 1343–51.

49. Apps R, Gardner L, Sharkey A M *et al.* A homodimeric complex of HLA-G on normal trophoblast cells modulates antigen-presenting cells via LILRB1. *Eur J Immunol* 2007; **37**: 1727–9.

50. Arnaiz-Villena A, Morales P, Gomez-Casado E *et al.* Evolution of MHC-G in primates: a different kind of molecule for each group of species. *J Reprod Immunol* 1999; **43**: 111–25.

51. Borges L, Hsu M L, Fanger N Kubin M, Cosman D. A family of human lymphoid and myeloid Ig-like receptors, some of which bind to MHC class I molecules. *J Immunol* 1997; **159**: 5192–6.

52. Colonna M, Navarro F, Bellon T *et al.* A common inhibitory receptor for major histocompatibility complex class I molecules on human lymphoid and myelomonocytic cells. *J Exp Med* 1997; **186**: 1809–18.

53. Colonna M, Samaridis J, Cella M *et al.* Human myelomonocytic cells express an inhibitory receptor for classical and nonclassical MHC class I molecules. *J Immunol* 1998; **160**: 3096–100.

54. Borges L, Cosman D. LIRs/ILTs/MIRs, inhibitory and stimulatory Ig-superfamily receptors expressed in myeloid and lymphoid cells. *Cytokine Growth Factor Rev* 2000; **11**: 209–17.

55. Allan D S, Colonna M, Lanier L L *et al.* Tetrameric complexes of human histocompatibility leukocyte antigen (HLA)-G bind to peripheral blood myelomonocytic cells. *J Exp Med* 1999; **189**: 1149–56.

56. Chapman T L, Heikeman A P, Bjorkman P J *et al.* The inhibitory receptor LIR-1 uses a common binding interaction to recognize class I MHC molecules and the viral homolog UL18. *Immunity* 1999; **11**: 603–13.

57. Shiroishi M, Tsumoto K, Amano K *et al.* Human inhibitory receptors Ig-like transcript 2 (ILT2) and ILT4 compete with CD8 for MHC class I binding and bind preferentially to HLA-G. *Proc Natl Acad Sci U S A* 2003; **100**: 8856–61.

58. Clements C S, Kjer-Nielsen L, Kostenko L *et al.* Crystal structure of HLA-G: a nonclassical MHC class I molecule expressed at the fetal-maternal interface. *Proc Natl Acad Sci U S A* 2005; **102**: 3360–5.

59. Gonen-Gross T, Achdout H, Arnon T I *et al.* The CD85J/leukocyte inhibitory receptor-1 distinguishes between conformed and beta 2-microglobulin-free HLA-G molecules. *J Immunol* 2005; **175**: 4866–74.

60. Shiroishi M, Kuroki K, Ose T *et al.* Efficient leukocyte Ig-like receptor signaling and crystal structure of disulfide-linked HLA-G dimer. *J Biol Chem* 2006; **281**: 10439–47.

61. Rajogopalan S, Long E O. A human histocompatibility leukocyte antigen (HLA)-G-specific receptor expressed on all natural killer cells. *J Exp Med* 1999; **189**: 1093–100.

62. Rajagopalan S, Bryceson Y T, Kuppusamy S P *et al.* Activation of NK cells by an endocytosed receptor for soluble HLA-G. *PLoS Biol* 2006; **4**:e9.

63. Chang C C, Ciubotariu R, Manavalan J S *et al.* Tolerization of dendritic cells by T(S) cells: the crucial role of inhibitory receptors ILT3 and ILT4. *Nat Immunol* 2002; **3**: 237–43.

64. Le Friec G, Laupeze B, Fardel O *et al.* Soluble HLA-G inhibits human dendritic cell-triggered allogeneic T-cell proliferation without altering dendritic differentiation and maturation processes. *Hum Immunol* 2003; **64**: 752–61.

65. Ristich V, Liang S, Zhang W, Wu J, Horuzsko A. Tolerization of dendritic cells by HLA-G. *Eur J Immunol* 2005; **35**: 1133–42.

66. Gardner L, Moffett A. Dendritic cells in the human decidua. *Biol Reprod* 2003; **69**: 1438–46.

67. Parham P. MHC class I molecules and KIRs in human history, health and survival. *Nat Rev Immunol* 2005; **5**: 201–14.

68. Gumperz J E, Parham P. The enigma of the natural killer cell. *Nature* 1995; **378**: 245–8.

69. Parham P. The genetic and evolutionary balances in human NK cell receptor diversity. *Semin Immunol* 2008; **20**: 311–6.

70. Kulkarni S, Martin M P, Carrington M. The Yin and Yang of HLA and KIR in human disease. *Semin Immunol* 2008; **20**:343–52.

71. Verma S, King A, Loke Y W *et al.* Expression of killer cell inhibitory receptors on human uterine natural killer cells. *Eur J Immuol* 1997; **27**: 979–83.

72. Sharkey A M, Gardner L, Hiby S *et al.* Killer Ig-like receptor expression in uterine NK cells is biased toward recognition of HLA-C and alters with gestational age. *J Immunol* 2008; **181**: 39–46.

73. Dokun H O, Kim S, Smith H R *et al.* Specific and nonspecific NK cell activation during virus infection. *Nat Immunol* 2001; **2**: 951–6.

74. Apps R, Gardner L, Hiby S E *et al.* Conformation of human leucocyte antigen-C molecules at the surface of human trophoblast cells. *Immunology* 2008; **124**: 322–8.

75. Moffett A, Hiby S E. How does the maternal immune system contribute to the development of pre-eclampsia? *Placenta* 2007; **28** (Suppl A): S51–S56.

76. Hiby S E, Walker J J, O'Shaughnessy K M *et al.* Combinations of maternal KIR and fetal HLA-C genes influence the risk of preeclampsia and reproductive success. *J Exp Med* 2004; **200**: 957–65.

77. Hiby S, Regan L, Lo W *et al.* Association of maternal killer-cell immunoglobulin-like receptors and parental

HLA-C genotypes with recurrent miscarriage. *Hum Reprod* 2008; **23**: 972–6.

78. Trowsdale J, Moffett A. NK receptor interactions with MHC class I molecules in pregnancy. *Semin Immunol* 2008; **20**: 317–20.

79. Held W. Tolerance and reactivity of NK cells: two sides of the same coin? *Eur J Immunol* 2008; **38**: 2930–3 [Review].

80. Sun J C, Beilke J N, Lanier L L. Adaptive immune features of natural killer cells. *Nature* 2009; **457**: 557–61.

81. Hanna J, Goldman-Wohl D, Hamani Y *et al.* Decidual NK cells regulate key developmental processes at the human fetal-maternal interface. *Nat Med* 2006; **12**: 1065–74.

82. Croy B A, van den Heuvel M J, Borzychowski A M *et al.* Uterine natural killers cells: a specialized differentiation regulated by ovarian hormones. *Immunol Rev* 2006; **214**: 161–85.

83. Ramsey E M, Houston M L, Harris J W *et al.* Interactions of the trophoblast and maternal tissues in three closely related primate species. *Am J Obstet Gynecol.* 1976; **124**: 647–52.

Placental angiogenesis

Christophe L. Depoix[1] and Robert N. Taylor[2]

[1]Laboratoire d'Obstétrique, Université Catholique de Louvain, Brussels, Belgium
[2]Department of Gynecology and Obstetrics, Emory University School of Medicine, Atlanta, GA, USA

Introduction

The placenta, an organ of fetal origin, is critical to the normal growth and development of a healthy baby. Among its manifold functions, the placenta maintains a complex interface between the fetal and maternal circulations allowing gas exchange, absorption of nutrients, and elimination of waste. As a result of these key transport functions, the placental circulation is a dynamic network of blood vessels that evolves and remodels throughout the course of pregnancy, responding to the growing needs of the embryo and fetus at each step of its development.

In this chapter, we will use a loose interpretation of 'placental angiogenesis' to include placental neovascular formation as well as transformation of the vessels during gestation. Classically, the *de novo* formation of blood vessels in the placental villi is called vasculogenesis [1], and occurs during the first trimester of pregnancy. Angiogenesis refers to the transformation of these blood vessels and their adaptation to the increasing transport needs of the fetus, and occurs from the second trimester to term. Another phenomenon critical for the development of the placenta involves the proper invasion of the uterine tissue by trophoblastic cells and the transformation of the maternal spiral arteries. Failure of this phenomenon leads to significant clinical complications of pregnancy like miscarriage, intrauterine growth restriction (IUGR), and preeclampsia (PE), as discussed in other chapters of this book.

Emphasis is placed on human tissues and we will use the clinical convention of gestational dating in weeks based on the last menstrual period (LMP); however, highly informative findings from mouse models and genetic knockout experiments are included where these are relevant to human placental physiology and disease.

Section I: developmental aspects of placental angiogenesis

Villous angiogenesis and villi formation

Human placentation starts just after the implantation of the blastocyst into the epithelium of the uterus about 3 weeks from the LMP. Following the hatching of the embryo from its *zona pellucida*, the trophectoderm penetrates and the blastocyst is quickly submerged below the endometrial surface epithelium. The trophoblasts proliferate rapidly, invade the endometrial stroma, and differentiate into two subpopulations of cells that form the placenta: an inner layer of proliferative cytotrophoblastic precursor cells and an outer layer of polynucleated differentiated cells called syncytiotrophoblasts [2].

By 4 weeks' gestation, the cytotrophoblasts proliferate and form the primary villi. Extravillous trophoblasts (EVT) invade the maternal tissues. They penetrate and fill the lumina of the spiral arteries, forming endovascular plugs. These plugs prevent maternal blood flow into the early developing placenta creating a hypoxic environment compared to the maternal tissues, postulated to promote cytotrophoblastic proliferation [3], and protect the developing fetal tissues from oxidative stress.

Growth and differentiation lead to the formation of three types of villi: primary, secondary, and tertiary [4]. At approximately 5 weeks, the core of the trophoblastic columns is filled with extra-embryonic mesenchyme and they are classified as secondary villi.

During the first month of human pregnancy, the villi remain avascular, but by 7 weeks' gestation, the tertiary villi progressively dominate and vasculogenic endothelial precursor cells give rise to primitive capillary tubes of the *decidua capsularis*. When these villi degenerate, the chorion becomes an avascular shell called *chorion laeve*. At the other pole, the tertiary villi associated with the *decidua basalis* proliferate forming the *chorion frondosum* or definitive placenta [5]. Unfortunately, less is known about the progressive angiogenesis of the placental bed during development.

> Primary and secondary villi are avascular. Tertiary villi, which first form at ~7 weeks' gestation and continue to form throughout pregnancy, have a vascular system

Structure of the placental plates

The placenta structurally provides a very intimate relationship between the maternal blood and fetal blood. Contact between the two blood circulations, while keeping them separate, is achieved by way of a complex architecture with three major structural components [6]:

- the chorionic plate includes the fetal side of the amnion, the chorion, and the rich chorionic blood vessels contiguous with the umbilical vessels;
- the intervillous space, containing 'floating' and 'anchoring' chorionic villi with fetal blood vessels organized in tree-like structures called placentomes, bathed in maternal blood;
- the basal plate of maternal endometrium (decidua) covered with a layer of syncytiotrophoblast and infiltrated by numerous EVT that extend into up to one-third of the myometrium.

The maternal blood enters the intervillous space through the uterine spiral artery openings. There, maternal blood flows across the surface of the villous trees and is returned to the maternal circulation through the endometrial veins [7].

From the fetal side, two umbilical arteries generally bring deoxygenated blood to the placenta. The blood flows into the heavily branched chorionic arteries and culminates in a complex arterio-capillary-venous system at the villous tip, where exchange between maternal and fetal blood contents takes place. Finally, fetal blood loaded with nutrients and oxygen diffusing from the maternal supply returns back to the fetus through chorionic veins draining into a single umbilical vein.

Structure of the placentome

Starting from the chorionic plate, a thick villous trunk gives rise to numerous stem villi. From 24 weeks' gestation onward, these outgrowths repeatedly develop into mature intermediate villi that do not duplicate themselves but instead grow by elongation. This elongation process ends up with the formation of the terminal villi, sites of gas and nutrient exchange [8].

Vasculogenesis

At about 5 weeks' gestation, vasculogenesis of the placental villi begins by a local *de novo* organization of pluripotent mesenchymal precursor cells inside the placental villous core. The mesenchymal cells differentiate into hemangiogenic stem cells, which give rise to angioblasts, progenitors of endothelial cells. The villi undergoing vasculogenesis are referred to as tertiary villi. Placental macrophages called Hofbauer cells, found in the villous core mesenchyme in close contact with the vasculogenic precursor cells, are thought to play a paracrine role in vasculogenesis [9]. Hofbauer cells secrete a variety of angiogenic growth factors that will be discussed in the detail in the following section.

> Hofbauer cells within the villous core secrete angiogenic proteins including vascular endothelial growth factors

The hemangioblastic cells are first organized into string-like aggregates of polygonal cells that form endothelial tubes by focal enlargement of centrally located intercellular clefts and fusion of these clefts to become a consolidated lumen. These endothelial tubes are surrounded by mesenchymal cells that differentiate to become pericytes. This developmental program is recapitulated when human umbilical vein endothelial cells (HUVEC) are cultured on Matrigel®-coated plates [10]. Confluent HUVEC (Fig. 7.1A) condense and form tubular bridges *in vitro* (Fig. 7.1B and C). Cross-sections of the tubular bridges reveal central lumina (Fig. 7.1D).

Early placental blood vessel formation from hematopoietic stem cells creates discontinuous capillary lumina in anticipation of their coalescence and connection to the umbilical cord vessels before these anastomose later to the embryonic circulation.

At around 9 weeks' gestation, the endothelial tubes fuse with each other and with the allantoic vessels leading to the establishment of a functional connection between embryonic and placental vascular beds. This

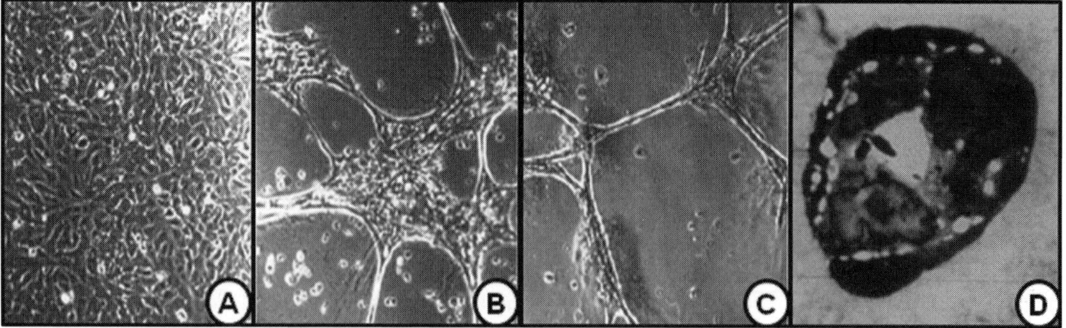

Fig. 7.1 (A) HUVEC grown for 48 hours on gelatin-coated plastic exhibit typical 'cobblestone' morphology. When the cells are cultured on Matrigel® for 8 hours (B) or 48 hours (C) they retract and form three-dimensional capillary-like bridges and tubules. (D) A high-power cross-section of the latter structure reveals a central lumen. Reproduced with permission from De Groot *et al.* 1995 [10]. See plate section for color version.

blood vessel formation happens in a relatively hypoxic environment. Up to 10 weeks' gestation, the oxygen tension within the developing placenta is <20 mmHg. Then, after 10–12 weeks' gestation, the endovascular cytotrophoblasts previously plugging the spiral arteries regress and maternal blood begins to flow into the intervillous space. By about 14 weeks, the pO_2 exceeds 50 mmHg [11,12]. Maternal blood flow starts in the periphery of the placenta and extends toward the center. The increase in oxygen tension reduces interstitial trophoblast proliferation and triggers the regression of peripheral villous capillaries. The mechanisms for endovascular trophoblastic 'deplugging' at the end of the first trimester are as yet unknown, but this phenomenon is associated with dispersion of the trophoblast cells and deeper migration into the spiral artery lumens. In third trimester placental sections, the frequency of apoptotic endovascular trophoblast cells was significantly increased in subjects with early-onset preeclampsia with IUGR compared with controls at term [13].

> A functional placental circulation does not form until 10–12 weeks' gestation. Prior to this time placental and embryonic cells are exposed to an oxygen tension <20 mmHg. The hypoxic environment appears to protect the growing products of conception from oxidative stress

Angiogenesis

Once blood vessels are formed within the tertiary villi, they begin to remodel and adapt to the changing needs of the growing embryo and fetus. Extensive transformation, leading to the formation of complex capillary networks, occurs up to the beginning of the third trimester. Capillary networks are formed throughout the second trimester first by branching angiogenesis, followed by non-branching angiogenesis. Branching angiogenesis actually decreases functional vessel length and resistance to blood flow and is achieved by lateral sprouting of vessel buds from existing vessels and/or by formation of transvascular pillars which partition one lumen into two or more lumina (intussusceptive angiogenesis) [14] (Fig. 7.2).

> Complex capillary networks within the placentome are generated by a combination of branching angiogenesis, intussusceptive angiogenesis, and vessel elongation

Non-branching angiogenesis consists of elongation of existing vessel segments by vascular endothelial cell proliferation and/or intercalation of endothelial progenitor cells.

Between 15 and 32 weeks' gestation, subtrophoblastic peripheral capillary regression and pericyte investment lead to the transformation of central capillaries into arteries and veins of the stem villi.

From 25 weeks to term, angiogenesis is predominantly non-branching and is characterized by an active and rapid lengthening of blood vessels, relative to the growth of the trophoblast layer. As a result, the latter cell layer becomes very thin, enhancing transport. The elongating blood vessels form loops and coils creating complex capillary plexi in the terminal villi, where fetal–maternal gas and nutrient exchange occur.

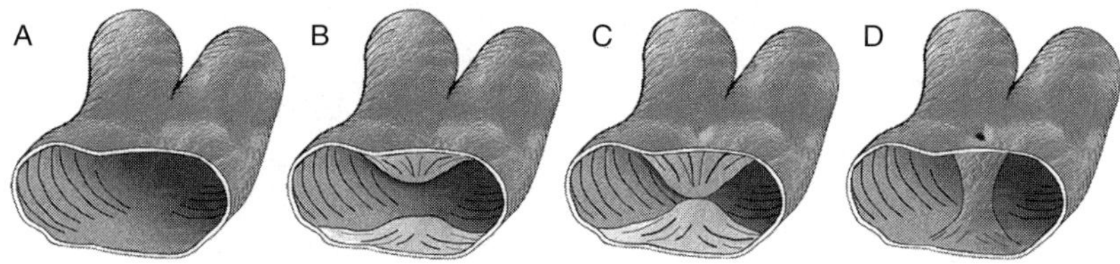

Fig. 7.2 Basic steps of intussusception: protrusion of opposing capillary walls into the lumen (A and B) and creation of a contact zone between the endothelial cells (C). After central perforation of the cellular bilayer, the fused endothelial cells form a transluminal cuff, invaded later by myofibroblasts or pericytes (D). Reproduced with permission from Kurz *et al.* 2003 [14].

Placental bed angiogenesis

The portion of the uterine mucosa directly in contact with the placenta is called the placental bed and is composed of the decidualized endometrium and the subjacent myometrium. The placental bed is perfused by approximately 100 endometrial spiral arteries [15]. These are highly specialized arterioles that present a unique morphology and undergo a critical transformation in pregnancy, with dilated walls and openings, allowing conversion of the maternal vessels from high resistance/low capacitance to low resistance/high capacitance blood conduits.

During cytotrophoblast proliferation and invasion of the endometrium in the first trimester of pregnancy, EVT reach and breach the spiral arteries. These endovascular cytotrophoblasts form plugs that block maternal blood from entering the intervillous space but some plasma filtrate penetrates. This plugging is restricted to the site of implantation creating a hypoxic environment favorable to villi development. Endovascular plugging does not occur away from the implantation site, which allows maternal blood to oxygenate the peripheral villi. This oxygenation is responsible for vascular regression in the villi leading to the formation of the smooth chorion.

Extravillous trophoblasts cause the spiral arteries to undergo a radical change in their structure, called 'physiological conversion' that increases the amount of maternal blood perfusing the placenta while decreasing the vascular resistance. First, there is a generalized remodeling of the arterial walls with disorganization of the vascular elastic fibers and smooth muscle cells, dilation of the lumen, followed by reduction in the number of smooth muscle cells, and deposition of fibrinoid material within the vessel walls. Finally, while it has been suggested that accelerated nitric oxide (NO) production by the trophoblasts may further dilate the arterial walls [16] some investigators failed to detect endovascular trophoblast NO synthase enzyme by immunohistochemistry [17]. During normal pregnancy, 'physiological conversion' results in a mean spiral arteriolar radius of 250 μm. In pregnancies complicated by PE, 'physiological conversion' is impaired, resulting in a mean spiral arteriolar radius of 100 μm. According to Poiseuille's law, this 60% decrement in vessel radius can account for a 40-fold increase in vascular resistance (Fig. 7.3).

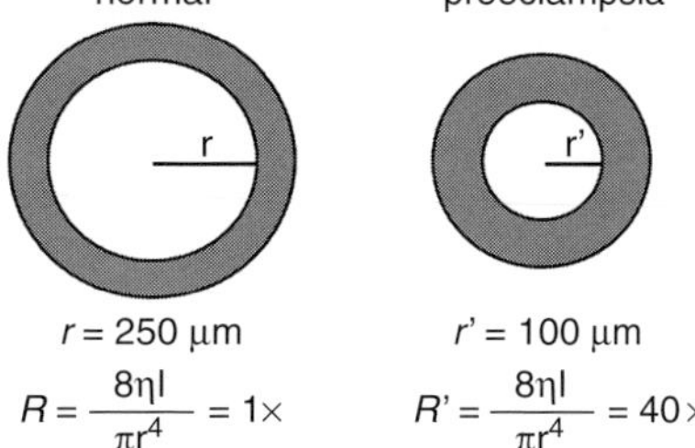

$r = 250\ \mu m$ $\qquad$ $r' = 100\ \mu m$

$$R = \frac{8\eta l}{\pi r^4} = 1\times \qquad R' = \frac{8\eta l}{\pi r^4} = 40\times$$

Fig. 7.3 In 1840 Jean Louis Marie Poiseuille derived a law to describe the non-turbulent flow of fluid through a tubular pipe. This phenomenon has been applied to vascular physiology and predicts that vessel resistance (*R*) is inversely proportional to the fourth power of its radius (*r*). Thus, a 60% reduction in spiral arteriolar radius (*r*) could generate a 40-fold increase in vascular resistance (*R'*).

> 'Physiological conversion' of the maternal spiral arterioles by invading extravillous trophoblasts is necessary to optimize blood flow to the placental bed. Failure of this transformation is associated with PE and IUGR

Section II: molecular aspects of placental angiogenesis

Placental angiogenesis is very complex and depends on an appropriate balance between pro-angiogenic and anti-angiogenic factors. Two of the best understood pro-angiogenic factors are the vascular endothelial growth factors (VEGFs) and the related protein, placental growth factor (PlGF). Other angiogenic factors also were identified in the placenta and are important in the formation and remodeling of placental blood vessels: angiopoietins 1 and 2 and their receptor

Tie-2, basic fibroblast growth factor (FGF-2), as well as the cytokine TGFβ will be discussed.

> Placental angiogenesis is regulated by a panoply of growth factors, among which VEGF, PlGF, FGF, angiopoietins 1 and 2 and TGFβ are the most prominent

Vascular endothelial growth factor-related proteins

Many factors modulate placental vascular development, but members of the VEGF family play a major role. The mammalian VEGF family consists of five members, VEGF-A, -B, -C, -D, and PlGF, all coded by different genes arising through evolutionary gene duplication. Recently, two new members have been identified with exogenous origins: VEGF-E identified in parapox and pseudocowpox viruses and VEGF-F found in some viper venoms [18,19].

VEGF-A and PlGF are expressed in the placenta throughout gestation and are responsible for neoangiogenesis observed during the implantation as well as the maintenance of placental vascularity during the pregnancy. These growth factors act on their target cells by binding to cell-surface tyrosine kinase receptors, VEGF receptor 1, and VEGF receptor 2 (previously known as Flt-1 and Flk-1/KDR, respectively) [20].

VEGF-A was the first VEGF identified and has been intensively studied. In the context of pregnancy, VEGF-A is a product of the endometrium and decidua, but it also is highly expressed in placental cytotrophoblast and Hofbauer cells, where it is responsible for the activation of the endothelial precursors to form angiogenic cords.

The human VEGF-A gene is located on chromosome 6. Alternative splicing of its mRNA leads to the production of a variety of VEGF protein isoforms, ranging in size from 121 amino acids to 206 amino acids. VEGF-A_{165} is the most abundantly secreted isoform. It forms homodimers that bind to VEGFR1 with a high affinity (Kd ~10 to 20 pM), but this receptor is not particularly effective in activating cellular responses. VEGF-A_{165} homodimers also bind with a lower affinity to VEGFR2 (Kd ~100 to 125 pM), which is the receptor responsible for their angiogenic activity. VEGF also binds to the transmembrane glycoproteins neuropilin-1 and neuropilin-2, shown to be coreceptors for several members of the semaphorin/collapsin family in the nervous system [21]. These coreceptors appear to modulate VEGF and PlGF binding to their cognate tyrosine kinase receptor dimers [22]. The receptors themselves, upon binding of VEGF, can form homodimers (R1-R1 and R2-R2) or heterodimers (R1-R2).

PlGF cDNA was first isolated by Maglione in 1991 from human placenta and found to share 42% amino acid homology with VEGF-A [23]. The human PlGF gene is located on chromosome 14. Four different PlGF isoforms arise by alternative splicing of a single pre-mRNA. Only PlGF-2 and -4 have heparin-binding domains. PlGF is highly expressed during pregnancy and while the placenta represents the primary organ secreting PlGF, it is also expressed in the lungs and the heart. Placental PlGF mRNA expression is predominantly localized to villous trophoblasts but PlGF protein is also noted in the cells of fetal stem vessels. The role of PlGF in placental angiogenesis is not well established presently. It is able to form homodimers or heterodimers with VEGF and bind to VEGFR1. The reported effects of PlGF binding to R1 are contradictory. In some cases, angiogenesis is suppressed while in other cases PlGF stimulates the proliferation of microvascular endothelial cells. Knockout mice for the PlGF gene are healthy and fertile but placental size is reduced [24]. In certain pathological conditions like tumor angiogenesis, ischemia, and skin wound healing, the absence of PlGF in knockout mice leads to impaired vascularization [25]. PlGF is a modulator of VEGF activity, synergistically increasing the effects of VEGF-A on endothelial cells *in vivo* [26]. *In vitro* experiments show that PlGF increases the proliferation and survival of isolated trophoblasts [27] as well as their production of NO and cell surface adhesion molecules.

VEGF and PlGF predominantly act through the VEGFR1 and R2 receptors that belong to the PDGFR tyrosine kinase family. Their structure consists of an amino terminal extracellular fragment containing seven immunoglobulin-like domains, a transmembrane fragment, a juxtamembrane fragment, and an intracellular fragment. This intracellular fragment has an interrupted tyrosine kinase domain, containing an insert of 70 amino acid residues. Upon binding of VEGF or PlGF dimers, the liganded receptors dimerize, which is followed by protein kinase activation and trans-autophosphorylation on tyrosine residues.

> Gene knockouts of VEGF-A, VEGFR1 and VEGFR2 all lead to angiogenic failure and embryonic lethality. PlGF knockout mice are viable but placental size is reduced

In the case of VEGFR2, the more important signaling molecule, phosphorylation promotes interactions with the SH2 domain of phospholipase C gamma (PLCγ) which is in turn tyrosine phosphorylated and activates the PKC-beta-c-Raf-MEK-MAP-kinase pathway [28]. VEGFR1 and VEGFR2 are both expressed in the placenta on angiogenic precursor cells and mature endothelium whereas R1 is also expressed on macrophages and trophoblasts.

The critical importance of these two receptors during placental angiogenesis has been revealed by knockout mouse experiments. VEGFR2 knockout mice die at embryonic day 8.0–8.5 from lack of vasculogenesis [29]. The VEGFR1 null mutation is also lethal and mice expressing mutated VEGFR1 die at about the same stage of development. Analysis of the embryos shows an excess of endothelial cells and disorganized tubules [30]. VEGFR2 is required for differentiation of hemangioblastic precursor cells into capillaries while VEGFR1 activation appears to be needed for formation of endothelial tubes by early endothelial cells.

Posttranscriptional modifications of the VEGFR1 mRNA lead to the synthesis and secretion of a soluble form of the receptor, sVEGFR1, also called sFlt-1 (soluble Fms-like tyrosine kinase 1) [31]. It is produced by HUVEC, trophoblasts, and monocytes [32,33]. This soluble form of the receptor possesses its VEGF binding domain but lacks the intracellular tyrosine kinase moiety. By its ability to bind to VEGF and PlGF with high affinity, sVEGFR1 adsorbs free VEGF and PlGF proteins in the serum and thus inhibits angiogenic activity and growth factor-mediated maintenance of endothelial cell function. Studies showing that the expression of VEGF, PlGF, and sVEGFR-1 are dysregulated in abnormal placentation associated with PE and IUGR are discussed below. VEGF null mice, and even heterozygotes with a single VEGF gene copy abrogated, die in early embryonic life, emphasizing the critical importance of this angiogenic factor [34]. In PlGF null mice, placental development and shape are abnormal and on average the placentae are reduced in size by >30% [24].

Like VEGF and PlGF, the VEGFRs are differentially regulated by hypoxia. The primary oxygen sensor in the cell is hypoxia-inducible factor 1 alpha (HIF-1α). Under high oxygen tension, cytoplasmic HIF-1α is rapidly ubiquitinated and degraded [35]. When the environment becomes hypoxic, ubiquitination is suppressed, HIF-1α accumulates in the cytoplasm and translocates to the nucleus where it dimerizes with aryl hydrocarbon receptor nuclear translocator (HIF-1β). This HIF-1α/HIF-1β heterodimer then binds to response elements located in the VEGF and VEGFR gene promoters. Early placentation *in vivo* is subject to low O_2 tensions consistent with HIF-1α activity. It is well accepted that hypoxia increases VEGF and sVEGFR-1 mRNA expression and protein secretion, whereas it decreases or inhibits the production of PlGF in trophoblasts [36,37]. The effect of hypoxia on PlGF expression seems to be cell-type dependent because in cultured fibroblasts, glioma cells and ischemic cardiomyocytes of normal mice, hypoxia stimulates the expression and secretion of PlGF. This effect appears to be mediated by metal transcription factor-1 (MTF-1) responsive elements located in the 5' UTR of the PlGF gene promoter [38]. MTF-1 expression was decreased in choriocarcinoma BeWo cells treated with cobalt chloride ($CoCl_2$) to mimic hypoxia while over-expression of HIF-1α had no effect on PlGF gene expression. MTF-1 expression was decreased in placental samples from preeclamptic patients relative to normal pregnancy. The decrease in PlGF gene expression and protein secretion could be due to down-regulation of MTF-1 by hypoxia.

A number of longitudinal studies measuring the concentrations of angiogenic factors in the serum of women with normotensive pregnancy and women with pregnancy complicated by PE showed that total VEGF and sVEGFR1 concentrations are increased in the blood of the latter group (Figure 7.4A and B) [39,40].

By contrast, while free PlGF concentrations follow the same pattern in normotensive and PE pregnancy, free PlGF concentrations are lower in PE (Fig. 7.4C) [41]. These differences between normotensive and preeclamptic women are even more accentuated when PE is accompanied by IUGR, which independently has features characteristic of defective placental vascularization [42]. All these changes are consistent with placental hypoxia in preeclampsia.

> Placental hypoxia results in increased total VEGF, sVEGFR1 and decreased PlGF production, phenomena that are observed in the maternal circulation of women with PE

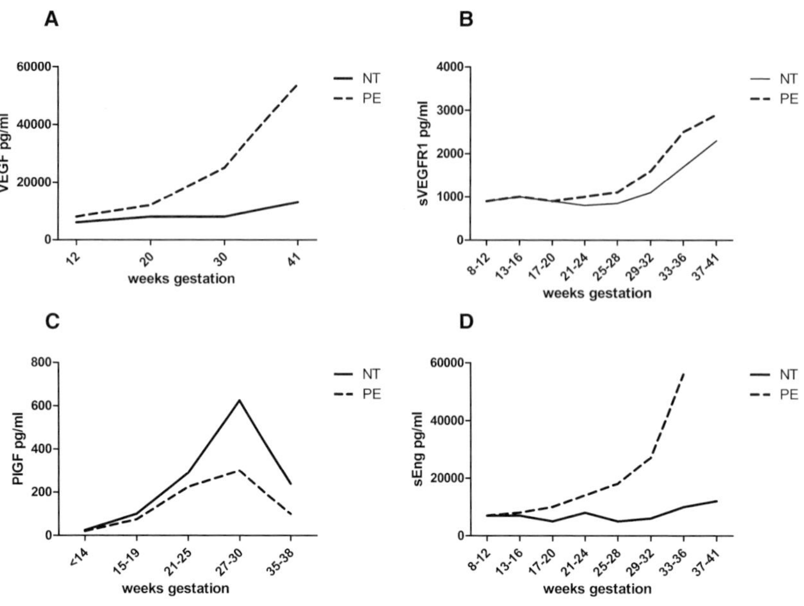

Fig. 7.4 Maternal serum concentrations of total VEGF (A), soluble (s)VEGFR1 (B), and soluble endoglin (sEng) (D) are higher across gestation in women destined to develop PE (dotted lines) relative to normotensive (NT) controls (solid lines). By contrast, circulating levels of free PlGF (C) are lower in women with PE (dotted line) than in normotensive (NT) controls (solid line). Modified from Hunter *et al.* 2000 [39], Levine *et al.* 2004 [40], Levine *et al.* 2006 [57], and Taylor *et al.* 2003 [41].

Angiopoietins 1 and 2 and their receptor Tie-2

In addition to proteins of the VEGF family, other factors also are required for vascular development. Angiopoietins 1 and 2 (Ang-1 and -2) and their receptor Tie-2 were shown to be important in the later stages of vasculogenesis and angiogenesis where they work in concert with VEGF-A as mediators of endothelial cell survival and vascular remodeling [43].

Both Ang-1 and Ang-2 bind to the cell surface tyrosine kinase receptor Tie-2. Ligation by Ang-1 induces phosphorylation of its intracellular moiety and activation of intracellular signaling pathways. Ang-1 is important for endothelial cell chemotaxis, survival, and association with pericytes to stabilize newly formed blood vessels. Ang-1 activity is counterbalanced by Ang-2 which binds to the same Tie-2 receptor but antagonizes its phosphorylation. The primary function of Ang-2 is to destabilize the vasculature and block vascular maturation; an effect of this modulation is to render the capillary more plastic and more responsive to sprouting angiogenesis signals by VEGF-A. Thus, it is well accepted that the ratio of Ang-1/Ang-2 plays an important balancing role in vasculogenesis/angiogenesis.

The presence of Tie-2 in cytotrophoblasts suggests that endothelial cells are not the only target of angiopoietins. Ang-2 enhances trophoblast DNA synthesis and NO release and Ang-1 is a chemotactic agent for trophoblasts, suggesting that these growth factors also may be important in the remodeling of the spiral arteries [44].

Like VEGF-A and PlGF, the angiopoietins are differentially regulated by hypoxia. It was reported that placental samples from pregnancies complicated by preeclampsia had reduced Ang-2 mRNA, potentially compromising the plasticity of placental vessels in these pregnancies [45].

Fibroblast growth factor-2

FGF-2 was the first angiogenic growth factor identified by Gospodarowicz in 1975 and finally purified in 1984 by Shing from bovine pituitary [46,47]. Within 2 years, FGF-2 was also isolated from human placenta [48].

FGF-2 is secreted by villous trophoblasts, as well as smooth muscle and endothelial cells of placental vessels. By binding to cell-surface receptors with tyrosine kinase activity it promotes endothelial cell proliferation and migration and stimulates the production of collagenase and plasminogen activator, which are needed to degrade the extracellular matrix. FGF-2 mRNA also has been detected in EVT where it is thought to play a role in the remodeling of spiral arteries and the elongation of the endometrial blood vessels during pregnancy [49].

Evidence from tumor angiogenesis studies indicates that FGF stimulates and potentiates angiogenic effects by increasing VEGF expression and controlling VEGFR2 signaling responsiveness [50]. FGF-2 stimulates vascular formation in embryoid bodies but not when the VEGFR2 gene is ablated. On the other hand, inhibiting VEGF-A with antibodies or VEGF-Traps [51] also inhibits FGF-induced angiogenesis. Knockout of FGF-1 in embryoid bodies also leads to impairment of VEGF expression and vascular formation which is rescued when VEGF is supplemented exogenously. These results have brought researchers to the conclusion that many FGF effects on vascular formation are upstream of VEGF.

Transforming growth factor β

Transforming growth factor β (TGFβ), the prototype of a superfamily of cytokines that includes activins, inhibins, and bone morphogenic peptides (BMP), was originally purified from human placenta. It has pleiotropic effects on human placental cell differentiation and proliferation and also for the invasiveness of trophoblasts into the endometrium [52]. The importance of TGFβ in vasculogenesis and angiogenesis is well known and has been demonstrated *in vivo* and *in vitro*. Knockout studies in mice of components of the TGFβ signaling pathway showed that TGFβ was important for the integrity of blood vessel walls [53].

> The physiological effects of TGFβ, its receptors, and modulators (e.g. endoglin) are not yet clearly defined in placental angiogenesis

There are three isoforms of TGFβ in mammalian tissues: β1, β2, and β3 with β1 thought to play the major role in vascular remodeling. Numerous studies showed that all three isoforms are expressed in the decidua and placenta; the cellular pattern of expression differing depending on the isoform studied.

TGFβ1 and -2 proteins are expressed in trophoblasts and especially in EVT during all trimesters of pregnancy, while TGFβ3 protein is produced only during the first trimester [54,55].

TGFβ binds to transmembrane receptors with serine/threonine kinase activities. Three types of receptors, type I, type II, and type III, exist as homo-oligomers, with type II being the most important signaling receptor. Phosphorylation of its serine/threonine residues allows interaction and phosphorylation of Smad mediator proteins that transduce the signal to the nucleus.

TβRIII consists of two proteins with a high degree of sequence homology: endoglin (Eng) and betaglycan. Their cytoplasmic domains have no kinase activity but present numerous serine and threonine residues. TβRIII do not appear to be required for TGFβ signal transduction but they seem to enhance the presentation of TGFβ to type I and type II receptors.

Recently, there has been great interest in placental endoglin, originally designated CD (cluster of differentiation) 105. It is a homodimeric transmembrane glycoprotein abundantly expressed by endothelial cells and syncytiotrophoblasts [56]. Endothelial cells that lack endoglin fail to migrate or proliferate and mutations in endoglin have been associated with hereditary hemorrhagic telangiectasia (Weber–Osler–Rendu syndrome). Elevated concentrations of serum soluble endoglin (sEng) are associated with PE [57,58] (Fig. 7.4D). Several studies showed that sEng inhibits TGFβ1 signaling, TGFβ1-mediated NO synthase activation in endothelial cells, endothelial cell proliferation, and capillary formation but the exact mechanism is not yet elucidated. As for sVEGFR1, which is postulated to inhibit angiogenic activity by sequestering free VEGF and PlGF, sEng is hypothesized to inhibit TGFβ signaling by binding to free TGFβ and preventing its ligation to membrane receptors.

Pregnancy-related diseases and placental angiogenesis

Placental pro- and anti-angiogenic factors are expressed in a timely manner to regulate vasculogenesis and angiogenesis. Dysregulation of placental angiogenesis often leads to pregnancy-related diseases.

Three common adverse pregnancy outcomes have been associated with defective placental vascularization: spontaneous abortion, IUGR, sometimes referred to as 'small-for-gestational age' (SGA), and PE. As noted elsewhere in this book, signs of PE include gestational hypertension and proteinuria with a wide range of severity. The placenta plays a critical role in PE as evidenced by the fact that its signs and symptoms disappear rapidly after the placenta is removed and can occur in complete molar pregnancies in which there is no fetal component. The exact causes of PE are not clearly defined but several studies of placental bed biopsies show shallow invasion of the maternal endometrium by EVT and reduced remodeling of the spiral arteries, which are thought to create a hypoxic placental environment. This hypothesis is consistent with the reported effects, detailed above, of hypoxia on placental expression of angiogenic growth factors and their binding proteins.

VEGF levels Total are increased while free PlGF levels are decreased in the serum of women who later develop PE compared to the serum levels of women with normotensive pregnancy (Figures 7.4A and C). At the same time, the anti-angiogenic factors sVEGFR1 and sEng are both increased in serum of women with PE (Figures 7.4B and D). Some of the differences in serum concentrations can be seen as early as 12 weeks' gestation, before the onset of any clinical manifestations of PE.

Further characterization of angiogenesis in placental development will better inform clinicians and scientists about healthy and pathological pregnancies. Biomarkers of these angiogenic processes, particularly PlGF, sVEGFR1 and sEng, promise to provide diagnostic and hopefully predictive non-invasive measures to identify mothers and their fetuses at risk for PE, IUGR, and other untoward complications (see also Chapter 21). Prudent utilization of these biomarkers should be based on a comprehensive understanding of the cellular and molecular events that dictate placental angiogenesis.

> Angiogenesis biomarkers are likely to become accurate predictors of human pregnancy pathophysiology

References

1. Risau W. Vasculogenesis, angiogenesis and endothelial cell differentiation during embryonic development. In: Feinberg R N, Sheror G K, Auerbach R, eds. *The development of the vascular system*. Philadelphia: Krager; 1991: pp. 58–68.
2. Duc-Goiran P, Mignot T M, Bourgeois C, *et al.* Embryo-maternal interactions at the implantation site: a delicate equilibrium. *Eur J Obstet Gynecol Reprod Biol* 1999; **83**(1): 85–100.
3. Genbacev O, Zhou Y, Ludlow J W, *et al.* Regulation of human placental development by oxygen tension. *Science* 1997; **277**(5332): 1669–72.
4. Kaufmann P, Mayhew T M, Charnock-Jones D S. Aspects of human fetoplacental vasculogenesis and angiogenesis. II. Changes during normal pregnancy. *Placenta* 2004; **25** (2–3): 114–26.
5. Jones C J, Jauniaux E. Ultrastructure of the materno-embryonic interface in the first trimester of pregnancy. *Micron* 1995; **26**(2): 145–173.
6. Benirschke K, Kaufmann P. Architecture of normal villous tree. In: *Pathology of the human placenta*, 4th ed. New York: Springer-Verlag; 2000; ch 7.
7. Ramsey E M, Martin C B Jr, Donner M W. Fetal and maternal placental circulations: simultaneous visualization in monkeys by radiography. *Am J Obstet Gynecol* 1967; **98**(3): 419–23.
8. Schuhmann R A. Placentone structure of the human placenta. *Bibl Anat* 1982; **22**: 46–57.
9. Seval Y, Korgun E T, Demir R. Hofbauer cells in early human placenta: possible implications in vasculogenesis and angiogenesis. *Placenta* 2007; **28**(8–9): 841–5.
10. de Groot C J, Chao V A, Roberts J M, Taylor R N. Human endothelial cell morphology and autacoid expression. *Am J Physiol* 1995; **268**(4 Pt 2): H1613–20.
11. Jauniaux E, Watson A L, Hempstock J, *et al.* Onset of maternal arterial blood flow and placental oxidative stress: a possible factor in human early pregnancy failure. *Am J Pathol* 2000; **157**(6): 2111–22.
12. Jauniaux E, Watson A, Burton G. Evaluation of respiratory gases and acid-base gradients in human fetal fluids and uteroplacental tissue between 7 and 16 weeks' gestation. *Am J Obstet Gynecol* 2001; **184**(5): 998–1003.
13. Kadyrov M, Kingdom J C, Huppertz B. Divergent trophoblast invasion and apoptosis in placental bed spiral arteries from pregnancies complicated by maternal anemia and early-onset preeclampsia/intrauterine growth restriction. *Am J Obstet Gynecol* 2006; **194**(2): 557–63.
14. Kurz H, Burri P H, Djonov V G. Angiogenesis and vascular remodeling by intussusception: from form to function. *News Physiol Sci* 2003; **18**: 65–70.
15. Pijnenborg R, Vercruysse L, Hanssens M. The uterine spiral arteries in human pregnancy: facts and controversies. *Placenta* 2006; **27**(9–10): 939–58.
16. Nanaev A, Chwalisz K, Frank H G *et al.* Physiological dilation of uteroplacental arteries in the guinea pig depends on nitric oxide synthase activity of extravillous trophoblast. *Cell Tissue Res* 1995; **282**(3): 407–21.
17. Lyall F, Bulmer J N, Kelly H *et al.* Human trophoblast invasion and spiral artery transformation: the role of nitric oxide. *Am J Pathol* 1999; **154**(4): 1105–14.
18. Roy H, Bhardwaj S, Yla-Herttuala S. Biology of vascular endothelial growth factors. *FEBS Lett* 2006; **580**(12): 2879–87.
19. Yamazaki Y, Morita T. Molecular and functional diversity of vascular endothelial growth factors. *Mol Divers* 2006; **10**(4): 515–27.
20. Sato Y, Kanno S, Oda N *et al.* Properties of two VEGF receptors, Flt-1 and KDR, in signal transduction. *Ann N Y Acad Sci* 2000; **902**: 201–5.
21. Fujisawa H, Kitsukawa T. Receptors for collapsin/semaphorins. *Curr Opin Neurobiol* 1998; **8**(5): 587–92.

22. Soker S, Takashima S, Miao H Q *et al.* Neuropilin-1 is expressed by endothelial and tumor cells as an isoform-specific receptor for vascular endothelial growth factor. *Cell* 1998; **92**(6): 735–45.

23. Maglione D, Guerriero V, Viglietto G *et al.* Isolation of a human placenta cDNA coding for a protein related to the vascular permeability factor. *Proc Natl Acad Sci U S A* 1991; **88**(20): 9267–71.

24. Tayade C, Hilchie D, He H *et al.* Genetic deletion of placenta growth factor in mice alters uterine NK cells. *J Immunol* 2007; **178**(7): 4267–75.

25. Carmeliet P, Moons L, Luttun A *et al.* Synergism between vascular endothelial growth factor and placental growth factor contributes to angiogenesis and plasma extravasation in pathological conditions. *Nat Med* 2001; **7**(5): 575–83.

26. Park J E, Chen H H, Winer J *et al.* Placenta growth factor. Potentiation of vascular endothelial growth factor bioactivity, in vitro and in vivo, and high affinity binding to Flt-1 but not to Flk-1/KDR. *J Biol Chem* 1994; **269**(41): 25646–54.

27. Athanassiades A, Lala P K. Role of placenta growth factor (PlGF) in human extravillous trophoblast proliferation, migration and invasiveness. *Placenta* 1998; **19**(7): 465–73.

28. Takahashi T, Yamaguchi S, Chida K *et al.* A single autophosphorylation site on KDR/Flk-1 is essential for VEGF-A-dependent activation of PLC-gamma and DNA synthesis in vascular endothelial cells. *EMBO J* 2001; **20**(11): 2768–78.

29. Shalaby F, Rossant J, Yamaguchi T P *et al.* Failure of blood-island formation and vasculogenesis in Flk-1-deficient mice. *Nature* 1995; **376**(6535): 62–6.

30. Fong G H, Rossant J, Gertsenstein M *et al.* Role of the Flt-1 receptor tyrosine kinase in regulating the assembly of vascular endothelium. *Nature* 1995; **376**(6535): 66–70.

31. Kendall R L, Thomas K A. Inhibition of vascular endothelial cell growth factor activity by an endogenously encoded soluble receptor. *Proc Natl Acad Sci U S A* 1993; **90**(22): 10705–9.

32. Helske S, Vuorela P, Carpen O *et al.* Expression of vascular endothelial growth factor receptors 1, 2 and 3 in placentas from normal and complicated pregnancies. *Mol Hum Reprod* 2001; **7**(2): 205–10.

33. Rajakumar A, Michael H M, Rajakumar P A *et al.* Extra-placental expression of vascular endothelial growth factor receptor-1 (Flt-1), and soluble Flt-1 (sFlt-1), by peripheral blood mononuclear cells (PBMCs) in normotensive and preeclamptic pregnant women. *Placenta* 2005; **26**(7): 563–73.

34. Ferrara N, Carver-Moore K, Chen H *et al.* Heterozygous embryonic lethality induced by targeted inactivation of the VEGF gene. *Nature* 1996; **380**(6573): 439–42.

35. Kaluz S, Kaluzova M, Stanbridge E J. Regulation of gene expression by hypoxia: integration of the HIF-transduced hypoxic signal at the hypoxia-responsive element. *Clin Chim Acta* 2008; **395**(1–2): 6–13.

36. Ahmed A, Dunk C, Ahmad S *et al.* Regulation of placental vascular endothelial growth factor (VEGF) and placenta growth factor (PIGF) and soluble Flt-1 by oxygen: a review. *Placenta* 2000; **21** (Suppl A): S16–S24.

37. Munaut C, Lorquet S, Pequeux C *et al.* Hypoxia is responsible for soluble vascular endothelial growth factor receptor-1 (VEGFR-1) but not for soluble endoglin induction in villous trophoblast. *Hum Reprod* 2008; **23**(6): 1407–15.

38. Nishimoto F, Sakata M, Minekawa R *et al.* Metal transcription factor-1 is involved in hypoxia-dependent regulation of placenta growth factor in trophoblast-derived cells. *Endocrinology* 2009; **150**: 1801–8.

39. Hunter A, Aitkenhead M, Caldwell C *et al.* Serum levels of vascular endothelial growth factor in preeclamptic and normotensive pregnancy. *Hypertension* 2000; **36**(6): 965–9.

40. Levine R J, Maynard S E, Qian C *et al.* Circulating angiogenic factors and the risk of preeclampsia. *N Engl J Med* 2004; **350**(7): 672–83.

41. Taylor R N, Grimwood J, Taylor R S *et al.* Longitudinal serum concentrations of placental growth factor: evidence for abnormal placental angiogenesis in pathologic pregnancies. *Am J Obstet Gynecol* 2003; **188** (1): 177–82.

42. Johns J, Jauniaux E. Placental haematomas in early pregnancy. *Br J Hosp Med (Lond)* 2007; **68**(1): 32–5.

43. Charnock-Jones D S. Soluble flt-1 and the angiopoietins in the development and regulation of placental vasculature. *J Anat* 2002; **200**(6): 607–15.

44. Schiessl B, Innes B A, Bulmer J N *et al.* Localization of angiogenic growth factors and their receptors in the human placental bed throughout normal human pregnancy. *Placenta* 2009; **30**(1): 79–87.

45. Zhang E G, Smith S K, Baker P N *et al.* The regulation and localization of angiopoietin-1, -2, and their receptor Tie2 in normal and pathologic human placentae. *Mol Med* 2001; **7**(9): 624–35.

46. Gospodarowicz D. Purification of a fibroblast growth factor from bovine pituitary. *J Biol Chem* 1975; **250**(7): 2515–20.

47. Shing Y, Folkman J, Sullivan R, *et al.* Heparin affinity: purification of a tumor-derived capillary endothelial cell growth factor. *Science* 1984; **223**(4642): 1296–9.

48. Ribatti D, Conconi M T, Nussdorfer G G. Nonclassic endogenous novel regulators of angiogenesis. *Pharmacol Rev* 2007; **59**(2): 185–205.

49. Ferriani R A, Ahmed A, Sharkey A *et al.* Colocalization of acidic and fibroblastic growth factor (FGF) in human placenta and the cellular effects of bFGF in trophoblast cell line JEG-3. *Growth Factors* 1994; **10**(4): 259–68.

50. Murakami M, Simons M. Fibroblast growth factor regulation of neovascularization. *Curr Opin Hematol* 2008; **15**(3): 215–20.

51. Rudge J S, Holash J, Hylton D *et al.* Inaugural article: VEGF Trap complex formation measures production rates of VEGF, providing a biomarker for predicting efficacious angiogenic blockade. *Proc Natl Acad Sci U S A* 2007; **104**(47): 18363–70.

52. Govinden R, Bhoola K D. Genealogy, expression, and cellular function of transforming growth factor-beta. *Pharmacol Ther* 2003; **98**(2): 257–65.

53. Pepper M S. Transforming growth factor-beta: vasculogenesis, angiogenesis, and vessel wall integrity. *Cytokine Growth Factor Rev* 1997; **8**(1): 21–43.

54. Bowen J M, Chamley L, Mitchell M D *et al.* Cytokines of the placenta and extra-placental membranes: biosynthesis, secretion and roles in establishment of pregnancy in women. *Placenta* 2002; **23**(4): 239–56.

55. Jones R L, Stoikos C, Findlay J K *et al.* TGF-beta superfamily expression and actions in the endometrium and placenta. *Reproduction* 2006; **132**(2): 217–32.

56. Bernabeu C, Conley B A, Vary C P. Novel biochemical pathways of endoglin in vascular cell physiology. *J Cell Biochem* 2007; **102**(6): 1375–88.

57. Levine R J, Lam C, Qian C *et al.* Soluble endoglin and other circulating antiangiogenic factors in preeclampsia. *N Engl J Med* 2006; **355**(10): 992–1005.

58. Luft F C. Soluble endoglin (sEng) joins the soluble fms-like tyrosine kinase (sFlt) receptor as a pre-eclampsia molecule. *Nephrol Dial Transplant* 2006; **21**(11): 3052–4.

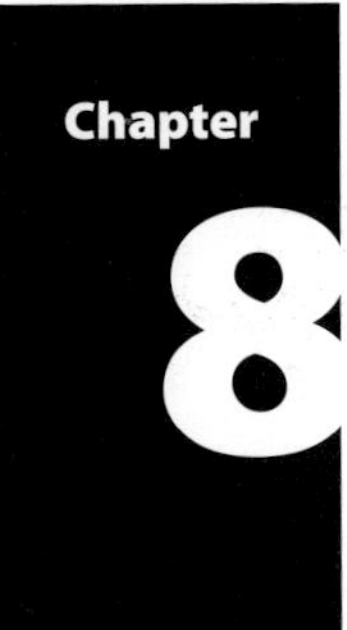

Oxygen delivery at the deciduoplacental interface

Eric Jauniaux[1] and Graham J. Burton[2]

[1]Academic Department of Obstetrics and Gynaecology, Institute for Women's Health, Royal Free and University College Hospitals, London, UK
[2]Centre for Trophoblast Research, University of Cambridge, UK

Introduction

Evolution for mammals living on dry land has been closely linked to adaptation to changes in oxygen (O_2) concentration in the environment over billions of years. O_2 was initially released as a by-product of photosynthesis following the emergence of the blue-green algae, and as atmospheric concentrations increased it became possible to support more complex, multicellular life forms, including the placental mammals [1]. In animals, O_2 has become essential for energy transformation of dietary proteins, carbohydrates, and fats into adenosine triphosphate (ATP). ATP molecules are the chemical energy required to conduct the cellular biochemical reactions essential to cellular life including protein biosynthesis, active transport of molecules through cellular membranes, and muscular contractions [2].

Most of the O_2 used during the oxidation of dietary organic molecules is converted into water through the activity of Complex IV of the mitochondrial electron transport chain. Around 1–2% of the O_2 consumed escapes this process, however, and is diverted into highly reactive oxygen free radicals (OFR) and other reactive O_2 species (ROS), mainly the superoxide ($O_2^{\cdot-}$), hydroxyl ($OH^{\cdot}$), peroxyl ($RO_2.$) and hydroperoxyl ($HO_2^{\cdot}$) anions [2]. ROS are constantly formed as a by-product of aerobic respiration and other metabolic reactions. The transfer of electrons from enzymes of the respiratory chain onto molecular O_2 results in the formation of $O_2^{\cdot-}$, at a rate dependent on the prevailing O_2 tension. Due to its charge, $O_2^{\cdot-}$ is membrane impermeable and remains within the mitochondrial matrix where it is detoxified by the enzyme manganese superoxide dismutase (MnSOD). SOD is present in all aerobic cells. In the cytoplasm, it is found as the copper/zinc form (Cu/ZnSOD). These enzymes convert $O_2^{\cdot-}$ to hydrogen peroxide (H_2O_2), which in turn is reduced to water by the antioxidant enzymes catalase (CAT) and glutathione peroxidase (GPX). In addition to the antioxidant enzymes, other molecules such as thiols, selenium, ceruloplasmin, taurine, lactoferrin and transferrin, and dietary antioxidant vitamins such as ascorbate (C) and α-tocopherol (E) play a crucial role in defense against ROS. When the production of OFR exceeds the cellular natural protection, indiscriminate damage can occur to proteins, lipids, and DNA [2]. Hence, oxygen is often referred to as the Janus gas, having both beneficial and potentially harmful actions.

Human early pregnancy is a challenging time. The most critical stages of embryonic development, including implantation, gastrulation, and establishment of the body plan take place before pregnancy is even manifested by the first missed menstrual period. Around one-third of clinical pregnancies are lost through spontaneous miscarriage [3], most of them within the first month after conception (6 weeks of gestation postmenstruation). This phenomenon is extremely rare in other mammalian species. For those pregnancies that continue, the exterior form of the fetus is complete and the rudiments of the major organ systems are in place by 10 weeks of gestation [2]. Until the last two decades remarkably little was known about the environment in which these key events take place, or the nutritional and metabolic pathways by which the embryo or early fetus is supported. The situation was transformed by the advent first of high-resolution ultrasound imaging, and subsequently of Doppler analysis of blood flow [4,5,6,7,8,9]. For the first time it became possible to visualize the early placenta developing and functioning *in vivo* in a non-invasive and reproducible way (Fig. 8.1). Equally importantly, ultrasound imaging allowed guided sampling and measurements to be performed from specific and identifiable sites within the fetoplacental unit,

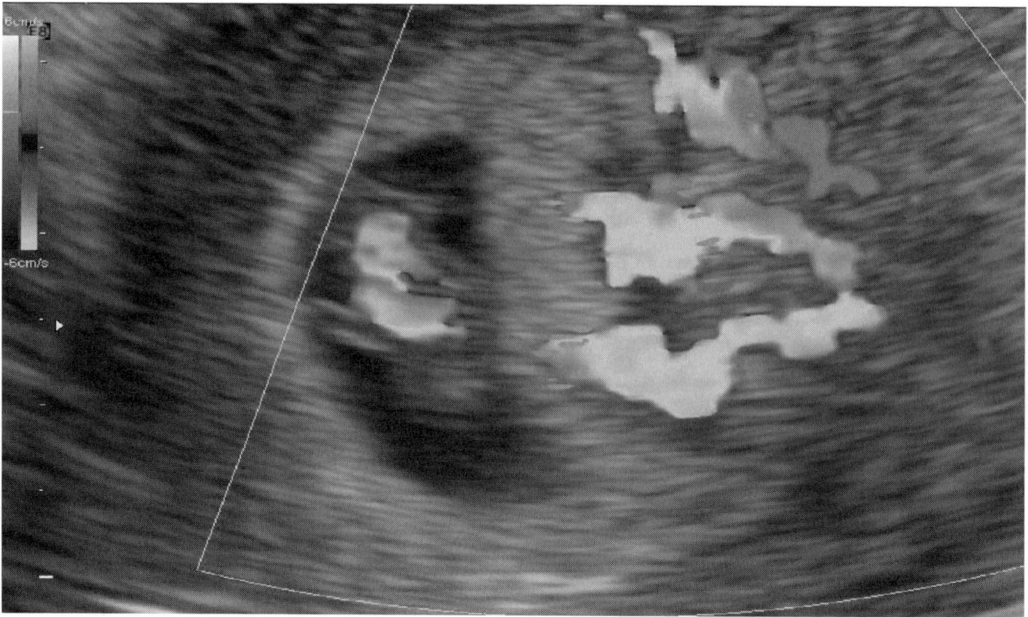

Fig. 8.1 Color flow mapping of the utero and umbilico-placental circulations at 7 weeks of gestation. See plate section for color version.

enabling a series of novel physiological and biochemical investigations to be performed from as early as 5 weeks of gestation [10,11,12,13,14,15,16,17]. The results obtained have necessitated a radical reappraisal of our understanding of early pregnancy, leading to a reassessment of the position of the human in relation to that of other mammals, and to a new appreciation of the pathophysiology of the commonest complications of human pregnancy.

In this chapter we have reviewed our work of the last two decades on the roles and distribution of O_2 inside the early human gestational sac and its impact on our understanding of the physiology of O_2 metabolism by the fetus during the first and early second trimesters of pregnancy.

The changing oxygen barriers of early human pregnancy

The mammalian fetus is exposed to major fluctuations in O_2 concentration from conception to delivery [1,3]. The O_2 tension in the oviduct and uterus of most mammalian species ranges between 11 and 60 mmHg which corresponds to approximately 1–9% O_2 [1]. These data indicate that the mammalian embryo and early fetus develops *in vivo* under low O_2 as opposed to the atmospheric O_2 tension of 21% (98 mmHg). Our data have shown that the human fetus is no exception to this universal rule and that the PO_2 measured within the human placenta *in vivo* increases from <20 mmHg at 7–10 weeks' gestation to >50 mmHg at 11–14 weeks [18,19,20,21]. At 13–16 weeks, we found that the fetal blood PO_2 is 24 mmHg, whereas during the second half of pregnancy the umbilical vein PO_2 ranges between 35 and 55 mmHg, which is relatively low compared to PO_2 values found in the maternal circulation throughout pregnancy [18,19,20,21,22].

The first trimester gestational sac has additional barriers to materno-fetal exchange compared to the definitive placenta of the second and third trimesters of pregnancy. These barriers and the remodeling of the first trimester gestational sac are closely linked to the development of the early fetus. At the end of the first trimester, two-thirds of the primitive placenta disappears, the exocoelomic cavity (ECC) is obliterated by the growth of the amniotic sac, and maternal blood flows progressively throughout the entire placenta [23]. These events bring the maternal blood closer to the fetal tissues, facilitating nutrient and gaseous exchanges between the maternal and fetal circulations.

The changing structure of human placental trophoblastic barrier

The human blastocyst implants with the polar trophectoderm cells overlying the inner cell mass establishing the initial contact with the uterine epithelial cells [24]. Gradually, as the conceptus moves into the superficial decidua, the layer of syncytiotrophoblast extends over the whole surface, forming a complete mantle. The trophectoderm of the human blastocyst gives rise to three main cell types: the syncytiotrophoblast which forms the epithelial covering of the villous tree and is the main endocrine component of the placenta; the villous cytotrophoblast cells which represent a germinative population that proliferate throughout pregnancy and fuse to generate the syncytiotrophoblast; and the extravillous trophoblast cells which are non-proliferative and invade into the maternal decidua. Until 16 weeks of gestation, the human placenta remains the largest tissue inside the gestational sac and its metabolic needs remain the highest of any fetal organ throughout the entire pregnancy. This is largely due to the combination of two highly energy-demanding cell processes, active transport and protein synthesis, which each account for approximately one-third of total placental oxygen consumption [25]. The apical and basal membranes of the syncytiotrophoblast are richly endowed with amino acid and other ATP-dependent transporters involved in active transport and the maintenance of ionic homeostasis. Equally, the syncytiotrophoblast produces large quantities of both steroid and peptide hormones throughout pregnancy, with secretion of human placental lactogen reaching 1 g per day towards term. The tissue therefore contains a large number of mitochondria, which are the primary source of OFR and have been implicated in the pathophysiology of complications such as preeclampsia [26]. In addition, folding of nascent proteins within the endoplasmic reticulum is an oxidative process that produces OFR as a by-product [27]. The syncytiotrophoblast is therefore a major site for the production of ROS during pregnancy.

Very little is known of the earliest stages of villous tissue development, mainly due to the inaccessibility of specimens. The chorionic villi, the basic structures of the early placenta, form during the 4th and 5th week postmenstruation [28] and surround the entire gestational sac until 8–9 weeks of gestation. Between the 3rd and 4th month, the villi at the implantation site become elaborately branched and form the definitive placenta, whereas the villi on the opposite pole degenerate to form the placental membranes, a process that appears to be linked with the onset of the maternal arterial circulation to the placenta as will be discussed later. This leaves the villi over the embryonic pole of the chorionic sac forming the discoid definitive placenta. The remainder of the chorionic membrane becomes the smooth chorion, or chorion laeve, and this transition is essential to allow for rupture of the extraembryonic membranes at birth.

The villous membrane accounts for nearly 90% of the total resistance to the diffusional exchange for O_2 [29]. The rate of diffusional exchange across the villous membrane is governed by the Fick equation, and a morphometric estimate (Dvm) of this can be generated as follows:

$$Dvm(cm^3.min^{-1}.mmHg^{-1}) = villous\ surface\ area + capillary\ surface\ area \times K/2 \times mean\ MTh$$

where K is the Krogh's diffusion coefficient and MTh is the harmonic mean thickness of the villous membrane, which includes the trophoblast, the villous stroma, and the endothelium of the fetal capillaries. We found that the MTh decreases slowly before 12 weeks with values ranging between 25 and 35 μm as compared with values <10 μm after 15 weeks [30].

Our experiments have shown that under ambient conditions (20–21% O_2), the first trimester syncytiotrophoblast degenerates rapidly despite excellent viability for the cytotrophoblast and stromal cell types [31]. The degenerative changes affect the cytoplasmic organelles and, in particular, the mitochondria and the microvilli. We also found that syncytiotrophoblast morphology and mitochondrial activity are retained when tissue of 8–10 weeks is placed in low O_2 (2%) and that the effects of ambient conditions are less marked when placental tissue of 14 weeks is used. The increase in intervillous PO_2, observed between 8 and 14 weeks of gestation, is accompanied by almost parallel increases in the activity and mRNA concentrations of the major antioxidant enzymes in the villous tissue [20].

Overall our data have shown that the placental syncytiotrophoblast is extremely sensitive to oxidative stress, partly because it is the outermost tissue of the conceptus and so is exposed to the highest concentrations of O_2 coming from the uterine circulation, and partly because it contains low levels of the principal antioxidant enzymes compared to other cell types in the placenta [32,33]. The reason for the latter is not understood. It may reflect depletion of the enzymes by the high rate of production of ROS within the syncytiotrophoblast described earlier. Alternatively, levels may be held low to enable the ROS produced to play key roles in signal transduction pathways. Although biological interest in ROS initially focused on their potentially harmful properties, as described earlier, it is now recognized that they act as important second messengers involved in the regulation of various homeostatic pathways [34]. In the placenta they have also been implicated in the control of cytotrophoblast cell fusion with the syncytiotrophoblast, for this is perturbed in cases of trisomy 21 where there is overexpression of the Cu/ZnSOD enzyme [35]. In this way placental development may be linked to the prevailing oxygen concentration. While this may be biologically attractive, the low levels of antioxidant defenses would appear to leave the syncytiotrophoblast peculiarly vulnerable to sudden changes in the intrauterine environment.

The rise and fall of the adnexial interface

The ECC is the largest anatomical space inside the gestational sac between 5 and 9 weeks of gestation and thus represents an important interface between the placenta and the fetal tissues. Until 12 weeks, when the amniotic membrane merges with the mesenchymal face of the chorionic plate, its composition is influenced mainly by the products of the villous trophoblast and secondary yolk sac (SYS) synthesis and metabolism [12]. We found that the exo-coelomic fluid (CF) has a lower pH, base excess, and bicarbonate concentration than maternal venous blood, and contains higher levels of CO_2, lactate and phosphate, and lower levels of protein, than the maternal serum [10,19,21,36,37]. These findings are consistent with a metabolic anaerobic acidotic status, which is mainly due to the accumulation of acidic bioproducts from placental metabolism in the ECC. We also detected high levels of polyols in the CF, indicating that the fetoplacental tissues may rely on primitive carbohydrate metabolic pathways involving non-phosphorylated sugars during early pregnancy when the oxygen concentration is low [14].

The CF has no O_2 consumption and should therefore allow diffusion more freely than an equivalent thickness of cells. However, as the CF does not contain an O_2 carrier, the total O_2 content must be low. Our *in vivo* experiments have shown that the mean coelomic PO_2 is approximately 20 mmHg during the first trimester and varies little between 7 and 10 weeks of gestation [19,20]. An O_2 gradient will inevitably exist between the source and the target. Measurements in human patients undergoing *in vitro* fertilization have shown that the PO_2 in follicular fluid falls as follicle diameter, assessed by ultrasound, increases [38]. Thus, diffusion across the ECC may be an important route of O_2 supply to the fetus before the development of a functional placental circulation, but it will maintain the early fetus in a low O_2 environment. The presence in the ECC of molecules with a well-established antioxidant role such as taurine, transferrin, vitamins A and C, and selenium support this concept [12,13]. This may serve as an additional protection for the fetal tissues from the potential damage by OFR released by the maternal tissues and placental metabolism during the crucial stages of embryogenesis and organogenesis.

The secondary yolk sac (SYS) is known to play a major role in the early embryonic development of all mammals, and in laboratory rodents, in particular, it has been demonstrated as one of the initial sites of hematopoiesis [39]. By contrast to the arrangement in most mammalian species, in all primates including the human, the SYS floats within the ECC lying between the placenta and the amniotic cavity. The SYS is directly connected to the embryonic gut, and possesses a rich vascular plexus at an earlier stage of pregnancy than placental villi. The inner cells of the SYS (endoderm) display morphological features typical of highly active synthetic cells and are known to synthesize several serum proteins in common with the fetal liver, such as alpha-fetoprotein (AFP), alpha$_1$-antitrypsin, albumin, prealbumin, and transferrin [12]. With rare exceptions, the secretion of most of these proteins is confined to the fetal compartments.

The external layer of the SYS (mesothelial) which lines the ECC has the appearance of an absorptive epithelium [40]. Our data showing a similar composition of the SYS and CF suggest that there is a free transfer for most molecules between the two corresponding compartments [41,42,43,44]. We have also demonstrated the presence of glycodelin and α-tocopherol transfer protein in the cytoplasm of the mesothelial layer and the presence of hCG in the yolk sac fluid although this molecule is not synthesized by the SYS. Around 28 days postovulation the chorionic vasculature is connected to the vascular plexus of the SYS via the vessels of connecting stalk, and both are connected with the primitive heart via the dorsal aorta. The rich vascular network of the SYS is most certainly the first part of the fetal adnexae to be perfused when the fetal heart starts to beat. Overall our data have

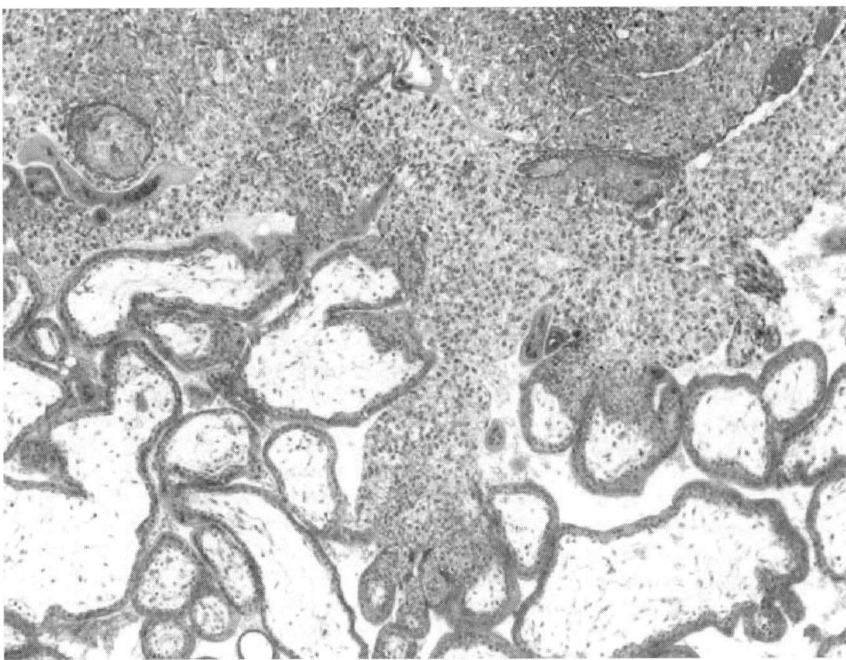

Fig. 8.2 Histological view of the materno-placental interface (deciduochorial) showing the cytotrophoblastic cell shell (hysterectomy specimen No H710: 4 mm embryo of 6 weeks of gestation, Boyd Collection, Department of Anatomy, University of Cambridge). See plate section for color version.

demonstrated that the human SYS plays also an important role in materno-fetal nutrient exchange prior to vascularization of the chorionic villi [7,8,9]. The main movement of molecules passes from the chorionic cavity to the SYS and subsequently to the embryonic gut and circulation. The circulation of the SYS contains the earliest form of fetal hemoglobin, which has a very high affinity for O_2. Thus it is likely that most of the O_2 molecules that diffuse through the ECC are also picked up by the SYS circulation.

The uterine glandular nesting layer

In all mammalian species the earliest nutrition of the conceptus is supplied by the secretions of the oviduct and subsequently the uterus, referred to as histiotrophic nutrition [45,46,47]. The importance of these secretions to normal development has been demonstrated in the sheep, where steroidal ablation of the endometrial glands results in failure of the conceptus to elongate and develop [45]. The duration of the phase of histiotrophic nutrition varies between species, being relatively long in those with epitheliochorial placentas where the conceptus remains within the uterine lumen throughout gestation.

In contrast, the human blastocyst becomes completely embedded in the uterine decidua between days 6 and 9, and in the past this has been taken as indicative of the end of the histiotrophic phase. The earliest specimen from the Boyd collection that we examined was from a 4 mm embryo, and so estimated to be of approximately 6 weeks' menstrual age (Fig. 8.2). We found that the endometrium beneath the conceptus is over 5 mm thick and contained highly active glands [46]. The distal portions of the spiral arteries are located between the decidual glands and thus the decidua does not constitute an additional O_2 barrier between the maternal and fetal tissue at any stage during pregnancy. However, we have demonstrated that the glands open through the developing basal plate of the placenta into the intervillous space, and that MUC-1 and glycodelin A (PP14), both proteins secreted by the uterine glands and whose mRNA is not expressed in the placenta, are phagocytosed by the syncytiotrophoblast [47,48,49]. We have further shown that the cytoplasm of the glandular epithelium is strongly immunopositive for α-tocopherol transfer protein and so is likely to be involved in the transfer of antioxidants in early pregnancy [13]. These findings demonstrate that the uterine glands are an important potential source of nutrients during organogenesis, when the metabolism of the gestational sac is essentially anaerobic and the O_2 tension within the fetus must be maintained at a low level for correct cell differentiation.

The formation of the placental hemochorial interface

Ample dilation of the uteroplacental circulation together with rapid villous angiogenesis are the key factors necessary to adequate placental development and function and subsequent fetal growth. The uterus loses its innervation during pregnancy [50] and the placenta and cord are not innervated at all [51]. These findings imply that the development of a low resistance to blood flow in the placental circulation is essentially the result of anatomical transformations and/or biochemically induced vasomotor mechanisms. Our comparison of Doppler ultrasound findings with anatomical and physiological features has suggested that the establishment of high-volume–low-resistance flow in both placental circulations is primarily the consequence of the considerable increase in the diameter of the corresponding vascular beds, the length of the vascular network and the blood viscosity having much smaller influences [5,6,7,8].

Development of the fetoplacental circulation

The development of the fetal vasculature begins during the third week post conception (5th week of pregnancy) with the *de novo* formation of hemangioblastic cell cords within the villous stromal core [52]. During the next few days connections form between neighboring tubes to form a plexus, and this ultimately unites with the allantoic vessels developing in the connecting stalk to establish the fetal circulation to the placenta. Around 28 days postovulation (6 completed weeks post-menstruation), the villous vasculature is connected with the primitive heart and the vascular plexus of the yolk sac via the vessels of connecting stalk [28].

Around the end of the 5th week of gestation, the primitive heart begins to beat and this pivotal phenomenon has been documented *in utero* as early as 36 days menstrual age [53]. From 6–9 weeks there is a rapid increase of the mean heart rate to a plateau in the second and third trimesters [8]. The fetoplacental circulation is theoretically established from around 8 weeks of gestation. However, it is questionable whether there is significant circulation through these early villous vessels and between the primitive placenta and the developing fetus during the first trimester. We and others have shown that the vast majority (>90%) of the fetal erythrocytes are nucleated at this stage [8]. These primitive erythrocytes are poorly deformable, ensuring that the resistance to flow is high and suggesting that a significant flow between the placenta and the fetus is only established towards the end of the first trimester, when the proportion of nucleated erythrocytes falls rapidly. This also supports our concept that most of the exchanges between the maternal and fetal circulation between 5 and 10 weeks take place via the ECC and the SYS [3], which has a much shorter pathway.

Development of the uteroplacental circulation

The human uterine vasculature is made of a complex vessel network which anastomoses with branches of the ovarian and vaginal arteries to establish a vascular arcade perfusing the internal genital organs [54]. The tortuous ascending uterine artery gives off approximately 8–10 arcuate branches which extend inwards for about one-third of the thickness of the myometrium and envelop the anterior and posterior walls of the uterus. From this network arise the radial arteries followed by the spiral arteries which enter the decidua. In addition to these main arteries, small basal arteries arise from the radials, which vasularize the basal layer of the endometrium in the non-pregnant uterus.

The basis of the adjustment of the maternal placental flow rates is the transformation of the uterine vasculature which is associated with the peripheral widening of the supplying arteries by tissue growth and remodeling of the arterial wall. It is a gradual process which starts at implantation and which is then linked to the trophoblastic infiltration of the endometrium and superficial myometrium. Anatomical and radiographic studies including uterine perfusion experiments have demonstrated that the uterine vascular network elongates and dilates steadily throughout pregnancy [55].

When the blastocyst attaches to the uterine wall, trophoblastic cells infiltrate the decidua from the proliferating tips of the anchoring villi and from the trophoblastic shell [56,57,58]. These cells can be first found both within and around the spiral arteries in the central area of the placenta. They gradually extend laterally, reaching the periphery of the placenta around mid-gestation. Depth-wise the changes normally extend as far as the inner third of the uterine myometrium within the central region of the placental bed, but the extent of invasion is progressively shallower towards the periphery.

Human placentation is also characterized by a remodeling of the spiral arteries. The architecture of their decidual and myometrial parts is disrupted with the loss of myocytes from the media and the internal elastic lamina and these essential arterial components are progressively replaced by fibrinoid material [56,58,59]. In normal pregnancies, the transformation of spiral arteries into uteroplacental arteries is described as being completed around mid-gestation. The main aim of these vascular changes is to optimize the distribution of maternal blood into a low-resistance uterine vascular network and ultimately inside the placental intervillous chamber. However, the physiological conversion may not be so important in terms of volume of intervillous blood flow but it may play a pivotal role in affecting the quality of that flow in terms of the perfusion pressure, the pulsatility and rate of blood flow, and the consistency of the flow.

Establishment of the intervillous circulation

For the authors of many ancient anatomy textbooks, the onset of the maternal circulation inside the placenta starts immediately after implantation when connections are established between the maternal capillaries, derived from the tips of the spiral arteries, and the trophoblast lacunae in between the primary stem villi. This is often indirectly evidenced by the appearance of erythrocytes within the lacunae, although Hertig and Rock remarked that they were not as numerous as might be expected if a true maternal circulation was established soon after implantation [24]. Boyd and Hamilton found no evidence of a true circulation inside the very early placenta and concluded in their book that a free circulation in the intervillous space is established late [28]. Whether these erythrocytes circulate through the lacunae is impossible to tell from static histological images, but if so any flow can only be of a slow capillary nature.

The work of Hustin and Schaaps has suggested that maternal arterial connections are only permanently established with the placenta at the end of the first trimester [60]. Our studies combining anatomical and *in vivo* investigations have confirmed that human placentation is in fact not truly hemochorial in early pregnancy [5,8,23]. Our review of the Boyd collection [46] of hysterectomy specimens with pregnancy *in situ* also demonstrated that soon after implantation, the extravillous trophoblast not only invades the uterine tissues but also forms a continuous shell at the level of the decidua [46]. The cells of this shell anchor the placenta to the maternal tissue but also form plugs in the tips of the uteroplacental arteries (Fig. 8.2). The shell and the plugs act like a labyrinthine interface that filters maternal blood, permitting a slow seepage of plasma but no true blood flow into the intervillous space. This is supplemented by secretions from the uterine glands, which are discharged into the intervillous space until at least 10 weeks [47,48,49]. The materno-placental interface is therefore better described as being of a deciduochorial nature during the first trimester.

The intervillous circulation in the definitive hemochorial placenta has been referred to as an open system compared to other circulatory beds where the blood is retained within arteries, through capillary beds to veins [61,62]. Because the spiral arteries open into essentially a large lake of blood and the intervillous space does not impose any impedance to flow, the human placenta has been considered to act as a large arteriovenous shunt. Recent data based on a combination of sonographic *in vivo* investigation, vascular casting and O_2 measurements have demonstrated conclusively that extensive shunting occurs within the myometrium under the placental bed [63]. Whether the formation of these shunts is related to trophoblast invasion is not clear, but they are not observed in the opposite wall of the uterus.

At the end of the first trimester, we found a burst of oxidative stress in the periphery of the early placenta [23]. The underlying uteroplacental circulation in this area is never plugged by the trophoblastic shell allowing limited maternal blood flow to enter the placenta from 8–9 weeks of gestation. We hypothesized that this leads to higher local O_2 concentrations at a stage of pregnancy when the trophoblast possesses low concentrations and activities of the main antioxidant enzymes superoxide dismutase, catalase, and glutathione peroxidase. We believe that focal trophoblastic oxidative damage and progressive villous degeneration trigger the formation of the fetal membranes [32], which is an essential developmental step enabling vaginal delivery in humans. Confirmation that there are striking regional differences in villous morphology at this stage of gestation has come also from our examination of archival placenta-*in-situ* specimens from the Boyd collection [46]. In a specimen of approximately 60 days's gestation the villi over the superficial pole of the chorionic sac (chorion laeve) were shorter than those on the deeper surface in contact with the decidua basalis, and were enmeshed in maternal erythrocytes. They were also avascular, consistent with down-regulation of angiogenic factors by hyperoxia, and the syncytiotrophoblast was thin and devoid of microvilli. By comparison, villi over the deep pole (chorion frondosum or definitive placenta) contain well-developed blood vessels and display a healthy two-layered trophoblastic covering. In later specimens, superficial villi regress further, being represented only by ghost-like structures with a collagenous core and a thin covering of trophoblast. We also found that the villi of the chorion laeve of a normal pregnancy are identical to the villi of the entire placenta in missed miscarriages where there is well demonstrated premature and excessive entry of maternal blood inside the placenta [64,65,66,67].

Conclusions

Overall our data have confirmed that the human placenta is not truly hemochorial until the end of the first trimester. Rather it is deciduochorial, being supported by tissue fluids and endometrial secretions. We have shown that it is essential that the placenta limits the transfer of O_2 between the mother and her fetus, but also to itself, until it has the enzyme battery necessary to metabolize the amount of free radicals normally found in adult tissues. The establishment of both the uteroplacental and the umbilical circulation has to concur with the placental capacity of dealing with the results of its own O_2 metabolism. The establishment of the maternal arterial circulation inside the placenta represents a major challenge to an ongoing pregnancy, most likely second only to that of implantation. Tapping into a high-pressure, high-velocity system is potentially hazardous, and recent evidence indicates that this must be carefully coordinated in order to succeed.

We found that the early placental villi are highly sensitive to oxidative stress, and this appears to be another major factor determining pregnancy outcome. To avoid these potential dangers a number of strategies appear to have evolved, both in the endometrium and during placental development. We have observed that the anatomical features of the early materno-fetal interface provide indirect evidence that the architecture of the human first trimester gestational sac limits, rather than facilitates, fetal exposure to O_2 to what is strictly necessary for its development during the period of organogenesis. Within this context, the human fetus has developed alternative nutritional routes involving mainly the ECC and SYS. During that period we have shown that the uterine glands are an important provider of maternal proteins to the fetal compartment indicating a histiotrophic rather than hemotrophic nutritional pathway. Towards the end of the first trimester the secretory activity in the endometrial glands wanes. Also, as one moves from the embryonic to the fetal stage of development there is a need for a switch to hemotrophic nutrition in order to support the rapid rate of growth that characterizes the latter. If it occurs too early or incorrectly then the conceptus may be dislodged and miscarry or the placental tissue may be severely damaged by the hemodynamic forces.

At the end of the first trimester the trophoblastic plugs are progressively dislocated, allowing maternal blood to flow progressively freely and continuously within the intervillous space. During the transitional phase of 10–14 weeks' gestation, two-thirds of the primitive placenta disappears, the ECC is obliterated by the growth of the amniotic sac and maternal blood flows progressively throughout the entire placenta. These events bring the maternal blood closer to the fetal tissues, facilitating nutrient and gaseous exchange between the maternal and fetal circulations. We have also found that O_2 plays a key role in remodeling the chorion frondosum and the formation of the definitive placenta, a role that was unsuspected by previous anatomists and placentologists but which is an essential step for human parturition.

References

1. Falkowski P G, Katz M E, Milligan A J *et al.* The rise of oxygen over the past 205 million years and the evolution of large placental mammals. *Science* 2005; **309**: 2202–4.
2. Burton G J, Hempstock J, Jauniaux E. Oxygen, early embryonic metabolism and free radical-mediated embryopathies. *Reprod Biomed Online* 2003; **6**: 84–96.
3. Jauniaux E, Poston L, Burton G J. Placental-related diseases of pregnancy: involvement of oxidative stress and implications in human evolution. *Hum Reprod Update* 2006; **12**: 747–55.
4. Jauniaux E, Campbell S, Vyas S. The use of color Doppler imaging for prenatal diagnosis of umbilical cord

anomalies: report of three cases. *Am J Obstet Gynecol* 1989; **161**: 1195–7.

5. Jauniaux E, Jurkovic D, Campbell S, Hustin J. Doppler ultrasound study of the developing placental circulations: correlation with anatomic findings. *Am J Obstet Gynecol* 1992; **166**: 585–7.
6. Jauniaux E, Jurkovic D, Campbell S, Kurjak A, Hustin J. Investigation of placental circulations by color Doppler ultrasound. *Am J Obstet Gynecol* 1991; **164**: 486–8.
7. Jurkovic D, Jauniaux E, Kurjak A *et al.* Transvaginal color Doppler assessment of utero-placental circulation in early pregnancy. *Obstet Gynecol* 1991; **77**: 365–9.
8. Jauniaux E, Jurkovic D, Campbell S. In vivo investigations of anatomy and physiology of early human placental circulations. *Ultrasound Obstet Gynecol* 1991; **1**: 435–45.
9. Jauniaux E, Zaidi J, Jurkovic D, Campbell S, Hustin J. Comparison of colour Doppler features and pathologic findings in complicated early pregnancy. *Hum Reprod* 1994; **9**: 243–7.
10. Jauniaux E, Jurkovic D, Gulbis B *et al.* Biochemical composition of coelomic fluid in early human pregnancy. *Obstet Gynecol* 1991; **78**: 1124–8.
11. Jauniaux E, Lees C, Jurkovic D, Campbell S, Gulbis B. Transfer of inulin across the first trimester human placenta. *Am J Obstet Gynecol* 1997; **176**: 33–6.
12. Jauniaux E, Gulbis B. Fluid compartments of the embryonic environment. *Hum Reprod Update* 2000; **6**: 268–78.
13. Jauniaux E, Cindrova-Davies T, Johns T *et al.* Distribution and transfer pathways of antioxidant molecules inside the first trimester human gestational sac. *J Clin Endocrinol Metab* 2004; **89**: 1452–8.
14. Jauniaux E, Hempstock J, Teng C, Battaglia F C, Burton G J. Polyol concentrations in the fluid compartments of the human conceptus during the first trimester of pregnancy: maintenance of redox potential in a low oxygen environment. *J Clin Endocrinol Metab* 2005; **90**: 1171–5.
15. Jauniaux E, Johns J, Gulbis B, Spasic-Boskovic O, Burton G J. Transfer of folic acid inside the first trimester gestational sac and the effect of maternal smoking. *Am J Obstet Gynecol* 2007; **197**: 58e1–58e6.
16. Jauniaux E, Pahal G S, Gervy C, Gulbis B. Blood biochemistry and endocrinology in the human fetus between 11 and 17 weeks of gestation. *Reprod Biomed On-line* 2000; **1**: 38–44.
17. Pahal G S, Jauniaux E, Kinnon C, Trasher A, Rodeck C H. Normal development of fetal hematopoiesis between eight and seventeen week's gestation. *Am J Obstet Gynecol* 2000; **183**: 1029–34.
18. Rodesch F, Simon P, Donner C, Jauniaux E. Oxygen measurements in the maternotrophoblastic border during early pregnancy. *Obstet Gynecol* 1992; **80**: 283–5.
19. Jauniaux E, Watson A, Ozturk O, Quick D, Burton G. In-vivo measurement of intrauterine gases and acid-base values early in human pregnancy. *Hum Reprod* 1999; **14**: 2901–4.
20. Jauniaux E, Watson A L, Hempstock J *et al.* Onset of maternal arterial blood flow and placental oxidative stress; a possible factor in human early pregnancy failure. *Am J Pathol* 2000; **57**: 2111–22.
21. Jauniaux E, Watson A L, Burton G J. Evaluation of respiratory gases and acid-base gradients in fetal fluids and uteroplacental tissue between 7 and 16 weeks. *Am J Obstet Gynecol* 2001; **184**: 998–1003.
22. Jauniaux E, Gulbis B, Burton G J. The human first trimester gestational sac limits rather than facilitates oxygen transfer to the foetus: a review. *Placenta-Trophoblast Res* 2003; **24**: S86–S93.
23. Jauniaux E, Hempstock J, Greenwold N, Burton G J. Trophoblastic oxidative stress in relation to temporal and regional differences in maternal placental blood flow in normal and abnormal early pregnancies. *Am J Pathol* 2003; **162**: 115–25.
24. Hertig A T, Rock J. The implantation and early human development of the human ovum. *Am J Obstet Gynecol* 1951; **61**: 8–14.
25. Carter A M. Placental oxygen consumption. Part I: in vivo studies: a review. *Placenta* 2000; **21**: S31–S7
26. Wang Y, Walsh S W. Placental mitochondria as a source of oxidative stress in pre-eclampsia. *Placenta* 1998; **19**: 581–6.
27. Tu B P, Weissman J S. Oxidative protein folding in eukaryotes: mechanisms and consequences. *J Cell Biol* 2004; **164**: 341–6
28. Boyd J D, Hamilton W J. *The human placenta.* Cambridge: Heffer and Sons; 1970.
29. Mayhew T M, Burton G J. Stereology and its impact on our understanding of human placental functional morphology. *Microsc Res Tech* 1997; **38**: 195–205.
30. Jauniaux E, Burton G J, Moscoso G J, Hustin J. Development of the early human placenta: a morphometric study. *Placenta* 1991; **12**: 269–76.
31. Watson A L, Palmer M E, Skepper J N, Jauniaux E, Burton G J. Susceptibility of human placental syncytiotrophoblast mitochondria to oxygen-mediated damage in relation to gestational age. *J Clin Endocrinol Metabol* 1998; **83**: 1697–705.
32. Watson A L, Palmer M E, Jauniaux E, Burton G J. Variations in expression of copper/zinc superoxide

dismutase in villous trophoblast of the human placenta with gestational age. *Placenta* 1997; **18**: 295–9.

33. Watson A L, Skepper J N, Jauniaux E, Burton G J. Changes in the concentration, localisation and activity of catalase within the human placenta during early gestation. *Placenta* 1998; **19**: 27–34.
34. Droge W. Free radicals in the physiological control of cell function. *Physiol Rev* 2002; **82**: 47–95.
35. Frendo J L, Therond P, Bird T *et al.* Overexpression of copper zinc superoxide dismutase impairs human trophoblast cell fusion and differentiation. *Endocrinology* 2001; **142**: 3638–48.
36. Jauniaux E, Jurkovic D, Gulbis B *et al.* Investigation of the acid-base balance of coelomic and amniotic fluids in early human pregnancy. *Am J Obstet Gynecol* 1994; **170**: 1359–65.
37. Gulbis B, Jauniaux E. Distribution of lactic dehydrogenase isoenzymes in coelomic fluid and fetal adnexae. *Placenta* 1996; **17**: 367–70.
38. Fischer B, Kunzel W, Kleinstein J, Gips H. Oxygen tension in follicular fluid falls with follicle maturation. *Eur J Obstet Gynecol Reprod Biol* 1992; **43**: 39–43.
39. Palis J. Ontogeny of erythropoiesis. *Curr Opin Hematol* 2008; **15**: 155–61.
40. Jones C P J, Jauniaux E. Ultrastucture of the materno-embryonic interface in the first trimester of pregnancy. *Micron* 1995; **2**: 145–73.
41. Gulbis B, Jauniaux E, Jurkovic D *et al.* Determination of protein pattern in embryonic cavities of early human pregnancies: a model to understand materno-embryonic exchanges. *Hum Reprod* 1992; **7**: 886–9.
42. Jauniaux E, Gulbis B, Jurkovic D *et al.* Protein and steroid levels in embryonic cavities of early human pregnancy. *Hum Reprod* 1993; **8**: 782–7.
43. Jauniaux E, Gulbis B, Jurkovic D *et al.* Relationship between protein levels in embryological fluids and maternal serum and yolk sac size during early human pregnancy. *Hum Reprod* 1994; **9**: 161–6.
44. Gulbis B, Jauniaux E, Cotton F, Stordeur P. Protein and enzyme pattern in the fluid cavities of the first trimester human gestational sac: relevance to the absorptive role of the secondary yolk sac. *Molec Hum Reprod* 1998; **4**: 857–62.
45. Gray C A, Taylor K M, Ramsey W S *et al.* Endometrial glands are required for preimplantation conceptus elongation and survival. *Biol Reprod* 2001; **64**: 1608–13.
46. Burton G J, Jauniaux E, Watson A L. Maternal arterial connections to the placental intervillous space during the first trimester of human pregnancy: the Boyd collection revisited. *Am J Obstet Gynecol* 1999; **181**: 18–24.
47. Burton G J, Hempstock J, Jauniaux E. Nutrition of the human fetus during the first trimester: a review. *Placenta-Trophoblast Res* 2001; **22**: S70–S6.
48. Burton G J, Watson A L, Hempstock J, Skepper J N, Jauniaux E. Uterine glands provide histiotrophic nutrition for the human fetus during the first trimester of pregnancy. *J Clin Endocrinol Metab* 2002; **87**: 2954–9.
49. Hempstock J, Cindrova-Davies T, Jauniaux E, Burton G J. Endometrial glands as a source of nutrients, growth factors and cytokines during the first trimester of human pregnancy: a morphological and immunohistochemical study. *Reprod Biol Endocrinol* 2004; **20**:58.
50. Morizaki N, Morizaki J, Hayashi R H, Garfield R E. A functional and structural study of the innervation of the human uterus. *Am J Obstet Gynecol* 1989; **160**: 218–28.
51. Reilly F D, Russell P T. Neurohistochemical evidence supporting an absence of adrenergic and cholinergic innervation in the human placenta and umbilical cord. *Anat Record* 1979; **188**: 277–86.
52. Charnock-Jones D S, Burton G J. Placental vascular morphogenesis. *Bailliere's Best Practice Research Clin Obstet Gynaecol* 2000; **14**: 953–68.
53. Hustin J, Jauniaux E. Curing the human embryo – curing the placenta. *Human Reprod* 1993; **8**: 1966–82.
54. Itskovitz J, Lindenbaum E S, Brandes J M. Arterial anastomosis in the pregnant human uterus. *Obstet Gynecol* 1980: **55**: 67–70.
55. Burchell C. Arterial blood flow in the human intervillous space. *Am J Obstet Gynecol* 1969; **98**: 303–11.
56. Pijnenborg R, Dixon G, Robertson W B, Brosens I. Trophoblastic invasion of human decidua from 8 to 18 weeks of pregnancy. *Placenta* 1980; **1**: 3–19.
57. Pijnenborg R, Bland J M, Robertson W B, Dixon G, Brosens I. The pattern of interstitial invasion of the myometrium in early human pregnancy. *Placenta* 1981; **2**: 303–16.
58. Pijnenborg R, Bland J M, Robertson W B, Brosens I. Uteroplacental arterial changes related to interstitial trophoblast migration in early human pregnancy. *Placenta* 1983; **4**: 397–414.
59. Pijnenborg R, Vercruysse L, Hanssens M. The uterine spiral arteries in human pregnancy: facts and controversies. *Placenta* 2006; **27**: 239–58.
60. Hustin J, Schaaps J P. Echographic and anatomic studies of the maternotrophoblastic border during the first trimester of pregnancy. *Am J Obstet Gynecol* 1987; **157**: 162–8.
61. Moll W, Kunzel W, Herberger J. Hemodynamic implications of hemochorial placentation. *Eur J Obstet Gynecol Reprod Biol* 1975; **5**: 67–74.

62. Moll W. Structure adaptation and blood flow control in the uterine arterial system after hemochorial placentation. *Eur J Obstet Gynecol Reprod Biol* 2003; **110**: S19–27.

63. Schaaps J P, Tsatsaris V, Giffin F *et al.* Shunting the intervillous space: new concepts in human uteroplacental vascularization. *Am J Obstet Gynecol* 2005; **192**: 323–32.

64. Hempstock J, Jauniaux E, Greenwold N, Burton G J. The contribution of placental oxidative stress to early pregnancy failure. *Hum Pathol* 2003; **34**: 1265–75.

65. Jauniaux E, Greenwold N, Hempstock J, Burton G J. Comparison of ultrasound and Doppler mapping of the intervillous circulation in normal and abnormal early pregnancies. *Fertil Steril* 2003; **79**: 100–6.

66. Greenwold N, Jauniaux E, Gulbis B *et al.* Relationships between maternal serum, endocrinology, placental karyotype and intervillous circulation in early pregnancy failure. *Fertil Steril* 2003; **79**: 1373–9.

67. Jauniaux E, Burton G J. Pathophysiology of histological changes in early pregnancy loss. *Placenta* 2005; **26**: 114–23.

Section 4 Chapter 9

Deep placentation

The junctional zone myometrium

Stephen R. Killick[1] and Piotr Lesny[2]

[1]The University of Hull and Hull York Medical School, Hull, UK
[2]Hull and East Yorkshire Hospitals NHS Trust and Hull York Medical School, Hull, UK

Introduction

In a book concerned with the placental bed it is no surprise that the majority of chapters concern themselves with the histology and biochemistry within the developing decidua and fetal placenta. These are, after all, the surfaces which are in direct apposition within the fetomaternal unit. There is evidence, however, that deeper layers within the uterine wall have a strong influence on the process of early implantation.

This chapter is concerned with the deeper zonal anatomy of the uterus and particularly with the role these areas have in controlling uterine movements. The endometrium does not contain any contractile tissue whereas these are, of course, the main histological components of the myometrium. There would appear to be structural and functional compartmentalization within the myometrium such that the outermost layer influences parturition and the ischemic pain of dysmenorrhea, whereas the innermost layer influences sperm transport and the placement of embryos prior to implantation.

Recognition of the uterine junctional zone

Since the earliest descriptions of uterine histological structure the uterus has been regarded as an organ with two structurally and histologically distinct layers, the myometrium and the endometrium; the former being responsible for the muscular contractions of parturition and the latter for cyclical histological changes culminating in the implantation of the embryo. Magnetic resonance (MR) was the first imaging modality to differentiate three distinct layers of uterine zonal architecture rather than two [1]. These three distinct layers were observed in women of reproductive age using T2-weighted MR images and consisted of an inner endometrial stripe of high signal intensity, an outer myometrium of medium signal intensity, and, seemingly between the endometrium and the myometrium, a low signal intensity junctional zone.

The structure of this intermediate junctional zone (JZ) initially created controversy as there was no difference between the JZ and the outer myometrial zone in terms of light microscopic appearances. However morphometric studies subsequently revealed that the JZ had a threefold greater nuclear area per unit area, a decreased cellular matrix per unit volume, and a lower water content [2,3,4,5].

The JZ can also be visualized as a subendometrial halo by transvaginal ultrasound [6] although ultrasound measurements of JZ thickness are consistently narrower when compared to MR and the border with the rest of the myometrium is less distinct. Nevertheless Tetlow *et al.* [7] confirmed that the JZ and subendometrial halo represent the same histological structure. Morphometric analysis demonstrated a greater total nuclear area in the subendometrial halo than in the outer myometrium, but no differences in individual nuclear size between the two zones. There was also greater staining specific for vascular endothelium in the JZ suggesting a raised blood perfusion in comparison with surrounding tissues. Such architecture increases the density of the JZ, altering its acoustic impedance to account for its echopenic appearance on ultrasound and decreasing the signal intensity with T2-weighted MR because of the decreased water content. The different ways in which these two methods create their images accounts for the different measurements, even though they are visualizing the same zone.

The morphology of the JZ suggests a distinct compartment of myometrium, tightly packed with muscle cells with an increased vascularity, designed as it were for a specific purpose. Embryological and physiological data also support this view. Noe *et al.* [8] highlighted the embryology, concluding that the JZ (the 'archimetrium') and endometrium have the same embryonic (paramesonephric) origin and should be treated as a separate functional entity, which they called the endometrial-subendometrial unit or 'archimetra'. They suggested that the outer myometrium of non-paramesonephric origin or 'neomyometrium' and the archimetra had completely different physiological functions. Physiological evidence comes from studies of the estrogen receptor (ER) and progesterone receptor (PR) expression in the myometrium [8,9]. The JZ exhibits a cyclical pattern of ER and PR expression that parallels that of the endometrium whereas the outer myometrium does not show cyclical ER and PR expression at all.

The JZ is hence responsive to changes in sex steroid levels, and undergoes a cycle of change which parallels the changes in endometrial thickness [10]. The JZ is thinner amongst patients using oral contraception [11], and when the level of sex steroids is low, either before menarche or after menopause, the zonal anatomy is indistinct, with low signal intensity from the entire myometrium [12]. During pregnancy the JZ increases in signal intensity and the zonal differences are less apparent. Postpartum normal zonal anatomy gradually reappears within a few months [13]. Suppression of ovarian steroids by gonadotropin-releasing hormone analogues creates an MR image of the uterus similar to that of postmenopausal women [14] whereas the treatment of postmenopausal women with hormonal replacement re-establishes premenopausal zonal anatomy [15].

The unique observation by Turnbull *et al.* [16] occurred fortuitously when one volunteer participating in a study designed to document the cyclical variations in uterine zonal anatomy was subsequently discovered to be pregnant. The images obtained 7 days postovulation showed a low signal intensity mass based in the JZ, presumably at the site of implantation, with thinning of the overlying endometrium. There was a clear loss of integrity and disruption of the junctional zone and reduction in signal intensity in the overlying myometrium (Fig. 9.1). Barton *et al.* [17] reported endometrial distension, an endometrial mass, and both junctional zone and myometrial disruption in patients with incomplete abortion of indeterminate gestational age but not in the case of ectopic pregnancy. It is most likely that the signal intensity changes and loss of normal zonal anatomy demonstrated by MR are due to the local changes in blood flow underlying the implantation site. These observations suggest that the interaction between the junctional zone and the endometrium plays an important part in the early implantation process.

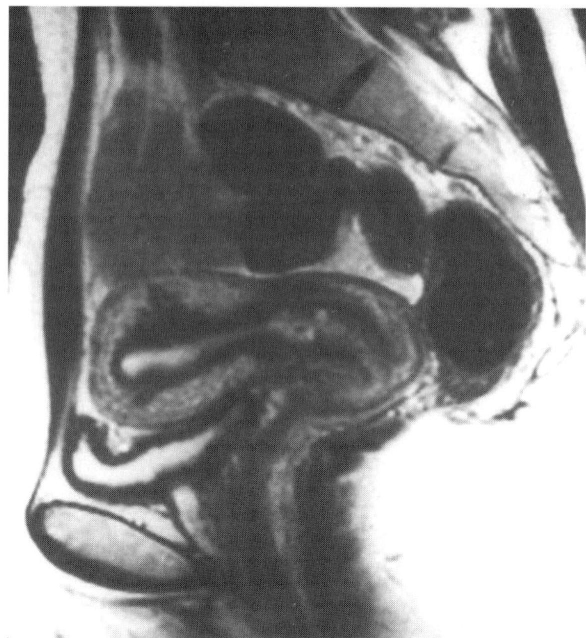

Fig. 9.1 Sagittal T2-weighted MR image of the uterus 7 days postovulation showing the probable site of a recent implantation. Note the low signal intensity mass based in the junctional zone, presumably at the site of implantation, with thinning of the overlying endometrium, disruption of the junctional zone, and reduction in signal intensity in the overlying myometrium. Reproduced with permission from Turnbull LW, Manton JD, Horsman A, Killick SR. Magnetic resonance imaging changes in the uterine zonal anatomy during a conception cycle. Br J Obstet Gynaecol 1995; 102: 330–1.

Consequently, attempts have been made to use MR and ultrasound to identify a favorable profile of uterine zonal anatomy which could predict a satisfactory outcome following IVF treatment. Turnbull *et al.* [18] described an association between the relative MR signal and successful implantation. Women with reduced contrast between the myometrium and the JZ were more likely to conceive. Lesny *et al.* [19] using ultrasound showed a more pronounced decrease in the JZ thickness throughout ovulation induction in patients who would later conceive. The highly significant differences between the JZ values at downregulation and at the time of embryo transfer between pregnant and non-pregnant groups suggested that this parameter could reflect uterine receptivity and that the responsiveness of the junctional zone could have an association with successful implantation (Fig. 9.2).

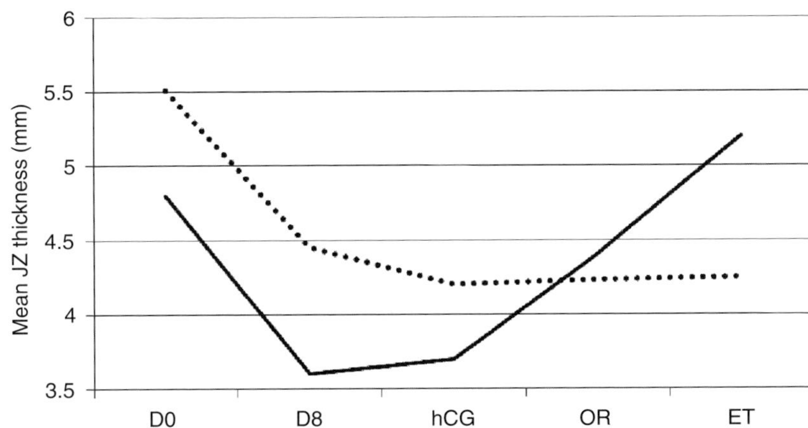

Fig. 9.2 Line drop plot of changes in junctional zone thickness during an IVF cycle. The solid line represents the pregnant group; the dotted line represents the non-pregnant group. D0 = day of downregulation, D8 = eighth day of ovulation induction; hCG = day of human chorionic gonadotropin injection; OR = day of oocyte retrieval; ET = day of embryo transfer. Reproduced with permission from Lesny P, Killick SR, Tetlow RL, Manton DJ, Robinson J, Maguiness SD. Ultrasound evaluation of the uterine zonal anatomy during in vitro fertilisation and embryo transfer. Hum Reprod 1999; 14: 1593–8.

Uterine junctional zone contractions

Advancements in real-time ultrasound scan technology and cine MR have provided an opportunity to move from an era of still photography to an era of moving video and digital images. It seems logical, in assessing the possible physiological role for a zone consisting of compacted myocytes, to look for muscular contractions.

A note on nomenclature

Various phrases have been used to describe the JZ contractions: endometrial movements [20], endometrial peristaltic movements [21], contractions of the inner third of myometrium [22], subendometrial myometrial contractions [23], uterine endometrial cavity movements [24], endometrial wavelike movements [25], and uterine contractions [26]. We prefer the terms 'junctional zone' (JZ) and 'junctional zone contractions' (JZC) to describe the subendometrial myometrium and its movements together with those of the adjacent endometrium [27,28].

A note on methodology

Jason Birnholz [20] was first to describe JZC using a 3.5 MHz transabdominal ultrasound transducer. Subsequent improvements in technique included the use of vaginal transducers [21] of greater frequency and resolving power [29,30,31] and video [22,23,24,29], then digital recordings[25,27,28,32,33]. Typical recordings are usually between 2 and 5 minutes with the images being viewed at 4–10 times normal speed.

Rapidly developing technology allows better images and the introduction of ever more complex classification of JZC [30,34]. However, the subjectivity of human observation of the resulting images remains a problem even though good intra- and interobserver error can be achieved by some [25,27,30,34,35].

The development of specialized computer programs [26,36,] has introduced some objectivity but no system has, so far, reached levels of reliability and ease of use to be universally useful [37,38]. Interestingly, invasive methods to measure intrauterine pressure within a non-pregnant uterus have been recently rejuvenated and improved by Buletti [39,40,41].

Classification of JZC

Waves of JZC can vary in a great many ways, including their frequency, their direction of travel, their distance of travel, their velocity of travel and their amplitude. It is evident that the technical ability of the ultrasound equipment used and the subjective processing of information will influence the reliability of the measurement of any of these parameters. Objective methods of measurement have been so far related to general contractility validated as number of contractions per minute [26,37] or as frequency expressed in Hz [38]. These analyses have been based on the change of brightness in a chosen ultrasound plane of observation or in a so-called region of interest.

The most frequently utilized classification is that of Ijland *et al.* [25] and relates to the direction of travel. They described five types of wave; no activity, waves travelling from cervix to fundus (cervico-fundal), waves travelling from fundus to cervix (fundo-cervical), opposing waves starting simultaneously at both the cervix and the fundus, and random waves originating at various foci. This group has recently added two more complex variations in the form of recoiling cervico-fundal waves and standing waves [30].

JZC during spontaneous cycles

As JZ architecture had previously been shown to be hormonally dependent it came as no surprise when the direction, amplitude, and frequency of JZC was found to show a recurring and predictable pattern throughout the ovarian cycle.

There is always some baseline activity in the JZ which takes the form of random contractions without any obvious coordination. With increasing estradiol levels during the early and mid-follicular phases the general level of activity rises and initially fundo-cervical waves are most prominent. From the mid-follicular phase onwards the dominance of cervico-fundal contractions becomes evident and activity culminates around the time of ovulation with the highest frequency and amplitude. After ovulation, under the influence of progesterone, there is a reduction in overall contractility, and the pattern of waveform changes to mainly opposing and random waves. The JZ and adjacent endometrium becomes increasingly quiescent after the mid luteal phase, when implantation would be expected to begin.

There have been a number of suggestions ascribing a physiological role to this changing pattern of contractions. It has been suggested that fundo-cervical waves during the follicular phase could facilitate cleansing of the uterine cavity, discharging any remains of menstruation and creating a barrier for ascending pathogens. During the lutual phase contractions could help provide a microenvironment favorable for the preimplantation embryo by facilitating supplies of nutrients and oxygen, or by spacing embryos in animals who have multiple implantation sites. Similarly it sounds logical that the still present cervico-fundal contractions during the luteal phase could facilitate blastocyst implantation near the fundus.

The most evident and proven physiological role for JZC is to enhance sperm transport around the time of ovulation, when uterine contractility is at its height and waves are almost exclusively cervico-fundal. This has been beautifully demonstrated in experiments by Kunz *et al.* [42]. They used transvaginal ultrasound and hysterosalpingoscintigraphy to detect the transport of technetium-labeled albumin placed at the external os of the uterine cervix. This model demonstrated that JZC in the late follicular phase can be responsible not only for rapid sperm transfer to the Fallopian tube but also preferentially toward the side of the dominant follicle. Such a mechanism, possibly under endocrine control of the leading follicle, could secure the highest number of spermatozoa at the site of fertilization. Their results regarding sperm transport were confirmed by further research [43] but tropism to the dominant follicle has been questioned [41].

JZC during assisted conception cycles

The frequent use of ultrasound during assisted conception cycles provides most of the information we have about JZC, with most data coming from the study of long protocol stimulation IVF cycles. It has been demonstrated that JZ contractility follows a similar pattern to the natural cycle but is more exaggerated throughout an IVF cycle. However, there have been a few differences. Our group has observed very strong but irregular contractions following oocyte retrieval, with cervico-fundal waves reaching their maximum frequency and velocity. Such activity following multiple puncture of ovarian follicles suggests the release of prostaglandins and other mediators of the inflammatory process, which might subsequently stimulate JZ contractility. The presence of prostaglandins in the ovarian vein [44], mediators of inflammatory reactions [45], and neuropeptides [46] has been described in animal models and during physiological ovulation. Subsequently, during the early luteal phase (2 and 3 days after oocyte retrieval) all our patients (oocyte donors) demonstrated increased contractility as compared to natural cycles. Similar results were reported by Ayoubi *et al.* [36] when the same patients were assessed during natural and IVF cycles. Whether the delayed establishment of uteroquiescence in IVF cycles is a lasting consequence of hyperactivity resulting from oocyte retrieval or from the effect of supraphysiological hormone levels remains to be answered. We observed decreasing activity by the fourth day after oocyte capture (6 days after the ovulatory trigger of hCG and prior to blastocyst transfer) which was also described by Fanchin *et al.* [47].

Implications of JZC for implantation

There is consensus starting to emerge that JZC at the time of implantation should be minimal. Excessive JZC have been shown to reduce implantation rates in both spontaneous and stimulated cycles [32,41,48]. The most significant research relating JZC to implantation was presented by Fanchin *et al.* [26]. They showed that a low frequency of JZC before embryo transfer (ET) during IVF cycles was associated with a higher implantation rate and a higher clinical and

Table 9.1. Differences in pregnancy rates between 50 consecutive patients treated with IVF who had less than 5 junctional zone contractions (JZC) in the 2 minutes immediately following embryo transfer (ET) as compared with patients who had more than 5 contractions in the 2 minutes following embryo transfer

	<5 JZC per 2 min after ET	>5 JZC per 2 min after ET
n	37	13
Clinical pregnancies	11	0
Pregnancy rate/ET (%)	29.7*	0*

* $P < 0.05$ by chi-squared.
Reproduced with permission from Killick S. Ultrasound and the receptivity of the endometrium. Reprod Biomed Online 2007;15: 63–67.

ongoing pregnancy rate. Our group [49] demonstrated a similar effect when assessing the JZC immediately after ET and linked it with a significantly lower clinical pregnancy rate if five or more contractions per minute were observed (Table 9.1).

Greater implantation rates are achieved during IVF if embryos are transferred later in the luteal phase, when they have reached the blastocyst stage about 5 days after fertilization [50]. The original interpretation of this fact was that this was purely a function of a more competent embryo, but, as JZC decrease with the duration of the luteal phase in both natural and stimulated cycles, the possibility that part of this effect is the result of JZC has been appreciated [51]. Classically, during IVF embryos are placed into the uterine cavity earlier (usually 2 days after fertilization) than would have been the case if they had descended from the Fallopian tube in a natural cycle [52,53]. They are hence transferred at the time when JZC are still intense. Transfer on day 5 or 6 is more physiological, the uterus is more quiescent, and the whole process better synchronized.

Using oocyte donors, who go through the IVF process up to but not including embryo transfer, we have been able to perform a series of studies in which we varied the technique of a mock embryo transfer 2 or 3 days after the act of donation [28]. Difficult embryo transfer or incorrect technique with touching the uterine fundus created turbulent contractions. These contractions moved mock embryos down to the cervix (fundo-cervical contractions) or up to the Fallopian tube (cervico-fundal contractions or strong random contractions at the wrong phase of the cycle). Interestingly, when we carried out the same experiment with the softer version of the same catheter, the mock embryos were moved to a lesser extent, and when we performed a mock transfer without touching the uterine fundus the increased contractility was not observed and the mock embryo remained in the same position. A similar effect of increased contractility was caused by the application of a tenaculum to the cervix [54] or the use of a transfer needle during transmyometrial embryo transfer [55]. It is now widely appreciated that JZC can be stimulated by mechanical stimulation and that atraumatic embryo transfer is a critical part of IVF treatment. Several strategies have been designed to avoid unnecessary uterine stimulation and facilitate higher implantation rates [51,56].

Appropriate circumstances must exist to allow for an initiation of dialog between the embryo and endometrium [57,58]. It is not difficult to imagine that if the embryo is moved from one place to another or at risk of being expelled through the cervix or pushed into the Fallopian tube proper contact is less likely to be possible. Once the embryo is positioned by diminishing cervico-fundal contractions within the fundal area of the uterus the process of adhesion, penetration, and invasion can occur. If this is so, and there appears to be enough evidence to suggest it is, then the quiescent endometrium is vital to allow adhesion of the embryo.

Progesterone appears to be a major controller of JZC during the luteal phase. Fanchin *et al.* [26] correlated a low frequency of contractions with a high progesterone level and a consequently higher pregnancy rate. The additional use of vaginal progesterone at the time of embryo transfer seemed to have a relaxing influence on JZC [59].

Indirect support for the role of progesterone as a possible regulator of JZ contractility has been provided by Mahmood *et al.* [60]. This group reported changes in epithelial ciliary beat frequency of the fallopian tube endosalpinx, which was significantly suppressed *in vitro* by progesterone. As the fallopian tube and the endometrial-subendometrial unit are of the same embryological origin, the archimetra, they may well share hormonal regulation.

An ectopic pregnancy would not be expected after IVF and ET when the embryos are transferred directly into the uterine cavity, avoiding the fallopian tube. However, not only was the first ever IVF pregnancy ectopic but some 4% of IVF pregnancies continue to be so, particularly when the fallopian tubes are diseased [61]. Our studies, using oocyte donors and appropriately small quantities of positive contrast ultrasound medium as mock embryos, demonstrated that pathological contractions during embryo transfer can relocate embryos from the uterus to the Fallopian tube and facilitate an ectopic or even a heterotopic pregnancy [28]. Further observation and a retrospective analysis of our IVF results led us to conclude that a difficult ET, where JZC are stimulated by greater mechanical stimulation, increases the risk of ectopic pregnancy [62,63]. This proved to be evident when a difficult ET was performed on day 2 after oocyte retrieval but not on day 3, suggesting an influence from decreasing JZC with time as discussed previously. It would be interesting to extrapolate these findings and investigate if abnormal contractions might be responsible for some ectopic pregnancies in the absence of tubal pathology in spontaneous cycles. The mechanism of echogenic contrast relocation from the uterine cavity has already been observed among patients with unexplained subfertility [41].

Once we accept that a certain pattern of JZC is associated with successful conception, the next step is whether abnormal contractility is associated with reduced fertility. Women with endometriosis show a significant increase in JZC and a disruption in the pattern of contractility in comparison to healthy controls [31]. Leyendecker's group [31] demonstrated a doubling of contraction frequency during the follicular and mid-luteal phases in endometriotic women and also that asynchrony in the late follicular phase compromised the mechanism of rapid sperm transport. Suppression of peristaltic activity during the periovulatory phase was also reported with the use of cine MRI [64]. Intrauterine pressure measurements have also demonstrated increased basal tone and an increased frequency and amplitude of contractions in women with endometriosis [40]. The evidence for disrupted sperm transport in women with endometriosis and/or adenomyosis is quite convincing but probably of more importance is the increased contractility or hyperperistalsis [65,66].

Alterations in JZ contractility have also been reported in uteruses with submucosal fibroids, which by definition arise from the JZ [67,68]. In cine MRI studies the JZC were altered by submucosal but not by intramural or subserosal leiomyomas [69] and abnormal contractility during the luteal phase and menstruation was also recorded in fibroid uteruses [70]. A clinical consequence of these observations is suggested by results from IVF treatment showing lower implantation rates in the presence of junctional zone fibroids [71].

Despite significant progress in understanding JZC, the physiological mechanism of their control is still elusive. Pharmacological suppression of contractions especially at the time of implantation is very tempting as a way of improving implantation rates and has the potential to revolutionize subfertility treatment. Hence many substances have been tried to alter contractility of uterine muscle *in vivo* [70,72,73] but attempts to treat patients before embryo transfer with prostaglandin synthetase inhibitors [74], ritodrine [75], diazepam [76], glyceryl trinitrate [77], and even embryo transfer under general anesthesia [78] were inconclusive or disappointing. The positive results with piroxicam (a COX inhibitor) and ritodrine (an anticholinergic) were not followed up or verified [79,80]. Our group have been unable to demonstrate any influence of diclofenac (a COX inhibitor), rofecoxib (a selective COX 2 inhibitor), or isosorbide (an NO donor) on contractions observed at the time of mock embryo transfer during the late luteal phase. The use of progesterone [60] has shown a reduction in JZC but even so its effect to improve pregnancy rates has been questioned [81]. Reduction in both sporadic and peristaltic contractions was demonstrated in cine MRI when hyoscine butylobromide (an anticholinergic agent) was given intravenously [82]. Serum oxytocin concentrations have been shown to increase following the use of a tenaculum during ET [83] and JZC increase with this procedure [54]. More recently Pierzynski *et al.* [37] have reported a successful pregnancy in a patient with multiple IVF treatment failures after reducing contractility with high doses of atosiban (a mixed vasopressin/oxytocin antagonist) (Fig. 9.3). Thus, in view of this evidence, the suppression of oxytocin receptors by highly selective treatment with atosiban or bartusiban may represent a new and long awaited opportunity.

There are also possible alternatives to medical treatment as uterine relaxation on the day of embryo transfer has been achieved by sacral surface electrical stimulation, and this may offer a much simpler and more practical solution [38].

The evidence of lesser contractility during the luteal phase of a natural cycle in comparison with conventional protocols used for subfertility treatment may add to the increasing popularity of alternative approaches to IVF. These include natural cycle IVF, minimal stimulation IVF, and *in vitro* maturation of oocytes ready for fertilization *in vitro* [84]. Historically,

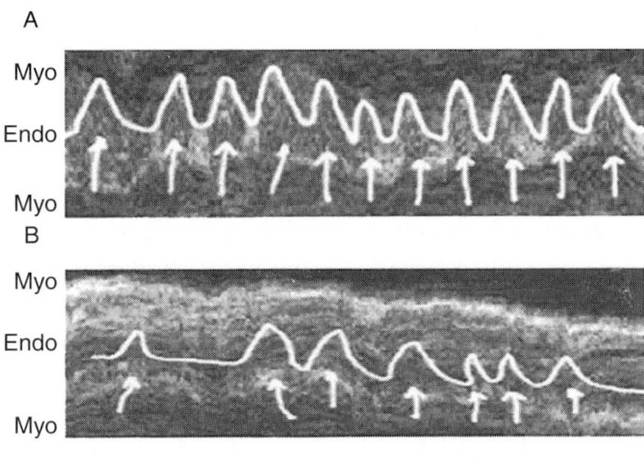

Fig. 9.3 Graphs showing the effect of an oxytocin antagonist on uterine junctional zone contractions. (A) before treatment, (B) after treatment with atosiban. Reproduced with permission from Pierzynski P, Reinheimer TM, Kuczynski W. Oxytocin antagonists may improve infertility treatment. Fertil Steril 2007; 88: 213.e19–22.

the first ever IVF pregnancy was ectopic and occurred in a stimulated cycle [85] whereas the IVF success story, Louise Brown, was conceived 2 years later during a natural monitored cycle. Was her mother's JZ contractility more quiescent to favor implantation?

There is no question that JZC represent a very exciting area of research. Although a lot has been achieved in recent years and a clearer picture is starting to emerge, our understanding of this biological phenomenon is still patchy. More basic research is needed. Even more urgently, a universal tool to assess and analyze JZC is required. We believe that it should be an ultrasound-based system. There is enough scientific and commercial interest to drive JZ research forward. At some point in the future it might be possible to simply measure contractions, and then diagnose and treat a patient accordingly.

References

1. Hricak H, Alpers C, Crooks L E *et al.* Magnetic resonance imaging of female pelvis: initial experience. *Am J Radiol* 1983; **141**; 1119–28
2. Lee J K T, Gersell D, Balfe D M *et al.* The uterus: in vitro MR-anatomic correlation of normal and abnormal specimens. *Radiology* 1985; **157**: 175–9.
3. McCarthy S, Scott G, Majumadar S *et al.* Uterine junctional zone: MR study of water content and relaxation properties. *Radiology* 1989; **171**: 241–3.
4. Scout L M, Flyn S D, Luthringer D J *et al.* Junctional zone of the uterus: correlation of MR imaging and histological examination of hysterectomy specimens. *Radiology* 1991; **179**: 403–7.
5. Brown H K, Stoll B S, Nicosia *et al.* Uterine junctional zone: correlation between histologic findings and MRI. *Radiology* 1991; **179**: 409–13.
6. Fleischer A C, Mendelson E B, Bohm-Velez M *et al.* Transvaginal and transabdominal sonography of the endometrium. *Semin Ultrasound CT MR* 1988; **9**: 81–101.
7. Tetlow R L, Richmond I, Manton D *et al.* Histological analysis of uterine junctional zone as seen by transvaginal ultrasound. *Ultrasound Obstet Gynaecol* 1999; **14**: 188–93.
8. Noe M, Kunz G, Herbertz M *et al.* The cyclic pattern of immunocytochemical expression of oestrogen and progesterone receptors in human myometrial and endometrial layers: characterisation of endometrial-subendometrial unit. *Hum Reprod* 1999; **14**: 190–7.
9. Richards P A, Tiltman A J. Anatomical variations of the oestrogen receptor in normal myometrium. *Virchovs Arch Abt A Pathol Anat* 1995; **427**: 303–7.
10. Wiczyk H P, Janus C L, Richards C J *et al.* Comparison of magnetic resonance imaging and ultrasound in evaluating follicular and endometrial development throughout the normal cycle. *Fertil Steril* 1988; **49**: 969–72.
11. McCarthy S, Tauber C, Gore J. Female pelvic anatomy: MR assessment of variation during the menstrual cycle and with the use of oral contraceptives. *Radiology* 1986; **160**: 119–23.
12. Brosens J J, De Souza N M, Barker F G. Uterine junctional zone: function and disease. *Lancet* 1995; **346**: 558–60.
13. Willms A B, Brown E D, Kettritz U I *et al.* Anatomic changes in the pelvis after uncomplicated vaginal delivery: evaluation with serial MR imaging. *Radiology* 1995; **195**: 91–4.
14. Zawin M, McCarthy S, Scoutt L *et al.* Monitoring therapy with gonadotropin-releasing hormone analogue: utility of MR imaging. *Radiology* 1990; **175**: 503–6.
15. Demas B E, Hricak H, Jaffe R B. Uterine MR imaging: effect of hormonal stimulation. *Radiology* 1986; **158**: 123–6.
16. Turnbull L W, Manton J D, Horsman A *et al.* Magnetic resonance imaging changes in the uterine zonal anatomy during a conception cycle. *Br J Obstet Gynaecol* 1995; **102**: 330–1.
17. Barton J W, McCarthy S M, Kohorn E I *et al.* Pelvic MR imaging findings in gestational trophoblastic disease, incomplete abortion and ectopic pregnancy. *Radiology* 1993; **186**: 163–8.

18. Turnbull L W, Rice C F, Horsman A *et al.* Magnetic resonance imaging and transvaginal ultrasound of the uterus prior to embryo transfer. *Hum Reprod* 1994; **9**: 2438–43.
19. Lesny P, Killick S R, Tetlow R L *et al.* Ultrasound evaluation of the uterine zonal anatomy during in vitro fertilisation and embryo transfer. *Hum Reprod* 1999; **14**: 1593–8.
20. Birnholz J C. Ultrasonic visualisation of endometrial movements. *Fertil Steril* 1984; **41**: 157–8.
21. Oike K, Obata S, Tagaki K *et al.* Observation of endometrial movements with transvaginal sonography. *J Ultrasound Med* 1988; **7**: 99.
22. De Vries K, Lyons E A, Ballard G *et al.* Contractions of the inner third of endometrium. *Am J Obstet Gynec* 1990; **162**: 678–82.
23. Lyons E A, Taylor P J, Zengh X H *et al.* Characterisation of subendometrial contractions throughout the menstrual cycle in normal fertile women. *Fertil Steril* 1991; **55**: 771–4.
24. Fukuda M, Fukuda K. Uterine endometrial cavity movements and cervical mucus. *Hum Reprod* 1994; **9**:1013–6.
25. Ijland M M, Evers J L H, Dunselman G A J *et al.* Endometrial wavelike movements during the menstrual cycle. *Fertil Steril* 1996; **65**: 746–9.
26. Fanchin R, Rhigini C, Olivennes F *et al.* Uterine contractions at the time of embryo transfer alter pregnancy rate after in vitro fertilisation. *Hum Reprod* 1998; **13**: 1968–74.
27. Lesny P, Killick S R, Tetlow L R *et al.* Uterine junctional zone contractions during assisted reproduction cycles. *Hum Reprod Update* 1998; **4**: 440–5.
28. Lesny P, Killick S R, Tetlow R L *et al.* Embryo transfer: can we learn anything new from the observation of junctional zone contraction? *Hum Reprod* 1998; **13**: 1540–6.
29. Abramowicz J S, Archer D F. Uterine endometrial peristalsis: a transvaginal ultrasound study. *Fertil Steril* 1990; **54**: 451–4.
30. Van Gestel I, Ijland M M, Evers J L H *et al.* Complex endometrial wave patterns in IVF. *Fertil Steril* 2007; **88**: 612–15.
31. Leyendecker G, Kunz G, Wildt L *et al.* Uterine peristalsis and dysperistalsis as dysfunction of the mechanism of rapid sperm transport in patients with endometriosis and infertility. *Hum Reprod* 1996; **11**: 1542–51.
32. Ijland M M, Evers J L H, Dunselman G A J *et al.* Relation between wavelike activity and fecundability in spontaneous cycles. *Fertil Steril* 1997; **67**: 492–6.
33. Ijland M M, Evers J L, Hoogland H J. Velocity of endometrial wavelike activity in spontaneous cycle. *Fertil Steril* 1997; **68**: 72–5.
34. Van Gestel I, Ijland M M, Hoogland H J *et al.* Endometrial waves in in vitro fertilisation cycles: a validation study. *Fertil Steril* 2005; **83**: 491–3.
35. Van Gestel, Ijland M M, Hoogland J H *et al.* Endometrial wavelike activity in non-pregnant uterus. *Hum Reprod Update* 2003; **9**: 131–8.
36. Ayoubi J M, Epiney M, Brioschi P A *et al.* Comparison of changes in uterine contractions frequency after ovulation in the menstrual cycle and in in vitro fertilisation cycles. *Fertil Steril* 2003; **79**: 1101–5.
37. Pierzynski P, Reinheimer T M, Kuczynski W. Oxytocin antagonists may improve infertility treatment. *Fertil Steril* 2007; **88**: 213.e19–22.
38. Fujii O, Murakami H, Murakawa Y *et al.* Uterine relaxation by sacral surface electrical stimulation on the day of embryo transfer. *Fertil Steril* 2008; **90**; 1240–2.
39. Bulletti C, Prefetto R A, Bazzocchi G *et al.* Electromechanical activities of human uteri during extra-corporeal perfusion with ovarian steroids. *Hum Reprod* 1993; **8**: 1558–63.
40. Bulletti C, de Ziegler D, Polli V *et al.* Characteristics of uterine contractility during menses in women with mild to moderate endometriosis. *Ferti Steril* 2002; **77**: 1156–61.
41. Bulletti C, De Ziegler D. Uterine contractility and embryo implantation. *Curr Opin Obstet Gynecol* 2006; **18**: 473–84.
42. Kunz G, Beil D, Deninger H *et al.* The dynamics of rapid sperm transport through the female genital tract: evidence from vaginal sonography of uterine peristalsis and hysterosalpingoscintigraphy. *Hum Reprod* 1996; **11**: 627–32.
43. Kissler S, Siebzehnruebl E, Kohl E *et al.* Uterine contractility and direct sperm transport assessed by hysterosalpingoscintigraphy (HSSG) and intrauterine pressure (IUP) measurement. *Acta Obstet Gynecol Scand* 2004; **83**: 369–74.
44. Wallach E E, Dharmarajan A M. Prostaglandins and ovulation. In: Sjoberg N O, Hamberger L, Janson P O, eds. *Local regulation of ovarian function.* Carnforth: Parthenon; 1992.
45. Espey L L. Ovulation as an inflammatory process. In: Sjoberg N O, Hamberger L, Janson P O, eds. *Local regulation of ovarian function.* Canforth: Parthenon; 1992.
46. Kannisto P, Jorgensen J, Liedberg F *et al.* Neuropeptides and ovulation. In: Sjoberg N O, Hamberger J, Janson P O, eds. *Local regulation of ovarian function.* Canforth: Parthenon; 1992.

47. Fanchin R, Ayoubi J M, Righini C *et al.* Uterine contractility decreases at the time of blastocyst transfer. *Hum Reprod* 2001; **16**; 1115–19.

48. Fusi L, Cloke B, Brosens J J. The uterine junctional zone. *Best Pract Res Clin Obstet Gynecol* 2006; **20**: 479–81.

49. Killick S. Ultrasound and the receptivity of the endometrium. *Reprod Biomed Online* 2007; **15**: 63–7.

50. Gardner D K, Vella P, Lane M *et al.* Culture and transfer of human blastocyst increases implantation rates and reduces the need for multiple embryo transfers. *Fertil Steril* 1998; **69**: 84–8.

51. Schoolcraft W B, Surrey E S, Gardner D K. Embryo transfer: techniques and variables affecting success. *Fertil Steril* 2001; **76**: 863–70.

52. Croxato H B, Ortiz M E, Diaz S *et al.* Studies on the duration of the egg transport by the human oviduct: ovum location at various intervals following luteinizing peak. *Am J Obstet Gynecol* 1978; **132**: 629–34.

53. Buster J, Bustillo M, Rodi I. Biologic and morphologic development of donated human ova recovered by nonsurgical uterine lavage. *Am J Obstet Gynecol* 1985; **153**: 211–17.

54. Lesny P, Killick S R, Robinson J *et al.* Embryo transfer and junctional zone contractions: is it safe to use a tenaculum? *Hum Reprod* 1999; **14**: 2367–70.

55. Biervliet F P, Lesny P, Maguiness S D *et al.* Transmyometrial embryo transfer and junctional zone contractions. *Human Reprod* 2002; **17**: 347–50.

56. Sallam H N. Embryo transfer: factors involved in optimizing the success. *Curr Opin Obstet Gynecol* 2005; **17**: 289–98.

57. Herrler A, von Rango U, Beier H M. Embryo-maternal signalling: how the embryo starts talking to its mother to accomplish implantation. *Reprod Biomed Online* 2003; **6**: 244–56.

58. Duc-Goiran P, Mignot T M, Bourgeois C *et al.* Embryo-maternal interactions at the implantation site: a delicate equilibrium. *Eur J Obstet Gynecol Reprod Biol* 1999; **83**: 85–100.

59. Fanchin R, Rhigini C, de Ziegler D *et al.* Effects of vaginal progesterone administration on uterine contractility at the time of embryo transfer. *Fertil Steril* 2001; **75**: 1136–40.

60. Mahmood T, Saridogan E, Smutna S *et al.* The effect of ovarian steroids on epithelial ciliary beat frequency in the human Fallopian tube. *Hum Reprod* 1998; **13**: 2991–4.

61. Marcus S F, Brinsden P R. Analysis of the incidence and risk factors associated with ectopic pregnancy following in vitro fertilisation and embryo transfer. *Hum Reprod* 1995; **10**: 199–203.

62. Lesny P, Killick S R, Robinson J *et al.* Transcervical embryo transfer as a risk factor for ectopic pregnancy. *Fertil Steril* 1999; **72**: 305–9.

63. Lesny P, Killick S R, Robinson J *et al.* Case report: ectopic pregnancy after transmyometrial embryo transfer. *Fertil Steril* 1999; **72**: 357–9.

64. Kido A, Togashi K, Nishino M *et al.* Cine MR imaging of uterine peristalsis in patient with endometriosis. *Eur Radiol* 2007; **17**: 1813–19.

65. Leyendecker G, Kunz G, Herbertz M *et al.* Uterine peristaltic activity and the development of endometriosis. *Ann N Y Acad Sci* 2004; **1034**: 338–55.

66. Kunz G, Beil D, Huppert P *et al.* Adenomyosis in endometriosis: prevalence and impact on fertility. Evidence from magnetic resonance imaging. *Hum Reprod* 2005; **20**: 2309–16.

67. Brosens J, Campo R, Gordts S *et al.* Submucus and outer myometrium leiomyomas are two distinct clinical entities. *Fertil Steril* 2003; **79**: 1452–54.

68. Gianaroli L, Gordts S, D'Angelo A *et al.* Effect of inner myometrium fibroid on reproductive outcome after IVF. *Reprod Biomed Online* 2005; **10**: 473–7.

69. Nishino M, Togashi K, Nakai A *et al.* Uterine contractions evaluated on cine MR imaging in patient with uterine leiomyomas. *Eur J Radiol* 2005; **53**: 142–6.

70. Morizaki N, Morizaki J, Hayashi R H *et al.* A functional and structural study of the innervation of human uterus. *Am J Obstet Gynecol* 1989; **160**: 218–28.

71. Orisaka M, Kurokawa T, Shukunami K *et al.* A comparison of uterine peristalsis in women with normal uteri and uterine leiomyoma by cine magnetic resonance imaging. *Eur J Obstet Gynecol Reprod Biol* 2007; **135**: 111–15.

72. Martinez-Mir M I, Estan L, Morales-Olivas F J *et al.* Effect of histamine and histamine analogues on human isolated myometrial strips. *Br J Pharmacol* 1992; **107**: 528–32.

73. Rudolph M I, Reinicke K, Cruz M A *et al.* Distribution of mast cells and the effect of their mediators on contractility in human endometrium. *Br J Obstet Gynaecol* 1993; **100**: 1125–9.

74. Poindexter A N, Thompson D J, Gibbons W E *et al.* Residual embryos in failed embryo transfer. *Fertil Steril* 1986; **46**: 262–7.

75. De Kretzer D, Dennis P, Hudson B. Transfer of human zygote. *Lancet* 1983; **1**: 728–9.

76. Meldrum D R, Chetkowski R, Steingold K A *et al.* Evolution of a highly successful in vitro and embryo transfer program. *Fertil Steril* 1987; **48**: 86–93.

77. Shaker A G, Fleming R, Jamieson M E *et al.* Assessment of embryo transfer after in vitro fertilisation: effects of glyceryl trinitrate. *Hum Reprod* 1993; **8**: 1426–8.

78. Diedrich K, Van der Ven H, Al Hasani A *et al.* Establishment of pregnancy related to embryo transfer techniques after IVF/ET. *Hum Reprod* 1989; **4**: 111–14.

79 Moon, Park S H, Lee J O. Treatment with piroxicam before embryo transfer increases the pregnancy rate after in vitro fertilisation and embryo transfer. *Fertil Steril* 2004; **82**: 816–20.

80. Tsirigotis M, Pelekanos M, Gilhespie S *et al.* Ritodrine use during the peri-implantation period reduces uterine contractility and improves implantation and pregnancy rates post-implantation. *ESHRE Conference*, June 25–28, 2000, Bologna, Italy: O–024.

81. Baruffi R, Mauri A L, Petersen C G *et al.* Effect of vaginal progesterone administration starting on the day of oocyte retrieval on pregnancy rates. *J Assist Reprod Genet* 2003; **20**: 517–20.

82. Nakai A, Togashi K, Kosaka K *et al.* Do anticholinergic agents suppress uterine peristalsis and sporadic myometrial contractions at cine MR imaging? *Radiology* 2008; **246**: 489–96.

83. Dorn C, Reisenberg J, Schlebusch H *et al.* Serum oxytocin concentration during embryo transfer procedure. *Eur J Obstet Gynecol Reprod Biol* 1999; **87**: 77–80.

84. Edwards R G. IVF, IVM, natural cycle IVF, a minimal stimulation IVF: time for a rethink. *Reprod Biomed Online* 2007; **15**: 106–19.

85. Steptoe P C, Edwards R G. Reimplantation of the human embryo with subsequent tubal pregnancy. *Lancet* 1976; **1**: 880–2.

Chapter

10 Endometrial and subendometrial blood flow and pregnancy rate of *in vitro* fertilization treatment

Ernest Hung Yu Ng and Pak Chung Ho

Department of Obstetrics & Gynaecology, The University of Hong Kong, Hong Kong Special Administrative Region, People's Republic of China

Introduction

Various causes of infertility can now be effectively treated by *in vitro* fertilization: embryo transfer (IVF-ET), which involves development of multiple follicles, oocyte retrieval, and embryo transfer after fertilization. Despite improvements in ovarian stimulation methods, culture media conditions, and the transfer technique of embryos, there has not been a significant increase in the implantation rates of cleaving embryos, which have remained steady at 20–25% for a long time.

Successful implantation depends on interaction between a good quality embryo and a receptive endometrium. Receptivity of the endometrium can be evaluated by the histological dating of an endometrial biopsy [1], endometrial cytokines in uterine flushing [2], the genomic study of a timed endometrial biopsy [3], or ultrasound examination of the endometrium [4]. Ultrasound examination of the endometrium is a non-invasive method to evaluate the endometrium during the peri-implantation period. Ultrasound parameters of endometrial receptivity include endometrial thickness, endometrial pattern, endometrial volume, and Doppler study of uterine arteries and the endometrium. Endometrial thickness and pattern have low positive predictive value and specificity for the IVF outcome [5,6] whereas endometrial volume measured by three-dimensional (3D) ultrasound is not predictive of pregnancy [7,8,9].

Angiogenesis plays a critical role in various female reproductive processes such as development of a dominant follicle, formation of a corpus luteum, growth of endometrium, and implantation [10,11]. Assessment of endometrial blood flow adds a physiological dimension to the anatomical ultrasound parameters and has drawn a lot of attention in recent years. A good blood flow toward the endometrium is usually considered an essential requirement for successful implantation. Jinno *et al.* [12] measured endometrial tissue blood flow in infertile patients by the intrauterine laser Doppler technique between days 4 and 6 of the luteal phase of a spontaneous cycle preceding IVF [12]. The chance of pregnancy in the subsequent IVF cycle was significantly higher in women with endometrial tissue blood flow of at least 29 ml/minute per 100 g of tissue than in women with lower values (42% vs 15%, respectively, $P < 0.05$). Endometrial blood flow was also superior to endometrial thickness, uterine pulsatility index (PI), and the histological dating of the endometrium in predicting the pregnancy.

Endometrial and subendometrial blood flow can now be non-invasively determined by two-dimensional (2D) or 3D ultrasound with color and power Doppler. This chapter reviews the role of endometrial and subendometrial blood flow determined by Doppler ultrasound in the prediction of pregnancy during IVF treatment.

Uterine blood flow

Doppler study of uterine vessels reflecting downstream impedance to flow is assumed in many studies to reflect the blood flow toward the endometrium. It is usually expressed as the pulsatility index (PI) and the resistance index (RI) (Fig. 10.1). PI is calculated as the peak systolic velocity (PSV) minus end-diastolic velocity divided by the mean whereas RI is the ratio of PSV minus end-diastolic velocity divided by PSV.

Goswamy *et al.* [13] first suggested that decreased uterine blood flow plays a role in subfertility. Subsequently, good uterine blood flow as shown by low PI or RI is correlated with successful IVF outcome [14,15,16,17]. Steer *et al.* [15] classified PI measured on the day of ET as low, medium, and high in the ranges of 0–1.99, 2.00–2.99, and 3.00, respectively, and reported a 35% implantation failure when PI was

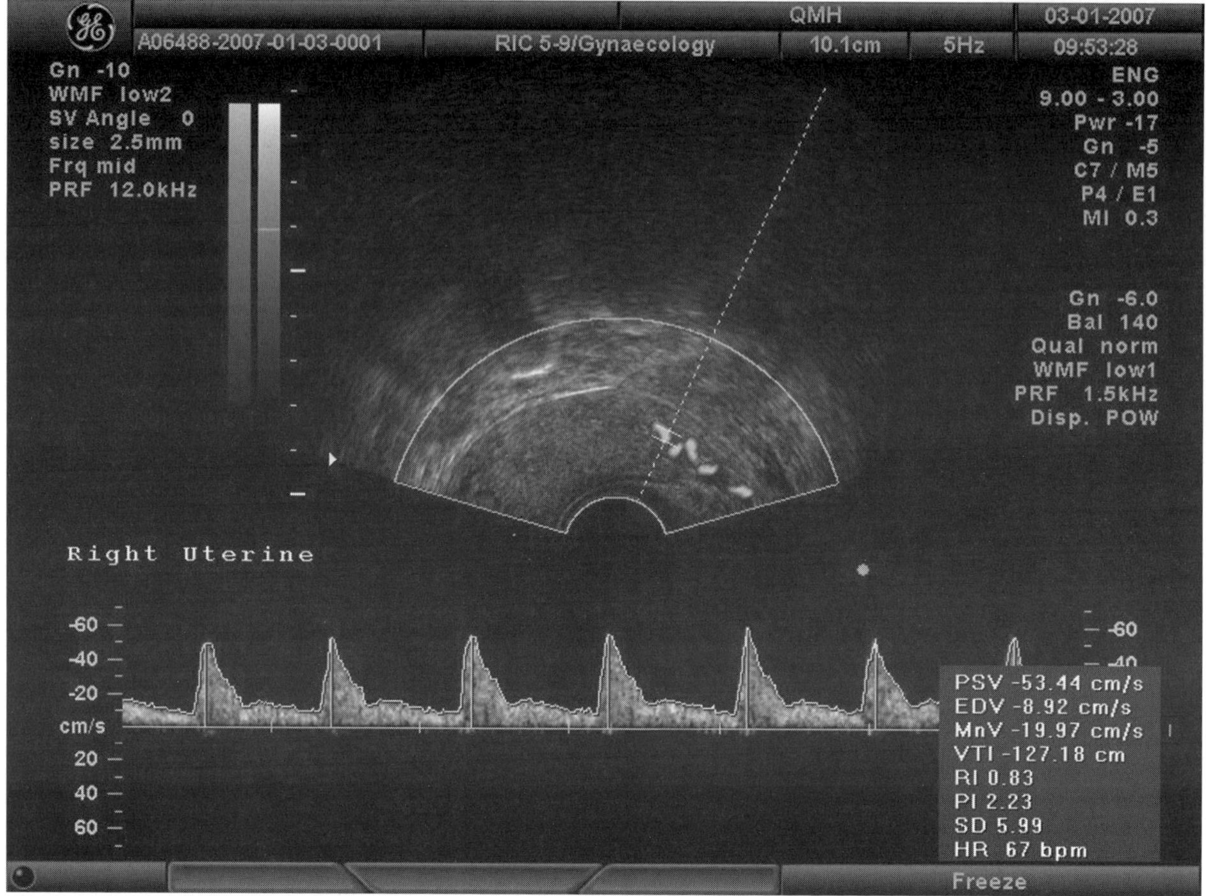

Fig. 10.1 Uterine blood flow measured by 2D Doppler ultrasound. See plate section for color version.

> 3.0. Using a PI upper limit of 3.0 [15] or 3.3 [16], the uterine Doppler flow indices have a high negative predictive value and sensitivity (in the ranges of 88–100% and 96–100%, respectively) and a relatively higher range of positive predictive value and specificity (44–56% and 13–35%, respectively) when compared with endometrial thickness and pattern [6].

Uterine Doppler study may not reflect the actual blood flow to the endometrium as the major compartment of the uterus is the myometrium and there is collateral circulation between uterine and ovarian vessels. We have correlated uterine blood flow assessed by 2D color Doppler and endometrial and subendometrial blood flow measured by 3D power Doppler in both stimulated and natural cycles [18]. Indeed, 2D Doppler study of uterine vessels is a poor reflection of subendometrial blood flow by 3D power Doppler during stimulated and natural cycles, and its measurement cannot reflect endometrial blood flow during stimulated cycles. Endometrial and subendometrial 3D Doppler flow indices were similar among patients with averaged uterine PI < 2.0, 2.0–2.99, and ≥ 3.0. Therefore, it is more logical to directly determine the endometrial and subendometrial blood flow.

Endometrial and subendometrial blood flow measured by 2D ultrasound

Endometrial blood flow comes from the radial artery, which divides after passing through the myometrial–endometrial junction to form the basal arteries that supply the basal portion of the endometrium, and the myometrial spiral arteries that continue up towards the endometrium. Kupesic and Kurjak [19] first reported endometrial blood flow measured by transvaginal color Doppler study during the peri-ovulatory period in patients undergoing donor insemination. Results were not correlated with the outcome of

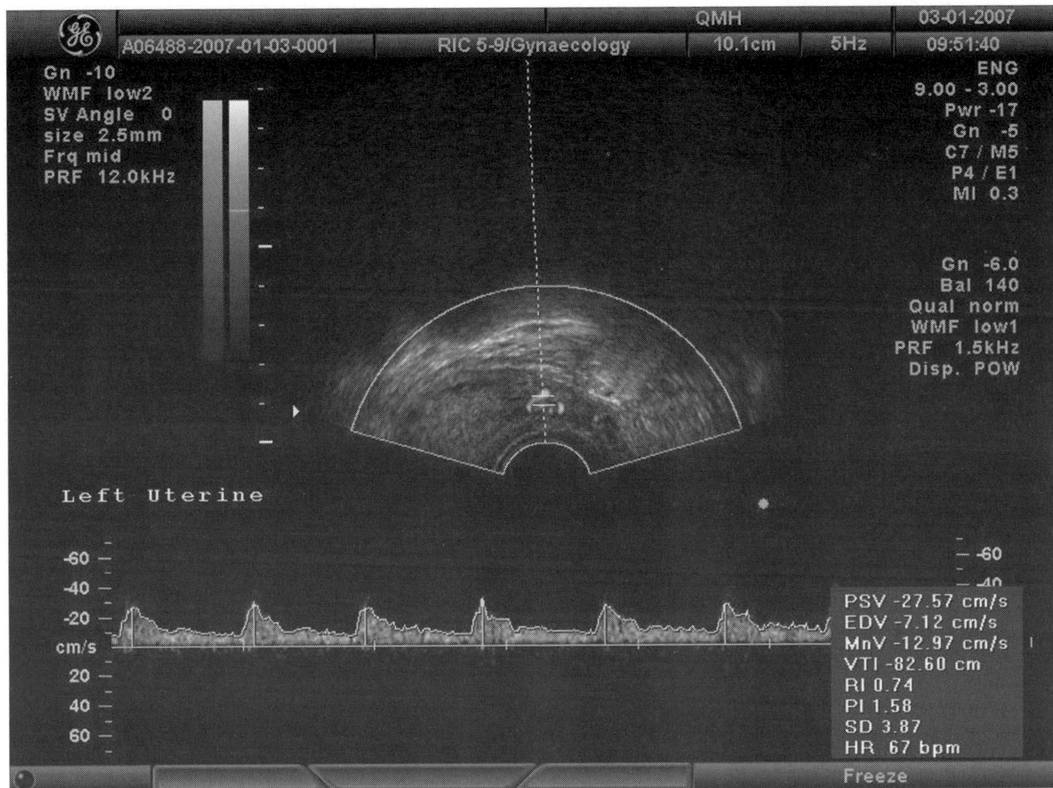

Fig. 10.1 (cont.)

the treatment. Subsequently, endometrial and subendometrial blood flow examined by color (Table 10.1) and power Doppler (Table 10.2) were correlated with implantation or pregnancy rates during IVF treatment. It appears that 2D Doppler flow indices of spiral arteries such as PI and PSV are not predictive of pregnancy [9,20,21], although Battaglia *et al.* [22] and Kupesic *et al.* [23] found significantly lower spiral artery PI in pregnant cycles than non-pregnant cycles.

Yang *et al.* [24] used computer software to measure the area and intensity of color signals present in the endometrium in a longitudinal axis, i.e. intraendometrial power Doppler area (EPDA). Significantly higher EDPAs were found in pregnant cycles than in non-pregnant cycles ($8.8\,mm^2$ vs $5.8\,mm^2$, respectively). Patients with EPDA $< 5\,mm^2$ had a significantly lower pregnancy rate (23.5% vs 47.5%; $P = 0.021$) and implantation rate (8.1% vs 20.2%; $P = 0.003$) than those with EPDA $\geq 5\,mm^2$. Contart *et al.* [25] graded endometrial blood flow by the visualization of power Doppler in the quadrants in the fundal region of the transverse plane but could not demonstrate any predictive value of such a grading system.

Presence of endometrial and subendometrial blood flow can be identified more easily with 2D Doppler ultrasound. Absent endometrial and subendometrial blood flow has been shown to be associated with no pregnancy [20,22] or a significantly lower pregnancy rate [26,27].

Endometrial and subendometrial blood flow measured by 3D ultrasound in IVF cycles

In combination with a 3D ultrasound, power Doppler provides a unique tool with which to measure the blood flow towards the whole endometrium and the subendometrial region. The built-in VOCAL® (Virtual Organ Computer-Aided Analysis) Imaging Program for the 3D power Doppler histogram can be used in the analysis to measure the endometrial volume and indices of blood flow within the endometrium (Fig. 10.2). Vascularization index (VI), which measures the ratio of the number of color voxels to the number of all the voxels, is thought to represent the presence of blood vessels (vascularity) in the endometrium, and this was expressed as a percentage (%) of the endometrial volume. Flow index (FI), the mean power Doppler signal

Table 10.1. Summary of studies of endometrial blood flow by 2D color Doppler

Study	IVF cycles	USS parameters	USS day	Results
Zaidi *et al.* (20)	96 cycles using a long protocol	Spiral PI and PSV Presence of endometrial and subendometrial flow	hCG	No difference in subendometrial PI and PSV between pregnant and non-pregnant cycles Absent subendometrial flow associated with no pregnancy
Battaglia *et al.* (22)	60 cycles	Uterine and spiral PI Presence of endometrial blood flow	OR	Uterine and spiral PI lower in pregnant than non-pregnant cycles Absent subendometrial flow associated with no pregnancy
Chien *et al.* (26)	623 cycles using ultrashort and ultralong protocols	Uterine and spiral PI and RI Presence of endometrial and subendometrial (<10 mm) blood flow	ET	Significantly lower implantation and pregnancy rates in patients without endometrial/subendometrial flow Presence of subendometrial flow 5.9 times more likely to become pregnant than those with absent flow

ET, embryo transfer; hCG, human chorionic gonadotropin; OR, oocyte retrieval; PI, pulsatility index; PSV, peak systolic velocity; USS, ultrasound.

Table 10.2. Summary of studies of endometrial blood flow by 2D power Doppler

Study	IVF cycles	USS parameter	USS day	Results
Yang *et al.* (24)	95 cycles using long and short protocols endometrium ≥ 10 mm	Intraendometrial power Doppler area (EDPA) < 5 mm^2; ≥ 5 mm^2	OR	Higher EPDA in pregnant cycles Lower implantation and pregnancy rates when EDPA < 5 mm^2
Yuval *et al.* (21)	156 cycles using a long protocol	PI and RI	OR and ET	No difference in any USS parameters between pregnant and non-pregnant cycles
Contart *et al.* (25)	185 cycles using a long protocol	Fundal region along transverse plan; Grades I, II, III, & IV according to visualization of power Doppler in the quadrants	hCG	Implantation and pregnancy rates similar in all grades of endometrial vascularity
Schild *et al.* (9)	135 cycles using a long protocol; first cycle only	PI and PSV of vessels in endometrium and subendometrial area (< 5 mm)	OR	No difference in spiral artery PI and PSV between pregnant and non-pregnant cycles Non-detectable spiral blood flow was not associated with a lower implantation rate
Maugey-Laulon *et al.* (27)	144 cycles using a long protocol	Presence of endometrial and subendometrial blood flow	ET	Absent endometrial and subendometrial flow associated with a lower pregnancy rate

ET, embryo transfer; hCG, human chorionic gonadotropin; OR, oocyte retrieval; PI, pulsatility index; PSV, peak systolic velocity; USS, ultrasound.

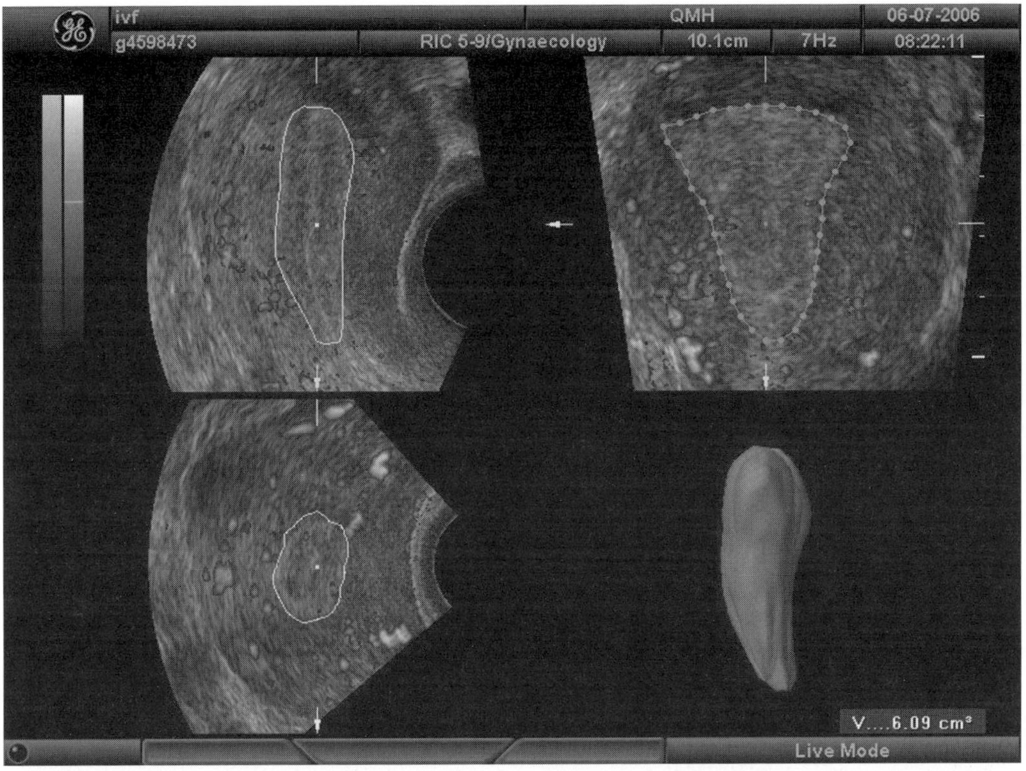

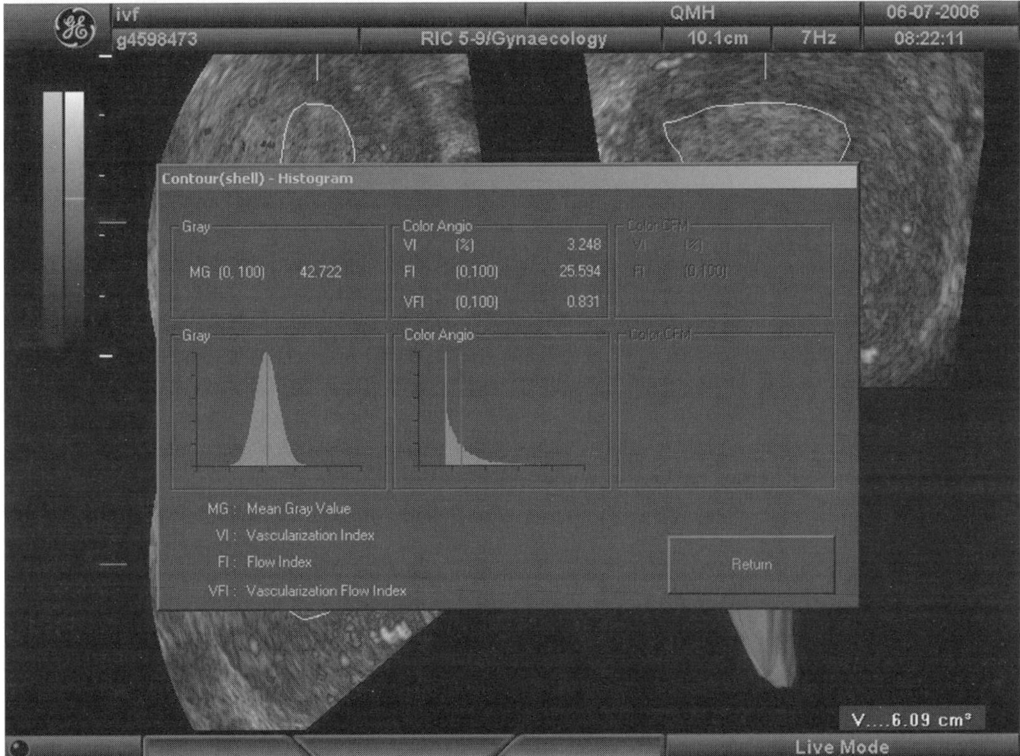

Fig. 10.2 Endometrial volume and blood flow measured by 3D Doppler ultrasound. See plate section for color version.

intensity inside the endometrium, is thought to express the average intensity of flow. Vascularization flow index (VFI) is a combination of vascularity and flow intensity [28].

Following the assessment of the endometrium itself, the subendometrium can be examined through the application of 'shell-imaging', which allows the user to generate a variable contour that parallels the originally defined surface contour. The VI, FI, and VFI of the subendometrial region are obtained accordingly (Fig. 10.3). The intraobserver and interobserver reliability of endometrial and subendometrial blood flow by 3D power Doppler has been confirmed to be high with all measurements obtaining an intraclass correlation of above 0.9 [29,30].

Studies addressing the role of endometrial and subendometrial blood flow measured by 3D Doppler in IVF treatment are summarized in Table 10.3. The first study was reported by Schild *et al.* [31], who measured the subendometrial blood flow after pituitary downregulation but prior to ovarian stimulation. Subendometrial VI, FI, and VFI were significantly lower in pregnant cycles than non-pregnant ones. Logistic regression analysis found that the subendometrial FI was the strongest predictive factor for the pregnancy outcome among other 3D Doppler flow indices. The authors suggested that a lesser degree of intrauterine vascularization and perfusion at the beginning of ovarian stimulation indicated a more favorable endometrial milieu. Another possibility is that lower subendometrial 3D Doppler flow indices may indicate a better functional downregulation of the endometrium following the use of a gonadotropin-releasing hormone agonist, which increases the chances of successful implantation. Unfortunately, there are no further studies to substantiate the findings of this interesting study.

Kupesic *et al.* [23] performed a 3D ultrasound examination on the day of blastocyst transfer, i.e. 5 days after oocyte retrieval, and found that subendometrial FI was significantly higher in pregnant cycles. Subendometrial VI and VFI were similar between pregnant and non-pregnant patients. Wu *et al.* [32] measured subendometrial blood flow on the day of human chorionic gonadotropin (hCG) administration and demonstrated that subendometrial VFI was significantly higher in the pregnant group. Subendometrial VI and FI were also similar between pregnant and non-pregnant cycles. Subendometrial VFI was superior to subendometrial VI, subendometrial FI, and endometrial volume in predicting the successful outcome in the receiver operating characteristics (ROC) curve analysis because areas under the ROC curve for VFI, VI, FI, and endometrial volume were 0.8912, 0.6011, 0.6373, and 0.6674, respectively. It has been further shown that the best predictive rate was achieved by a subendometrial VFI cutoff value of > 0.24.

On the day of oocyte retrieval, Dorn *et al.* [33] compared the subendometrial blood flow before and after intravenous administration of Levovist, which is a contrast agent and consists of 99.9% D-galactose. All subendometrial 3D Doppler flow indices after the administration of the contrast agent were significantly higher than those without the contrast agent. However, all subendometrial 3D Doppler flow indices with and without the contrast agent were comparable between pregnant and non-pregnant cycles. The results of this study suggested that the use of 3D power Doppler ultrasound under a contrast agent during IVF treatment provided no additional advantage over the conventional 3D power Doppler ultrasound examination.

Järvelä *et al.* [34] determined endometrial and subendometrial VI after gonadotropin stimulation but before hCG administration and again on the day of oocyte retrieval. There were no differences between those who conceived and those who did not conceive in endometrial and subendometrial VI on either day examined. Endometrial and subendometrial VI decreased after hCG injection in the pregnant and non-pregnant groups. The weaknesses of this study included the small number of subjects and variation in the day of ultrasound examinations after gonadotropin stimulation. The ultrasound examination after gonadotropin stimulation was performed on the day of hCG administration in 18 out of 35 (51.4%), 1 day before the hCG injection in 12 (34.3%), and 2 days before the hCG injection in 5 (14.3%) patients.

We have published the largest study involving 451 transfer cycles [35]. Patients in the pregnant group had significantly lower uterine RI, endometrial VI, and VFI than those in the non-pregnant group. Endometrial thickness, endometrial volume, endometrial pattern, uterine PI, endometrial FI, and subendometrial VI, FI, and VFI were similar between the non-pregnant and pregnant groups. The number of embryos replaced and endometrial VI were the only two predictive factors for pregnancy in a logistic multiple regression analysis. ROC curve analysis revealed that the area under the curve was around

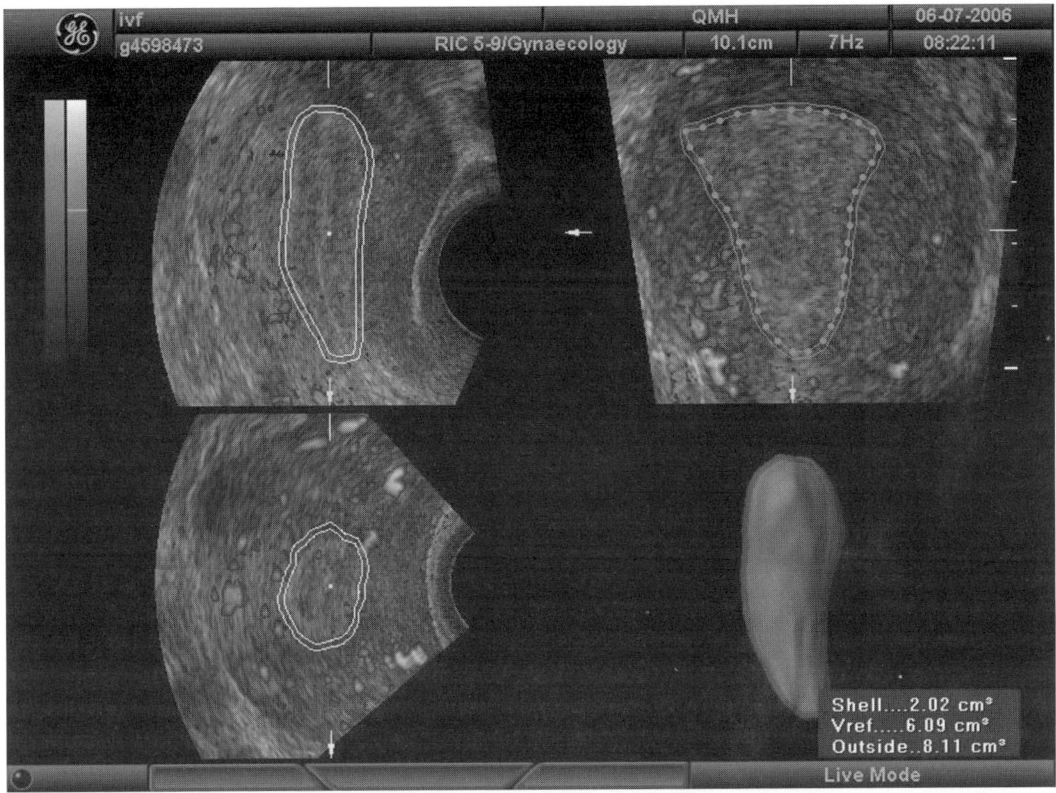

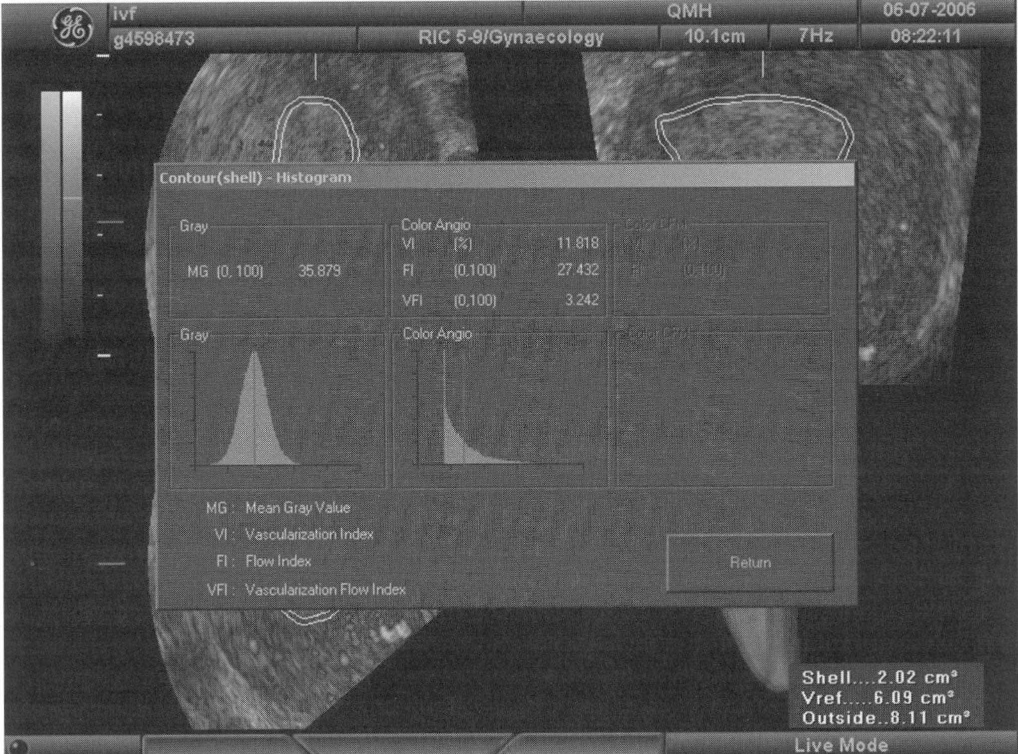

Fig. 10.3 Subendometrial volume and blood flow measured by 3D Doppler ultrasound. See plate section for color version.

Table 10.3. Summary of studies of endometrial and subendometrial blood flow by 3D power Doppler ultrasound

Study	IVF cycles	Inclusion/exclusion criteria	USS day	Results
Schild *et al.* (31)	75 cycles using a long protocol ET 2 days after OR	Inclusion criteria – downregulation confirmed (endometrium < 5 mm; no ovarian cyst of > 2.5 cm; serum estradiol < 60 pg/ml)	Before stimulation	Subendometrial VI, FI, and VFI lower in pregnant than non-pregnant cycles Subendometrial FI is the strongest predictive factor for IVF in logistic regression analysis
Kupesic *et al.* (23)	89 cycles using a long protocol Blastocyst transfer 5 days after OR	Inclusion criteria – serum FSH < 10 IU/l, no fibroid, ovarian cysts and ovarian endometriosis	ET (hCG +7)	Higher subendometrial FI in pregnant cycles
Wu *et al.* (32)	54 cycles; first cycles only (details of ovarian stimulation and ET not given)	Inclusion criteria – age < 38 yr, normal uterine cavity, serum FSH < 15 IU/l, ≥ 2 good-quality embryos	hCG	Subendometrial VFI higher in pregnant cycles
Dorn *et al.* (33)	42 cycles using a long protocol	Exclusion criteria – polycystic ovary syndrome, endometrium < 6 mm, gynecological surgery	OR	No difference in subendometrial VI, FI, and VFI between pregnant and non-pregnant cycles
Järvelä *et al.* (34)	35 cycles using a long protocol ET 2 days after OR	Exclusion criteria – uterine fibroids, endometriosis, single ovary, previous operation on uterus or salpingectomy	After stimulation and OR	No difference in endometrial and subendometrial VI between pregnant and non-pregnant cycles on both days
Ng *et al.* (35)	451 cycles using a long protocol; first cycle only ET 2 days after OR	Inclusion criteria – normal uterine cavity on scanning	OR	Endometrial VI and VFI lower in pregnant cycles
Ng *et al.* (38)	193 cycles Frozen-thawed embryo transfer cycles	Inclusion criteria – normal uterine cavity	LH +1	No difference in endometrial and subendometrial 3D Doppler flow indices between pregnant and non-pregnant cycles
Mercè *et al.* (40)	80 cycles using a long protocol	Inclusion criteria – first cycle, normal uterine cavity, serum FSH < 10 IU/l, regular cycles, non-smokers	hCG	Higher endometrial VI, FI, and VFI in pregnant cycles
Ng *et al.* (48)	293 cycles using a long protocol ET 2 days after OR	Inclusion criteria – first cycle, normal uterine cavity	OR and ET	No difference in endometrial and subendometrial 3D Doppler flow indices on the 2 days and changes in these indices between pregnant and non-pregnant cycles

ET, embryo transfer; FI, flow index; hCG, human chorionic gonadotropin; OR, oocyte retrieval; USS, ultrasound; VI, vascularization index; VFI, vascularization flow index.

0.5 for all ultrasound parameters for endometrial receptivity. In a subgroup analysis of patients with good prognosis defined as patients aged ≤ 35 years with endometrial thickness > 8 mm, transfer of ≥ two good-quality embryos, and the availability of frozen embryo(s), there were no significant differences between the non-pregnant and pregnant groups in all endometrial and subendometrial 3D Doppler flow indices.

In our study [35], endometrial and subendometrial blood flow was absent in 31 patients and 23 patients, respectively. Twenty patients had no endometrial and subendometrial blood flow. Implantation and pregnancy rates were higher in patients without endometrial and subendometrial blood flow than those with endometrial and subendometrial blood flow, although the difference did not reach statistical significance. This finding is contradictory to those obtained by 2D

Doppler ultrasound, which suggested that absent endometrial and subendometrial blood flows were associated with no pregnancy [20,22] or much reduced pregnancy rate [26,27].

The age of women, their smoking habits, their types of infertility and parity, and causes of subfertility had no effect on all endometrial and subendometrial 3D Doppler flow indices [36]. Endometrial blood flow was negatively affected by serum estradiol concentration on the day of hCG administration. Indeed, we found that endometrial and subendometrial 3D Doppler flow indices in the stimulated cycles were significantly lower than those in the natural cycles of the same patients undergoing IVF treatment [37].

We have also examined the role of the endometrial and subendometrial blood flow in the prediction of pregnancy during frozen-thawed embryo transfer cycles using natural or clomiphene-induced cycles [38]. Endometrial thickness, endometrial volume, endometrial pattern, uterine PI, uterine RI, and endometrial and subendometrial 3D Doppler flow indices were comparable between the non-pregnant and pregnant groups. On the other hand, endometrial and subendometrial blood flow was significantly higher in pregnant patients with livebirth following IVF and frozen-thawed embryo transfer treatment [39].

More recently, Mercè *et al.* [40] found that endometrial 3D power Doppler flow indices were statistically significantly higher in the pregnant group. The area under the ROC curve was statistically significant for endometrial VI, FI, and VFI when no grade 1 embryos or only one were transferred but not when two or three grade 1 embryos were transferred.

Differences among studies on endometrial blood flow measured by 3D ultrasound in IVF cycles

Kupesic *et al.* [23], Wu *et al.* [32], and Mercè *et al.* [40] found significantly higher subendometrial blood flow in pregnant cycles while Dorn *et al.* [33] and Järvelä *et al.* [34] could not demonstrate any differences in endometrial and subendometrial 3D power Doppler indices. The pregnant group had significantly lower endometrial blood flow in our study [35]. We published the largest study (n = 451) while a much smaller number of subjects ranging from 35 to 89 was evaluated by others [23,32,33,34,40]. These studies clearly varied in patients' characteristics (Table 10.3), the machine setting, selection of the subendometrial region, and the day of ultrasound examination.

The 3D power Doppler flow indices are affected by the machine setting such as gain, signal power, pulse repetition frequency, etc. [41,42]. It is important to maintain the same Doppler settings in studies to facilitate intersubject comparison but it may be difficult to compare among studies because of different Doppler settings in different studies. In the studies of Kupesic *et al.* [23], Wu *et al.* [32] and Dorn *et al.* [33], 3D Doppler flow indices of the endometrial region were not given. The subendometrial region is considered to be within 1 mm [35], 5 mm [23,32], or 10 mm [34] of the originally defined myometrial–endometrial contour. Dorn *et al.* [33] did not give the details of the subendometrial shell. We reported endometrial and subendometrial blood flows separately and the subendometrial region was defined as a shell within 1 mm of the myometrial–endometrial interface. Only the myometrium immediately underlying the endometrium exhibits a cyclic pattern of steroid receptor expression similar to that of the endometrium [43].

Ultrasound examination was performed on the day of hCG administration [32,40], oocyte retrieval [33,34,35], and blastocyst transfer [23]. There is still no consensus as to when the ultrasound examination for assessing endometrial receptivity in IVF treatment should be done. The day of the ultrasound examination in these studies was chosen for logistic reasons and did not take into consideration the physiological changes of endometrial blood flow throughout the menstrual cycle [44,45].

Changes of endometrial vascularity in the luteal phase

Ultrasound examination was performed only once in the above studies. However, endometrial blood flow changes throughout the menstrual cycle [44,45]. Fraser *et al.* [44] determined endometrial blood flow through the menstrual cycle in non-pregnant women with the use of the clearance of radiolabeled xenon133 following its instillation into the uterine cavity. There was a significant elevation in the middle to late follicular phase, followed by a substantial fall and a secondary slow luteal phase rise that was maintained until the onset of menstruation. Similarly, Raine-Fenning *et al.* [45] showed that endometrial and subendometrial blood flow by 3D ultrasound increased during the proliferative phase, peaking around 3 days prior to ovulation before decreasing to a nadir 5 days postovulation.

Hypoxia in the endometrium may play a beneficial role for implantation as the expression of vascular endothelial growth factor is upregulated by hypoxia [46] and relatively low oxygen tension was present around the blastocyst during the time of implantation [47]. The degree of change in endometrial perfusion from the late follicular phase through to the early luteal phase may be a more important determinant of endometrial receptivity.

We have evaluated endometrial and subendometrial blood flow on the days of hCG administration and ET and the percentage change in endometrial and subendometrial vascularity between these 2 days in the prediction of pregnancy during IVF treatment [48]. Patients in non-pregnant and pregnant groups had comparable 3D Doppler flow indices of endometrial and subendometrial regions measured on either day. Percentage changes in endometrial and subendometrial 3D Doppler flow indices were also similar. Again, none of the ultrasound parameters was predictive of pregnancy in a multiple logistic regression analysis and the ROC curve analysis.

Conclusion

Ultrasound examination of the endometrium provides a non-invasive method to assess endometrial receptivity during IVF treatment. Doppler study of uterine vessels is a poor reflection of endometrial and subendometrial blood flow as demonstrated by 3D power Doppler ultrasound. Doppler flow study of spiral arteries is again not predictive of pregnancy. The role of endometrial and subendometrial blood flow assessed by 3D power Doppler ultrasound in predicting pregnancy is still controversial and more studies are warranted.

References

1. Noyes R W, Hertig A T, Rock J. Dating the endometrial biopsy. *Fertil Steril* 1950; **1**: 3–25.
2. Lédée-Bataille N, Laprée-Delage G, Taupin J L *et al.* Concentration of leukaemia inhibitory factor (LIF) in uterine flushing fluid is highly predictive of embryo implantation. *Hum Reprod* 2002; **17**: 213–8.
3. Horcajadas J A, Pellicer A, Simón C. Wide genomic analysis of human endometrial receptivity: new times, new opportunities. *Hum Reprod Update* 2007; **13**: 77–86.
4. Ng E H Y, Ho P C. The role of ultrasound parameters in the prediction of pregnancy during in vitro fertilization treatment. *Expert Rev Obstet Gynaecol* 2008; **3**: 503–14.
5. Turnbull L W, Lesny P, Killick S R. Assessment of uterine receptivity prior to embryo transfer: a review of currently available imaging modalities. *Hum Reprod Update* 1995; **1**: 505–14.
6. Friedler S, Schenker J G, Herman A, Lewin A. The role of ultrasonography in the evaluation of endometrial receptivity following assisted reproductive treatments: a critical review. *Hum Reprod Update* 1996; **2**: 323–35.
7. Raga R, Bonilla-Musoles F, Casan E M, Klein O, Bonilla F. Assessment of endometrial volume by three-dimensional ultrasound prior to embryo transfer: clues to endometrial receptivity. *Hum Reprod* 1999; **14**: 2851–4.
8. Yaman C, Ebner T, Sommergruber M, Polz W, Tews G. Role of three-dimensional ultrasonographic measurement of endometrium volume as a predictor of pregnancy outcome in an IVF-ET program: a preliminary study. *Fertil Steril* 2000; **74**: 797–801.
9. Schild R L, Knoblock C, Dorn C *et al.* Endometrial receptivity in an in vitro fertilization program as assessed by spiral artery blood flow, endometrial thickness, endometrial volume, and uterine artery blood flow. *Fertil Steril* 2001; **75**: 361–6.
10. Abulafia O, Sherer D M. Angiogenesis of the ovary. *Am J Obstet Gynecol* 2000; **182**: 240–6.
11. Smith S K. Regulation of angiogenesis in the endometrium. *Trends Endocrinol Metab* 2001; **12**: 147–51.
12. Jinno M, Ozaki T, Iwashita M *et al.* Measurement of endometrial tissue blood flow: a novel way to assess uterine receptivity for implantation. *Fertil Steril* 2001; **76**: 1168–74.
13. Goswamy R K, Williams G, Steptoe P C. Decreased uterine perfusion: a cause of infertility. *Hum Reprod* 1988; **3**: 955–9.
14. Sterzik K, Grab D, Sasse V *et al.* Doppler sonographic findings and their correlation with implantation in an in vitro fertilization program. *Fertil Steril* 1989; **52**: 825–8.
15. Steer C V, Campbell S, Tan S L *et al.* The use of transvaginal color flow imaging after in vitro fertilization to identify optimum uterine conditions before embryo transfer. *Fertil Steril* 1992; **57**: 372–6.
16. Coulam C B, Bustillo M, Soenksen D M, Britten S. Ultrasonographic predictors of implantation after assisted reproduction. *Fertil Steril* 1994; **62**: 1004–10.
17. Serafini P, Batzofin J, Nelson J, Olive D. Sonographic uterine predictors of pregnancy in women undergoing ovulation induction for assisted reproductive treatments. *Fertil Steril* 1994; **62**: 815–22.
18. Ng E H Y, Chan C C W, Tang O S, Yeung W S B, Ho P C. Relationship between uterine blood flow and endometrial

and subendometrial blood flow during stimulated and natural cycles. *Fertil Steril* 2006 ;**85**: 721–7.

19. Kupesic S, Kurjak A. Uterine and ovarian perfusion during periovulatory period assessed by transvaginal color Doppler. *Fertil Steril* 1993;**60**: 439–43.
20. Zaidi J, Campbell S, Pittrof F R, Tan S L. Endometrial thickness morphology, vascular penetration and velocimetry in predicting implantation in an IVF program. *Ultrasound Obstet Gynecol* 1995; **6**: 191–8.
21. Yuval Y, Lipitz S, Dor J, Achiron R. The relationship between endometrial thickness, and blood flow and pregnancy rates in in-vitro fertilization. *Hum Reprod* 1999; **14**: 1067–71.
22. Battaglia C, Artini P G, Giulini S *et al.* Colour Doppler changes and thromboxane production after ovarian stimulation with gonadotrophin-releasing hormone agonist. *Hum Reprod* 1997; **12**: 2477–82.
23. Kupesic S, Bekavac I, Bjelos D, Kurjak A. Assessment of endometrial receptivity by transvaginal color Doppler and three-dimensional power Doppler ultrasonography in patients undergoing in vitro fertilization procedures. *J Ultrasound Med* 2001; **20**: 125–34.
24. Yang J H, Wu M Y, Chen C D *et al.* Association of endometrial blood flow as determined by a modified colour Doppler technique with subsequent outcome of in-vitro fertilization. *Hum Reprod* 1999; **14**: 1606–10.
25. Contart P, Baruffi R L, Coelho J *et al.* Power Doppler endometrial evaluation as a method for the prognosis of embryo implantation in an ICSI program. *J Assist Reprod Genet* 2000; **17**: 329–34.
26. Chien L W, Au H K, Chen P L, Xiao J, Tseng C R. Assessment of uterine receptivity by the endometrial-subendometrial blood flow distribution pattern in women undergoing in vitro fertilization-embryo transfer. *Fertil Steril* 2002; **78**: 245–51.
27. Maugey-Laulon B, Commenges-Ducos M, Jullien V *et al.* Endometrial vascularity and ongoing pregnancy after IVF. *Eur J Obstet Gynecol Reprod Biol* 2002; **104**: 137–43.
28. Pairleitner H, Steiner H, Hasenoehrl G, Staudach A. Three-dimensional power Doppler sonography: imaging and quantifying blood flow and vascularization. *Ultrasound Obstet Gynecol* 1999; **14**: 139–43.
29. Raine-Fenning N J, Campbell B K, Clewes J S, Kendall N R, Johnson I R. The reliability of virtual organ computer-aided analysis (VOCAL) for the semiquantification of ovarian, endometrial and subendometrial perfusion. *Ultrasound Obstet Gynecol* 2003; **22**: 633–9.
30. Raine-Fenning N J, Campbell B K, Clewes J S, Kendall N R, Johnson I R. The interobserver reliability of three-dimensional power Doppler data acquisition within the female pelvis. *Ultrasound Obstet Gynecol* 2004 ;**23**: 501–8.
31. Schild R L, Holthanus S, Alquen J D *et al.* Quantitative assessment of subendometrial blood flow by three-dimensional-ultrasound is an important predictive factor of implantation in an in-vitro fertilization programme. *Hum Reprod* 2000; **15**: 89–94.
32. Wu H M, Chiang C H, Huang H Y *et al.* Detection of the subendometrial vascularization flow index by three-dimensional ultrasound may be useful for predicting the pregnancy rate for patients undergoing in vitro fertilization-embryo transfer. *Fertil Steril* 2003; **79**: 507–11.
33. Dorn C, Reinsberg J, Willeke C *et al.* Three-dimensional power Doppler ultrasound of the subendometrial blood flow under the administration of a contrast agent (Levovist). *Arch Gynecol Obstet* 2004; **270**: 94–8.
34. Järvelä I Y, Sladkevicius P, Kelly S *et al.* Evaluation of endometrial receptivity during in-vitro fertilization using three-dimensional power Doppler ultrasound. *Ultrasound Obstet Gynecol* 2005; **26**: 765–9.
35. Ng E H Y, Chan CC W, Tang O S, Yeung W S B, Ho P C. The role of endometrial and subendometrial blood flow measured by three-dimensional power Doppler ultrasound in the prediction of pregnancy during in vitro fertilization treatment. *Hum Reprod* 2006; **21**: 164–70.
36. Ng E H Y, Chan C C W, Tang O S, Yeung W S B, Ho P C. Factors affecting endometrial and subendometrial blood flow measured by three-dimensional power Doppler ultrasound during in vitro fertilization treatment. *Hum Reprod* 2006; **21**: 1062–9.
37. Ng E H Y, Chan C C W, Tang O S, Yeung W S B, Ho P C. Comparison of endometrial and subendometrial blood flow measured by three-dimensional power Doppler ultrasound between stimulated and natural cycles in the same patients. *Hum Reprod* 2004; **19**: 2385–90.
38. Ng E H Y, Chan C C W, Tang O S, Yeung W S B, Ho P C. The role of endometrial and subendometrial vascularity measured by three-dimensional power Doppler ultrasound in the prediction of pregnancy during frozen-thawed embryo transfer cycles. *Hum Reprod* 2006; **21**: 1612–7.
39. Ng E HY, Chan C C W, Tang O S, Yeung W S B, Ho P C. Endometrial and subendometrial vascularity is higher in pregnant patients with live birth following ART than in those who suffer a miscarriage. *Hum Reprod* 2007; **22**: 1134–41.
40. Mercè L T, Barco M J, Bau S, Troyano J. Are endometrial parameters by three-dimensional ultrasound and power Doppler angiography related to in vitro

fertilization/embryo transfer outcome? *Fertil Steril* 2008; **1**: 111–7.

41. Raine-Fenning N J, Nordin N M, Ramnarine K V *et al.* Evaluation of the effect of machine settings on quantitative three-dimensional power Doppler angiography: an in-vitro flow phantom experiment. *Ultrasound Obstet Gynecol* 2008; **32**: 551–9.
42. Schulten-Wijman M J, Struijk P C, Brezinka C, De Jong N, Steegers E A. Evaluation of volume vascularization index and flow index: a phantom study. *Ultrasound Obstet Gynecol* 2008; **32**: 560–4.
43. Noe M, Kunz G, Herbertz M, Mall G, Leyendecker G. The cyclic pattern of the immunocytochemical expression of oestrogen and progesterone receptors in human myometrial and endometrial layers: characterization of the endometrial-subendometrial unit. *Hum Reprod* 1999; **14**: 190–7.
44. Fraser I S, McCarron G, Hutton B, Macey D. Endometrial blood flow measured by xenon 133 clearance in women with normal menstrual cycles and dysfunctional uterine bleeding. *Am J Obstet Gynecol* 1987; **156**: 158–66.
45. Raine-Fenning N J, Campbell B K, Kendall N R, Clewes J S, Johnson I R. Quantifying the changes in endometrial vascularity throughout the normal menstrual cycle with three-dimensional power Doppler angiography. *Hum Reprod* 2004; **19**: 330–8.
46. Sharkey A M, Day K, McPherson A *et al.* Vascular endothelial growth factor expression in human endometrium is regulated by hypoxia. *J Clin Endocrinol Metab* 2000; **85**: 402–9.
47. Graham C H, Postovit L M, Park H, Canning M T, Fitzpatrick T E. Adriana and Luisa Castellucci award lecture 1999: role of oxygen in the regulation of trophoblast gene expression and invasion. *Placenta* 2000; **21**: 443–50.
48. Ng E H Y, Chan C C W, Tang O S, Yeung W S B, Ho P C. Changes in endometrial and subendometrial blood flows in IVF. *Reproductive BioMedicine Online* 2009; **18**: 269–75.

Chapter 11

Deep trophoblast invasion and spiral artery remodeling

Robert Pijnenborg[1] and Ivo Brosens[2]

[1]Katholieke Universiteit Leuven, Department Woman & Child, University Hospital Leuven, Leuven, Belgium
[2]Leuven Institute for Fertility and Embryology, Leuven, Belgium

The discovery of deep trophoblast invasion and associated vascular remodeling

After a period of confusion about the different cell types in the placenta and placental bed (see Chapters 1 and 2), it was eventually well established that extravillous trophoblastic cells are not retained within the basal plate, but invade deeply into the uterine wall including the subendometrial or junctional zone (JZ) myometrium. Painstaking observations on large tissue sections of complete pregnant uteri with placentas still attached supported the trophoblastic nature of interstitial and endovascular migratory cells because of their histological continuity with the cytotrophoblastic shell [1,2,3]. Regarding the origin of the endovascular cells Hamilton and Boyd had listed several possibilities of their being: (1) modified endothelial cells, (2) other maternal vascular cells, (3) wandering interstitial cells breaking through the vessel wall, or (4) cells derived from the cytotrophoblastic shell showing retrograde ('antidromic') migration along the vessel lumen [1]. Although early microscopists favored the first two scenarios, later investigators definitely ascribed a trophoblastic origin to these cells [4], which was amply confirmed later on by applying immunohistochemical staining methods. Although some investigators nowadays still hold that a local 'intravasation' by interstitial trophoblasts is the most likely pathway of vascular invasion [5], Hamilton and Boyd [1] clearly preferred the fourth possibility of a retrograde intravascular migration from the cytotrophoblastic shell, emphasizing that it is by examination of placentae *in situ* that this scenario emerges as the most likely one.

Research on trophoblast invasion received a substantial boost by the clinical finding of placental hypoperfusion in hypertensive pregnancies, indicating a link which had not been considered before (Chapters 2 and 3). At the time of the discovery of the 'physiological changes' of spiral arteries in the pregnant uterus, Brosens *et al.* suggested that these changes result from the destructive action of the invading trophoblasts on the vascular smooth muscle and the elastic membrane [6]. It became clear, however, that also a maternal contribution has to be considered in both the decidua and the JZ myometrium (Chapter 4). Based upon histological studies of well-timed early pregnant hysterectomy specimens as well as numerous third-trimester placental bed biopsies, we distinguished four main steps in spiral artery remodeling: (1) decidua-associated remodeling, (2) the intraluminal appearance of migratory endovascular trophoblasts, (3) their intramural incorporation and trophoblast-associated remodeling, and (4) maternal re-endothelialization and other maternal tissue repair processes (Fig. 11.1) [7]. In this chapter we will reiterate our main findings regarding the successive remodeling steps.

Spiral artery remodeling as a multistep process

Step one: decidua-associated remodeling

During the decidualization of the endometrium, starting in the late luteal phase of the menstrual cycle, morphological alterations occur in the spiral arteries, presumably under progesterone control. This early vascular remodeling involves the perivascular as well as the intimal layers. Perivascular sheaths of swollen decidual cells ('Streeter's columns') appear as early as postovulatory day 11 [3]. According to Brettner, some of the swollen perivascular cells are derived from vascular smooth muscle [8]. Craven and colleagues described intimal (endothelial) and medial vacuolization as well as vascular smooth muscle disorganization in the decidua of early abortion samples (9 ± 3 weeks since the last menstrual period, LMP) [9].

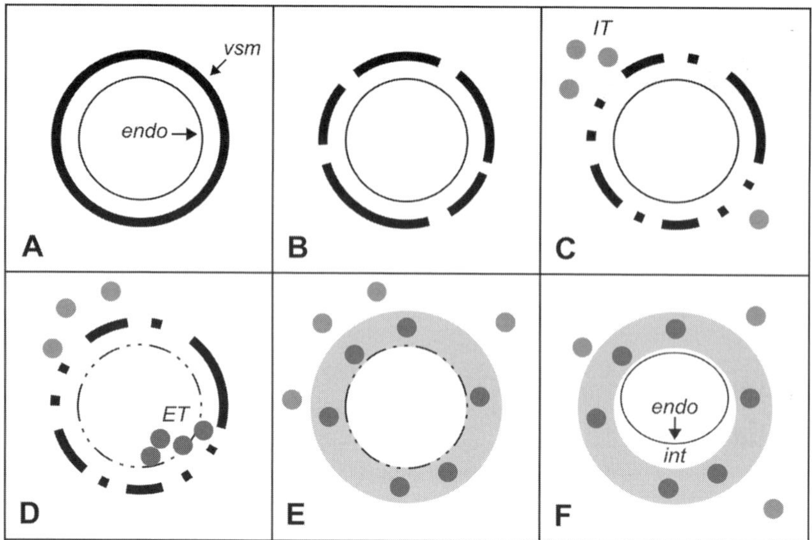

Fig. 11.1 Diagrammatic representation of spiral artery remodeling steps. A: unmodified spiral artery (*endo*, endothelium; *vsm*, vascular smooth muscle). B: step one, decidua-associated remodeling with disorganization of vascular smooth muscle. C: step two, interstitial trophoblast (*IT*) invasion enhances vascular smooth muscle disorganization. D: endovascular trophoblast (*ET*) temporarily replaces the endothelium. E: step 3, intramural incorporation of endovascular trophoblast and deposition of fibrinoid, replacing the vascular smooth muscle. F: step 4, re-endothelialization and intimal thickening (*int*).

Unfortunately they unintentionally confused the literature by referring to this process as a 'physiological change', the term previously introduced to specifically describe trophoblast-associated vascular changes [7]. Angiogenic growth factors (VEGFs, PlGF, angiopoietins) are presently considered to be potentially important inducers of this early remodeling. Such molecules can be released by various cell types in the decidualized endometrium, but especially by the uterine natural killer (uNK) cells [10].

Early vascular changes, preceding endovascular migration, also occur in the JZ myometrium. Endothelial vacuolization, edema of the vessel wall, disintegration of the elastica, and changes in the smooth muscle cells have been described (Fig. 11.2) [11,12] and can be considered as an extension of the decidualization process initiated in the endometrium. Unfortunately, myometrial vascular changes have only been studied from the 8th week onwards (since LMP), at a time when this JZ compartment is already being invaded by interstitial trophoblast, which precludes an easy discrimination between the decidua-associated changes and those induced by the trophoblast. This invasion pathway into the JZ myometrium precedes the appearance of intravascular cells in this tissue compartment for a period of about 6 weeks [12]. Certain vascular alterations, such as intimal vacuolation, can also be observed outside the placental bed, i.e. in the myometrial compartment underlying the decidua vera, while vascular smooth muscle disorganization and loss of elastica in the placental bed myometrium are more closely related to the presence of interstitial trophoblast. It is not yet clear which cell types may release angiogenic factors in the JZ myometrium since uNK cells are reported to be absent from this tissue compartment [13]. A recent immunohistochemical study demonstrated the presence of VEGFs as well as angiopoietins in both interstitial and endovascular trophoblasts from 8 weeks onwards [14]. It is therefore not inconceivable that the lack of angiogenesis-stimulating uNK cells in the JZ myometrium is amply compensated by the presence of interstitially invading trophoblast, preceding the arrival of endovascular trophoblasts.

Step two: trophoblast invasion and intra-arterial migration

In early pregnancy, invasion of the decidua by trophoblast is initiated by the disintegration of the trophoblastic shell, and subsequently replenished by the cell columns of the anchoring villi [15]. Invasion follows an interstitial and an endovascular course, the latter occurring in spiral arteries but never in veins. Interstitial, but not endovascular, trophoblasts subsequently fuse to form multinuclear giant cells [16]. Although giant cells are by their size the most striking interstitial cells, the mononuclear cytotrophoblasts seem to be the most invasive, occupying extensive areas of the uterine wall within a relatively short time. Oddly enough, in their extensive review of the subject Boyd and Hamilton [17] ignored the

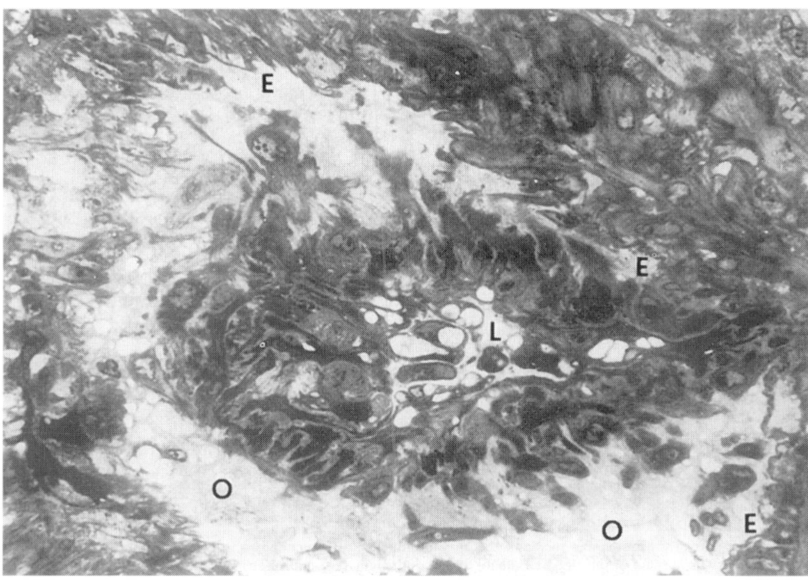

Fig. 11.2 Decidua-associated remodeling of spiral artery in the junctional zone myometrium at 14 weeks (*L*, lumen; *O*, edema; *E*, internal elastic lamina). Reproduced with permission from Brosens *et al.* [11], Copyright Elsevier (1975).

mononuclear trophoblast invasion and focused on the giant 'wandering cells', probably because Hertig's observations on early postimplantation stages seemed to indicate that the primary invasive cells are multinuclear [18]. In consequence, by focusing on giant cells they missed the overwhelming numbers of basophilic mononuclear cells in between the dispersed smooth muscle elements of the JZ myometrium. Quantitative studies indicated that their distribution shifts from a peak density at the center of the placental bed (weeks 8–14 since LMP) toward a biphasic distribution (weeks 16–18), thus following a ring-like pattern toward the periphery of the placental bed [19]. It is thought that, after their fusion to giant cells, these cells have lost some of their invasive potential. Interstitial invasion of stromal tissues obviously requires the secretion of proteolytic enzymes, particularly matrix metalloproteinases for digesting intercellular matrix components [20,21]. During endometrial decidualization, selective breakdown of some extracellular matrix components occurs independently of any trophoblast action, probably allowing easier penetration of the decidualized tissue [22]. It is not clear whether a similar matrix degradation also occurs spontaneously in the JZ myometrium, as an extension of the endometrial decidualization process. The loosening of the inner myometrium is likely to be amplified by the action of invading interstitial trophoblast, which also contributes to the disorganization of spiral artery smooth muscle [12].

In the human, interstitial invasion of decidua and JZ myometrium precedes spiral artery invasion for a period of several weeks. In early pregnancy mononuclear trophoblasts plug the outlets of spiral arteries at the basal plate, and thus create a low oxygen environment for the developing placenta and fetus [23,24,25] (see also Chapter 8). The exact time period when the intraluminal migration of endovascular trophoblast is initiated is not known. Following the early plugging stage [1,23,26], endovascular trophoblast may be found at various depths in the decidua from 8 weeks onwards [27]. After 10 weeks the whole length of the decidual spiral arteries may contain trophoblast, even reaching the most superficial vascular sections in the JZ myometrium (Fig. 11.3). Using a catching metaphor, Ramsey compared the appearance of sheets of trophoblastic cells migrating along the distended luminal surface to the dripping of wax down the side of a candle [28]. Deep invasion of the myometrial segments of the spiral arteries is not seen before 15 weeks [12] (Figs. 11.3 and 11.4). The several weeks' delay of the arrival of endovascular trophoblasts in the JZ myometrium compared to the decidua provided the inspiration for the 'two wave hypothesis' of endovascular migration [12] (see also Chapter 4). Since the decidual spiral artery segments are usually rather thin-walled, some interstitial cells may 'intravasate' into the arteries at this level, which is the more likely since in the decidua these trophoblasts are often densely clustered around the vessels. This perivascular aggregation by

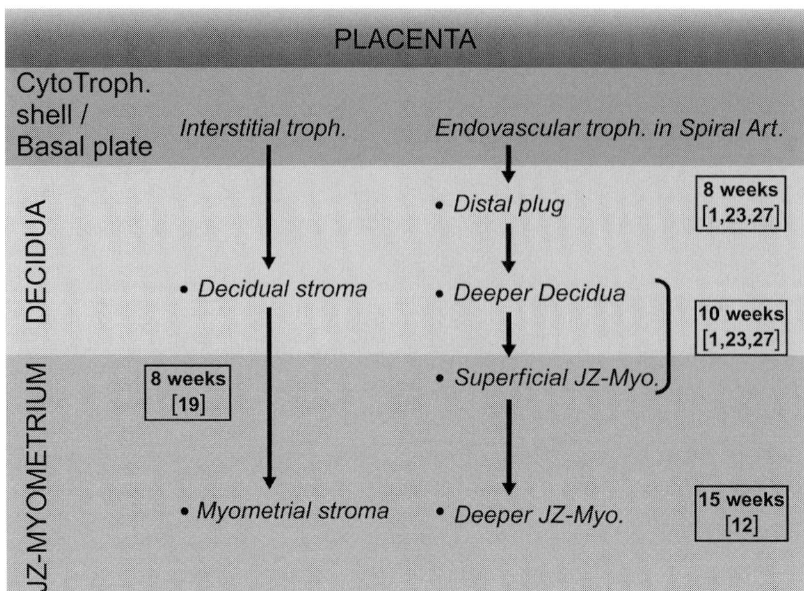

Fig. 11.3 Diagrammatic representation of the timing of interstitial and endovascular trophoblast invasion of the decidua and the junctional zone (JZ) myometrium.

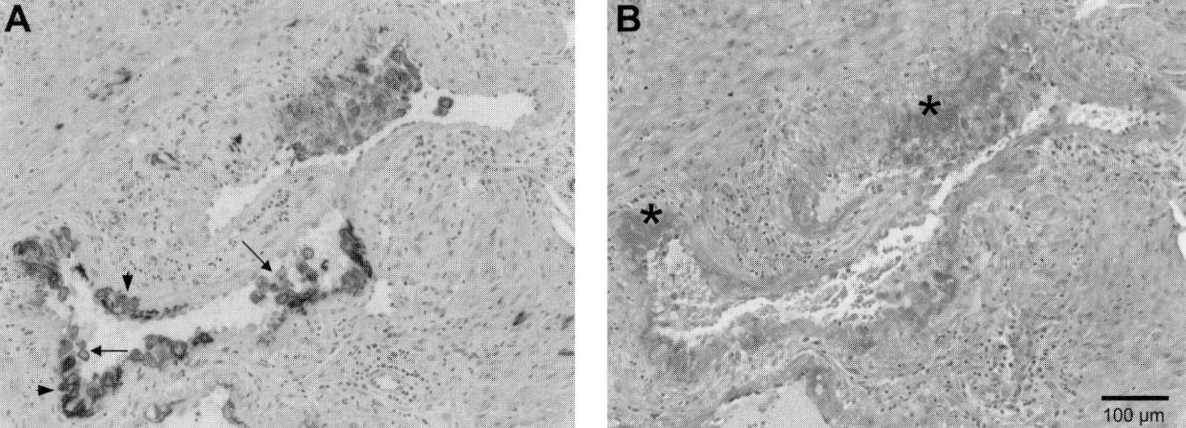

Fig. 11.4 Section of a myometrial spiral artery at 15 weeks, immunostained for cytokeratin (A), showing endovascular trophoblast in the artery lumen (arrowed), and PAS (periodic acid Schiff) to reveal fibrinoid in the vessel wall (B, asterisks). Some of the trophoblasts are being embedded into the vessel wall (arrowheads).

interstitial trophoblast is not so striking in the JZ myometrium, where interstitial trophoblasts are more evenly spread. Furthermore, the thicker vessel walls in this region, compared to the decidua, may well impede 'intravasation'. This, together with frequent observations of continuous 'streaks' of luminal trophoblast in accordance with Ramsey's 'candle wax dripping', made us believe that most of the endovascular trophoblasts appearing deep in the JZ myometrial spiral arteries must have migrated from the decidual segments following an intravascular route.

Step three: trophoblast-associated remodeling

While the previous step merely involves the appearance of intraluminal trophoblasts, in the next remodeling step the trophoblasts are incorporated into the arterial wall. By this process the maternal spiral artery is effectively converted – at least temporarily – into a 'fetal' blood vessel. This vascular incorporation is initiated by the penetration of the endothelium. Electron microscopic studies have shown that intraluminal trophoblasts penetrate between healthy endothelial cells and cross the underlying basement membrane [29]. The question as to whether the endothelium is ever completely replaced has never been adequately answered however. It is not inconceivable that the persistence of endothelial streaks between invading trophoblasts may have fuelled the idea that endovascular trophoblast may acquire an endothelial phenotype [30], a concept that was eagerly supported by some but criticized by other investigators [31,32].

Co-culture experiments of trophoblast and explanted arterial segments revealed that trophoblasts are able to induce apoptosis in endothelial and vascular smooth muscle cells [33,34,35] (see also Chapter 14). Possibly the previously described smooth muscle disorganization (step 1) facilitates trophoblast penetration of the arterial wall, which might be enhanced by matrix metalloproteinase secretion by intraluminal trophoblast [36]. This smooth muscle penetration ultimately leads to its replacement by trophoblast embedded within a fibrinoid matrix, probably secreted by the trophoblasts themselves [29] although plasma proteins also may be precipitated in this material. During the replacement of the vascular smooth muscle the elastica also disappears, and the spiral artery thus becomes 'physiologically changed'. Indeed, following the muscular loss the vessel no longer shows vasomotor activities and must therefore be passively distended by the increasing maternal flow, while the disappearance of the elastica precludes a rebounding of the artery to its initial size. Intramural trophoblasts subsequently acquire a characteristic spider-like shape, possibly related to an increasing accumulation of fibrinoid material between extending cell processes. As a rule such cells remain mononuclear or at the most may become binuclear, which sets them apart from the differentiation pathway observed in the interstitial trophoblast.

Step four: re-endothelialization and other maternal repair responses

The first reports about physiological changes in the placental bed were still cautious regarding the possible derivation of the intramural fibrinoid-embedded cells from intraluminal trophoblast [7,37]. Indeed, a different – seemingly maternal – tissue layer is often positioned between the fibrinoid-embedded cells in the wall and the vessel lumen. Infiltration by inflammatory cells or thrombus formation with recanalization

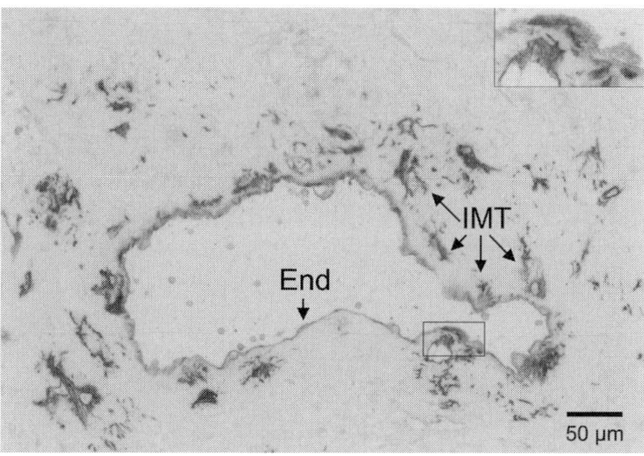

Fig. 11.5 Cytokeratin (black)/CD31 (grey) double immunostaining of a remodeled spiral artery, illustrating endothelial repair (*End*) after intramural incorporation of the trophoblast (*IMT*). The insert is a high-power picture showing a trophoblastic cell very close to the lumen, covered by a very thin layer of endothelium. Reproduced with permission from Pijnenborg *et al.* [7], Copyright Elsevier (2006). See plate section for color version.

have been considered as likely consequences of endothelial damage caused by penetrating trophoblast. Although it is stated in the literature over and over again that the endothelium is replaced by trophoblast during the remainder of the pregnancy, re-endothelialization definitely occurs, as shown by double immunostaining for trophoblast and endothelial cell markers (Fig. 11.5). A restored endothelial lining is indeed present in the large majority of remodeled spiral arteries in third trimester placental bed biopsies [38]. It is not known whether the maternal vascular lining is repaired by endothelial remnants which were still present after the intramural invasion, or whether a new endothelial covering may be derived from circulating endothelial progenitor cells [39].

The presence of patches of thickened intima is a regular feature of remodeled spiral arteries, but it does not consistently occur in all vessels. Intima thickening may result from maternal repair processes, possibly also after retraction of a blood clot adhering to a damaged segment of the vessel wall. Such cushions of connective tissue may be more common in bends of vessels which follow an extremely spiral course, suggesting an effect of shear forces created by turbulent flow. A characteristic feature of such thickened intimae is the presence of α-actin-immunopositive myointimal cells, which are thought to act as precursor cells for postpartum repair of the vascular smooth muscle (Fig. 11.6).

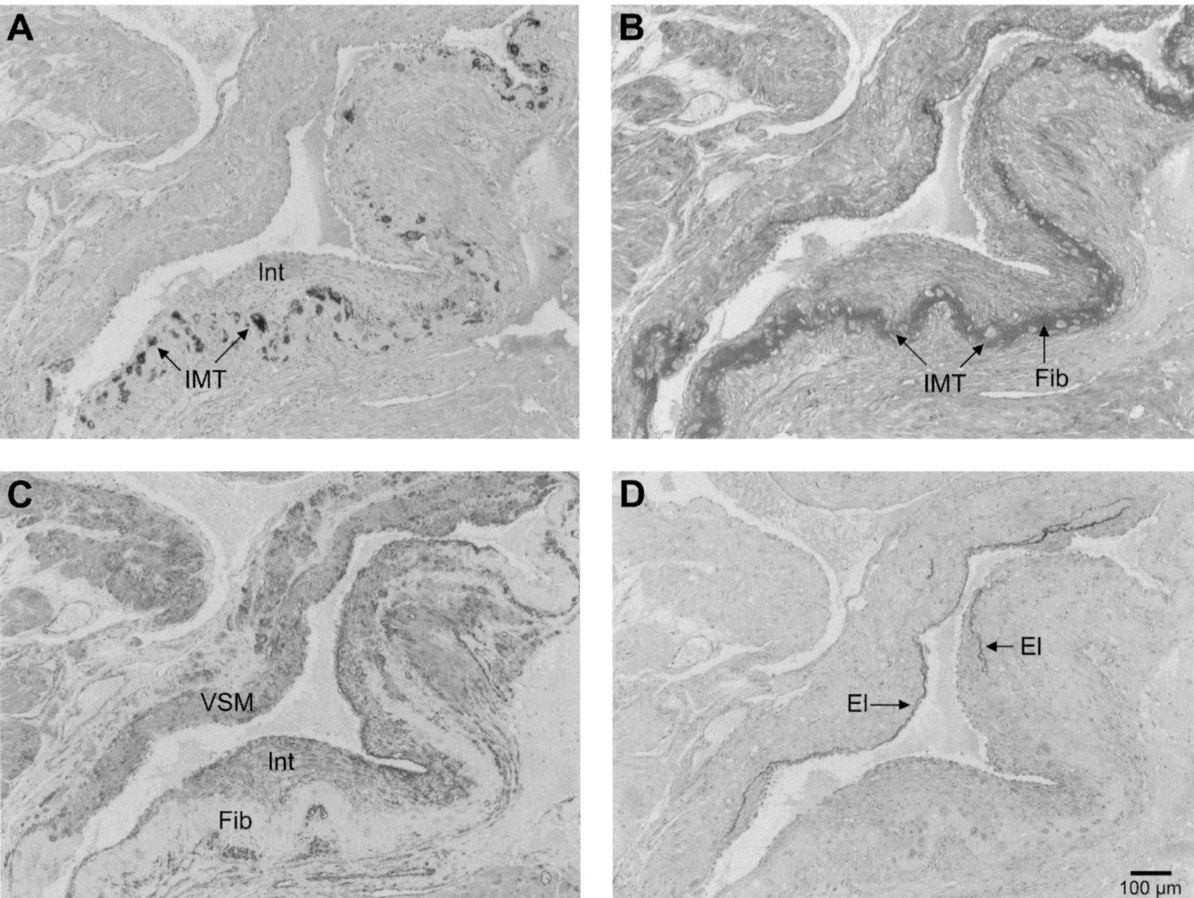

Fig. 11.6 Partial vascular remodeling in parallel sections stained (A) for cytokeratin, (B) with PAS to show the fibrinoid, (C) for α-actin, and (D) with acid orcein to show the elastica. (A) shows intramural trophoblast (*IMT*) partially covered by an intimal cushion (*Int*). (B) illustrates intramural trophoblast (*IMT*) incorporation in fibrinoid (*Fib*). (C) shows α-actin-immunopositive vascular smooth muscle (*VSM*) at the non-invaded part of the vessel, as well as α-actin-immunopositive myointimal cells in the intima (*Int*) overlying the unstained fibrinoid (*Fib*). In (D) the elastica (*El*) is obvious in the non-invaded parts of the vessel, ending abruptly at the beginning of the fibrinoid zone. Reproduced with permission from Pijnenborg *et al.* [7], Copyright Elsevier (2006).

Spiral artery remodeling related to uteroplacental flow

The extensive investigations of Jauniaux and colleagues have contributed a lot to our present understanding of the uteroplacental flow in early pregnancy [24,25] (see also Chapter 8). It seems therefore appropriate to relate the time-course of the vascular remodeling process to the new insights in uteroplacental flow changes during this pregnancy period. The curve representing changes in intervillous oxygen tension has a sigmoid shape, showing a steep rise in the 10–12 weeks period (Fig. 11.7) [25]. Preceding this marked rise, oxygen levels gradually increase from the earliest studied period (7 weeks) onwards. 'Revisiting' the Boyd collection, Burton [26] described the absence of connecting channels between spiral arteries and the intervillous space at 7 weeks and their appearance at 8 weeks. From that period onwards, the endovascular plugs of endovascular trophoblast at the arterial outlets gradually disintegrate, endovascular trophoblasts appear at different levels in the decidual spiral artery segments, and from 10 weeks onwards their invasion can be extended over the whole thickness of the decidua [27]. The 7–10 weeks early rise of intervillous flow apparently occurs simultaneously with the decidua-associated remodeling and endovascular trophoblast migration into the decidual segments, but it is obviously impossible to draw conclusions about causality. Deeply invaded endovascular trophoblasts were observed in the

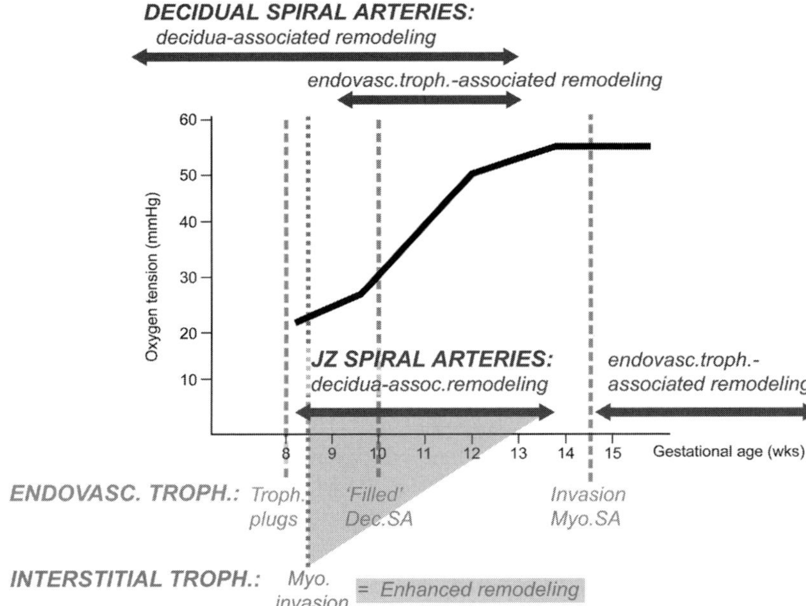

Fig. 11.7 Placental oxygen tension curve (redrawn from Jauniaux *et al.* 2000 [25]), with indications of successive steps in endovascular and interstitial invasion in the decidua and the junctional zone (JZ) myometrium. Interstitial invasion is associated with enhanced decidua-associated remodeling (shaded triangle) in the myometrial spiral arteries (SA).

myometrial segments from 15 weeks onwards [12], well after the steep 10–12 weeks rise in placental oxygen (Fig 11.7). Therefore this deep invasion 'wave' itself cannot be the cause but may occur as a response to the rising placental oxygen/intervillous flow. On the other hand, the preceding vascular remodeling of the myometrial segments does occur during the 8–14 weeks period and may therefore play a role in accommodating the vessels to the increasing flow. Subsequent intramural incorporation of the invaded trophoblast is associated with complete removal of the smooth muscle and elastica layers, thus transforming the vessels into the widely opened rigid tubes which are able to continuously deliver high volumes of blood to the intervillous space. The early remodeling steps in the myometrial segments may therefore provide an essential preparation for the steep rise of uteroplacental flow, while the subsequent trophoblast-associated remodeling stabilizes the vessels to sustain this increased flow.

Topology of vascular remodeling in the placental bed

In the previous paragraph, spiral artery remodeling has been described as a straightforward process occurring in all the spiral arteries throughout the placental bed. It has to be questioned how far this is true. We already alluded to cell density gradients of interstitial trophoblast from the center to the margins of the placental bed [18]. Since at 18 weeks one-third of the placental bed spiral arteries showed deep endovascular invasion into their myometrial segments, it was tentatively suggested that during the remainder of pregnancy the non-invaded vessels also might be gradually invaded and remodeled [11]. However, this 8–18 weeks period may delimit the time of maximal invasion, which thereafter might gradually decline. In Doppler studies at 17–20 weeks, Matijevic and colleagues found higher impedance to flow in spiral arteries in the periphery than in the central placental bed [40], but did not see a tendency of change during the studied time period. Unfortunately, few complete placental beds have ever been studied histologically at term. Only Brosens [41] reported observations on the extent of spiral artery remodeling in a complete hysterectomy specimen with attached placenta at the end of a normal pregnancy, noting an absence of vascular remodeling at the periphery of the placental bed, thus indicating a lateral gradient of diminished invasion depth near the placental edge. In a major review Robertson and colleagues discussed briefly the topological problem of distinguishing peripheral from central placental bed biopsies, suggesting the paucity of interstitial giant cells in the myometrium as a useful criterion [42]. Another useful feature for recognizing peripheral parts of the placental bed is the presence of stacks of endometrial glands, which tend to be pushed aside by the growing placenta. Robertson *et al.* concluded that also in normal pregnancy vascular remodeling may be restricted to the decidual spiral artery segments in the most peripheral parts of the placental bed.

In preeclampsia, trophoblast-associated remodeling is restricted to decidual spiral arteries throughout the placental bed [43]. Khong and colleagues reported that even decidual segments may show defective remodeling [44]. This observation is suggestive for a gradient of failed invasion starting already at the decidual compartment rather than an abrupt hindrance to deeper myometrial invasion. In a rare specimen of a complete placental bed of a preeclamptic woman at term, Brosens saw physiological changes in myometrial segments in a few vessels only at the very center of the placental bed [41], indicating a dramatic shift in the lateral gradient of diminished invasion depth, which in normal cases is only visible near the placental periphery. This observation once again highlights the potential difficulty in interpreting trophoblast invasion in a placental bed biopsy of uncertain location.

Impaired spiral artery remodeling

Spiral artery conversion is obviously important for safeguarding an adequate maternal blood supply to the placenta. It is well documented that maternal placental perfusion is seriously impaired in preeclampsia, and several studies have indicated a relationship between abnormal Doppler flow patterns and impaired placental bed invasion and vascular remodeling [45,46,47,48,49]. Although the precise mechanism of defective remodeling is still unknown, it seems logical to consider possible defects in each of the successive steps of vascular remodeling.

Step one: failed decidua-associated remodeling?

The idea that a decidualization defect, which would include a failure of the first step in vascular remodeling, may prevent subsequent invasion and further vascular change, is attractive but there is still a paucity of supporting data (Chapter 4). This defect may already be present during the late luteal phase of the cycle, and it has been argued that repeated cycles of menstrual shedding of decidualizing endometrium may act as a preconditioning for successful implantation and deep placentation [50]. Decidualization of the endometrium is associated with an infiltration by uNK cells, which are now considered to be major effector cells for local trophoblast–uterine interaction (Chapter 6). Since uNK cells seem to be important agents for vascular smooth muscle remodeling in mice, Croy [51] hypothesized that a deficiency of these cells might similarly lead to defective early remodeling in human spiral arteries and thus create a high risk of preeclampsia. This has been confirmed by a recent quantitative study of leucocyte populations in the placental bed decidua in preeclampsia as well as fetal growth restriction [62]. However, recent evidence revealed that uNK cell-associated defects of trophoblast invasion may be due to disturbed ligand–receptor interactions between the two cell types, rather than lower or higher cell numbers [52]. Uterine NK cells are apparently absent in the JZ myometrium [13], but their angiogenic action might be taken over by interstitially invading trophoblast [14]. Defective early remodeling may theoretically result from impaired interstitial invasion, but there is no consensus about possible defects of this invasion pathway in preeclampsia [6].

Step two: failed trophoblast migration?

As suggested in Chapter 4, a failed integrin-shift had been regarded as a likely mechanism for disturbed intra-arterial migration of trophoblast [53]. Also a failure of the trophoblast to acquire an endothelial phenotype had been advocated as a possible factor in failed migration [54]. In addition to the question of adhesion molecules, there is also a report of disturbed HLA-G expression by extravillous trophoblast, which may impair fetal–maternal interaction [55] leading to macrophage attack and/or induction of apoptosis [56,57], thus preventing deeper migration. None of these proposed mechanisms has been completely convincing so far. On the other hand, if trophoblast migration is indeed regulated by uteroplacental flow, an impaired rise in blood flow, as a result of defective decidualization and disturbed angiogenesis, might be considered as possible causes of defective invasion.

Step three: failed trophoblast-associated remodeling?

Failure of trophoblast-associated vascular remodeling may also result from impaired intramural incorporation of endovascular trophoblast and/or lack of fibrinoid deposition. Failed penetration of the arterial wall may be caused by an impaired production or secretion of proteinases. Although there is evidence that proteinase secretion is reduced in cultured trophoblast of preeclamptic placentae [58], the study was performed on villous trophoblast isolated from term pregnancies, which cannot be representative for extravillous trophoblast of the active invasion period. Since trophoblast-associated vascular remodeling presumably also depends on the clearing of vascular smooth muscle by apoptosis induction (Chapter 15) [34,35], this process might be inadequate in preeclampsia because of defective trophoblast signaling. Also this particular aspect merits further investigation. Finally, defects in fibrinoid deposition could be postulated. Unfortunately, nothing is known about the existence of possible factors which might stimulate or inhibit the formation of this intramural material of unknown composition. A definite feature of failed remodeling is the maintenance of the vascular smooth muscle and elastica. Robertson and colleagues suggested that hypertension-associated hyperplasia of smooth muscle may interfere with the normal physiological change of the spiral arteries [37,42]. When this condition is present subclinically before pregnancy, the preexisting media hyperplasia might also interfere with early decidua-associated remodeling.

Step four: increased maternal inflammatory responses?

Since trophoblast invasion inevitably induces maternal tissue repair responses as indicated by the presence of inflammatory cells even in normal pregnancies, it is not inconceivable that in certain conditions such responses may become somewhat unsettled. A maternal 'overreaction' might theoretically lead to the elimination of invading trophoblast. The presence of high numbers of maternal inflammatory cells in some trophoblast-invaded areas has been described before [59], but such rather dramatic pictures are not exclusively associated with preeclampsia. It is not unlikely that the acute atherosis lesion (Chapter 3) may be the result of such 'overreaction', with heavy infiltration by macrophages (lipophages) [60] and local tissue destruction, including elimination of invaded trophoblast. Occasionally remnants of trophoblast may indeed be found in such vessels [61].

Conclusions

Deep trophoblast invasion and spiral artery remodeling of the inner 'junctional zone' myometrium is a feature of normal human pregnancy, while in preeclampsia and maybe in other pregnancy complications this process may be seriously impaired. Whether or not a failed vascular remodeling of myometrial spiral arteries is to be regarded as the primary pathogenic mechanism is a different matter, since we are still largely ignorant about the regulation of early trophoblast invasion. Further research should therefore be directed to unravel the mechanisms of the different steps in the remodeling process using a variety of approaches, including the use of experimental animals (see Chapter 13). It is not unlikely that different pathogenic pathways – related to the subsequent remodeling steps – may lead to a common manifestation of the disease, which has long been considered as a disease of theories. Also, with the growing awareness of a possible link between subfertility and pregnancy complications, these considerations might be valuable for the future management of human reproductive failure.

References

1. Hamilton W J, Boyd J D. Development of the human placenta in the first three months of gestation. *J Anat* 1960; **94**: 297–328.
2. Hamilton W J, Boyd J D. Trophoblast in human utero-placental arteries. *Nature* 1966; **212**: 906–8.
3. Harris J W S, Ramsey E M. The morphology of human uteroplacental vasculature. *Contrib Embryol* 1966; **38**: 43–58.
4. Grosser O. Die Placenta maternal. In: *Frühentwicklung, Eihautbildung und Placentation des Menschen und der Säugetiere*. München: Verlag von JF Bergmann; 1927: pp. 363–71.
5. Kaufmann P, Black S, Huppertz B. Endovascular trophoblast invasion: implications for the pathogenesis of intrauterine growth retardation and preeclampsia. *Biol Reprod* 2003; **69**: 1–7.
6. Brosens I, Robertson W B, Dixon H G. The physiological response of the vessels of the placental bed to normal pregnancy. *J Pathol Bacteriol* 1967; **93**: 569–79.
7. Pijnenborg R, Vercruysse L, Hanssens M. The uterine spiral arteries in human pregnancy: facts and controversies. *Placenta* 2006; **27**: 939–58.
8. Brettner A. Zum Verhalten der Sekundären Wand der Uteroplacentargefässe bei der Decidualen Reaksion. *Acta Anat* 1964; **57**: 367–76.
9. Craven C M, Morgan T, Ward K. Decidual spiral artery remodelling begins before cellular interaction with cytotrophoblasts. *Placenta* 1998; **19**: 241–52.
10. Li X F, Charnock-Jones S, Zhang E *et al.* Angiogenic growth factor messenger ribonucleic acids in uterine natural killer cells. *J Clin Endocr Metab* 2001; **86**: 1823–34.

11. Brosens I A. Discussion. *Eur J Obstet Gynec Reprod Biol* 1975; **5**: 47–65.

12. Pijnenborg R, Bland J M, Robertson W B, Brosens I. Uteroplacental arterial changes related to interstitial trophoblast migration in early human pregnancy. *Placenta* 1983; **4**: 397–414.

13. Bulmer J N, Lash G E. Human uterine natural killer cells: a reappraisal. *Mol Immunol* 2005; **42**: 511–21.

14. Schiessl B, Innes B A, Bulmer J N *et al.* Localization of angiogenic growth factors and their receptors in the human placental bed throughout normal human pregnancy. *Placenta* 2009; 30: 79–87.

15. Damsky C H, Fitzgerald M L, Fisher S J. Distribution patterns of extracellular matrix components and adhesion receptors are intricately modulated during first trimester cytotrophoblast differentiation along the invasive pathway, in vivo. *J Clin Invest* 1992; **89**: 210–22.

16. Coutifaris C, Kao L C, Sehdev H M *et al.* E-cadherin expression during the differentiation of human trophoblasts. *Development* 1991; **113**: 767–777.

17. Boyd J D, Hamilton W J. The giant cells of the pregnant human uterus. *J Obstet Gyn Br Emp* 1960; **67**: 208–18.

18. Hertig A T, Rock J, Adams E C. A description of 34 human ova within the first 17 days of development. *Am J Anat* 1956; **98**: 435–94.

19. Pijnenborg R, Bland J M, Robertson W B, Dixon G, Brosens I. The pattern of interstitial trophoblastic invasion of the myometrium in early human pregnancy. *Placenta* 1981; **2**: 303–16.

20. Nawrocki B, Polette M, Maquoi E, Birembaut B. Expression of matrix metalloproteinases and their inhibitors during human placental development. *Trophoblast Res* 1997; **10**: 97–113.

21. Huppertz B, Kertschanska S, Demir A Y, Frank H G, Kaufmann P. Immunohistochemistry of matrix metalloproteinases (MMP), their substrates, and their inhibitors (TIMP) during trophoblast invasion in the human placenta. *Cell Tissue Res* 1998; **291**: 133–48.

22. Aplin J D, Charlton A J, Ayad S. An immunohistochemical study of human endometrial extracellular matrix during the menstrual cycle and first trimester of pregnancy. *Cell Tissue Res* 1988; **253**: 231–40.

23. Hustin J, Schaaps J P. Echocardiographic and anatomic studies of the maternotrophoblastic border during the first trimester of pregnancy. *Am J Obstet Gynecol* 1987; **157**: 162–8.

24. Rodesch F, Simon P, Donner C, Jauniaux E. Oxygen measurements in endometrial and trophoblastic tissues during early pregnancy. *Obstet Gynecol* 1992; **80**: 283–5.

25. Jauniaux E, Watson A L, Hempstock J *et al.* Onset of maternal arterial blood flow and placental oxidative stress. *Am J Pathol* 2000; **157**: 2111–22.

26. Burton G J, Jauniaux E, Watson A L. Maternal arterial connections to the placental intervillous space during the first trimester of human pregnancy: the Boyd collection revisited. *Am J Obstet Gynecol* 1999; **181**: 718–24.

27. Pijnenborg R, Dixon G, Robertson W B, Brosens I. Trophoblast invasion of human decidua from 8 to 18 weeks of pregnancy. *Placenta* 1980; **1**: 3–19.

28. Ramsey E M, Donner M W. *Placental vasculature and circulation.* Stuttgart: Georg Thieme; 1980: p. 12.

29. De Wolf F, De Wolf-Peeters C, Brosens I, Robertson W B. The human placental bed: electron microscopic study of trophoblastic invasion of spiral arteries. *Am J Obstet Gynecol* 1980; **137**: 58–70.

30. Zhou Y, Fisher S J, Janatpour M J *et al.* Human cytotrophoblasts adopt a vascular phenotype as they differentiate: a strategy for successful endovascular invasion? *J Clin Invest* 1997; **99**: 2139–51.

31. Pijnenborg R, Vercruysse L, Verbist L, Van Assche F A. Interaction of interstitial trophoblast with placental bed capillaries and venules of normotensive and pre-eclamptic pregnancies. *Placenta* 1988; **19**: 569–75.

32. Lyall F, Bulmer J N, Duffie E *et al.* Human trophoblast invasion and spiral artery transformation: the role of PECAM-1 in normal pregnancy, preeclampsia, and fetal growth restriction. *Am J Pathol* 2001; **158**: 1713–21.

33. Ashton S V, Whitley G St J, Dash P R *et al.* Uterine spiral artery remodeling involves endothelial apoptosis induced by extravillous trophoblasts through Fas/FasL interactions. *Artioscler Thromb Vasc Biol* 2005; **25**: 102–8.

34. Harris L K, Keogh R J, Wareing M *et al.* Invasive trophoblasts stimulate vascular smooth muscle cell apoptosis by a Fas ligand-dependent mechanism. *Am J Pathol* 2006; **169**: 1863–74.

35. Keogh R J, Harris L K, Freeman A *et al.* Fetal-derived trophoblasts use the apoptotic cytokine tumor necrosis factor-α-related apoptosis-inducing ligand to induce smooth muscle cell death. *Circ Res* 2007; **100**: 834–41.

36. Fernandez P L, Merino M J, Nogales F F *et al.* Immunohistochemical profile of basement membrane proteins and 72 kilodalton Type IV collagenase in the implantation placental site. *Lab Invest* 1992; **66**: 572–9.

37. Robertson W B, Brosens I, Dixon G. Uteroplacental vascular pathology. *Eur J Obstet Gynecol Reprod Biol* 1975; **5**: 47–65.

38. Khong T Y, Sawyer I H, Heryet A R. An immunohistologic study of endothelialization of uteroplacental vessels in human pregnancy. *Am J Obstet Gynecol* 1992; **167**: 751–6.

39. Robb A O, Mills N L, Newby D E, Denison F C. Endothelial progenitor cells in pregnancy. *Reproduction* 2007; **133**: 1–9.

40. Matijevic R, Meekins J W, Walkinshaw S A *et al.* Spiral artery blood flow in the central and peripheral areas of the placental bed in the second trimester. *Obstet Gynecol* 1995; **86**: 289–92.

41. Brosens I. The utero-placental vessels at term – the distribution and extent of physiological changes. *Trophoblast Res* 1988; **3**: 61–7.

42. Robertson W B, Khong T Y, Brosens I *et al.* The placental bed biopsy: review from three European centers. *Am J Obstet Gynecol* 1986; **155**: 401–12.

43. Brosens I, Robertson W B, Dixon H G. The role of the spiral arteries in the pathogenesis of pre-eclampsia. *Obstet Gynecol Annu* 1972; **1**: 177–91.

44. Khong T Y, De Wolf F, Robertson W B, Brosens I. Inadequate maternal vascular response to placentation in pregnancies complicated by pre-eclampsia and by small-for-gestational age infants. *Br J Obstet Gynaecol* 1986; **93**: 1049–59.

45. Aardema M W, Oosterhof H, Timmer A, van Rooy I, Aarnoudse J G. Uterine artery Doppler flow and uteroplacental vascular pathology in normal pregnancies and pregnancies complicated by pre-eclampsia and small for gestational age fetuses. *Placenta* 2001; **22**: 405–11.

46. Lin S, Shimizu I, Suehara N, Nakayama M, Aono T. Uterine artery Doppler velocimetry in relation to trophoblast migration into the myometrium of the placental bed. *Obstet Gynecol* 1995; **85**: 760–5.

47. Olofsson P. A high uterine pulsatility index reflects a defective development of placental bed spiral arteries in pregnancies complicated by hypertension and fetal growth retardation. *Eur J Obstet Gynecol Reprod Biol* 1993; **49**: 161–8.

48. Sagol S, Özkinay E, Öztekin K, Özdemir N. The comparison of uterine artery Doppler velocimetry with the histopathology of the placental bed. *Aust NZ J Obstet Gynaecol* 1999; **39**: 324–9.

49. Voigt H J, Becker V. Doppler flow measurements and histomorphology of the placental bed in uteroplacental insufficiency. *J Perinat Med* 1992; **20**: 139–47.

50. Brosens J J, Parker M G, McIndoe A, Pijnenborg R, Brosens I A. A role for menstruation in preconditioning the uterus for successful pregnancy. *Am J Obstet Gynecol*, in press.

51. Croy B A, Ashkar A A, Minhas K, Greenwood J D. Can murine uterine natural killer cells give insights into the pathogenesis of preeclampsia? *J Soc Gynecol Invest* 2000; 7: 12–20.

52. Moffett A, Hiby S E. How does the maternal immune system contribute to the development of pre-eclampsia? *Placenta* 2007; **28** (**Suppl A**): S51–S56.

53. Zhou Y, Damsky C H, Chiu K, Roberts J M, Fisher S J. Preeclampsia is associated with abnormal expression of adhesion molecules by invasive cytotrophoblasts. *J Clin Invest* 1993; **91**: 950–60.

54. Zhou Y, Damsky C H, Fisher S J. Preeclampsia is associated with failure of human cytotrophoblasts to mimic a vascular adhesion phenotype. *J Clin Invest* 1997; **99**: 2152–64.

55. Goldman-Wohl D S, Ariel I, Greenfield D *et al.* Lack of human leukocyte antigen-G expression in extravillous trophoblasts is associated with pre-eclampsia. *Mol Human Reprod* 2000; **6**: 88–95.

56. DiFederico E, Genbacev O, Fisher S J. Preeclampsia is associated with widespread apoptosis of placental cytotrophoblasts within the uterine wall. *Am J Pathol* 1999; **155**: 293–301.

57. Reister F, Kingdom J, Frank H G *et al.* Maternal leukocyte sub-populations impair trophoblast invasiveness in preeclampsia. *Hypertens Pregnancy* 2002; **21** (**Suppl 1**): 7.

58. Graham C H, McCrae K R. Altered expression of gelatinase and surface-associated plasminogen activator activity by trophoblast cells isolated from placentas of preeclamptic patients. *Am J Obstet Gynecol* 1996; **175**: 555–62.

59. Pijnenborg R, Vercruysse L, Hanssens M, Van Assche F A. Trophoblast invasion in pre-eclampsia and other pregnancy disorders. In: Lyall F, Belfort M, eds. *Pre-eclampsia: etiology and clinical practice.* Cambridge: Cambridge University Press; 2007: pp. 3–19.

60. Hanssens M, Pijnenborg R, Keirse M J N C *et al.* Renin-like immunoreactivity in uterus and placenta from normotensive and hypertensive pregnancies. *Eur J Obstet Gynecol Reprod Biol* 1998; **81**: 177–84.

61. Meekins J W, Pijnenborg R, Hanssens M, McFadyen I R, Van Assche F A. A study of placental bed spiral arteries and trophoblast invasion in normal and severe pre-eclamptic pregnancies. *Br J Obstet Gynaecol* 1994; **101**: 669–74.

62. Williams P J, Bulmer J N, Searle R F *et al.* Altered decidual leucocyte populations in the placental bed in pre-eclampsia and foetal growth restriction: a comparison with late pregnancy. *Reproduction* 2009; **138**: 177–184.

Comparative anatomy and research models

Comparative anatomy and placental evolution

Anthony M. Carter[1] and Robert D. Martin[2]

[1]Cardiovascular and Renal Research, University of Southern Denmark, Odense, Denmark
[2]Department of Anthropology, The Field Museum, Chicago, Illinois, USA

The orders of mammals

Comparative studies of placentation across mammals have been greatly facilitated by the availability of phylogenetic trees for the entire range of placental mammals based on molecular data. Such trees have clarified major subdivisions among placentals and indicated likely phylogenetic relationships between orders. The availability of well-supported trees has greatly enhanced our capacity to reconstruct the evolution of features lacking fossil evidence, as is the case for virtually every character involved in reproduction. Broad-based studies of DNA sequences in mammals over the past decade (notably [1,2,3,4,5]) have progressively yielded molecular trees with many consistent features. A consensus supertree combining results from > 2500 partial trees and including most mammal species is particularly informative [6]. Molecular results are broadly compatible with traditional subdivisions of placental mammals into ~ 18 orders based on anatomical evidence from extant and fossil forms (Table 12.1). However, they also present a number of hitherto unexpected features. For instance, DNA-based trees have repeatedly yielded four previously unidentified high-level clusters (superorders) of placental mammals: Afrotheria, Euarchontoglires, Laurasiatheria, and Xenarthra.

Afrotheria is a novel assemblage including aardvarks, certain insectivores, elephant-shrews, hyraxes, elephants, and sirenians. One notable consequence of this assemblage is that it splits the order previously known as 'Insectivora'. Tenrecs, golden moles, and otter shrews are now often allocated to the separate order Afrosoricida within Afrotheria. The cluster Euarchontoglires combining Euarchonta (tree-shrews, colugos, primates) with Glires (lagomorphs, rodents) was less unexpected. However, inclusion of colugos as close relatives of primates had not been clearly indicated by anatomical evidence and was not widely acknowledged. It has long been suggested that tree-shrews (order Scandentia) may be related to primates, and Simpson [7] included them in the order Primates in his influential classification of mammals. But the balance of molecular evidence now indicates that colugos are actually the sister group of primates [8,9]. The proposed assemblage Laurasiatheria also fits well with many conclusions drawn from anatomical studies. It includes the remaining part of the former order 'Insectivora' along with bats, carnivores, pangolins, odd-toed ungulates (perissodactyls), even-toed ungulates (artiodactyls), and cetaceans. Insectivores included in Laurasiatheria (hedgehogs, moles, shrews, solenodons) are now often allocated to the new order Eulipotyphla. In this connection, it is worth noting that 'insectivores' exhibit unusual diversity in fetal membranes [10,11]. DNA-based studies have consistently indicated an additional key innovation within Laurasiatheria: cetaceans (whales and dolphins) are embedded within artiodactyls as the sister group to hippopotamuses. Accordingly, the previous orders Artiodactyla and Cetacea are often combined into the single order Cetartiodactyla. This is now supported by morphological evidence [12]. The fourth cluster of placental mammals indicated by DNA sequence data, Xenarthra, is by far the smallest and contains only New World anteaters, armadillos, and sloths. It is notable that these xenarthrans were previously often grouped with pangolins (members of Laurasiatheria) and aardvarks (Tubulidentata) in the assemblage 'Edentata'. It now seems that the main character once believed to link these various mammals – virtual loss of teeth – evolved

Table 12.1. Orders of mammals generally recognized on morphological grounds

Common name	Order	Notes
Insectivores	Insectivora	Now split into Afrosoricida and Eulipotyphla
Bats	Chiroptera	
Carnivores	Carnivora	Includes seals and sea-lions
Pangolins	Pholidota	Formerly part of 'Edentata'
Odd-toed ungulates	Perissodactyla	
Even-toed ungulates	Artiodactyla	
Whales and dolphins	Cetacea	
Rabbits, hares, and pikas	Lagomorpha	
Rodents	Rodentia	
Tree-shrews	Scandentia	Formerly included in Primates
Colugos	Dermoptera	
Primates	Primates	
Elephant-shrews	Macroscelidea	Formerly included in Insectivora
Aardvarks	Tubulidentata	
Hyraxes	Hyracoidea	
Elephants	Proboscidea	
Sea-cows and manatees	Sirenia	
Sloths, anteaters, and armadillos	Xenarthra	Formerly part of 'Edentata'

convergently in Afrotheria, Laurasiatheria, and Xenarthra. The only assemblage that lacks toothless representatives is Euarchontoglires.

Types of placentation

Having established a general phylogenetic framework, it is possible to proceed to comparisons of placenta types across mammals. A good starting-point is the simple scheme proposed by Grosser [13], recognizing three main types of definitive placenta according to the relationship established between the chorion (the outermost fetal membrane) and the uterine wall (Fig. 12.1). This classification has been widely used as a basis for comparative studies (e.g. [14,15,16]). The most superficial, epitheliochorial type of placenta lacks significant invasion of the uterine lining (endometrial epithelium), which remains intact and provides the contact surface for the chorion. With a non-invasive placenta of this type, an extensive area of the chorion is in close contact with the uterine lining, so the placenta is diffuse. Conspicuously developed glands in the uterine wall are a prominent feature of epitheliochorial placentae. Outlets of uterine glands are typically clustered to interface with special absorptive areas of the chorion (vesicles or areolae). These absorptive areas facilitate transfer of particular nutrients (e.g. iron, lipid) from the uterus to the fetus [14,17]. The other two placenta types in Grosser's [13] classification both involve invasion of the uterine wall. Initial invasion of the uterine wall would erode only the superficial layer of endometrial epithelium, bringing the chorion into contact with underlying maternal connective tissue. Although not recognized in Grosser's [13] classification, this type of placentation (syndesmochorial placenta) was added to the list for a while, but electron microscopy then generally eliminated it from consideration because it is never found in the interhemal regions [18]. Deeper penetration of the uterine wall brings the chorion into contact with maternal blood vessels (endotheliochorial placenta). It is interesting, incidentally, that invasion of the uterine epithelium leading to formation of an endotheliochorial placenta begins with penetration into the orifices of uterine glands [19]. The third, most invasive placenta type arises through erosion of the walls of maternal blood vessels, leading to direct contact between the chorion and maternal blood (hemochorial placenta). Moderately invasive (endotheliochorial) and highly invasive (hemochorial) placenta types both differ from the epitheliochorial type in being more localized. They are limited to specific regions of the chorion, either an encircling band (zonary placenta) or one or two circular or oval patches (discoid placenta). Endotheliochorial and hemochorial placentae also differ from the epitheliochorial type in the shedding of maternal tissue at birth.

The three basic placenta types defined by Grosser [13] on grounds of increasing invasiveness (epitheliochorial, endotheliochorial, and hemochorial) have routinely served as a basis for comparative discussions. However, refinements are both possible and justified. Ultrastructural studies revealed that intervening membranes can become quite thin, thus considerably

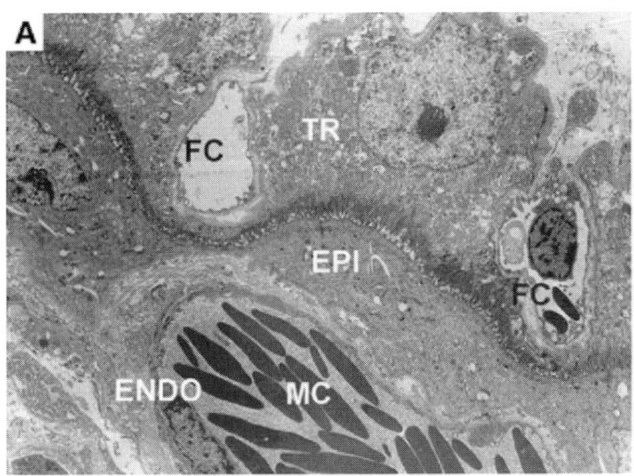

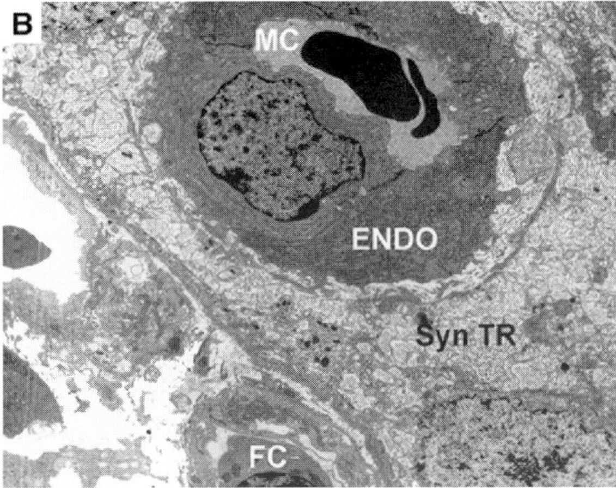

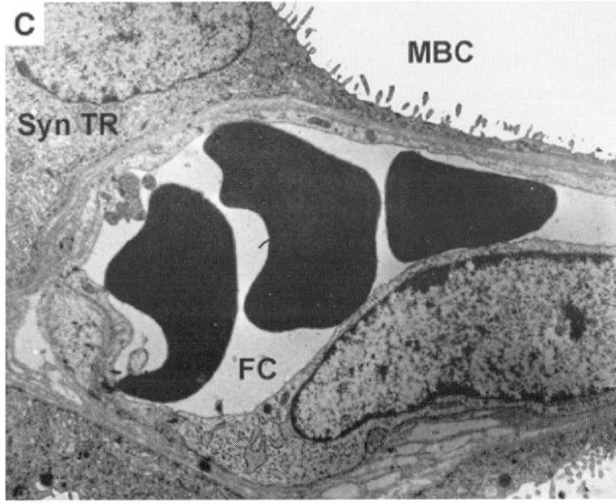

Fig. 12.1 Three main types of placentation can be defined by reference to the tissue layers in the interhemal barrier. (A) Epitheliochorial placentation in a camelid (kindly provided by Dr. Karl Klisch, Medical School Hannover). (B) Endotheliochorial placentation in the three-toed sloth (*Bradypus tridactylus*). (C) Hemochorial placentation in the degu (*Octodon degus*). ENDO, maternal endothelial cells; EPI, uterine epithelium; FC, fetal capillary including the vessel endothelium; MBC, maternal blood channel; MC, maternal capillary; Syn TR, syncytial trophoblast; TR, trophoblast cells. Reproduced with permission from Mess & Carter [24] © 2007 Elsevier Inc.

reducing the diffusion distance between maternal and fetal bloodstreams [20]. Recognition of finer differences permits expansion of Grosser's original classification to six main types of definitive placenta: synepitheliochorial (e.g. ruminant artiodactyls); epitheliochorial (e.g. strepsirrhine primates, pangolins, non-ruminant artiodactyls, cetaceans, perissodactyls); endotheliochorial (e.g. carnivores, elephants, sloths, some bats); hemotrichorial (e.g. most myomorph rodents); hemodichorial (e.g. lagomorphs, colugos, most bats); hemomonochorial (e.g. higher primates, hystricomorph rodents). It is also important to note that placentation and associated fetal membranes involve a complex of fine details that should be considered in any comprehensive analysis [21]. Mossman [10,11,22] appropriately emphasized the relationships of fetal membranes, rather than focusing exclusively on the placenta.

One immediately striking finding is that placenta type is relatively conservative within large groups of placental mammals. In two-thirds of placental mammal orders (11 out of 18), all species so far studied uniformly exhibit just one of the three basic placenta types recognized in Grosser's [13] classification (Table 12.2). This indicates that a basic pattern became established early in the evolution of each of these orders, with the degree of placental invasiveness remaining stable thereafter. It seems highly likely, for

Table 12.2. Distribution of placenta types among mammals

Placenta type	Superorder	Order
Epitheliochorial	Laurasiatheria	Artiodactyla[a]
		Cetacea[a]
		Perissodactyla
		Pholidota
	Euarchontoglires	Primates (strepsirrhines)
Endotheliochorial	Laurasiatheria	Carnivora (except hyenas)
		Chiroptera (some)
		Eulipotyphla (shrews; moles)
	Euarchontoglires	Rodentia (few)
		Scandentia
	Afrotheria	Afrosoricida (otter shrews)
		Proboscidea
		Sirenia
		Tubulidentata
	Xenarthra	Xenarthra (sloths)[b]
Hemochorial	Laurasiatheria	Carnivora (hyenas)
		Chiroptera (most)
		Eulipotyphla (hedgehogs)
	Euarchontoglires	Rodentia (most)
		Lagomorpha
		Primates (haplorhines)
		Dermoptera
	Xenarthra	Xenarthra (armadillos; anteaters)[b]
	Afrotheria	Hyracoidea
		Afrosoricida (tenrecs; golden moles)
		Macroscelidea

[a] These 2 orders are now commonly combined into the single order Cetartiodactyla.
[b] Some split the Xenarthra into 2 separate orders: Pilosa (anteaters and sloths) and Cingulata (armadillos). However, this does not reflect the division according to type of placenta. Furthermore, a molecular supertree for mammals [6] indicates an unresolved trichotomy for anteaters, armadillos, and sloths.
After Carter & Enders [15] and Mess & Carter [21].

example, that placentation was epitheliochorial in ancestral perissodactyls, endotheliochorial in ancestral carnivores, and hemochorial in ancestral lagomorphs. Indeed, extraordinary fossil evidence supports this inference in the case of perissodactyls [23]. Almost all (six out of seven) of the remaining placental orders containing species with two alternative types of placentation show either the endotheliochorial or the hemochorial condition, and one type usually predominates. For instance, the great majority of carnivores have endotheliochorial placentae, but hyenas differ in having hemochorial placentae. Among eulipotyphlan insectivores, shrews and most moles have endotheliochorial placentae while hedgehogs have hemochorial placentae. Among afrosoricidan insectivores, tenrecs and golden moles have hemochorial placentae whereas otter shrews have endotheliochorial placentae. The nature of placentation in bats has often been misunderstood since Mossman [10] indicated that most bat families are characterized by endotheliochorial placentation. However, although members of various bat families initially have endotheliochorial placentae, many show a transition to a hemochorial state in late pregnancy [21,24]. Given that in most bats the placenta is hemochorial at term, that is the majority condition accepted here [25]. Among xenarthrans, placentation is hemochorial in armadillos and anteaters and endotheliochorial in sloths. Similarly, the placenta is hemochorial in most rodents but endotheliochorial in some. Overall, it is noteworthy that endotheliochorial and hemochorial placentae are both represented in all four superorders of placental mammals – Afrotheria, Euarchontoglires, Laurasiatheria, and Xenarthra [15,16]. By contrast, epitheliochorial placentation occurs in only two superorders: Euarchontoglires and Laurasiatheria.

Primates differ starkly from all other placental mammal orders because the two extreme kinds of placentation are represented, while the moderately invasive (endotheliochorial type) is not. Lemurs and lorisiforms (strepsirrhines) have the least invasive, epitheliochorial type of placenta, whereas tarsiers and simians (haplorhines) all have the most invasive, hemochorial type (Fig. 12.2). This sharp dichotomy in placentation between two major subgroups of primates became evident toward the end of the nineteenth century and led several early authors to see strepsirrhines and haplorhines as two entirely separate groups of mammals. It was repeatedly suggested that the order Primates should be restricted to haplorhines

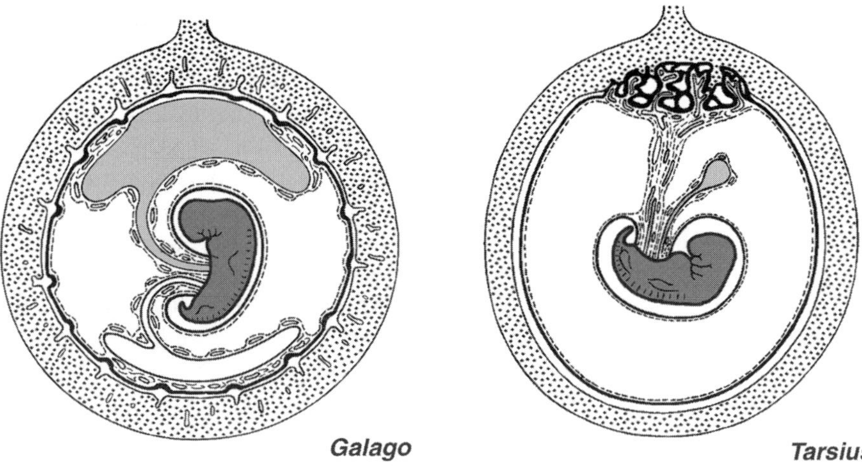

Fig. 12.2 Diagrams illustrating fetal membranes and placentation in strepsirrhine and haplorhine primates: dwarf bush baby (*Galago demidoff*) and spectral tarsier (*Tarsius spectrum*). The chorion is shown as a thick black line, while the fetus is shaded in dark gray. The diffuse epitheliochorial type of placenta in strepsirrhines is associated with pronounced development of uterine glands and the presence of chorionic vesicles (shown as indentations in the chorion). Haplorhines have a contrasting discoidal, hemochorial type of placenta and only weakly developed uterine glands. In strepsirrhines, the yolk sac (light gray) and its blood vessels are prominent early in pregnancy, but are progressively replaced by the allantois (white). In haplorhines, the yolk sac is typically poorly developed and its vessels are not involved in placentation; the allantois develops only as a vestigial stalk-like structure, but its blood vessels play an exclusive role in the placental circulation. (From Martin [34]; adapted from Mossman [10].)

(i.e. tarsiers, monkeys, apes, and humans). Discussions of the relationship between tarsiers and other primates have hence often emphasized placentation [10,26,27, 28,29,30]. Placentation and other reproductive features together provide crucial evidence that tarsiers shared a common ancestry with higher primates (monkeys, apes, and humans). At the same time, the dichotomy between strepsirrhines and haplorhines indicates that these two primate subgroups diverged very early in placental mammal evolution.

Given that DNA-based trees now indicate a link between primates, tree-shrews, and colugos in the assemblage Euarchonta, the placentation of the latter is of particular interest. Tree-shrews in fact have an unusual condition with twin pads on the endometrial wall serving as attachment sites for discoidal, endotheliochorial placentae [31,32,33]. There is no obvious connection between the placentation of tree-shrews and that of any primate [29,34]. Unfortunately, little is known about the placentation of colugos. Hitherto, this obscure group of Southeast Asian mammals, containing only two monospecific genera (*Cynocephalus*, *Galeopithecus*), has received scant attention. This must now change in view of the fact that colugos may be the sister group of primates. Preliminary information indicates that colugos have a hemochorial type of placenta [35,36], but there is as yet nothing to suggest a specific connection with primates.

Evolution of placentation in mammals

Reliable inference of the primitive condition is an essential starting-point for successful reconstruction of the evolution of placentation in placental mammals. In fact, each of the three main placenta types identified by Grosser [13] has been favored by different authors as the ancestral condition for placentals (reviewed by Martin [29,34]). In recent decades, the dominant interpretation – notably promoted by Luckett [27,28,37,38] – has been that epitheliochorial placentation is primitive. However, several authors identified the hemochorial condition as primitive. Only a small minority supported the interpretation that endotheliochorial placentation was the ancestral condition for placentals. It is striking that the leading contenders for the primitive placental condition have thus been the two extremes: non-invasive epitheliochorial or highly invasive hemochorial. This issue continues to be a subject of active discussion [39].

At first sight, it seems quite reasonable to suggest that the non-invasive epitheliochorial type of placenta is ancestral for placental mammals. The transition from egg-laying (ovipary) to intrauterine development and live birth (vivipary) undoubtedly involved a stage in which the egg was simply retained in the uterus to develop there (ovovivipary). Placentation would have evolved from an initial condition involving only superficial contact between the retained developing egg and the uterine lining. Modern marsupials provide an approximate parallel to this hypothetical non-invasive stage in the evolution of placentation in placentals. In all marsupials, some degree of fetal development takes place within the uterus, but the chorion is virtually surrounded by a shell membrane throughout all or most of pregnancy. Despite the presence of the shell membrane, however, marsupials typically have a rudimentary yolk-sac placenta [40]. Indeed, a few (e.g. the bandicoot, *Perameles*) show limited invasion of the endometrium, and the allantois is involved in vascularization of the placenta along with the yolk sac.

Like many other areas of biology, interpretation of the evolution of placentation has been insidiously influenced by the *Scala naturae*, in which extant species are arranged on an ascending phylogenetic scale. Accordingly, a sequence progressing from egg-laying monotremes through ovoviviparous marsupials to fully viviparous placentals has often been equated with the actual evolutionary sequence for placentation. The *Scala naturae* encourages a dangerous tendency to regard extant forms as ‘frozen ancestors’ that have remained unchanged since they diverged from more advanced lineages. Thus, placentation in marsupials has often been seen as a frozen condition corresponding to that in the common ancestor of marsupials and placentals. But marsupials have followed a long independent evolutionary trajectory since they diverged from placentals at least 125 million years ago (mya). Marsupials are alternative mammals, not inferior mammals [41]. It is exceedingly unlikely that reproduction in marsupials has remained totally unchanged for more than 125 mya, and we need to consider the possibility that emphasis on pouch development has led to evolutionary reduction of intrauterine development [19,29,34,39]. It must also be remembered that a considerable time elapsed between the initial divergence between marsupials and placentals and the subsequent emergence of a common ancestor of extant placentals. In other words, a long stem lineage preceded the crown radiation. It is therefore entirely possible that an original ovoviviparous condition in the common ancestor of marsupials and placentals had already given rise to invasive placentation by the time the common ancestor of crown placentals emerged.

In another influential example of the *Scala naturae*, Hill [26] inferred a step-wise progression in the evolution of placentation and fetal membranes among extant primates. His inferred sequence passed through the following stages: (1) ‘lemuroid’ (strepsirrhines); (2) ‘tarsioid’ (tarsiers); (3) ‘pithecoid’ (New and Old World monkeys); (4) ‘anthropoid’ (apes and humans). Hill [26] proposed that invasiveness of the placenta increased through this sequence, accompanied by progressively earlier development of the chorioallantoic circulation. His series started with non-invasive epitheliochorial placentation in strepsirrhines and showed a distinct shift to hemochorial placentation in the tarsioid stage. Thereafter, hemochorial placentation became increasingly invasive in passing through the pithecoid to the anthropoid (i.e. hominoid) stages. Large-bodied hominoids (great apes and humans) exhibit interstitial implantation of the blastocyst in a small cavity in the uterine wall, and establishment of the chorioallantoic circulation is especially rapid.

Luckett [27,28] refined and elaborated the evolutionary progression proposed by Hill [26], advocating epitheliochorial placentation as the primitive condition for placental mammals. An additional persuasive argument advanced by Luckett is that in species with an epitheliochorial placenta fetal membranes exhibit a shared array of other features. He argued that such uniform sharing of characters could not have arisen through convergent evolution, so epitheliochorial placentation must be primitive for placental mammals. Luckett [27,28] claimed that, by contrast, placental mammals with hemochorial or endotheliochorial placentae all show divergent specializations, indicating multiple independent evolution of those placenta types during mammalian evolution. According to Luckett's reconstruction, every single feature of placentation and fetal membrane relationships in strepsirrhine primates is primitive. However, there are in fact certain differences in fetal development between mammals with epitheliochorial placentation. Moreover, some mammals with endotheliochorial placentation (e.g. carnivores, tree-shrews) show all of the primitive features inferred for epitheliochorial placentation by Luckett other than non-invasiveness [34]. Indeed, the endotheliochorial placenta of tree-shrews is more primitive than the epitheliochorial placenta of strepsirrhines in that the yolk sac remains prominent throughout gestation.

Comparison of the condition of the offspring at birth (neonate type) and of gestation periods in mammals yields a crucial additional perspective on the evolution of placentation. Pioneering studies by Portmann [42,43] revealed that two distinct types of neonates can be recognized according to the degree of development at birth: altricial (poorly developed) and precocial (well developed). Whereas all marsupials have hyper-altricial neonates, placentals may have either altricial or precocial neonates. Among placentals, every major group (i.e. order or at least suborder) is usually characterized by either altricial or precocial neonates. Insectivores (both afrosoricidans and eulipotyphlans), tree-shrews, colugos, carnivores, lagomorphs, and two out of three rodent suborders (myomorphs, sciuromorphs) generally have altricial neonates; artiodactyls, cetaceans, perissodactyls, hyraxes, elephants, sirenians, hystricomorph rodents, elephant-shrews, bats, and primates typically have precocial neonates. In view of the clear distinction between altricial and precocial neonates, it is notable that tree-shrews [29] and colugos [44] have altricial neonates whereas primates uniformly produce precocial neonates. Neonate type is correlated with several other key features including gestation period, litter size, neonatal brain size, and the duration of postnatal life-history phases [29,30]. All of these features are scaled to body size. Moreover, small-bodied mammals tend to breed rapidly and produce altricial neonates, while large-bodied mammals typically breed slowly and give birth to precocial neonates.

Ancestral placentals were almost certainly small-bodied, so they were probably altricial, producing multiple litters after relatively short gestations. Developmental evidence supports this inference [45]. In altricial neonates, the eyes and ears are closed over at birth and open during postnatal development. Fusion of eyelids and sealing of ears also takes place during fetal development of precocial mammals, but reopening occurs around the time of birth. It is as if an ancestral nest phase had been absorbed into gestation. Evidence from birds neatly confirms this interpretation. Primitive birds were seemingly precocial, with the altricial condition being a secondary development, and transient fusion of the eyelids does not occur during development of precocial birds within the egg. Given the small body size inferred for ancestral placentals, it is notable that placenta type is associated with body size [34] (Fig. 12.3). Whereas hemochorial placentation is prevalent among small-bodied mammals (modal body mass = 237 g), epitheliochorial placentation is mainly found in large-bodied mammals (modal body mass = 52.5 kg). Endotheliochorial placentation is found across a particularly wide spectrum of body sizes, ranging from the smallest known mammals (certain bats and shrews) up to elephants, such that modal body mass (9.6 kg) is intermediate. Accordingly, placentation in ancestral placentals was surely more likely to have been invasive (endotheliochorial or hemochorial) than epitheliochorial.

Recognition of the fundamental distinction between altricial and precocial neonates is indispensable for interpreting the scaling of gestation period to maternal body size in placental mammals [34,46,47]. Although both altricial and precocial mammals show a scaling exponent of ~ 0.15, there is a clear grade distinction between them. For a given maternal body size, gestation periods are some four times longer in precocial than in altricial species. Residual values calculated across placentals using an exponent value of 0.15 are clearly bimodal, reflecting the basic dichotomy between altricial and precocial species. Groups characterized by altricial neonates (e.g. eulipotyphlan and afrosoricidan insectivores, carnivores, tree-shrews, lagomorphs, myomorph and sciuromorph rodents) uniformly have relatively short gestations; those typified by precocial neonates (e.g. artiodactyls, cetaceans, perissodactyls, hystricomorph rodents, primates) have comparatively long gestations.

Kihlström [48] noted that in mammals with intermediate invasiveness of the placenta (endotheliochorial or labyrinthine hemochorial) gestation periods are consistently shorter, relative to maternal body mass, than in those with either non-invasive epitheliochorial or highly invasive villous hemochorial placentation. This suggests that intermediate invasiveness of the placenta is primitive for placental mammals, given that the seemingly primitive altricial neonates are associated with relatively short gestations. Non-invasive epitheliochorial placentation is essentially restricted to mammals with precocial neonates and relatively long gestations, so this type of placenta is highly unlikely to be primitive. The sole potential exception is the American mole (*Scalopus*), reported to have epitheliochorial placentation combined with relatively short gestation and altricial neonates [49]. However, the *Scalopus* placenta may be endotheliochorial as in the European mole (*Talpa*) [50,51].

Divergent evolution of non-invasive and highly invasive placentation from an ancestral, moderately invasive type requires multiple convergence. However, it is important to recognize two additional factors: (1) a localized invasive placenta is always associated with a large expanse of 'free' chorion; (2) the degree of development of uterine glands during

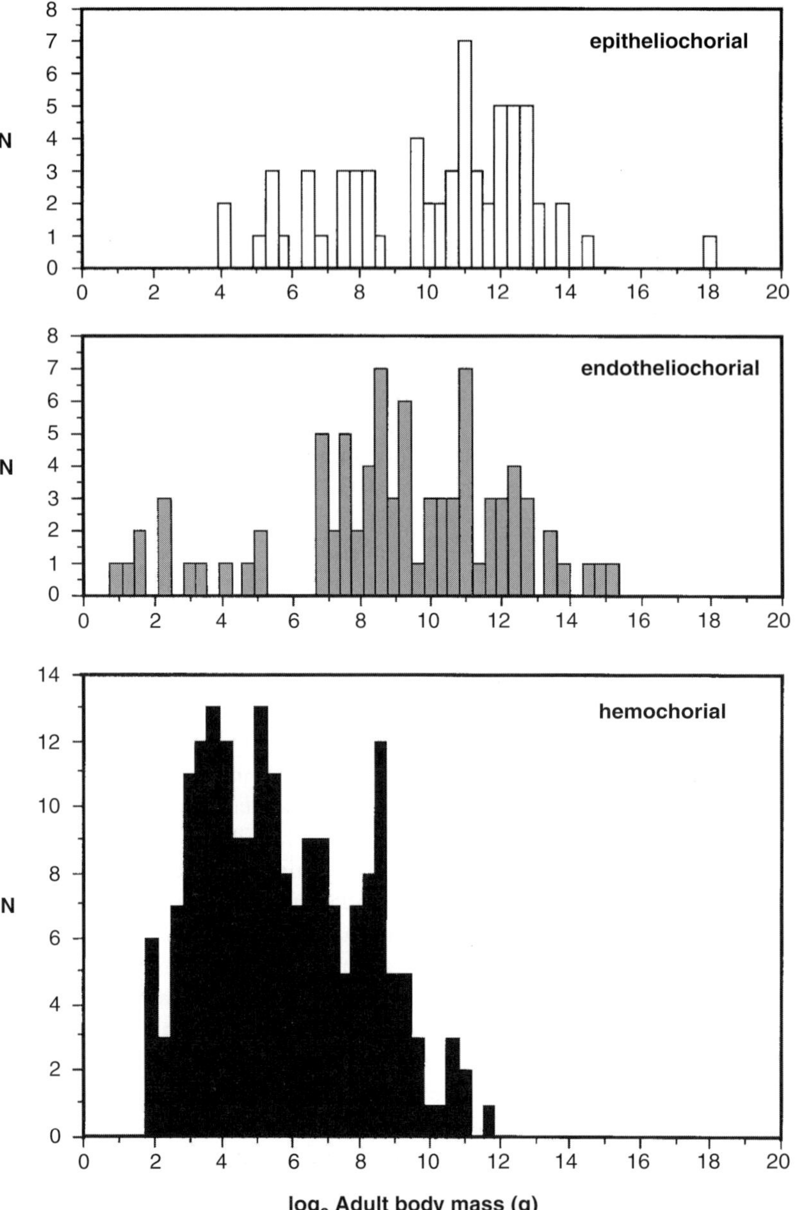

Fig. 12.3 Frequency distributions for body mass of placental mammal species according to placenta type: epitheliochorial (n = 84), endotheliochorial (n = 65), or hemochorial (n = 199). Body mass is shown on a logarithmic scale for ease of representation. (Adapted from Martin [34].)

gestation increases as invasiveness of the placenta decreases. This indicates a trade-off between proximity to maternal blood (maximal with a localized, highly invasive placenta) and absorption of uterine milk (maximal with a diffuse, non-invasive placenta). One can hence infer an ancestral condition for placental mammals in which a localized, moderately invasive placenta was combined with a vascularized 'free' area of chorion serving a general absorptive function, perhaps through specialized chorionic areas (vesicles or areolae). Approximate models for this hypothetical ancestral condition are provided by certain insectivores such as the eulipotyphlan European mole and afrosoricidan tenrecs, and also by tree-shrews [34].

The proposal that epitheliochorial placentation evolved from a more invasive ancestral condition is in fact supported by embryological evidence from certain strepsirrhine primates. Invasive features in early gestation have been reported for certain bushbaby species. Hill [26] suggested that a modified endotheliochorial zone in the placenta of *Galago demidoff* represents an intermediate stage in the evolutionary transition from epitheliochorial to hemochorial placentation, but it could be a retained primitive feature instead. It eventually emerged that the lesser mouse lemur (*Microcebus*), in addition to having an initial invasive attachment comparable to that of *G. demidoff*, retains an endotheliochorial zone in its definitive placenta [52,53].

Fundamental reappraisal of the evolution of placentation in placental mammals has recently resulted from analyses of the distribution of character states using the scaffold provided by comprehensive DNA-based trees (e.g. [2]). On this basis, Carter & Enders [15] concluded that the probable evolutionary sequence was from endotheliochorial to hemochorial or epitheliochorial placentae. Epitheliochorial placentation was interpreted as a secondary specialization that evolved twice, once in Laurasiatheria and once in strepsirrhine primates. Vogel [16] similarly inferred that invasive placentation (endotheliochorial or hemochorial) was present at all basal nodes in the placental mammal tree and that epitheliochorial placentation is hence not primitive but secondary. He differed from Carter & Enders [15] in accepting a third separate origin of epitheliochorial placentation in *Scalopus*. More detailed cladistic reconstructions of the evolution of placentation and fetal membranes based on molecular trees were conducted subsequently [21,54]. Mess & Carter [21] inferred that the ancestral condition for placentation in placental mammals was endotheliochorial, whereas Wildman *et al.* [54] concluded that it was hemochorial. Elliot & Crespi [55] also superimposed placenta types on a molecular tree and concluded that the ancestral condition was hemochorial. However, they combined endotheliochorial and epitheliochorial types in their analysis, so separate determination of the endotheliochorial condition as ancestral was simply excluded *a priori*. Despite somewhat divergent conclusions, all recent studies that have reconstructed the evolution of placentation on DNA-based trees concord in identifying the epitheliochorial condition as secondary. The consensus interpretation is that the ancestral condition of the placenta was either moderately or markedly invasive.

Simple application of the sister-group principle [29] also indicates that ancestral placentals had invasive placentation. Epitheliochorial placentation occurs only in some members of the apparently monophyletic cluster containing Laurasiatheria and Euarchontoglires. Xenarthra and Afrotheria, which both branched off prior to the common ancestor of that cluster, have only invasive placentation (endotheliochorial or hemochorial). This indicates that some kind of invasive placentation is probably primitive for placental mammals. The sister-group principle also indicates that invasive placentation was ancestral for Euarchontoglires. Lagomorphs, rodents, tree-shrews, and colugos, which all branched away prior to the common ancestry of primates, uniformly have invasive placentation (hemochorial in most; endotheliochorial in some). Thus invasive placentation is indicated as the likely ancestral condition for primates.

Implications of different ancestral character states for the evolution of placenta type have been examined relative to the consensus supertree for placental mammals generated by Bininda-Emonds *et al.* [6], assuming no reversals [34] (Fig. 12.4). If endotheliochorial placentation is taken as primitive, •11 character state transitions (3 to epitheliochorial and 8 to hemochorial) are needed to explain the distribution of placenta types among orders of placental mammals. If hemochorial placentation is taken as primitive, •13 transitions are needed (3 double changes through endotheliochorial to epitheliochorial and 7 single changes to endotheliochorial), whereas if epitheliochorial placentation is taken as the primitive condition •17 transitions are needed (6 double changes from epitheliochorial to hemochorial, 3 single changes to endotheliochorial and 2 subsequent changes to hemochorial). Proposing epitheliochorial as the ancestral condition is hence the least parsimonious solution by a large margin. Among invasive placenta types, endotheliochorial placentation is somewhat more parsimonious as the ancestral condition than hemochorial placentation.

Practical implications of differences in placentation have been little explored [56], and limited understanding of functional aspects has been a major obstacle to progress [16]. In fact, Mossman [10,11,22] emphasized the conservative nature of fetal membranes and placentation, stating that they are particularly useful indicators of evolutionary relationships among mammals because they are not exposed to external selective factors. It is certainly the case that characters involved in fetal development provide valuable clues to evolutionary relationships among mammals, but it is nevertheless important to explore the functional significance of different forms of placentation.

One major functional conclusion that has often been drawn is that differences in efficiency distinguish

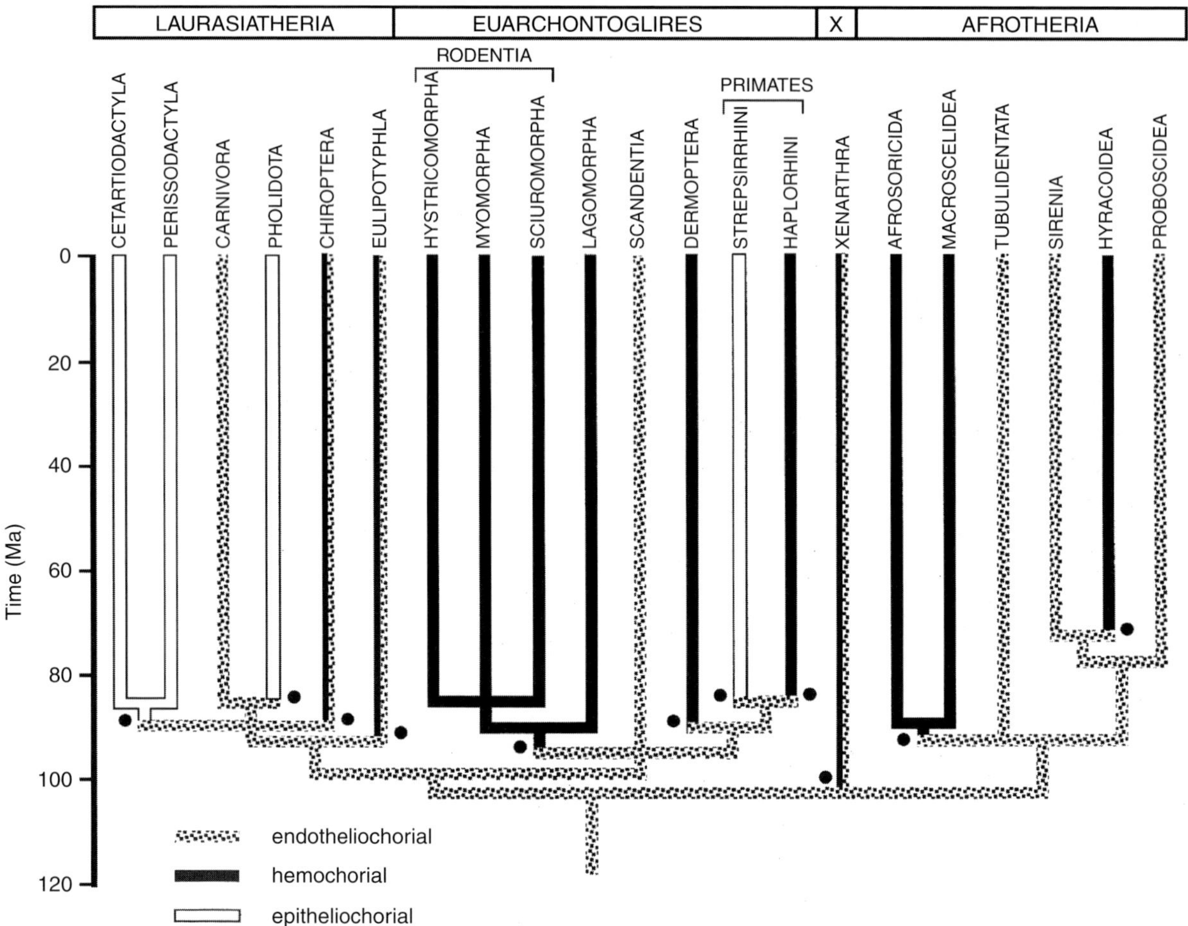

Fig. 12.4 Character state changes (black dots) required, assuming no reversals, if the endotheliochorial placenta type is ancestral for placental mammals. Consensus molecular phylogeny from Bininda-Emonds *et al.* [6]. (Adapted from Martin [34].)

the three basic types of placenta recognized by Grosser [13]. It is widely assumed that an epitheliochorial placenta is necessarily relatively inefficient because it presents the greatest number of potential barriers to diffusion between maternal and fetal bloodstreams. This assumption has bolstered the interpretation that epitheliochorial placentation is primitive. Conversely, the hemochorial placenta type has commonly been seen as most efficient, and hence most advanced, because potential barriers to diffusion between maternal and fetal bloodstreams are minimal. According to this view, the stark dichotomy between epitheliochorial placentae in strepsirrhine primates and hemochorial placentae in haplorhines reflects a major difference in placental efficiency.

Apparent support for the inference that the strepsirrhine placenta is less efficient came from the finding that primates show a parallel dichotomy in the scaling of neonate mass to maternal body mass [57]. A clear grade shift separates strepsirrhines from haplorhines, with the latter giving birth to neonates that are some three times heavier relative to given maternal mass. This grade shift is not due to any clear divergence between strepsirrhines and haplorhines in the scaling of gestation periods, although a few lemurs do have unusually short pregnancies [29,30,58]. It seems reasonable to attribute this difference in relative size of neonates to lower rates of nutrient supply across the non-invasive epitheliochorial placenta of strepsirrhines [57]. However, simple scaling analyses can only reveal correlations; demonstration of underlying causal relationships requires careful testing. Examination of scaling of neonate mass to maternal body mass across placental mammals generally reveals that relative neonate size in all primates is in fact intermediate [30,34,47,58]. Comparison is of course complicated by the fact that relative gestation length is much longer in precocial mammals such as primates. The expectation is that relative neonate size should be markedly smaller in altricial mammals. However, it is valid to compare primates directly with artiodactyls, cetaceans, and perissodactyls, as all produce precocial offspring after similarly lengthy gestations, relative to maternal body mass [58,59]. Neonates of artiodactyls, cetaceans, and perissodactyls turn out to be relatively heavier than those of all primates, including haplorhines. Yet those non-primate mammals uniformly have non-invasive epitheliochorial placentation broadly similar to that of strepsirrhine primates.

The production of relatively large neonates by artiodactyls, cetaceans, and perissodactyls with non-invasive epitheliochorial placentation clearly clashes with the interpretation that this type of placenta necessarily limits rates of fetal development. Moreover, some lemurs (e.g. *Microcebus*, *Varecia*) produce neonates comparable in size to those of other strepsirrhines of similar maternal body mass despite having relatively short gestation periods [34]. Analyses that simultaneously take into account neonatal body mass, maternal body mass, and gestation period show that inferred rates of individual fetal development in these lemurs are higher than in many haplorhines [59]. Scaling analyses also indicate that lower rates of fetal growth in other strepsirrhines may be connected with relatively low basal metabolic rates rather than with placental efficiency as such.

A straightforward ratio between neonate mass and gestation period provides a coarse indication of fetal growth per unit of time. This is admittedly a stark oversimplification, as fetal mass increases approximately according to the cube of time elapsed through most of gestation [46]. Nonetheless, the neonate mass: gestation ratio serves as an informative maternal investment index (MII), giving a crude average figure for resources transferred across the placenta during gestation. The clear expectation from the notion that non-invasive placentation is relatively inefficient is that MII values should be generally lower than with invasive placentation and should increase with endotheliochorial placentation and even more with hemochorial placentation. However, a plot of MII values against gestation period showed no difference in the scaling relationship according to placenta type [16]. Similarly, a plot of MII values against adult body mass for 348 placental mammal species showed no distinction between species according to placenta type [34]. Because gestation period is a confounding variable, a more satisfactory approach is to plot residual values for neonate mass against residuals for gestation period (both determined relative to adult body mass). This reveals the relationship between neonate mass and gestation after excluding effects of adult body mass. There is once again no separation according to placenta type [34]. Indeed, this analysis clearly reveals that species with epitheliochorial placentation generally produce relatively large neonates after relatively long gestation periods (Fig. 12.5). Many other mammals with either endotheliochorial or hemochorial placentae overlap completely with species having

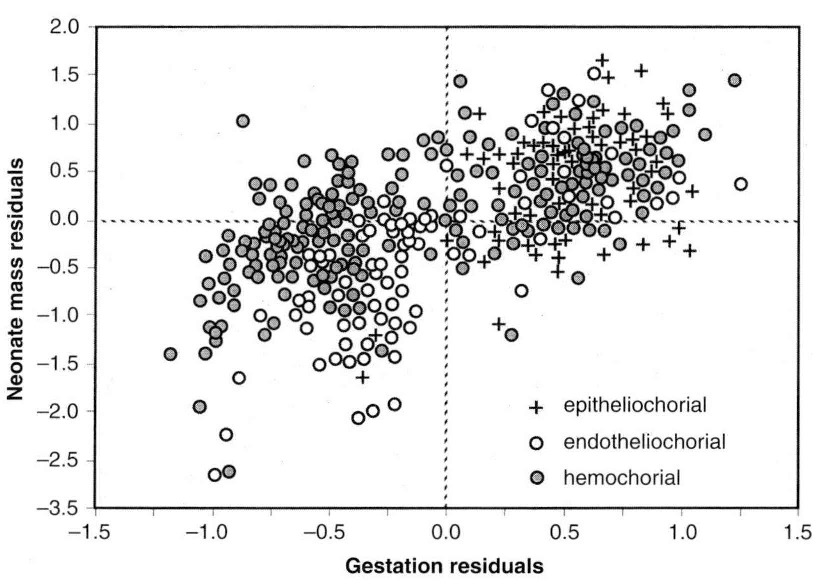

Fig. 12.5 Plot of residual values for neonate mass against residuals for gestation period, both calculated relative to mean adult body mass, for 348 placental mammal species. It is clearly evident that species with epitheliochorial placentation tend to have relatively large neonates and long gestation periods. Conversely, species with relatively small neonates and short gestation periods typically have endotheliochorial or hemochorial placentation. (Adapted from Martin [34].)

epitheliochorial placentation. By contrast, epitheliochorial placentation is almost lacking among species with relatively short gestation periods, which typically have either endotheliochorial or hemochorial placentation and predominantly have relatively small neonates. Among mammals with relatively short gestation periods, there is an interesting tendency for species with endotheliochorial placentation to have relatively small neonates compared to those with hemochorial placentation. This may indicate that a hemochorial placenta is advantageous for producing relatively large neonates during a relatively short gestation period.

The basic conclusion from broad comparisons of placental mammals – namely, that epitheliochorial placentation is not correlated with relatively smaller neonates relative to gestational time – is somewhat unexpected. The surface area of epitheliochorial placentae is generally smaller, relative to adult body size, than that of hemochorial placentae [16,60,61]. The only known exception occurs in ruminant artiodactyls, in which a special cotyledonary structure of the chorion is associated with an increase in surface area to match that found with invasive placentation. Overall, comparative evidence indicates that resources can be transmitted across an epitheliochorial placenta at a rate comparable to that occurring with invasive placentae, despite the fact that the surface area available for transfer is often smaller. One possibility is that active transport is more important with non-invasive placentation.

Because the developing brain requires a rich oxygen supply, it has often been suggested that highly invasive (hemochorial) placentation is essential for evolution of a relatively large brain (e.g. see Leutenegger [57]). This is coupled with the notion that hemochorial placentation is necessarily more advanced. Comparisons of primates also provide apparent support for this interpretation: haplorhines, with hemochorial placentae, typically have relatively larger brains than strepsirrhines, with epitheliochorial placentae. Once again, however, comparisons across mammals generally fail to confirm the inference based on primates alone. Humans have the largest relative brain size among mammals, but the largest values among non-primates are found in dolphins, which have relatively larger brains than monkeys and apes. In fact, as already noted, dolphins produce notably large neonates, and their brain size at birth actually exceeds that in humans. So the non-invasive epitheliochorial placentation of dolphins clearly does not preclude development of a large brain [30]. Moreover, the aye-aye (*Daubentonia*) – a strepsirrhine primate – has a relative brain size within the range of monkeys and apes, showing that epitheliochorial placentation does not necessarily limit brain development even among primates. So there is no clear evidence that placenta type limits brain size.

Placentation in Old World monkeys and apes

Having considered the general background to evolution of the placenta in primates, it is now possible to focus specifically on catarrhines (Old World monkeys, apes, and humans). The human placenta at term, together with those of apes and Old World monkeys, is remarkable in two respects. First, the maternal blood flows through an extensive intervillous space, whereas in labyrinthine hemochorial placentae it is confined to narrow channels lined by trophoblast. Second, blood is delivered to the intervillous space through the grossly widened orifices of the spiral arteries, whose walls have been greatly transformed due to invasion by the fetal trophoblast. Each of these features occurs in other mammals but not in combination. Thus, armadillos and anteaters have a villous hemochorial placenta formed as the fetal villi grow into a preexisting network of blood sinuses in the uterine wall [62]. Trophoblast invasion of uterine arteries occurs in many mammals and, compared to primates, reaches even further in hystricomorph rodents [63] and some bats [64].

In a labyrinthine placenta, the fetal capillaries and maternal blood channels are arranged in parallel but with fetal and maternal blood flowing in opposite directions. This allows for countercurrent exchange, which is a more efficient way of supplying oxygen than a multivillous system such as that of the human placenta. Theoretical analysis reveals, however, that the difference is not substantial when the oxygen transport capacity of the blood is high [65]. Transport capacity is a rather complex function, but the prime determinant is the rate of maternal placental blood flow [56]. Indeed the key to understanding the evolution of a villous hemochorial placenta from a labyrinthine one is that it allows for very high rates of maternal placental blood flow and oxygen delivery toward term. This is the solution adopted by haplorhine primates to facilitate development of precocial neonates with large brains.

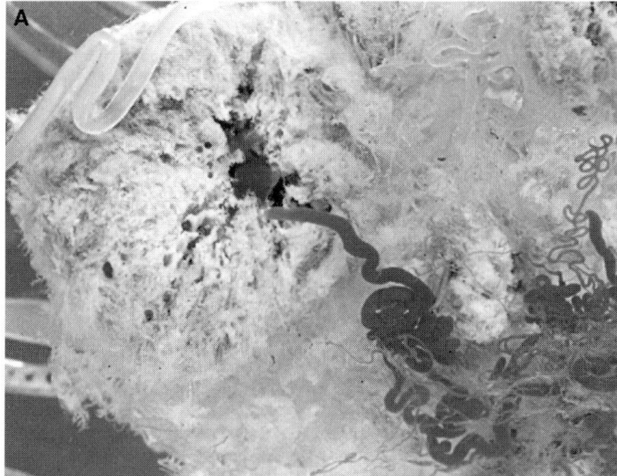

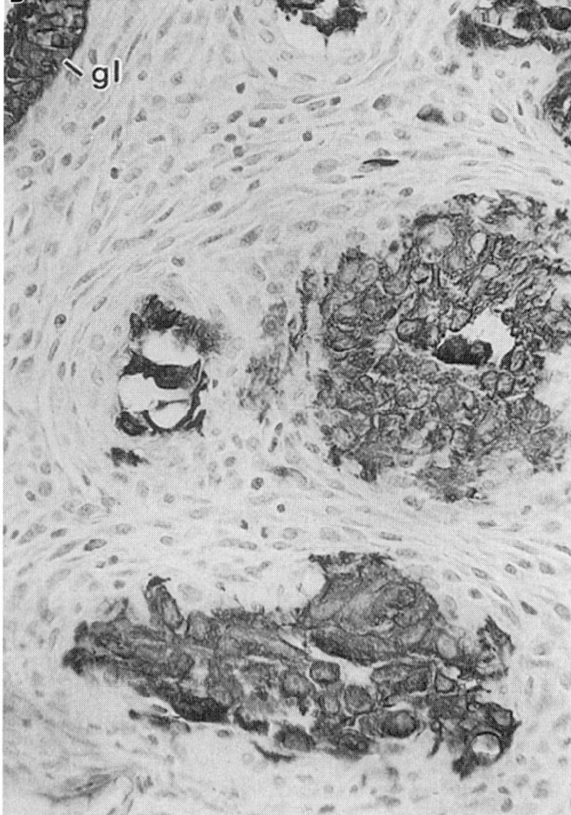

Fig. 12.6 Placentation in Old World monkeys. (A) The basic functional unit of the placenta demonstrated by vascular casts using two colors of plastic. A uterine spiral artery (dark gray) opens at the center of a fetal cotyledon (white). A loop of injection catheter appears at top left. Carnegie monkey 7B (*M. mulatta*) on day 159 of pregnancy. Courtesy of the late Dr. Elizabeth M. Ramsey. (B) Trophoblast invasion of a spiral artery can be seen in this day 7 implantation site of *M. fascicularis*. Cross-sections of three coils of a spiral artery are shown. The cytokeratin-positive trophoblast cells (black) have apparently intruded into the vessel wall. Courtesy of Dr. Allen C. Enders. Reproduced with permission from Enders *et al.* [73] © 1996 S. Karger AG, Basel.

Architecture of the intervillous space

The functional unit of the catarrhine placenta is a villous tree, with the villi housing the fetal capillaries, and a maternal spiral artery opening into a space at the center of the tree. This can be visualized both in the rhesus monkey (*Macaca mulatta*; Fig. 12.6A) and in the human placenta [66] by making injection casts with differently colored plastic.

There are 10–12 large villous trees (fetal cotyledons) and 40–50 medium to small ones in the human placenta and they are formed at around 40–50 days postovulation [67]. Each primary villus originates at the chorionic plate. It divides into second- and third-order villi and some of the latter form anchoring villi that secure the tree to the basal plate. The fetal placental circulation is established quite early but the maternal circulation does not appear until the cotyledons are formed, since the arteries initially are plugged with trophoblast. There is still dispute as to when maternal circulation is established in the human placenta [68]. It can be detected as early as 20 days' gestation in a catarrhine monkey *Macaca fascicularis* [69] and in humans may be responsible for formation of a cavity in the middle of the fetal cotyledon. It does appear that the rate of blood flow in the intervillous space is low throughout the first trimester of human pregnancy.

Based on limited material, the architecture of the intervillous space in chimpanzee and gorilla is identical to that of human placenta [70]. Development of the villous placenta in *M. mulatta* has been described in great detail by Elizabeth Ramsey, and in a comparison with human placenta it was concluded that any differences were of minimal importance from a physiological standpoint [71].

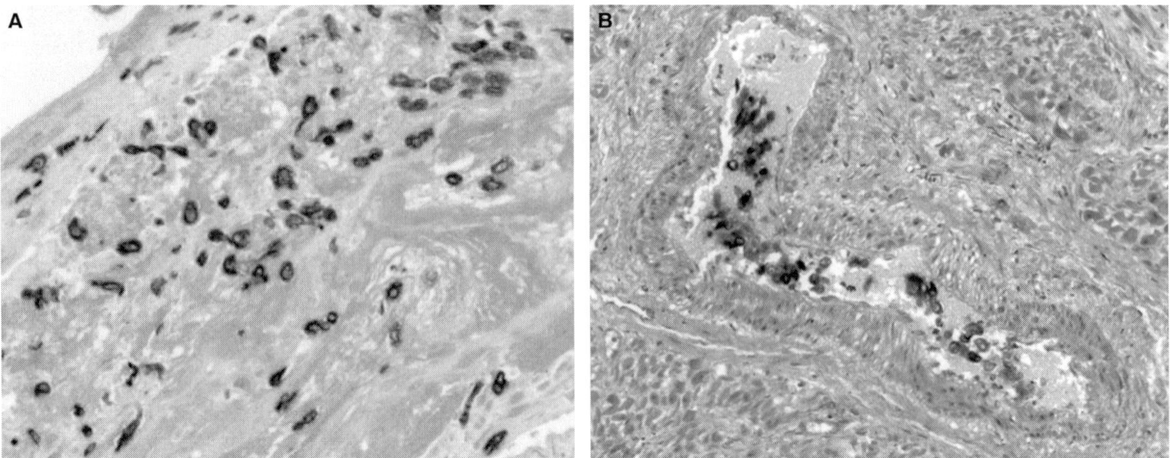

Fig. 12.7 Trophoblast invasion of the uterine wall in great apes. (A) Trophoblast invasion by the interstitial route in a gorilla (*G. gorilla*). The cytokeratin-positive trophoblast cells are darkly stained. (B) Trophoblast invasion by the endovascular route in the inner third of the myometrium in a chimpanzee (*P. troglodytes*). The cytokeratin-positive trophoblast cells in the lumen are darkly stained.

Trophoblast invasion of the uterine arteries

As described in the preceding chapter, remodeling of the spiral arteries commences during decidualization of the endometrium in the late luteal phase of the cycle. Continuation of this process and disorganization of the tunica media is associated with the migration of extravillous trophoblast by the interstitial route. A second wave of migration occurs by the endovascular route and is followed by loss of the vessel endothelium and incorporation of trophoblasts into the vessel wall, where they become embedded in a matrix of fibrinoid material. This process is thought to be causally associated with widening of the spiral arteries and their conversion of these vessels into low-resistance channels. It affects the vessels through the entire depth of the endometrium and the inner third of the myometrium. Once this phase has been completed there is some degree of vascular repair, notably re-establishment of the endothelium [72].

The initial stages of implantation are remarkably similar in Old World monkeys and man, although in Old World monkeys a large part of the blastocyst remains in the uterine cavity, whereas in humans the blastocyst is pulled just beneath the surface. Despite this more superficial implantation, the trophoblast of the monkey is initially more aggressive and it appears in spiral arteries beneath the placenta earlier than has been seen in the human [73] (Fig. 12.6B). However, in contrast to this rapid invasion by the endovascular route, there is little or no interstitial trophoblast. The difference arises as cytotrophoblasts spread out from the anchoring villi to form a trophoblastic shell. In *M. mulatta* and the baboon (*Papio anubis*, *P. cynocephalus*) this shell is continuous, slightly thicker than in the human placenta, and sharply delineated from the underlying endometrium [73,74]. In human placenta the shell is much less uniform and the extravillous trophoblast can be seen streaming off into the endometrium. The paucity of interstitial trophoblast cells in the monkey is an important difference from human placentation. Perhaps associated with this, transformation of the arteries never reaches as far as the myometrium, although there is a strong resemblance in the way spiral arteries are invaded and transformed within the endometrial layer [75,76].

The deeper invasion of trophoblast in the human is sometimes linked to the occurrence of preeclampsia, which affects about 5% of pregnancies. It is often stated, with Chez [77] as the authority, that preeclampsia is a uniquely human disease. In point of fact this has never been documented and the unique changes of the renal glomeruli associated with preeclampsia can be induced by uterine artery ligation in the pregnant baboon (*P. hamadryas*) [78]. They have been seen to arise spontaneously in the chimpanzee [79] and cases of eclampsia have been observed in captive gorillas [80].

These observations led one of us (AC) to ask whether the routes and depth of trophoblast invasion in great apes were similar to those in human pregnancy. This had not been a focus of attention in early studies of primate placentation and the more recent literature described only the delivered placenta. Fortunately, a number of gravid uteri of the common chimpanzee (*Pan troglodytes*) and Western gorilla (*Gorilla gorilla*), of known provenance, were available in the Hill Collection. It was possible to show that trophoblast invasion in both species occurs by both the interstitial and endovascular routes (Fig. 12.7). Moreover, in keeping with this close resemblance to the human condition, trophoblast invasion and transformation of the arterial wall occurred in the inner third of the myometrium.

Thus, as had been predicted [30], the deeper invasion of the uterine wall found in the human is shared by our closest relatives. It allows a further increase in blood flow and oxygen supply to the placenta and may well be important for prenatal brain development [30]. In contrast, placentation in gibbons resembles that of Old World monkeys (Carter, Pijnenborg, and Vercruysse, unpublished data). It has yet to be established whether the orangutans (*Pongo* spp.) represent an intermediate state.

Placentation in tarsiers and New World monkeys

The architecture of the placenta is notably different in New World monkeys (platyrrhines), which diverged from catarrhines at least 40 mya [81]. In platyrrhines proliferation of the trophoblast continues until much later in gestation and connections persist between the villi, which form an interconnecting network of slender trabeculae or strands [26,36]. Only at a late stage of fetal development are branched villi found within a more or less continuous intervillous space. The arrangements for maternal blood supply are also very different in platyrrhines. Enlarged maternal capillaries, originating in the compact basal decidua, wend their way through the trophoblast and the maternal blood reaches the intertrabecular spaces through gaps in the walls of these intraplacental vessels [26]. A trabecular network is also a feature of the tarsier placenta, but an intervillous space does not occur at any stage of gestation [26].

Wislocki [36] regarded the placenta of the spider monkey *Ateles geoffroyi* as a stage in the evolution of a villous hemochorial placenta. To illustrate an intermediate between the platyrrhine placenta and a true labyrinthine placenta, such as that of rodents, Wislocki [36] chose the Sunda colugo *Galeopithecus variegatus*. He described the labyrinth of this placenta as a comb-like structure containing maternal blood lacunae. In numerous places adjacent channels became confluent to form irregular sinusoids which, ‘instead of being themselves enclosed, now appear to be the enclosing medium for the fetal tissue’, i.e. something approaching the intertrabecular space of platyrrhines. In an independent study of the same species, Starck [35] also characterized the colugo placenta as a theoretically important intermediate between labyrinthine and villous placentation.

Conclusions

Ancestral placental mammals were almost certainly small-bodied and probably gave birth to multiple litters of altricial young after relatively short gestations. Several lines of reasoning lead us to conclude that the common ancestor of living placentals had a moderately invasive placenta of the endotheliochorial type. From this the less invasive epitheliochorial type evolved at least twice and the more highly invasive hemochorial placenta many times. Whatever the forces driving this evolution, there is no evidence to support the assumption that one placental type is more efficient than the other. An epitheliochorial placenta has a greater number of tissue layers between maternal and fetal bloodstreams, yet in ruminant artiodactyls it is able to support long gestation periods ending in delivery of large precocial neonates. Dolphins have diffuse epitheliochorial placentae, and they produce neonates with brains that are relatively larger than those of newborn monkeys and apes. In catarrhine primates, with hemochorial placentae, development of a villous rather than labyrinthine type, supplied by greatly dilated uterine arteries, enables a high rate of oxygen delivery to a relatively compact placenta. This may be an alternative strategy to produce a precocial neonate with a large brain, although arguably it is a less effective one as brain development has to be completed postnatally. This was acknowledged by Portmann [42,43] when he characterized human babies as secondarily altricial. To round out the picture it may be noted that elephants [82] and manatees [83] have endotheliochorial placentae and also deliver large precocial young after a long gestation.

References

1. Murphy W J, Eizirik E, Johnson W E *et al.* Molecular phylogenetics and the origins of placental mammals. *Nature* 2001; **409**: 614–18.

2. Murphy W J, Eizirik E, O'Brien S J *et al.* Resolution of the early placental mammal radiation using Bayesian phylogenetics. *Science* 2001; **294**: 2348–51.
3. Springer M S, Murphy W J, Eizirik E, O'Brien S J. Placental mammal diversification and the Cretaceous-Tertiary boundary. *Proc Natl Acad Sci U S A* 2003; **100**: 1056–61.
4. Springer M S, Stanhope M J, Madsen O, de Jong W W. Molecules consolidate the placental mammal tree. *Trends Ecol Evol* 2004; **19**: 430–8.
5. Arnason U, Adegoke J A, Gullberg A *et al.* Mitogenomic relationships of placental mammals and molecular estimates of their divergences. *Gene* 2008; **421**: 37–51.
6. Bininda-Emonds O R P, Cardillo M, Jones K E *et al.* The delayed rise of present-day mammals. *Nature* 2007; **446**: 507–12.
7. Simpson G G. The principles of classification and a classification of mammals. *Bull Am Mus Nat Hist* 1945; **85**: 1–350.
8. Janecka J E, Miller W, Pringle T H *et al.* Molecular and genomic data identify the closest living relative of primates. *Science* 2007; **318**: 792–4.
9. Martin R D. Colugos: obscure mammals glide into the evolutionary limelight. *J Biol* 2008; **7**: 1–5.
10. Mossman H W. *Vertebrate fetal membranes*. London/New Brunswick, NJ: Macmillan/Rutgers University Press; 1987.
11. Mossman H W. Classics revisited: comparative morphogenesis of the fetal membranes and accessory uterine structures. *Placenta* 1991; **12**: 1–5.
12. Geisler J H, Uhen M D. Morphological support for a close relationship between hippos and whales. *J Vert Paleontol* 2003; **23**: 991–6.
13. Grosser O. *Vergleichende Anatomie und Entwicklungsgeschichte der Eihäute und der Placenta*. Vienna: Wilhelm Braumüller; 1909.
14. King B F. Development and structure of the placenta and fetal membranes of nonhuman primates. *J Exp Zool* 1993; **266**: 528–40.
15. Carter A M, Enders A C. Comparative aspects of trophoblast development and placentation. *Reprod Biol Endocrinol* 2004; **2**: 1–15.
16. Vogel P. The current molecular phylogeny of eutherian mammals challenges previous interpretations of placental evolution. *Placenta* 2005; **26**: 591–6.
17. King B F. Comparative studies of structure and function in mammalian placentas with special reference to maternal-fetal transfer of iron. *Am Zool* 1992; **32**: 331–42.
18. Steven D H. Anatomy of the placental barrier. In: D H Steven, ed. *Comparative placentation: essays in structure and function*. London: Academic Press; 1975: pp. 25–57.
19. Pijnenborg R, Robertson W B, Brosens I. Morphological aspects of placental origin and phylogeny. *Placenta* 1985; **6**: 155–62.
20. Wooding F B P, Flint A P F. Placentation. In: Lamming G E, ed. *Marshall's physiology of reproduction*, Part I, Volume III. London: Chapman & Hall; 1994: pp. 233–460.
21. Mess A, Carter A M. Evolutionary transformations of fetal membrane characters in Eutheria with special reference to Afrotheria. *J Exp Zool B Mol Dev Evol* 2006; **306**: 140–63.
22. Mossman H W. Comparative morphogenesis of the fetal membranes and accessory uterine structures. *Contrib Embryol Carnegie Inst* 1937; **26**: 129–246.
23. Franzen J L. A pregnant mare with preserved placenta from the middle Miocene maar of Eckfeld, Germany. *Palaeontographica Abt B* 2006; **278**: 27–35.
24. Mess A, Carter A M. Evolution of the placenta during the early radiation of placental mammals. *Comp Biochem Physiol A* 2007; **148**: 769–79.
25. Carter A M, Mess A. Evolution of the placenta and associated reproductive characters in bats. *J Exp Zool B Mol Dev Evol* 2008; **310**: 428–49.
26. Hill J P. The developmental history of the primates. *Phil Trans R Soc Lond B* 1932; **221**: 45–178.
27. Luckett W P. Ontogeny of the fetal membranes and placenta: their bearing on primate phylogeny. In: Luckett W P, Szalay F S, eds. *Phylogeny of the primates*. New York: Plenum Press; 1975: pp. 157–82.
28. Luckett W P. Cladistic relationships among primate higher categories: evidence of the fetal membranes and placenta. *Folia Primatol (Basel)* 1976; **25**: 245–76.
29. Martin R D. *Primate origins and evolution: a phylogenetic reconstruction*. New Jersey: Princeton University Press; 1990.
30. Martin R D. Human reproduction: a comparative background for medical hypotheses. *J Reprod Immunol* 2003; **59**: 111–35.
31. Hill J P. On the placentation of *Tupaia*. *J Zool (Lond)* 1965; **146**: 278–304.
32. Kaufmann P, Luckhardt M, Elger W. The structure of the tupaia placenta. 2. Ultrastructure. *Anat Embryol (Berl)* 1985; **171**: 211–21.
33. Luckhardt M, Kaufmann P, Elger W. The structure of the tupaia placenta. 1. Histology and vascularization. *Anat Embryol (Berl)* 1985; **171**: 201–10.
34. Martin R D. Evolution of placentation in primates: implications of mammalian phylogeny. *Evol Biol* 2008; **35**: 125–45.
35. Starck D. Ontogenie und Entwicklungsphysiologie der Säugetiere. In: Kükenthal W, ed. *Handbuch der Zoologie*, vol. 8. Berlin: de Gruyter; 1959: pp. 1–276.

36. Wislocki G B. Remarks on the placentation of a platyrrhine monkey (*Ateles geoffroyi*). *Am J Anat* 1925; **36**: 467–87.

37. Luckett W P. The comparative development and evolution of the placenta in primates. *Contrib Primatol* 1974; **3**: 142–234.

38. Luckett W P. Uses and limitations of mammalian fetal membranes and placenta for phylogenetic reconstruction. *J Exp Zool* 1993; **266**: 514–27.

39. Pijnenborg R, Vercruysse L. Thomas Huxley and the rat placenta in the early debates on evolution. *Placenta* 2004; **25**: 233–7.

40. Freyer C, Zeller U, Renfree M B. The marsupial placenta: a phylogenetic analysis. *J Exp Zool A Comp Exp Biol* 2003; **299**: 59–77.

41. Renfree M B. Marsupials: alternative mammals. *Nature* 1981; **293**: 100–1.

42. Portmann A. Die Ontogenese der Säugetiere als Evolutionsproblem. II. Zahl der Jungen, Tragzeit und Ausbildungsgrad der Jungen bei der Geburt. *Biomorphosis* 1938/1939; **1**: 109–26.

43. Portmann A. Nesthocker und Nestflüchter als Entwicklungszustände von verschiedener Wertigkeit bei Vögeln und Säugern. *Rev Suisse Zool* 1939; **46**: 385–90.

44. Lim N. *Colugo: the flying lemur of South-East Asia.* Singapore: Draco; 2007.

45. Weber R. Transitorische Verschlüsse von Fernsinnesorganen in der Embryonalperiode bei Amnioten. *Rev Suisse Zool* 1950; **57**: 19–108.

46. Martin R D, MacLarnon A M. Gestation period, neonatal size and maternal investment in placental mammals. *Nature* 1985; **313**: 220–3.

47. Martin R D, Genoud M, Hemelrijk C K. Problems of allometric scaling analysis: examples from mammalian reproductive biology. *J Exp Biol* 2005; **208**: 1731–47.

48. Kihlström J E. Period of gestation and body weight in some placental mammals. *Comp Biochem Physiol A* 1972; **43**: 673–9.

49. Prasad M R N, Mossman H W, Scott G L. Morphogenesis of the fetal membranes of an American mole, *Scalopus aquaticus*. *Am J Anat* 1979; **155**: 31–68.

50. Carter A M. Placentation in an American mole *Scalopus aquaticus*. *Placenta* 2005; **26**: 597–600.

51. Carter A M, Enders A C. Placentation in mammals once grouped as insectivores. *Int J Dev Biol* 2010; **54**: 483–493.

52. Reng R. Die Placenta von *Microcebus murinus* Miller. *Z Saugetierkd* 1977; **42**: 201–4.

53. Strauss F. The ovoimplantation of *Microcebus murinus* Miller (Primates, Lemuroidea, Strepsirhini). *Am J Anat* 1978; **152**: 99–110.

54. Wildman D E, Chen C, Erez O *et al.* Evolution of the mammalian placenta revealed by phylogenetic analysis. *Proc Natl Acad Sci U S A* 2006; **103**: 3203–8.

55. Elliot M, Crespi B J. Placental invasiveness mediates the evolution of hybrid inviability in mammals. *Am Nat* 2006; **168**: 114–20.

56. Carter A M. Evolution of factors affecting placental oxygen transfer. *Placenta* 2009; **30** Suppl A: S19–S25.

57. Leutenegger W. Maternal-fetal weight relationships in primates. *Folia Primatol (Basel)* 1973; **20**: 280–93.

58. Martin R D. The evolution of human reproduction: a primatological perspective. *Yearb Phys Anthropol* 2007; **50**: 59–84.

59. Martin R D, MacLarnon A M. Comparative quantitative studies of growth and reproduction. *Symp Zool Soc Lond* 1988; **60**: 39–80.

60. Baur R. Morphometry of placental exchange area. *Adv Anat Embryol Cell Biol* 1977; **53**: 1–65.

61. Baur R. Morphometric data and questions concerning placental transfer. *Placenta Suppl* 1981; **2**: 35–44.

62. Enders A C. Development and structure of the villous haemochorial placenta of the nine-banded armadillo (*Dasypus novemcinctus*). *J Anat* 1960; **94**: 34–45.

63. Mess A, Zaki N, Kadyrov M, Korr H, Kaufmann P. Caviomorph placentation as a model for trophoblast invasion. *Placenta* 2007; **28**: 1234–8.

64. Badwaik N K, Rasweiler J J 4th, Muradali F. Co-expression of cytokeratins and vimentin by highly invasive trophoblast in the white-winged vampire bat, *Diaemus youngi*, and the black mastiff bat, *Molossus ater*, with observations on intermediate filament proteins in the decidua and intraplacental trophoblast. *J Reprod Fertil* 1998; **114**: 307–25.

65. Metcalfe J, Bartels H, Moll W. Gas exchange in the pregnant uterus. *Physiol Rev* 1967; **47**: 782–838.

66. Freese U E. The uteroplacental vascular relationship in the human. *Am J Obstet Gynecol* 1961; **101**: 8–16.

67. Reynolds S R. Formation of fetal cotyledons in the hemochorial placenta: a theoretical consideration of the functional implications of such an arrangement. *Am J Obstet Gynecol* 1966; **94**: 425–39.

68. Carter A M. When is the maternal placental circulation established in man? *Placenta* 1997; **18**: 83–7.

69. Simpson N A, Nimrod C, De Vermette R, Fournier J. Determination of intervillous flow in early pregnancy. *Placenta* 1997; **18**: 287–93.

70. Wislocki G B. Gravid reproductive tract and placenta of the chimpanzee. *Am J Phys Anthropol* 1933; **18**: 81–92.

71. Ramsey E M, Harris J W S. Comparison of uteroplacental vasculature and circulation in the rhesus

monkey and man. *Contrib Embryol Carnegie Inst* 1966; **38**: 59–70.

72. Pijnenborg R, Vercruysse L, Hanssens M. The uterine spiral arteries in human pregnancy: facts and controversies. *Placenta* 2006; **27**: 939–58.
73. Enders A C, Lantz K C, Schlafke S. Preference of invasive cytotrophoblast for maternal vessels in early implantation in the macaque. *Acta Anat (Basel)* 1996; **155**: 145–62.
74. Pijnenborg R, D'Hooghe T, Vercruysse L, Bambra C. Evaluation of trophoblast invasion in placental bed biopsies of the baboon, with immunohistochemical localisation of cytokeratin, fibronectin, and laminin. *J Med Primatol* 1996; **25**: 272–81.
75. Ramsey E M, Houston M L, Harris J W. Interactions of the trophoblast and maternal tissues in three closely related primate species. *Am J Obstet Gynecol* 1976; **124**: 647–52.
76. Blankenship T N, Enders A C. Modification of uterine vasculature during pregnancy in macaques. *Microsc Res Tech* 2003; **60**: 390–401.
77. Chez R A. Nonhuman primate models of toxemia of pregnancy. In: Lindheimer M D, Katz A I, Zuspan F P, eds. *Hypertension in pregnancy*. New York: John Wiley & Sons; 1976: pp. 421–4.
78. Makris A, Thornton C, Thompson J *et al.* Uteroplacental ischemia results in proteinuric hypertension and elevated sFLT-1. *Kidney Int* 2007; **71**: 977–84.
79. Stout C, Lemon W B. Glomerular capillary swelling in a pregnant chimpanzee. *Am J Obstet Gynecol* 1969; **105**: 212–5.
80. Thornton J G, Onwude J L. Convulsions in pregnancy in related gorillas. *Am J Obstet Gynecol* 1992; **167**: 240–1.
81. Steiper M E, Young N M. Primate molecular divergence dates. *Mol Phylogenet Evol* 2006; **41**: 384–94.
82. Allen W R. Ovulation, pregnancy, placentation and husbandry in the African elephant (*Loxodonta africana*). *Phil Trans R Soc Lond B Biol Sci* 2006; **361**: 821–34.
83. Carter A M, Miglino M A, Ambrosio C E *et al.* Placentation in the Amazonian manatee (*Trichechus inunguis*). *Reprod Fertil Dev* 2008; **20**: 537–45.

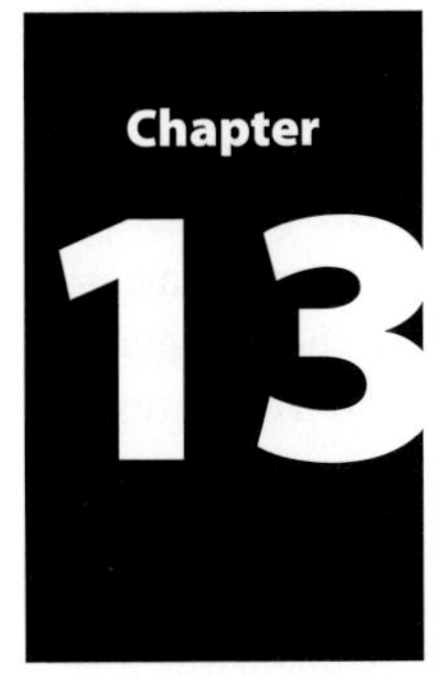

Animal models of deep trophoblast invasion

Robert Pijnenborg and Lisbeth Vercruysse

Katholieke Universiteit Leuven, Department Woman & Child, University Hospital Leuven, Leuven, Belgium

Hemochorial placentation and trophoblast invasion

From the very beginning of anatomical investigation, animal models were extensively used for elucidating the structure and function of the various organs of the human body. For studies of fetal development such an approach was essential, since specimens of pregnant human uteri were extremely difficult to obtain. In the meantime, investigators became increasingly aware of major species differences, particularly in reproductive organs and not least in placental structure. Because of the growing impact of evolutionary thinking in the late nineteenth century, biologists took advantage of interspecies similarities and differences for tracing phylogenetic trees and clarifying the origin of viviparous reproduction. In this context Hubrecht had taken up the study of hedgehog placentation in the late 1880s (see Chapter 1) [1], although he certainly did not consider this animal to be a 'model' for the human. Nevertheless, he was delighted when in 1899 Peters described a similar development of trophoblast in the earliest human implantation site available at that time (Fig. 13.1) [2]. The fact that both investigators had been dealing with a hemochorial type of placenta was a lucky coincidence, since the existence of different histological types was not yet fully appreciated. In 1909 Grosser introduced his well-known histological terminology, which was based upon Strahl's classification of different placenta types according to the progressive elimination of maternal tissue layers [3], and only then investigators had a firm basis for studies on comparative placentology, offering a rationale for the selection of appropriate animal models for human placentation.

The hemochorial type of placenta occurs in different eutherian taxa, having evolved independently in the four superorders of eutherian mammals [4] (Chapter 12). In order to get access to the maternal blood, trophoblast has to penetrate the uterine epithelium and the endometrial (decidual) stroma, which implies that trophoblast invasion is an essential feature of hemochorial placentation. Depending on the species, trophoblasts may also invade deeper layers of the decidua and even the myometrium, where they may further interact with the vasculature. A recurrent feature of hemochorial placentation is the transformation of the endometrium into decidua, which is thought to play a role in the regulation of trophoblast invasion. In the less invasive endotheliochorial placenta, the trophoblast never acquires a direct contact with maternal blood. In such placentas scattered 'decidual cells' have been described, but it is not clear in how far their sporadic appearance can be compared to the extensive decidualization which is associated with deeply invasive hemochorial placentas. Since invasive placental types (either endotheliochorial or hemochorial) are now considered as the most probable ancestral forms [5] (Chapter 12), the evolution of an epitheliochorial structure must have necessitated either the loss of invasive properties of the trophoblast, or the elaboration of a resistant uterine epithelium for curtailing trophoblast invasion. The latter scenario is supported by the finding that isolated trophoblasts of pig placentas still show intrinsic invasive properties if transplanted to ectopic sites [6]. In this context also the uterine invasion by 'endometrial cup' trophoblast in horses and related species [7] might be considered as a legacy of an ancestral invasive placenta type. Decidualization of the endometrial stroma as a means for controlling – and even protecting – trophoblast invasion, would therefore have become redundant in species with epitheliochorial placentation. It is not unlikely that in horses the absence of a decidua may be responsible for the hostile leukocytic milieu and the destruction of endometrial cup trophoblast at the end of the first trimester [7].

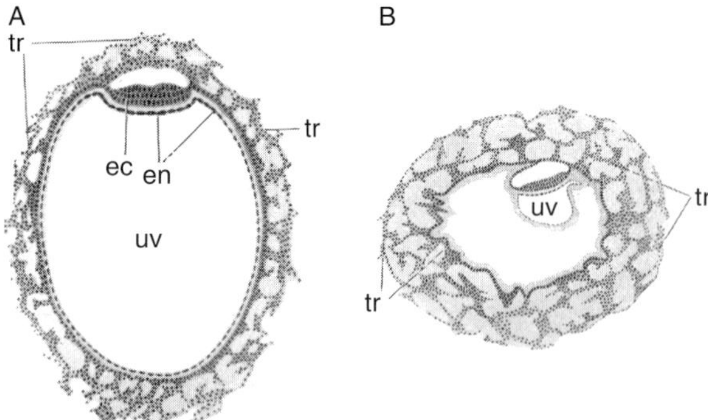

Fig. 13.1 (A) Hubrecht's schematical outline of the tissue layers in the postimplantation hedgehog blastocyst, showing maternal blood-filled spaces in the trophoblastic wall. (B) Hubrecht's redrawing of Peters' embryo, showing analogous blood-filled lacunae (after Hubrecht 1909 [55]).

Since hemochorial placentation usually involves an early access to maternal blood, this placental type has been regarded as a useful adaptation for a strategy of rapid reproduction with short gestational periods as seen in small mammals. This is clearly not applicable to 'higher' primates with long gestations which deliver precocial young. It is tempting to speculate that in this case the hemochorial condition may carry a higher risk for pregnancy complications because of potentially injurious interactions between invading trophoblast and uterine tissues during these prolonged pregnancies. The severity of the risk would of course depend on factors such as the degree of decidualization, the intensity or depth of trophoblast invasion, and the efficiency of maternal tissue repair. In searching for appropriate animal models, investigators might therefore consider using non-human primates as a first choice, but this will carry inevitable and sometimes insurmountable logistical problems. Most investigators therefore tend to turn to laboratory rodents with short gestational periods as being the most convenient for planning short-term research programs. In spite of their short gestations, they are valuable for studying trophoblast invasion and vascular remodeling, in the first place because of their hemochorial condition, but in the second place because of the similarity of at least some of the vascular remodeling steps to the human. Various patterns of trophoblast invasion have been described in different species [8], the most studied being listed in Table 13.1. It should be clear that not a single species can be used as a straightforward model covering all aspects of vascular remodeling in the human (described in Chapter 11).

Following the main theme of this book the following questions might be approached by studying selected animal models: (1) How are the spiral arteries prepared for invasion? (2) What is the trigger for initiating vascular invasion? (3) What regulates the depth of vascular invasion? (4) What is the exact impact of endovascular trophoblast on vascular remodeling? (5) Is interstitial trophoblast involved in vascular remodeling? Apart from these basic questions about mechanisms of vascular change, we also want to understand the reasons for failed invasion and/or impaired vascular remodeling in pregnancy complications such as preeclampsia. In the last part we will discuss possible vascular remodeling defects after experimental induction of preeclampsia-like conditions in laboratory animals.

Decidua-associated vascular remodeling

In most menstruating non-human primates, as in the human, endometrial decidualization occurs spontaneously in the late luteal phase of the menstrual cycle, and may be regarded as an essential preparation for trophoblast invasion and placental development. In the human, decidual swelling starts in perivascular sheaths surrounding the spiral arteries (Streeter's columns), and gradually spreads throughout the endometrial stroma. The time-course of the process is controlled by ovarian steroids (estrogen and progesterone), allowing implantation to occur only within a narrow 'window' during the late luteal phase of the cycle. However, in most other mammals with hemochorial placentation decidualization does not occur spontaneously, but is directly induced by implanting blastocysts and is therefore spatially restricted to the implantation sites. The implantation-associated decidualization-induction is not trophoblast-specific, however, since it can also be induced by aspecific stimuli applied during the 'implantation window', such as needle scratching or intrauterine oil injection, which provoke discrete swellings ('deciduomata') around the scattered oil droplets or scratched areas [9]. Menstruation in primates results from the shedding of decidualized endometrium which is no longer maintained because of the falling progesterone levels at the end of the cycle. Apart from primates, menstruation only occurs in some bat species but the occurrence of spontaneous decidualization during their cycle has not been properly investigated. In rodents, decidual swelling is not initiated in perivascular

Table 13.1. Trophoblast invasion in eutherian mammals

Species	Invasion pathway		Invasion extent		Refs
	Interstitial	Endovascular	Decidual	Deep	
Primates					
Human	+	+	+	+	[38, 16, 21]
Rhesus monkey	(+)	+	+	– /?	[15, 32]
Baboon	(+)	+	+	–	[15, 33]
Rodents					
Mouse	+	–	+	–	[28, 29, 30, 31]
Rat	+	+	+	+	[26, 39, 13, 40]
Golden hamster	?	+	+	+	[19, 14]
Guinea-pig	+	+	+	+	[53, 35, 42, 45]

sheaths around spiral arteries, but begins in the antimesometrial endometrial stroma, where the blastocyst makes its first contact, and proceeds toward the mesometrial part of the uterus where the placenta will develop. In mice, rats, and hamsters the decidua has a restricted lifespan, and shows progressive regression starting in the antimesometrial decidua approximately 1 week after its formation. Because of this pattern of regression, which coincides with the expansion of the gestational sac, Billington [10] postulated that healthy decidua restricts trophoblast invasion which only would proceed after the spontaneous onset of decidual necrosis. This hypothesis fitted well with the results of Kirby's transplantation experiments of ectoplacental cone trophoblast into various ectopic sites, showing the least invasion in a decidualized uterus [11]. In the human such spontaneous decidual regression apparently does not occur, as indicated by the maintenance of a well-developed decidua parietalis (decidua vera) during the whole pregnancy period.

In the human, the first stage of the spiral artery remodeling is closely associated with the decidualization process (Chapter 11), in which also uterine natural killer (uNK) cells, as producers of angiogenic factors, are involved (Chapter 6). In rats, mice, and hamsters decidualization also involves perivascular sheaths of the spiral arteries in the mesometrial decidua and the mesometrial triangle, which is an extension of decidual tissue beyond the inner (circular) myometrium (Fig. 13.2). During this process uNK cells appear within these decidualized compartments and tend to cluster around the spiral arteries, as clearly seen in hamsters and rats. Studies on uNK cell-deficient mice suggested that these cells must be directly responsible for the thinning of the vascular smooth muscle as part of the decidua-associated (trophoblast-independent) vascular remodeling [12]. A similar muscular thinning was observed in induced deciduomata in rats, while in implantation sites the vascular smooth muscle is partly removed, apparently by the deeply invading trophoblast in that species [13]. In pregnant golden hamsters it was observed that in deciduomata, induced in a previously ligated non-pregnant uterine horn, the decidualized arterial walls underwent necrosis at the time trophoblast normally invades this tissue [14]. While these hamster data seem to support Billington's barrier hypothesis, necrosis of decidualized arterial walls coinciding with trophoblast invasion does not occur in the rat [13] and has never been observed in the human. Ramsey and colleagues therefore emphasized that the decidual barrier hypothesis is not applicable to our own species [15]. On the contrary, their comparative study including rhesus monkeys and baboons revealed that in the human, where the deepest invasion occurs, decidualization is most pronounced.

The trigger for initiating vascular invasion

Little information is available about the exact time when vascular invasion starts in the human. At

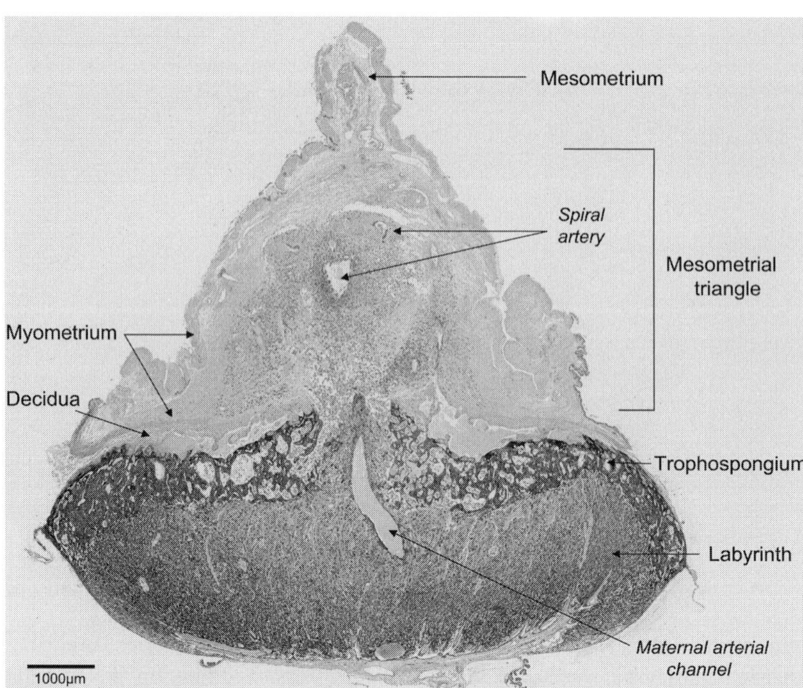

Fig. 13.2 Rat placenta attached to the uterine wall at day 18 of pregnancy. Cytokeratin immunostaining.

8 weeks of pregnancy endovascular invasion of the decidual spiral arteries is on its way [16], while before that time no direct arterial connections with the intervillous space have been seen [17]. In rhesus monkeys, endovascular trophoblasts appear in spiral arteries very early after implantation [18] (see Fig. 12.6B). Although some of the illustrations in the quoted paper suggest plugging, trophoblasts were also seen in deeper arterial sections in all specimens examined. These observations did not reveal any specific mechanism which might have triggered this endovascular migration.

Observations in some rodent species have been more revealing, especially in the golden hamster. Following the pioneering studies by Orsini [19], this species was considered as a good candidate for investigating deep trophoblast invasion in spiral arteries. Also after grafting ectoplacental cones into ectopic sites, hamster trophoblast showed a predilection for endovascular invasion [20]. The latter paper was even quoted by Hamilton & Boyd [21] for providing support to the then still disputed idea that intravascular cells in human spiral arteries could indeed be trophoblastic. A peculiarity of the hamster is that not only trophoblasts derived from the ectoplacental cone – which represents the placental primordium – but also mural trophoblastic giant cells of the original blastocyst wall have strong invasive properties. Furthermore, the actual time-course of invasion seems to suggest a role of hemodynamics in initiating the intravascular migration. While in a non-pregnant rodent uterus the main blood supply is provided via circumferential and radial arteries, this is shifted in early pregnancy toward the spiral arteries which enter the uterus at the insertion site of the mesometrium (Fig. 13.3) [22]. It cannot be a mere coincidence that precisely during the early circumferential flow predominance, mural trophoblastic giant cells (derived from the wall of the blastocyst) retrogradely migrate into these vessels, while after the flow-shift toward the spiral arteries the latter vessels are invaded by placenta-derived trophoblasts. It is interesting, however, that the actual migration of the trophoblasts into the spiral arteries is preceded by a plugging phase, when the most distal lumina are obliterated by a non-invasive type of trophoblastic cell derived from the placental surface (day 10) (Fig. 13.4). During dissolution of the plugs transplacental maternal channels appear (day 11), seemingly created by maternal blood flowing into the placenta, which is followed by migration of endovascular trophoblasts in the corresponding decidual (day 12) and mesometrial triangle

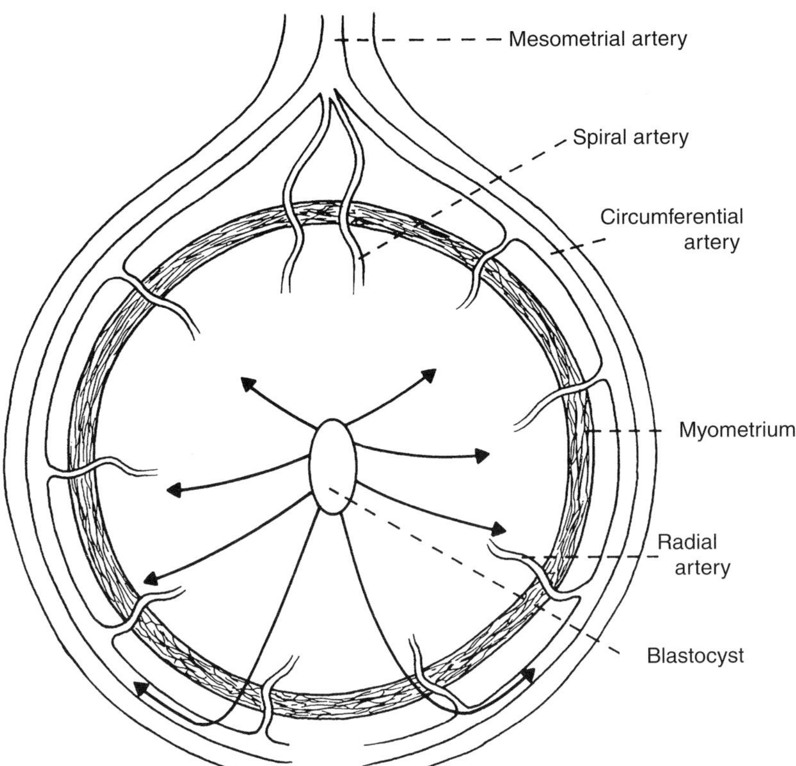

Fig. 13.3 Diagram of the arterial blood supply of the hamster uterus, with indication of endovascular invasion of the radial-circumferential-mesometrial arteries by trophoblastic giant cells.

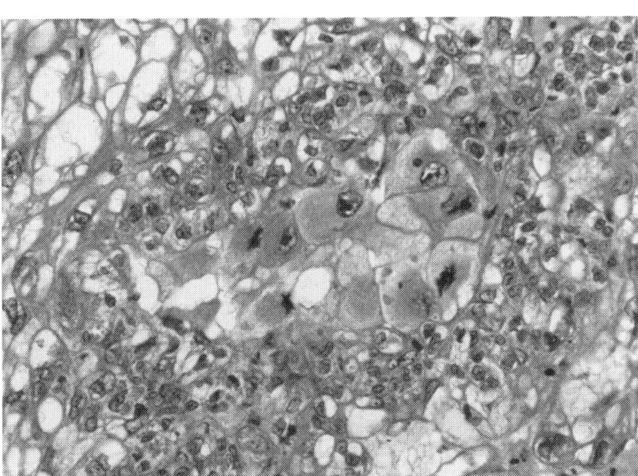

Fig. 13.4 Plugged decidual spiral artery near the placental surface (trophospongium) in the golden hamster at day 10. Reproduced from Pijnenborg *et al.* [14], © Society for Reproduction and Fertility (1974). Reproduced with permission.

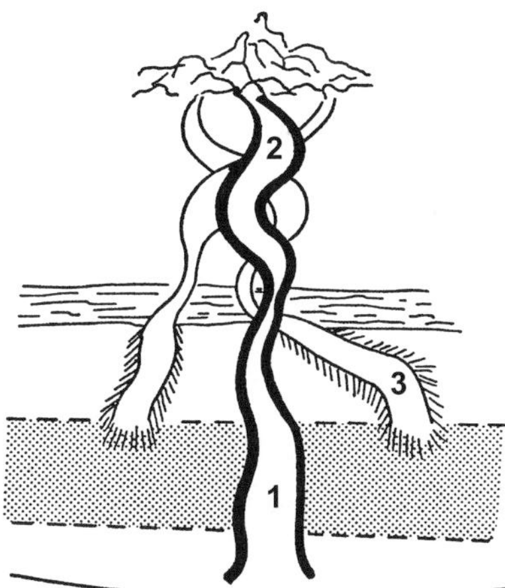

Fig. 13.5 Diagram showing necrotizing non-invaded spiral arteries, not communicating with a transplacental maternal arterial channel, in an ovariectomized pregnant hamster treated with progesterone only. The transplacental maternal arterial channel 1 communicates with spiral artery 2. Spiral artery 3 ends blindly and does not communicate with a maternal channel. Reproduced from Pijnenborg *et al.* [23], © Society for Reproduction and Fertility (1975). Reproduced with permission.

(day 13) spiral artery segments [14]. The putative impact of hemodynamics was supported by the finding of defective transplacental channel formation in ovariectomized progesterone-only treated hamsters, in which the corresponding spiral arteries were not invaded by trophoblast [23]. Instead, these non-invaded decidualized spiral artery walls underwent necrosis as previously described in deciduomata (Fig. 13.5).

Such a clear link between the opening of transplacental arterial channels and the start of endovascular invasion has not been observed in the rat, where quite early in gestation (day 9–10) spiral artery lumina in the decidua may contain endovascular trophoblast, but without forming real plugs [24]. Extension of the endovascular invasion into the mesometrial triangle has been seen at day 15 [13], but the exact starting time for this deeper invasion has not been established.

The literature on trophoblast invasion in the mouse remained obscure for a long time. In his pioneering 1892 study on rodent placentation, Duval describes the invasion of mouse trophoblast into maternal blood sinuses, which he considered as a mechanism for placental growth into the decidua, resulting in the capture of decidual cell islands (now known to be glycogen cells of trophoblastic origin) into the trophospongium [25]. This erroneous interpretation was based on an unfortunate overgeneralization of his discovery of endovascular trophoblast in rat spiral arteries [26]. In another early classic paper, Jenkinson [27] denied the presence of endovascular trophoblast in mice, considering the big intravascular cells as swollen endothelia and disputing Duval's earlier interpretations. Relevant information can be gleaned from more recent literature [28,29], but only Adamson [30] and Hemberger [31] made a systematic description of vascular invasion in mice. Both papers, concurring with our own limited (unpublished) observations, seem to indicate an early perivascular rather than an endovascular pathway of invasion (Fig. 13.6), followed by replacement of the endothelium in the most distal arterial segments. This implies a completely different mechanism triggering the invasion, in which hemodynamics cannot be considered as the main regulatory factor.

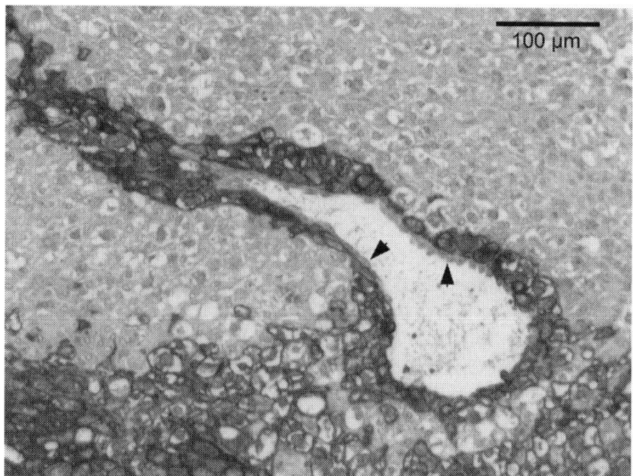

Fig. 13.6 Mouse spiral artery at day 14, communicating with a maternal arterial channel penetrating the superficial trophospongium (bottom). The artery shows perivascular trophoblast migration outside an intact endothelial layer (arrowed). Cytokeratin immunostaining.

This overview indicates that arterial invasion may be triggered by different mechanisms, even in closely related species such as rats and mice. Since the actual trigger for trophoblast invasion in the human is still unknown, it is impossible to consider any of the rodent species studied so far as the proper model for what might happen in early human pregnancy.

The depth of spiral artery invasion

In her seminal paper comparing invasion depth in primates, Ramsey noted that in rhesus monkeys and baboons invasion is restricted to the decidua, which is in marked contrast with the deep invasion in the human [15]. Although doubts have been expressed about the decidua-restricted invasion in the rhesus macaque [32], the limited invasion in the baboon has been confirmed [33]. These findings obviously raise questions about mechanisms controlling invasion depth and the possible relevance of deep invasion for placental function. The latter is obviously important for understanding situations with restricted vascular remodeling in the human such as preeclampsia, where trophoblast invasion of the myometrial segments seems to be impaired [34].

In the common laboratory rodents deep arterial invasion occurs in rats [24,13], hamsters [19,14], and guinea-pigs [35] (Table 13.1). In all these cases endovascular trophoblast moves beyond the decidua and the thinned circular myometrial layer, ending up in the mesometrial triangle or even – in the guinea-pig – deep in the mesometrium. In mice, however, the preferred animal model in most research areas applying to the human, vascular invasion is entirely restricted to the decidua.

Invasion depth may depend on the degree of intrinsic invasiveness of the cells and/or mechanisms for arresting the invasion, and it is difficult to determine the dominating process in each species. The appearance of a fibrinoid layer between migrating cells and vessel wall suggests deposition of adhesive substances, which may result from specific interactions between the trophoblast and the cellular components in the vessel wall. Substances such as fibronectin, laminin, and collagen IV are likely components of this 'fibrinoid', but species differences in its composition have been reported [33]. It is possible – but not

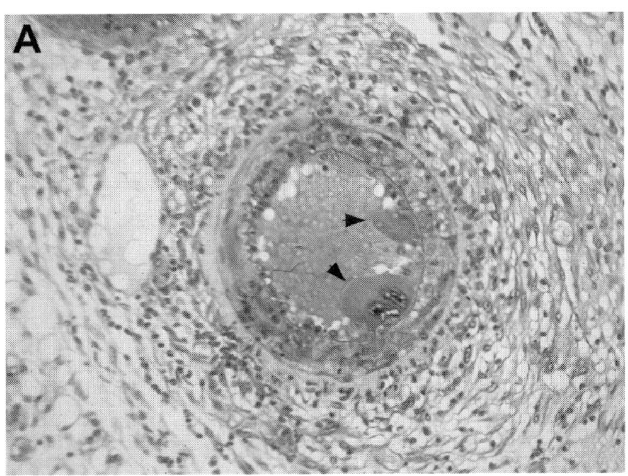

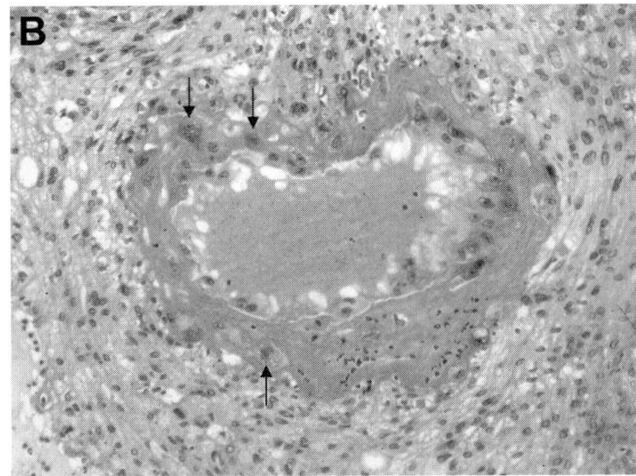

Fig. 13.7 (A) Mesometrial spiral artery of a golden hamster containing intraluminal giant cells (arrowheads), surrounded by inflammatory cells. (B) Section of a remodeled spiral artery at day 15, showing fibrinoid-embedded trophoblast (arrowed); reproduced from Pijnenborg *et al.* [14], © Society for Reproduction and Fertility (1974). Reproduced with permission.

proven – that the extent of the decidua-associated vascular remodeling and associated extracellular matrix changes are involved and may thus regulate the depth of endovascular invasion. Later in pregnancy increasing amounts of fibrinoid may lead to a complete embedding of endovascular trophoblasts, as seen in the human and in the baboon [33]. In the rat the fibrinoid of the invaded spiral arteries remains relatively thin [13], and in late pregnancy thick fibrinoid deposits with completely embedded trophoblasts can only be seen at the junction of the spiral arteries with the transplacental arterial channels in the thinned decidual layer.

Some experimental manipulations have led to changes in invasion depth. Alpha-macroglobulin-deficient mice showed deficiencies in decidualization and uNK cell differentiation, and this was associated with deeper trophoblast invasion, albeit not as far as the myometrium [36]. Keeping in mind that in mice the invasion is not really endovascular, this finding may indicate a role of perivascular uNK cells in controlling invasion depth. In a completely different experiment, pregnant rats exposed to a low oxygen environment from days 8.5 to 9.5 showed a marked increase of endovascular, but not interstitial, invasion in the mesometrial triangle, resulting in a significant dilatation of the vessels [37]. Although not explicitly stated in the paper, the illustrations seem to indicate a virtually complete covering of all the arterial cross-sections of the triangle by trophoblast, including the vessels at the top, suggesting increasing depth of invasion.

Trophoblast-associated vascular remodeling

Already in the pioneering days of placental bed research, the loss of vascular smooth muscle and elastica were recognized as functionally the most significant characteristics of the 'physiologically changed' spiral arteries in the human [38]. The similarity of such changes with vascular alterations in other species was noticed first in the golden hamster (Fig. 13.7B) [14], but the lack of immunohistochemical technology at that time precluded detailed histological analysis. One striking feature of the hamster was that these changes typically occur within the spiral arteries, which had previously undergone decidual change. They do not occur in the circumferential and mesometrial arteries, which do not decidualize and are invaded earlier in pregnancy by trophoblastic giant cells (see previous section). This means that they lack the typical fibrinoid embedding of the trophoblast as described in the spiral arteries, but undergo intense inflammatory cell infiltration (Fig. 13.7A). The only alterations in giant cell-invaded mesometrial arteries are the fragmentation of the elastica and a perivascular fibrosis at the end of pregnancy, the latter obviously resulting from the local inflammation.

Application of immunohistochemical techniques to the deeply invaded rat spiral arteries revealed a close similarity to the human: after the arrival of endovascular trophoblast, the underlying endothelial layer shows fragmentation and subsequently disappears, while a fibrinoid layer is deposited underneath

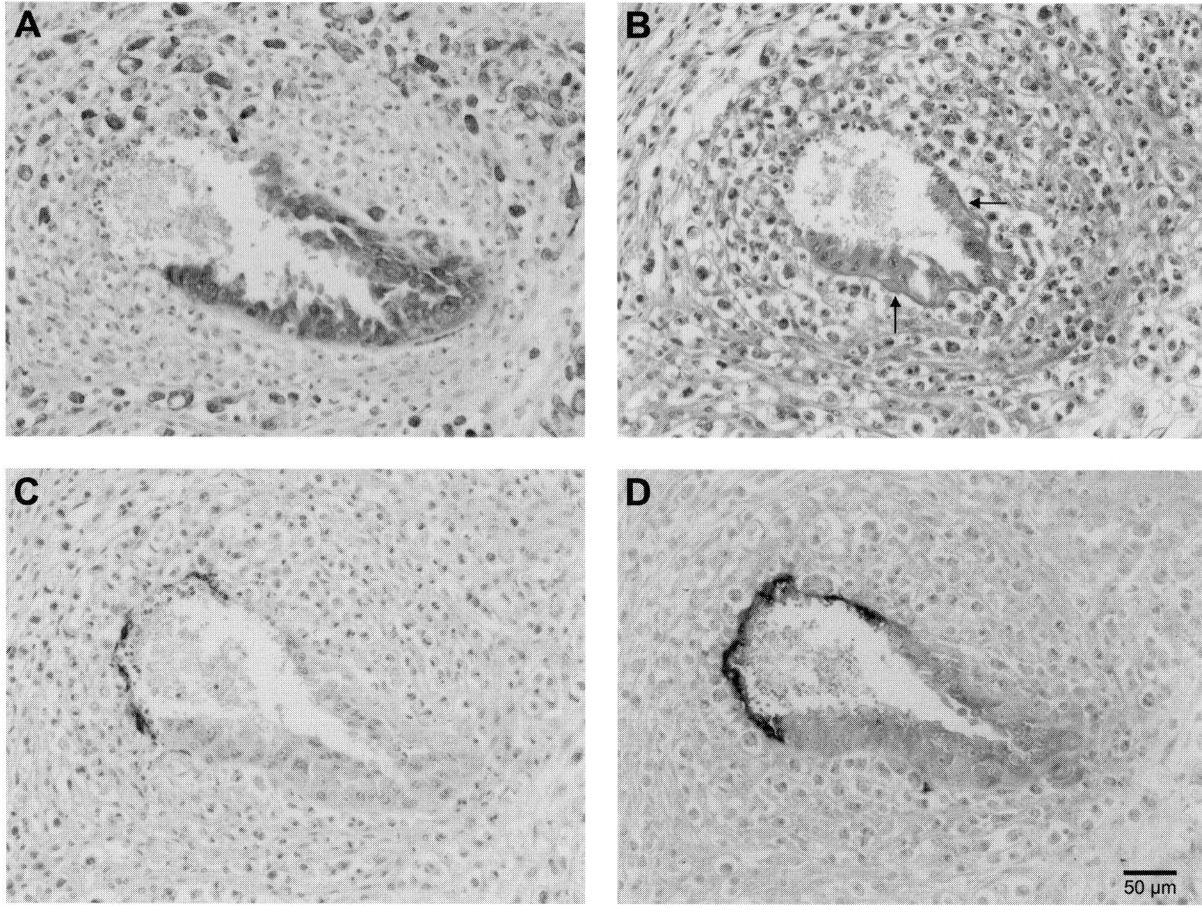

Fig. 13.8 Invaded spiral artery in the mesometrial triangle of a rat at day 18, showing the presence of trophoblast (A: cytokeratin immunostaining), fibrinoid (B: PAS staining), vascular smooth muscle breakdown (C: alpha-actin immunostaining) and endothelial replacement (D: CD31 immunostaining). The arrows in B indicate the PAS-positive fibrinoid layer underneath the endovascular trophoblast. Reproduced with permission from Caluwaerts *et al.* [13], Copyright Elsevier (2005).

the trophoblast. Endothelial loss, and also subsequent fragmentation and even loss of vascular smooth muscle, is mainly a focal event, which is closely associated with the overlying endovascular trophoblast (Fig. 13.8). At day 21, just before parturition, the endovascular trophoblasts have sunk into the vessel wall which has meanwhile restored its endothelial lining [13]. In the rat there is no suggestion of any thrombotic event during this process, or of intimal thickening as described in the human (Chapter 11).

In the mouse, some endothelial replacement by the perivascular trophoblast was described for day 13.5 [30], but unfortunately no data were provided about a possible endothelial repair, which might occur near the end of pregnancy. Other features of vascular remodeling, particularly the thinning of vascular smooth muscle, also occur upstream in the vessels at a distance from the invading trophoblast and are therefore merely the result of decidua-associated remodeling as described earlier.

The role of interstitial trophoblast in vascular remodeling

In the human most of the invading trophoblast follows an interstitial pathway which precedes endovascular invasion and includes the junctional zone of the myometrium. Interstitial trophoblast is also involved in spiral artery remodeling, although its actual impact is still under discussion (Chapter 11). In rhesus monkeys and baboons, however, very little interstitial invasion seems to occur, and trophoblast-associated remodeling must be effected chiefly by endovascular trophoblast [15,32]. This paucity of interstitial trophoblast, restricted to the most distal layers of the decidua basalis, is related to the persistence of an intact cytotrophoblastic shell at the placental–decidual border during the whole pregnancy period, in contrast to the human where early disintegration of the shell heralds the beginning of trophoblast invasion.

In the hamster, spiral artery sections in the mesometrial triangle are not contained within an extensive decidualized stromal tissue as in the rat, but are suspended within a very loose connective tissue. Following the endovascular invasion of the spiral arteries, interstitial basophilic cells appear within these intervascular tissue spaces, while they are absent in deciduomata induced in contralateral ligated uterine horns. Although these cells have not been identified immunohistochemically, it is almost certain that they are of trophoblastic origin [14]. Because of their late arrival, it is not likely that they play a role in the onset of vascular remodeling in the mesometrial triangle. It was not possible to distinguish morphologically similar interstitial cells in the decidua.

In the rat both decidua and mesometrial triangle are invaded by interstitial trophoblast which originates from the glycogen cells in the trophospongial compartment of the placenta [39,40]. Since also in this species interstitial invasion occurs after the endovascular invasion – in contrast to what happens in the human – trophoblast-associated vascular remodeling must be mainly effected by the endovascular trophoblast, although in later stages interstitial trophoblasts approach the spiral artery lumina very closely [13], where they gradually replace degenerating uNK cells in the perivascular regions [39]. In the mouse the situation seems to be different. Although in this species spiral artery invasion is mainly perivascular, molecular marker studies indicated a different origin of the perivascular trophoblasts compared to the 'real' interstitially invading cells [41]. As in the rat, the latter cells originate from the trophospongial glycogen cells, but their invasion barely covers the whole thickness of the decidual layer. The shallowness of both perivascular and interstitial invasion precludes a major impact on the vascular remodeling in the deeper decidua and mesometrial triangle.

Of all rodent species the deepest invasion has been observed in guinea-pigs [35]. By focusing on endovascular trophoblast Hees [42] challenged the idea that trophoblast could provide the initial trigger for vascular changes, since deep invasion was thought to be initiated only around the fifth week of pregnancy, after the breakdown of the elastica membrane in the mesometrial arteries. Later studies revealed however that during the initial vascular dilatation before day 30, interstitial trophoblasts are already present in the vicinity of these blood vessels. These cells were found to express endothelial as well as macrophage nitric oxide synthase, thought to be responsible for the early vascular remodeling [43]. A close analogy with the early spiral artery disorganization by interstitial trophoblast in the human (see Chapter 11) was therefore suggested. Extrapolation of these findings to our own species was not successful however, since in the human extravillous trophoblasts do not seem to express nitric oxide synthase [44]. Further studies on guinea-pigs and other related hystricomorph species would certainly be worthwhile, since comparative studies in this rodent group may reveal subtle differences in timing and types of cellular interaction [45], broadening our views on possible mechanisms regulating invasion and remodeling.

Trophoblast invasion in animal models for preeclampsia

At this stage we should consider the situation in animal models for preeclampsia, which in the human is associated with restricted endovascular trophoblast invasion and inadequate spiral artery remodeling [34]. We are still uncertain as to whether impaired trophoblast invasion could be a primary defect triggering subsequent steps leading to preeclampsia, or may be a consequence of some different – maybe maternal – defect in decidualization or maternal blood supply. For exploring this problem, various experimental strategies may be followed. When in search for an animal model, it seems appropriate to focus on species with deep endovascular invasion, in which one may try to interfere with some of the steps in the vascular remodeling process. Ideally, one should aim to devise an experimental method for specifically reducing endovascular trophoblast invasion and look for subsequent vascular defects and the appearance of preeclampsia-like symptoms. Such techniques are presently not established.

Based upon the idea that preeclampsia may result from uteroplacental underperfusion, uteroplacental ischemia has been induced to study subsequent effects on pregnancy. Several experimental approaches have been followed to achieve this, the most popular being vascular ligation which indeed may induce preeclampsia-like symptoms [46,47]. So far, the only study focusing on trophoblast invasion in such RUPP (reduced uteroplacental perfusion) models was performed in the rhesus monkey [48]. While this species normally does not show deep invasion [15], the big surprise was that in ligated animals interstitial, but not endovascular, trophoblasts showed deeper invasion, including the inner myometrium. The authors suggested that ligation-induced hypoxia might play a role in inducing deeper invasion, although later *in vitro* studies on human trophoblast indicated a need for high oxygen for inducing invasion [49]. In laboratory rodents, nobody has specifically looked at the effect of RUPP on trophoblast invasion so far.

Tinkering with blood pressure regulation may be another fruitful approach. A most intriguing example is the preeclamptic double transgenic rat, obtained by crossing a human angiotensinogen gene-carrying female with a human renin gene-carrying male [50]. When such animals become pregnant, they develop the typical preeclampsia symptoms of hypertension and proteinuria, although the blood pressure will drop near the end of pregnancy. An exciting observation was also the sporadic appearance of vascular lesions, not unlike acute atherosis, in some of the spiral arteries. It is not clear, however, whether these lesions are completely comparable with the real vasculopathies in human preeclampsia. Surprisingly enough, a significantly deeper invasion of endovascular trophoblast was found in the preeclamptic animals compared to controls, but this was associated with a decreased degradation of vascular smooth muscle [51]. The histological finding of deeper invasion in this model was supported by decreased resistance indices revealed by Doppler studies [52]. It is not known in how far this deeper invasion might be the result of a compensatory mechanism to overcome an impaired (decidua-associated?) early vascular remodeling. Such unexpected findings highlight our poor understanding of the regulation of the invasion process and associated vascular changes. Elucidating these processes should stand high on the priority list of future research on animal models for normal and preeclamptic pregnancies.

Concluding remarks

There cannot be any doubt that the study of factors controlling the depth of trophoblast invasion in different species provides a source of inspiration for further studies in the human. A comparative approach may indeed be very rewarding, not only by studying different species, but even different strains of the common laboratory animals such as mice and rats, an aspect which unfortunately has not received sufficient attention so far. Furthermore one should always consider that invasion depth and spiral artery remodeling are the result of a close interaction between trophoblast and the uterine environment. Decidualization is one important factor, and it is by no means certain as to whether decidualization in rapidly reproducing small rodents and the more slowly reproducing primates plays a similar role in restricting or promoting trophoblast invasion (see Chapter 4). Also the succession of vascular remodeling steps, the events triggering trophoblast invasion, and of course invasion depths show marked species differences (Table 13.2). Decidua-associated remodeling of spiral arteries seems to be a common feature for the decidual arterial segments, but its possible extension into the myometrium has not been studied in non-human primates. Endovascular plugging by trophoblast has only been observed in the human and in hamsters so far. If plugging was indeed absent in other species, this would indicate different relationships between trophoblast invasion and blood flow and/or oxygen supply, which may restrict the validity of these species as models. Fibrinoid deposition and intramural trophoblast replacement of vascular smooth muscle seem to be common features in most experimental animals, but the occurrence of endothelial repair has not been studied in most cases. There are important differences in the depth of invasion, which should be taken into account if one wants to focus specifically on trophoblast-associated vascular remodeling in deeper compartments of the placental bed. In such cases it is equally important to evaluate the extent of preceding decidua-associated remodeling in the presence or absence of uNK cells. The investigation of deep trophoblast invasion and associated remodeling would of course be particularly relevant for studies on animal models of preeclampsia. We have previously considered that defective deep vascular remodeling in preeclampsia may have different causes, as indeed also each of the subsequent remodeling steps might be impaired [54] (Chapter 11). The ideal experimental animal will probably remain elusive, since it seems unlikely that an identical sequence of remodeling steps will be found in any other species, except maybe in our closest anthropoid relatives (Chapter 12).

Table 13.2. Remodeling steps in different species

Species	Human	Rhesus	Baboon	Mouse	Rat	Hamster	Guinea-pig
Decidua-associated vascular remodeling							
Decidua	+	+	+				
Myometrium	+	?	?				
Meso. triangle				+	+	+	?
Trophoblast-associated vascular remodeling							
Trophoblast invasion							
– Plugs	+	?	?	–	?	+	?
– Endovascular migration	+	+	+	–	+	+	?
– Deep invasion myometrium	+	–	–				
– Deep invasion meso. triangle				–	+	+	+
Vascular remodeling							
– Fibrinoid + media replacement	+	+	+	+	+	+	± ?
– Endothelial repair	+	?	?	?	+	?	?

Acknowledgment

We wish to thank Anthony Carter for his critical comments on this chapter.

References

1. Hubrecht AA W. Studies in mammalian embryology. 1. The placentation of *Erinaceus europaeus*, with remarks on the phylogeny of the placenta. *Q J Microsc Sci* 1889; **30**: 283–404.
2. Peters H. *Ueber die Einbettung des menschlichen Eies und das früheste bisher bekannte menschliche Placentationsstadium*. Leipzig und Wien: Franz Deuticke; 1899.
3. Grosser O. *Vergleichende Anatomie und Entwicklungsgeschichte der Eihäute und der Placenta*. Vienna: Wilhelm Braumüller; 1909.
4. Carter A M. Evolution of the placenta and fetal membranes seen in the light of molecular phylogenetics. *Placenta* 2001; **22**: 800–7.
5. Carter A M, Mess A. Evolution of the placenta in Eutherian mammals. *Placenta* 2007; **28**: 259–62.
6. Samuel C A, Perry J S. The ultrastructure of pig trophoblast transplanted to an ectopic site in the uterine wall. *J Anat* 1972; **113**: 139–49.
7. Allen W R. Fetomaternal interactions and influences during equine pregnancy. *Reproduction* 2001; **121**: 513–27.
8. Carter A M. Animal models of human placentation. *Placenta* (28, Suppl A) *Trophoblast Res* 2007; **2**: S41–S47.
9. De Feo V J. Decidualization. In: Wynn R M, ed. *Cellular biology of the uterus*. Amsterdam: North Holland Publishing Company; 1967: pp. 191–290.
10. Billington W D. Biology of the trophoblast. *Adv Reprod Physiol* 1971; **5**: 27–66.
11. Kirby D R S, Cowell T P. Trophoblast-host interactions. In: Fleischmajer R, Billingham R E, eds. *Epithelial-mesenchymal interactions*. Baltimore: Williams & Wilkins; 1968: pp. 64–77.
12. Greenwood J D, Minhas K, Di Santo J P *et al.* Ultrastructural studies of implantation sites from mice deficient in uterine natural killer cells. *Placenta* 2000; **21**: 693–702.
13. Caluwaerts S, Vercruysse L, Luyten C *et al.* Endovascular trophoblast invasion and associated structural changes in uterine spiral arteries of the pregnant rat. *Placenta* 2005; **26**: 574–84.
14. Pijnenborg R, Robertson W B, Brosens I. The arterial migration of trophoblast in the uterus of the golden hamster, *Mesocricetus auratus*. *J Reprod Fert* 1974; **40**: 269–80.

15. Ramsey E M, Houston M L, Harris J W S. Interactions of the trophoblast and maternal tissues in three closely related primate species. *Am J Obstet Gynecol* 1976; **124**: 647–52.
16. Pijnenborg R, Dixon G, Robertson W B, Brosens I. Trophoblastic invasion of human decidua from 8 to 18 weeks of pregnancy. *Placenta* 1980; **1**: 3–19.
17. Burton G J, Jauniaux E, Watson A L. Maternal arterial connections to the placental intervillous space during the first trimester of human pregnancy: the Boyd collection revisited. *Am J Obstet Gynecol* 1999; **181**: 718–24.
18. Blankenship T N, Enders A C. Trophoblast cell-mediated modifications to uterine spiral arteries during early gestation in the macaque. *Acta Anat* 1997; **158**: 227–36.
19. Orsini M W. The trophoblastic giant cells and endovascular cells, associated with pregnancy in the hamster, *Cricetus auratus*. *Am J Anat* 1954; **94**: 273–330.
20. Billington W D. Vascular migration of transplanted trophoblast in the golden hamster. *Nature* 1966; **211**: 988–9.
21. Hamilton W J, Boyd J D. Trophoblast in human utero-placental arteries. *Nature* 1966; **212**: 906–8.
22. Young A. The vascular architecture of the rat uterus during pregnancy. *Trans Roy Soc Edinb* 1956; **63**: 167–83.
23. Pijnenborg R, Robertson W B, Brosens I. The role of ovarian steroids in placental development and endovascular trophoblast migration in the golden hamster. *J Reprod Fert* 1975; **44**: 43–51.
24. Bridgman J. A morphological study of the development of the placenta of the rat. II. A histological and cytological study of the development of the chorioallantoic placenta of the white rat. *J Morphol* 1949; **83**: 195–224.
25. Duval M. *Le placenta des rongeurs*. Paris: Felix Alcan; 1892, 640.
26. Pijnenborg R, Vercruysse L. Mathias Duval on placental development in mice and rats. *Placenta* 2006; **27**: 109–18.
27. Jenkinson J W. Observations on the histology and physiology of the placenta of the mouse. *Tijdschr Nederl Dierk Vereen* 1902; **1**: 124–98.
28. Redline R W, Lu C Y. Localization of fetal major histocompatibility complex antigens and maternal leukocytes in murine placenta. *Lab Invest* 1989; **61**: 27–36.
29. Georgiades P, Ferguson-Smith A C, Burton G J. Comparative developmental anatomy of the murine and human definitive placentae. *Placenta* 2002; **23**: 3–19.
30. Adamson S L, Lu Y, Whiteley K J *et al.* Interactions between trophoblast cells and the maternal and fetal circulation in the mouse placenta. *Develop Biol* 2002; **250**: 358–73.
31. Hemberger M, Nozaki T, Masutani M *et al.* Differential expression of angiogenic and vasodilatory factors by invasive trophoblast giant cells depending on depth of invasion. *Developmental Dynamics* 2003; **227**: 185–91.
32. Blankenship T N, Enders A C, King B F. Trophoblastic invasion and the development of uteroplacental arteries in the macaque: immunohistochemical localization of cytokeratins, desmin, type IV collagen, laminin and fibronectin. *Cell Tissue Res* 1993; **272**: 227–36.
33. Pijnenborg R, D'Hooghe T, Vercruysse L *et al.* Evaluation of trophoblast invasion in placental bed biopsies of the baboon, with immunohistochemical localisation of cytokeratin, fibronectin, and laminin. *J Med Primatol* 1996; **25**: 272–81.
34. Brosens I, Robertson W B, Dixon H G. The role of spiral arteries in the pathogenesis of preeclampsia. In: Wynn R M, ed. *Obstetrics and gynecology annual*. New York: Appleton-Century-Crofts; 1972: pp. 177–91.
35. Verkeste C M, Slangen B F M, Daemen M *et al.* The extent of trophoblast invasion in the preplacental vasculature of the guinea-pig. *Placenta* 1998; **19**: 49–54.
36. Esadeg S, He H, Pijnenborg R, Van Leuven F, Croy B A. Alpha-2 macroglobulin controls trophoblast positioning in mouse implantation sites. *Placenta* 2003; **24**: 912–21.
37. Rosario G X, Konno T, Soares M J. Maternal hypoxia activates endovascular trophoblast cell invasion. *Dev Biol* 2008; **314**: 362–75.
38. Brosens I, Robertson W B, Dixon H G. The physiological response of the vessels of the placental bed to normal pregnancy. *J Path Bact* 1967; **93**: 569–79.
39. Ain R, Canham L N, Soares M J. Gestation stage-dependent intrauterine trophoblast cell invasion in the rat and mouse: novel endocrine phenotype and regulation. *Dev Biol* 2003; **260**: 176–90.
40. Vercruysse L, Caluwaerts S, Luyten C *et al.* Interstitial trophoblast invasion in the decidua and mesometrial triangle during the last third of pregnancy in the rat. *Placenta* 2006; **27**: 22–33.
41. Simmons D G, Cross J C. Determinants of trophoblast lineage and cell subtype specification in the mouse placenta. *Dev Biol* 2005; **284**: 12–24.
42. Hees H, Moll W, Wrobel K H, Hees I. Pregnancy-induced structural changes and trophoblastic invasion in the segmental mesometrial arteries of the guinea pig. *Placenta* 1987; **8**: 609–26.
43. Nanaev A K, Chwalisz K, Frank H G *et al.* Physiological dilation of uteroplacental arteries in the guinea pig

depends on nitric oxide synthase activity of extravillous trophoblast. *Cell Tissue Res* 1995; **282**: 407–21.

44. Lyall F, Bulmer J N, Kelly H, Duffie E, Robson S C. Human trophoblast invasion and spiral artery transformation: the role of nitric oxide. *Am J Pathol* 2000; **154**: 1105–14.
45. Mess A, Zaki N, Kadyrov M, Korr H, Kaufmann P. Caviomorph placentation as a model for trophoblast invasion. *Placenta* 2007; **28**: 1234–8.
46. Conrad K P. Animal models of pre-eclampsia: do they exist? *Fetal Med Rev* 1990; **2**: 67–88.
47. Podjarny E, Baylis C, Losonczy G. Animal models of preeclampsia. *Semin Perinatol* 1999; **23**: 2–13.
48. Zhou Y, Chiu K, Brescia R J *et al.* Increased depth of trophoblast invasion after chronic constriction of the lower aorta in rhesus monkeys. *Am J Obstet Gynecol* 1993; **169**: 224–9.
49. Genbacev O, Zhou Y, Ludow J W, Fisher S J. Regulation of human placental development by oxygen tension. *Science* 1997; **277**: 1669–72.
50. Dechend R, Gratze P, Wallukat G *et al.* Agonistic autoantibodies to the AT1 receptor in a transgenic rat model of preeclampsia. *Hypertension* 2005; **45**: 742–6.
51. Geusens N, Verlohren S, Luyten C *et al.* Endovascular trophoblast invasion, spiral artery remodelling and uteroplacental haemodynamics in a transgenic rat model of pre-eclampsia. *Placenta* 2008; **29**: 614–23.
52. Verlohren S, Niehoff M, Hering L *et al.* Uterine vascular function in a transgenic preeclampsia rat model. *Hypertension* 2008; **51** (part 2): 547–53.
53. Davies J, Dempsey E W, Amoroso E C. The subplacenta of the guinea pig: development, histology and histochemistry. *J Anat* 1961; **95**: 457–73.
54. Pijnenborg R, Vercruysse L, Hanssens M. The uterine spiral arteries in human pregnancy: facts and controversies. *Placenta* 2006; **27**: 939–58.
55. Hubrecht A A W. *Die Säugetierontogenese in ihrer Bedeutung für die Phylogenie der Wirbeltiere.* Jena: Gustav Fischer Verlag; 1909: pp. 12–13.

Chapter 14

Trophoblast–arterial interactions *in vitro*

Judith E. Cartwright and Guy St. J. Whitley

Division of Basic Medical Sciences, St. George's, University of London, London, UK

Importance of studying trophoblast–arterial interactions

Uterine spiral arteries are remodeled extensively in the early part of pregnancy. This remodeling results in large dilated vessels with an increased blood flow, a change of crucial importance for delivering an increased blood supply to the developing fetus. In pregnancy complications such as preeclampsia this remodeling is incomplete. These alterations in the vessel properties occur as a result of remodeling of the vessel wall. In a remodeled vessel trophoblasts have invaded into the medial layer and replaced the vascular smooth muscle layer. The endothelium is temporarily replaced with trophoblast, although it is restored later in pregnancy. The lumen of the remodeled vessel is dilated and there is deposition of a fibrinoid material in the vessel wall. These changes were termed 'physiological change' [1]. Some changes to the vessel occur during decidualization (prior to trophoblast invasion) such as endothelial vacuolation and vascular smooth muscle swelling. Trophoblasts invade by two routes – the interstitial and endovascular paths – and are positioned such that they can influence both the vascular cells and the surrounding matrix. It is postulated that the interstitial trophoblast prepares the vessel for subsequent endovascular invasion, although the relative importance of each trophoblastic subtype remains to be clarified. The hypotheses regarding different roles of the trophoblast are extensively reviewed by Pijnenborg *et al.* 2006 [2]. It is clear that trophoblasts play an active role in the remodeling events that occur in the decidual and inner myometrial spiral arteries.

Studies of spiral arteries have been confined primarily to immunohistochemical analysis of placental bed biopsies while *in vitro* studies have been hampered by the lack of suitable human models to directly examine cellular interactions during trophoblast invasion. In recent years a number of groups have attempted to address this through the development of *in vitro* coculture and explant models and, using these, have gained valuable insights into the challenging question of how spiral arteries are remodeled in early pregnancy. In this chapter we will review the cell models currently available to study spiral artery remodeling and indicate how the move from simple cocultures through to more complex 3D explant models can address some of the questions that cannot be answered by histological studies alone. We will discuss the advantages and disadvantages of each approach and highlight the fact that valuable mechanistic insights into these important events have been acquired through imaginative use of culture models.

What are the problems in modeling the placental bed/spiral arteries *in vitro*?

Although the driving force behind much of the research in this area is to increase our understanding of pregnancy complications such as recurrent miscarriage, preeclampsia, and intrauterine growth restriction, we know surprisingly little about the cellular and molecular mechanisms behind the events that take place in the early weeks of a normal human pregnancy. Much of this is due to the lack of appropriate animal models. Human tissue can be obtained from first trimester therapeutic terminations of pregnancy and from both normal and complicated pregnancies at term. Clearly due to ethical considerations both these approaches have limitations and they merely give snapshots of dynamic events that occur slowly over a number of weeks. Interventional studies directed at establishing mechanisms at a cellular or molecular level are completely impossible.

There are many difficulties in investigating mechanisms that may be at fault early in complicated pregnancies. Changes that occur during spiral artery remodeling will be initiated in the first trimester of pregnancy, but when tissue is obtained at this stage it is not known if it would have developed normally or not. Tissue obtained at term from pregnancies known to be normal or preeclamptic will not give much information about the changes that occur in the first trimester.

In recent years two approaches have been used to address these problems which will have an impact on experimentation in this field. First trophoblasts have been isolated from chorionic villous samples obtained for diagnostic purposes from ongoing pregnancies [3,4]. Second, Doppler ultrasound sonography has been used to identify pregnancies with high bilateral uterine artery resistance in the first trimester indicating an increased risk of preeclampsia. Application of this method to women undergoing terminations of pregnancy has allowed access to tissue from pregnancies characterized as at 'high risk' or 'low risk' of preeclampsia had the pregnancy progressed to term [5,6].

Complicating the matter further, spiral artery remodeling involves not only the vascular cells and trophoblast but also immune and decidual cells. There are therefore potentially many possible interactions between multiple cell types that should be considered in any *in vitro* model of this process.

Modeling trophoblast–arterial interactions *in vitro*

What cell types can be used to model these events?

Trophoblast

First trimester placental tissue is available from therapeutic terminations of pregnancy following ethical approval and informed consent. Cytotrophoblasts can be isolated from this tissue using modifications of the original method published by Kliman *et al.* [7] for term placenta. The combination of enzymic digestion, density gradient centrifugation, and negative selection of contaminating cells will give highly pure, although somewhat limited numbers of cytotrophoblasts [8]. These cells can, depending on culture conditions, be further differentiated into syncytiotrophoblast following culture directly on plastic for 72 hours or extravillous trophoblast if cultured on Matrigel™ for 48 hours [9,10].

Chorionic villous explants cultured on collagen I or Matrigel™ will produce outgrowths of HLA-G and cytokeratin-7 positive extravillous trophoblasts over time (use and methodologies are reviewed in detail in [10,11]). These cultures can be used for the isolation of RNA, whole-mount antibody staining, observation of invasive outgrowth [12], manipulation using siRNA [13], or assessment of morphological changes using time-lapse microscopy [6]. Although they are a good source of pure extravillous trophoblast the numbers of cells that can be obtained are low and because of low proliferation rates they can be difficult to subculture.

Isolates of trophoblast from term placentae yield many more cells; over 250 million cells can be obtained from 50 g of placental villous tissue [14]. Cells can be isolated from pregnancies that are clinically normal and from pregnancies where there were clinical complications. However, cells obtained from the third trimester are not the most appropriate model when studying early differentiated trophoblast functions such as invasion as they will behave differently from first trimester cells. Of particular relevance to modeling spiral artery interactions is the recent finding that interactions with vascular cells are different depending on the gestational age of the trophoblasts used [15].

A number of extravillous trophoblast cell lines have been generated from first trimester tissue either spontaneously from outgrowths or following genetic manipulation of the cells to extend their lifespan (reviewed and discussed in [16,17,18]). These can be a good model if cultured appropriately and used in conjunction with primary cultures. As will be discussed in detail later removal of any cell from its 3D environment can alter the expression of genes and proteins. Hence, criticism of cell lines may be no more valid than criticism of a primary isolate taken from its normal environment and further cultured. Confirmation of results in both primary and cell line cultures is therefore important.

Endothelial cells

Vascular endothelial cells line the lumen of all blood vessels including the spiral artery. During early gestation, invading endovascular trophoblasts interdigitate and ultimately displace the endothelial cells. As the pregnancy progresses the endothelial cells begin to repopulate the vessel. Being able to study the interactions of endothelial cells with the extravillous trophoblast will give some insight into an important aspect of the mechanism of remodeling. Until relatively recently the most commonly used endothelial cells in vascular biology were those isolated from the human umbilical vein. Chosen primarily for their availability and relative ease of isolation these cells have been used in numerous studies. However, it is known that endothelial cells from different vascular beds can behave differently from each other and that these differences may be retained in culture. To address this problem endothelial cells have been isolated from term decidua [19] and this method has been modified for use on first trimester decidual tissue [20]. Cells isolated in this way are a mixture of both arterial and venous endothelial cells and are likely to have a similarly mixed phenotype. More recently, endothelial cells have also been isolated from spiral arteries dissected from non-placental bed biopsies obtained at term; however, to date cell yields have been low (Cartwright & Whitley, unpublished data). Again it should be recognized that, as with trophoblasts obtained at term, endothelial cells obtained at this time may be different from those that might be isolated from first trimester spiral arteries.

To reduce variability and to overcome the relatively low proliferation of primary endothelial cells a number of groups have produced and characterized endothelial cells from different vascular beds [21]. Most have used transfection with a plasmid encoding the SV40 protein T-antigen [22,23] but more recently an endometrial endothelial cell line has been reported which used telomerase-mediated transfection [24]. Our experience would indicate that the cell lines produced in this way are phenotypically stable over many passages and have retained many of the endothelial cell markers expressed by the parent cells [25].

Vascular smooth muscle cells

Unlike muscle cells from other tissues, vascular smooth muscle cells (VSMC) are not terminally differentiated. Depending on the local environment VSMC can switch between a differentiated contractile phenotype and a de-differentiated synthetic phenotype. In a healthy quiescent vessel the VSMC grow very slowly and exhibit a contractile phenotype expressing specific contractile proteins such as smooth muscle α-actin, smooth muscle myosin heavy chain, calponin, and smooth muscle 22α (SM22α) but do not generally proliferate. However, in response to culture *in vitro* they can adopt a more synthetic phenotype resulting in the downregulation of contractile proteins and the increased synthesis of components of the extracellular matrix such as elastin [26]. It is unclear how long the synthetic phenotype is maintained in prolonged culture. *In vitro* a differentiated phenotype can be induced by the addition of factors such as ascorbate and insulin-like growth factor or the inhibition of the intracellular signaling molecule mTOR [27].

Efforts have been made to make and characterize human VSMC lines for studies in a number of physiological [28,29,30] and pathological situations [31]. These lines have been made by targeting the retinoblastoma gene with the E6/E7 of human papilloma virus or p53 with the SV40 protein T-antigen. VSMC lines produced in this way tend to exhibit a synthetic phenotype under normal growth conditions and therefore careful choice of the conditions is needed if a fully differentiated VSMC is required.

Simple coculture studies

Simple coculture is applicable to many different cell types, does not necessarily need large cell numbers for experiments, is useful when conducting experiments with primary cells, and is easy to manipulate to investigate mechanisms (Fig. 14.1A).

There are difficulties in interpretation that have to be overcome when two cell types are grown together in monolayer culture; for example, how to distinguish between the two cell types? In recent years this has been overcome with the use of cell-permeable fluorescent dyes such as CellTracker™ from Molecular Probes which, once in the cell, undergo modification to form a membrane-impermeant product. These are largely non-toxic and can be used for prolonged periods in culture. An alternative approach is to transfect cells with plasmids that encode a fluorescent protein such as the enhanced green fluorescent protein. Both approaches enable the cultures to be monitored by live cell fluorescent microscopy.

Using this approach we have shown that primary extravillous trophoblast and trophoblast cell lines can induce both endothelial and VSMC apoptosis, and we were the first to suggest that apoptotic events may be important in spiral artery remodeling [20,28]. Morphological changes can be easily monitored in cocultures over time using time-lapse microscopy. When cells undergo apoptosis there is a distinct series of changes to their appearance when viewed by phase contrast microscopy: the cells round up, become phase-bright, and membrane blebs and blisters appear. The time point at which each cell starts to undergo apoptosis can be scored, allowing sensitive measurement of the kinetics of the apoptotic response. These experiments are easily manipulated with blocking antibodies, and the simple nature of the cocultures means that defined manipulations can be carried out

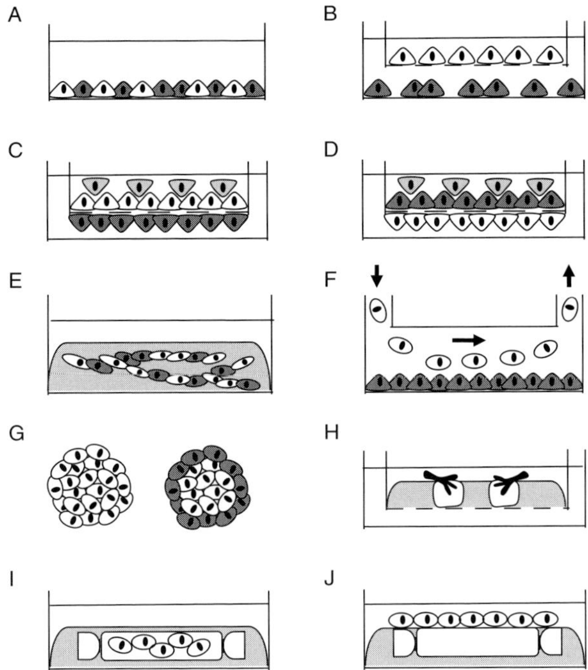

Fig. 14.1 *In vitro* models of trophoblast–arterial interactions. (A) Monolayer coculture of trophoblast with either endothelial cells or VSMC. The two cell types are distinguished by labeling with fluorescent dyes [20,28]. (B) Cocultured cells are separated by a microporous transwell filter allowing soluble factors to diffuse through to the target cell [20,28]. (C and D) Endothelial cells and VSMC are grown on either side of a collagen-coated microporous membrane to mimic vessel structure [38]. Trophoblasts added to interact with the endothelial cells could mimic endovascular interactions while interstitial events could be modeled by adding trophoblasts to interact with VSMC. (E) Coculture of trophoblast with endothelial cells in Matrigel^{TM} leads to the formation of tube-like structures consisting of a mixture of cell types [36]. (F) The effect of flow on trophoblast interactions with monolayers of endothelial cells can be examined using a parallel plate flow chamber [48]. (G) Trophoblast grown on non-adherent plates or at zero gravity form 3D spheroids [54,55]. Endothelial cells and VSMC cocultured as 3D spheroids organize with a VSMC core and a layer of endothelial cells on the surface [56]. (H) Explant cultures in Matrigel^{TM} of first trimester villi at low oxygen tension in contact with sections of decidua parietalis from the same patient [61]. Extravillous trophoblasts invade and interact with the decidual blood vessels. (I and J) Non-placental bed spiral arteries isolated at term are either perfused with fluorescently labeled trophoblasts to model endovascular invasion prior to culture in fibrin gels or cultured with trophoblast to model interstitial invasion [58,59].

to block or activate signaling within a particular cell type prior to coculture. This approach allowed us to identify a role for Fas/FasL in trophoblast-induced endothelial apoptosis [20] and also a role for Fas/FasL and TRAIL in VSMC apoptosis [28,30]. An advantage of this approach is that relatively few cells are required, which is ideal for primary isolates such as decidual endothelial cells [20], and advances in time-lapse microscopy mean that subtle changes can be monitored over a long period.

A role for soluble factors in the remodeling process can be identified by physically separating the two cell types whilst allowing the diffusion of soluble factors. This is most readily achieved using microporous filters (Fig. 14.1B). If the target cell is grown in the well while the effecter cell is grown on the filter the fate of the target cell can be monitored by time-lapse microscopy. Using this method we were able to identify that soluble FasL was in part responsible for trophoblast-induced endothelial cell apoptosis [20].

The induction of apoptosis in the spiral artery, as part of a normal adaptation to pregnancy, seems conceptually appealing when we consider the nature of the apoptotic process and its established role in normal development. Apoptosis is an asynchronous process that occurs physiologically over an extended period of time, in keeping with the gradual remodeling of vessels. Apoptotic cells can be rapidly removed by neighboring phagocytic cells (either professional phagocytes such as macrophages, or amateur phagocytes which are essentially any other cell type under the right conditions) thus preventing any associated inflammatory response. It is interesting to note here that trophoblasts can be phagocytic and can degrade matrix components and other cell types [32,33].

The extracellular matrix plays an important role in regulating cellular behavior [34]. It has been known for a number of years that endothelial cells grown on Matrigel^{TM} migrate together and form capillary-like structures. In cross section some of these structures are seen to have a lumen [35]. Aldo *et al.* [36] have developed a similar culture system to investigate trophoblast interactions with endothelial cells. In these studies a human endometrial endothelial cell line (HEEC) formed tube-like structures when cultured on Matrigel^{TM}. When first trimester trophoblast cells (either the HTR-8 cell line or primary trophoblasts) were added to the preformed tubes trophoblasts migrated toward the structures and integrated with the endothelial cells (Fig. 14.1E). Studies in our laboratory have additionally shown that when trophoblasts and endothelial cells are added in culture simultaneously on Matrigel^{TM}, the resulting tube-like structures consist of a mixture of trophoblast and endothelial cells (McCormick, Whitley, & Cartwright, unpublished observations). Growing cells on matrices can help to re-establish some of the differentiated functions that might otherwise be lost in a simple coculture system; however, these matrices also have limitations. For example, most are extracted from animals or cultured cells and will therefore be variably contaminated with soluble components such as growth factors which could affect experimental reproducibility and confound the dissection of individual signaling events. The development of synthetic scaffolds may help to address this problem [37].

In a normal arteriole, luminal endothelial cells are separated from the underlying smooth muscle cells by a basement membrane consisting of collagen IV and elastin fibers. The glycoproteins laminin and fibronectin are also present and help bind the cells to the matrix. To mimic this structure, endothelial cells and VSMC have been grown on either side of a collagen-coated microporous membrane and it has been suggested that this model functions similarly to a vessel *in vivo* [38]. Adaptation of this approach may provide an excellent model to examine how trophoblasts interact with the endothelial cells and VSMC (Fig. 14.1C and 1D).

In addition to starting to dissect the apoptotic events involved in vessel remodeling coculture studies of trophoblast with vascular cells have given other valuable information regarding cellular interactions. Studies of the adhesive interactions between trophoblast and endothelial cells have demonstrated a role for β1 integrins [39], vitronectin receptors [40], VCAM-1, α4β1 [41], and MUC1 [42] while Chen *et al.* [43,44] have demonstrated that the activation status of the endothelial cells can influence the nature of their interaction with trophoblast. An important factor to consider is the ability of the trophoblast cells to migrate and invade in a directional manner toward the vessels in order to facilitate remodeling. We have begun to dissect this chemoattraction using live cell image analysis methods which allow quantitative assessment of the behavior of two cell types in coculture [45]. In coculture, trophoblasts migrated more than in the absence of VSMC and showed directionality of movement toward VSMC. Development of this analysis will allow the role of specific chemoattractant factors to be examined.

Modeling hemodynamic factors involved in spiral artery remodeling

The hemodynamic changes that take place in spiral arteries during pregnancy are considerable [46]. Trophoblastic plugging and remodeling events which alter vessel structure all influence the shear and mechanical stresses on the vascular cells. Shear stress and the vessel deformation are important regulators of vascular cell function. Although the VSMC may also be influenced by shear stress they are exposed more to mechanical stretch. In many vessels including the unmodified spiral artery this will be experienced in pulses and the extent to which it affects VSMC will depend on their degree of differentiation [47].

Modeling the effects of these stresses on trophoblast interactions with vascular cells has largely been unexplored. However, recent developments in cell culture techniques mean that such studies can now begin. Using a parallel plate flow chamber and video microscopy Soghomonians *et al.* [48] have examined trophoblast migration and concluded that migration under flow was regulated by endothelial cells (Fig. 14.1F). In addition, this group have begun to dissect the adhesive interactions that are influenced by flow conditions [49,50]. It will be informative to repeat these studies in the presence of VSMC, and to this end a study co-culturing endothelial cells and VSMC on either side of microporous membranes has been combined with flow [51].

Modeling the complex 3D environment

It is often assumed that cell monolayers reflect the physiology of real tissues. However, studies comparing cell behavior when grown in monolayer (i.e. 2D) versus a more 3D environment have shown that there are significant differences in cell behavior, including gene expression, growth, morphogenesis, motility, and differentiation (reviewed in [52]). Consequently there has been a push towards 3D cultures in cell biology. Use of these techniques in the study of tumorigenesis has been at the forefront, but such an approach may also be highly relevant in our quest for knowledge of uteroplacental cell biology. A number of different approaches can be taken to examine cell culture in 3D including explant cultures, cellular spheroids, and microcarrier cultures; however, experimental analysis can be a significant problem (reviewed in [53]).

Spheroid cultures can be formed by growing cells in the absence of an adhesive matrix, on non-adherent plates, or at zero gravity and studies have shown that 3D growth of trophoblasts in this way alters their gene expression and increases their invasive behavior [54, 55]. Korff *et al.* [56] demonstrated that when endothelial cells and VSMC were cocultured as 3D spheroids the cells organized such that the VSMC formed the core while the endothelial cells were on the surface, thus mimicking the vascular cells of a vessel (Fig. 14.1G). Combining this approach with the trophoblast cultures could be useful for studying the process of remodeling; indeed Baal *et al.* have recently reported a three-dimensional, three-component spheroidal coculture model with trophoblasts, villous stromal cells, and endothelial precursor cells which could be adapted for this purpose [57].

Ex vivo models

To move further toward a more 3D model of events occurring in spiral artery remodeling we have described an *ex vivo* model of spiral artery invasion and remodeling, developed using spiral artery explants, extravillous trophoblast cell lines, and primary cytotrophoblasts [58, 59]. In this model, non-placental bed spiral arteries isolated at term are either perfused with fluorescently labeled trophoblasts to model endovascular invasion or cultured with trophoblast to model interstitial invasion (Fig. 14.1I and J). A number of factors can be studied using this model including the interactions between trophoblasts and vascular cells, alteration of expression of markers during invasion, the effect of growth factors and oxygen tension on invasion, and the cellular and molecular events occurring during vascular remodeling. In addition, invasion of non-placental bed spiral arteries from preeclamptic and growth-restricted pregnancies can be compared to arteries from normal pregnancies at similar gestational age.

Using this approach we have shown that trophoblasts are capable of interacting with cells in the vessel wall, with invasion occurring both interstitially and endovascularly [58]. Extension of these studies by Crocker *et al.* [60], who investigated culture at different oxygen tensions, showed that when the extravillous trophoblast/vessel cultures were maintained at 17% oxygen for 3 days, both endovascular and interstitial invasion occurred, with endovascular invasion being more extensive. Breakdown of the vessel wall could be observed where trophoblast aggregates had attached. However, at 3% oxygen tension there was less invasion by either route. A comparison with omental vessels taken from the same patient at cesarean section or non-pregnant myometrial vessels obtained at hysterectomy showed limited invasion, suggesting that some of the decidua-associated changes prior to trophoblast invasion are important in priming the vessels for subsequent invasion.

Loss of the endothelium can be mimicked effectively in this vessel model. Perfusion of trophoblasts (either SGHPL-4 cell line or primary first trimester extravillous trophoblasts) into the lumen of dissected spiral arteries led to loss of endothelial cells after 4 days of culture, as determined by staining cryosectioned vessels for vWF, a specific endothelial marker [20]. The expression of the apoptotic marker cleaved PARP in these vessels indicated apoptosis was the mode of cell death. Inhibiting Fas/FasL interactions using a blocking antibody prevented endothelial apoptosis, confirming the coculture results [20].

The effects of trophoblast and trophoblast-derived factors on spiral artery VSMC were assessed using a modification of this model. To facilitate direct interactions between trophoblasts and VSMC, the endothelium of the dissected spiral artery was removed by passing a bubble of air through the vessel. Perfusion of the vessels with trophoblasts (primary extravillous, SGHPL-4 cells, or BeWo cell lines) induced apoptotic changes in the VSMC [28,29]. Addition of recombinant human TRAIL or a Fas-activating antibody induced VSMC apoptosis, and blocking Fas/FasL interactions prevented trophoblast induction of VSMC apoptosis in the vessel; these observations confirmed the coculture studies implicating these two pro-apoptotic cytokines [28,30]. The relative importance to the remodeling process of interstitial versus endovascular cells, soluble versus cell-associated pro-apoptotic factors, and the extent of redundancy within the system with regard to the involvement of multiple pro-apoptotic cytokines remain to be determined.

The advantages of this model are that the vessels are unmodified by trophoblasts and it is easy to identify non-placental bed uterine areas at cesarean section. Comparisons can be made between normal and preeclamptic vessels, and the relative roles of interstitial versus endovascular invasion elucidated. The system is amenable to use with manipulated trophoblast cells and function-blocking antibodies. Limitations that should be taken into account are that these are term vessels so care must be taken when extrapolating results to remodeling in the first trimester, and also that dissection of intact vessels which are sufficiently undamaged to allow perfusion is technically challenging.

Other groups have taken alternative approaches to models of these events. Dunk *et al.* [61] cultured first trimester villous explants at low oxygen tension in contact with sections of decidua parietalis from the same patient (Fig. 14.1H). In these studies extravillous trophoblast columns invaded the decidua and decidual blood vessels showed morphological disruption. Explant cultures such as these will preserve the cytoarchitecture and cellular differentiation of the original tissue and have advantages in that the tissue is from the first trimester. Care must be taken in this model to dissect decidua parietalis since the decidua basalis would already have some trophoblast-dependent changes occurring. In addition it would prove difficult to manipulate this system to identify mechanisms and, since the tissue is obtained in the first trimester, comparisons between normal and preeclamptic pregnancies have so far proven impossible. Use of first trimester tissue classified by uterine artery Doppler ultrasound as more likely to have come from a pregnancy that would have developed preeclampsia [6] may be informative in this model.

Red-Horse *et al.* [62] developed an *in vivo* model where chorionic villi were implanted into the mammary fat pads of *Scid* mice for 3 weeks. Their studies showed that trophoblasts invaded and interacted with the vessels, disrupting the arterial integrity and inducing apoptosis in the endothelial and smooth muscle layers of the arteries (but not veins). This is an innovative approach, although the events are cross-species and the vessels in mammary fat pads may not be representative of those in the placental bed.

Conclusions

Spiral artery remodeling is a multistep process taking place over a period of weeks. Consequently, this phenomenon must be tightly regulated to prevent sudden loss of vessel integrity. Determining how trophoblasts interact with cells of the maternal vessels is critical, since defects in vessel remodeling have been identified in pathological complications of pregnancy that compromise both maternal and fetal health.

Considerable advances in our understanding have been made in the last few years through the development of *in vitro* human coculture and explant models which build on previous immunohistochemical studies. A number of mechanisms may be responsible for the changes to vascular cells, in addition to the apoptotic ones that we and others have demonstrated, and it is likely that many precisely orchestrated processes will have a role to play. Only continued investigation will give a clearer mechanistic picture.

Our experience in developing *in vitro* models suggests an approach of starting with a simple system and building up the biological complexity when the conditions have been fully optimized. In addition, careful consideration of the scientific question to be addressed when choosing an appropriate model is crucial. It can be all too easy to be critical of the models that are being used in this field. As long as experimenters are aware of the limitations of their model, then progress will be made. This may result from a cumulative weight of evidence from many sources rather than the one perfect experiment which, in this challenging yet fascinating field, placental biologists know is usually impossible to carry out.

References

1. Brosens I, Robertson W B, Dixon H G. The physiological response of the vessels of the placental bed to normal pregnancy. *J Pathol Bacteriol* 1967; **93**(2): 569–79.
2. Pijnenborg R, Vercruysse L, Hanssens M. The uterine spiral arteries in human pregnancy: facts and controversies. *Placenta* 2006; **27**(9–10): 939–58.
3. Seeho S K, Park J H, Rowe J, Morris J M, Gallery E D. Villous explant culture using early gestation tissue from ongoing pregnancies with known normal outcomes: the effect of oxygen on trophoblast outgrowth and migration. *Hum Reprod* 2008; **23**(5): 1170–9.
4. Campbell S, Park J H, Rowe J *et al.* Chorionic villus sampling as a source of trophoblasts. *Placenta* 2007; **28**(11–12): 1118–22.
5. Prefumo F, Sebire N J, Thilaganathan B. Decreased endovascular trophoblast invasion in first trimester pregnancies with high-resistance uterine artery Doppler indices. *Hum Reprod* 2004; **19**(1): 206–9.
6. Whitley G S, Dash P R, Ayling L J *et al.* Increased apoptosis in first trimester extravillous trophoblasts from pregnancies at higher risk of developing preeclampsia. *Am J Pathol* 2007; **170**(6): 1903–9.
7. Kliman H J, Nestler J E, Sermasi E, Sanger J M, Strauss J F 3rd. Purification, characterization, and in vitro differentiation of cytotrophoblasts from human term placentae. *Endocrinology* 1986; **118**(4): 1567–82.
8. Frank H G, Genbacev O. Cell culture models of human trophoblast: primary culture of trophoblast – a workshop report. *Placenta* 2000; **21**(Suppl A): S120–S2.
9. Tarrade A, Lai Kuen R, Malassine A *et al.* Characterization of human villous and extravillous trophoblasts isolated from first trimester placenta. *Lab Invest* 2001; **81**(9): 1199–211.
10. Miller R K, Genbacev O, Turner M A *et al.* Human placental explants in culture: approaches and assessments. *Placenta* 2005; **26**(6): 439–48.

11. Aplin J D. In vitro analysis of trophoblast invasion. *Methods Mol Med* 2006; **122**: 45–57.
12. Aplin J D, Haigh T, Jones C J, Church H J, Vicovac L. Development of cytotrophoblast columns from explanted first-trimester human placental villi: role of fibronectin and integrin α5β1. *Biol Reprod* 1999; **60**(4): 828–38.
13. Forbes K, Desforges M, Garside R, Aplin J D, Westwood M. Methods for siRNA-mediated reduction of mRNA and protein expression in human placental explants, isolated primary cells and cell lines. *Placenta* 2009; **30**: 124–9.
14. Petroff M G, Phillips T A, Ka H, Pace J L, Hunt J S. Isolation and culture of term human trophoblast cells. *Methods Mol Med* 2006; **121**: 203–17.
15. Kalkunte S, Lai Z, Tewari N *et al.* In vitro and in vivo evidence for lack of endovascular remodeling by third trimester trophoblasts. *Placenta* 2008; **29**(10): 871–8.
16. Whitley G S. Production of human trophoblast cell lines. *Methods Mol Med* 2006; **121**: 219–28.
17. Shiverick K T, King A, Frank H *et al.* Cell culture models of human trophoblast II: trophoblast cell lines – a workshop report. *Placenta* 2001; **22**(Suppl A): S104–6.
18. Sullivan M H. Endocrine cell lines from the placenta. *Mol Cell Endocrinol* 2004; **228**(1–2): 103–19.
19. Grimwood J, Bicknell R, Rees M C. The isolation, characterization and culture of human decidual endothelium. *Hum Reprod* 1995; **10**(8): 2142–8.
20. Ashton S V, Whitley G S, Dash P R *et al.* Uterine spiral artery remodeling involves endothelial apoptosis induced by extravillous trophoblasts through Fas/FasL interactions. *Arterioscler Thromb Vasc Biol* 2005; **25**(1): 102–8.
21. Bouis D, Hospers G A, Meijer C, Molema G, Mulder N H. Endothelium in vitro: a review of human vascular endothelial cell lines for blood vessel-related research. *Angiogenesis* 2001; **4**(2): 91–102.
22. Fickling S A, Tooze J A, Whitley G S. Characterization of human umbilical vein endothelial-cell lines produced by transfection with the early region of Sv40. *Exp Cell Res* 1992; **201**(2): 517–21.
23. Purdie K J, Whitley G S, Johnstone A P, Cartwright J E. Hepatocyte growth factor-induced endothelial cell motility is mediated by the upregulation of inducible nitric oxide synthase expression. *Cardiovasc Res* 2002; **54**(3): 659–68.
24. Krikun G, Mor G, Lockwood C. The immortalization of human endometrial cells. *Methods Mol Med* 2006; **121**: 79–83.
25. Cartwright J E, Whitley G S, Johnstone A P. The expression and release of adhesion molecules by human endothelial-cell lines and their consequent binding of lymphocytes. *Exp Cell Res* 1995; **217**(2): 329–35.
26. Owens G K, Kumar M S, Wamhoff B R. Molecular regulation of vascular smooth muscle cell differentiation in development and disease. *Physiol Rev* 2004; **84**(3): 767–801.
27. Arakawa E, Hasegawa K, Irie J *et al.* L-ascorbic acid stimulates expression of smooth muscle-specific markers in smooth muscle cells both in vitro and in vivo. *J Cardiovasc Pharmacol* 2003; **42**(6): 745–51.
28. Harris L K, Keogh R J, Wareing M *et al.* Invasive trophoblasts stimulate vascular smooth muscle cell apoptosis by a fas ligand-dependent mechanism. *Am J Pathol* 2006; **169**(5): 1863–74.
29. Harris L K, Keogh R J, Wareing M *et al.* BeWo cells stimulate smooth muscle cell apoptosis and elastin breakdown in a model of spiral artery transformation. *Hum Reprod* 2007; **22**(11): 2834–41.
30. Keogh R J, Harris L K, Freeman A *et al.* Fetal-derived trophoblast use the apoptotic cytokine tumor necrosis factor-alpha-related apoptosis-inducing ligand to induce smooth muscle cell death. *Circ Res* 2007; **100**(6): 834–41.
31. Bennett M R, Macdonald K, Chan S W, Boyle J J, Weissberg P L. Cooperative interactions between RB and p53 regulate cell proliferation, cell senescence, and apoptosis in human vascular smooth muscle cells from atherosclerotic plaques. *Circ Res* 1998; **82**(6): 704–12.
32. Choy M Y, Manyonda I T. The phagocytic activity of human first trimester extravillous trophoblast. *Hum Reprod* 1998; **13**(10): 2941–9.
33. Chen Q, Stone P R, McCowan L M, Chamley L W. Interaction of Jar choriocarcinoma cells with endothelial cell monolayers. *Placenta* 2005; **26**(8–9): 617–25.
34. Kleinman H K, McGarvey M L, Hassell J R *et al.* Basement membrane complexes with biological activity. *Biochemistry* 1986; **25**(2): 312–8.
35. Folkman J, Haudenschild C. Angiogenesis by capillary endothelial cells in culture. *Trans Ophthalmol Soc UK* 1980; **100**(3): 346–53.
36. Aldo P B, Krikun G, Visintin I *et al.* A novel three-dimensional in vitro system to study trophoblast-endothelium cell interactions. *Am J Reprod Immunol* 2007; **58**(2): 98–110.
37. Tsang V L, Bhatia S N. Fabrication of three-dimensional tissues. *Adv Biochem Eng Biotechnol* 2007; **103**: 189–205.
38. Burch M G, Pepe G J, Dobrian A D, Lattanzio F A Jr, Albrecht E D. Development of a coculture system and use of confocal laser fluorescent microscopy to study human microvascular endothelial cell and mural cell interaction. *Microvasc Res* 2005; **70**(1–2): 43–52.

39. Thirkill T L, Hendren S R, Soghomonians A *et al.* Regulation of trophoblast β1-integrin expression by contact with endothelial cells. *Cell Commun Signal* 2004; **2**(1): 4.
40. Douglas G C, Thirkill T L, Blankenship T N. Vitronectin receptors are expressed by macaque trophoblast cells and play a role in migration and adhesion to endothelium. *Biochim Biophys Acta* 1999; **1452**(1): 36–45.
41. Cartwright J E, Balarajah G. Trophoblast interactions with endothelial cells are increased by interleukin-1 [beta] and tumour necrosis factor-α and involve vascular cell adhesion molecule-1 and α4β1. *Exp Cell Res* 2005; **304**(1): 328–36.
42. Thirkill T L, Cao T, Stout M *et al.* MUC1 is involved in trophoblast transendothelial migration. *Biochim Biophys Acta* 2007; **1773**(6): 1007–14.
43. Chen Q, Stone P R, McCowan L M, Chamley L W. Activated endothelial cells resist displacement by trophoblast in vitro. *Placenta* 2007; **28**: 743–7.
44. Chen Q, Stone P R, McCowan L M, Chamley L W. Phagocytosis of necrotic but not apoptotic trophoblasts induces endothelial cell activation. *Hypertension* 2006; **47**(1): 116–21.
45. Hamzic E, Cartwright J E, Keogh R J *et al.* Live cell image analysis of cell-cell interactions reveals the specific targeting of vascular smooth muscle cells by fetal trophoblasts. *Exp Cell Res* 2008; **314**(7): 1455–64.
46. Pijnenborg R. Uterine haemodynamics as a possible driving force for endovascular trophoblast migration in the placental bed. *Medical Hypotheses* 2000; **55**(2): 114–8.
47. Haga J H, Li Y S, Chien S. Molecular basis of the effects of mechanical stretch on vascular smooth muscle cells. *J Biomech* 2007; **40**(5): 947–60.
48. Soghomonians A, Barakat A I, Thirkill T L, Douglas G C. Trophoblast migration under flow is regulated by endothelial cells. *Biol Reprod* 2005; **73**(1): 14–9.
49. Cao T C, Thirkill T L, Wells M, Barakat A I, Douglas G C. Trophoblasts and shear stress induce an asymmetric distribution of icam-1 in uterine endothelial cells. *Am J Reprod Immunol* 2008; **59**(2): 167–81.
50. Soghomonians A, Barakat A I, Thirkill T L, Blankenship T N, Douglas G C. Effect of shear stress on migration and integrin expression in macaque trophoblast cells. *Biochim Biophys Acta* 2002; **1589**(3): 233–46.
51. Wang H Q, Huang L X, Qu M J *et al.* Shear stress protects against endothelial regulation of vascular smooth muscle cell migration in a coculture system. *Endothelium* 2006; **13**(3): 171–80.
52. Yamada K M, Cukierman E. Modeling tissue morphogenesis and cancer in 3D. *Cell* 2007; **130**(4): 601–10.
53. Pampaloni F, Reynaud E G, Stelzer E H. The third dimension bridges the gap between cell culture and live tissue. *Nat Rev Mol Cell Biol* 2007; **8**(10): 839–45.
54. LaMarca H L, Ott C M, Honer Z U *et al.* Three-dimensional growth of extravillous cytotrophoblasts promotes differentiation and invasion. *Placenta* 2005; **26**(10): 709–20.
55. Korff T, Krauss T, Augustin H G. Three-dimensional spheroidal culture of cytotrophoblast cells mimics the phenotype and differentiation of cytotrophoblasts from normal and preeclamptic pregnancies. *Exp Cell Res* 2004; **297**(2): 415–23.
56. Korff T, Kimmina S, Martiny-Baron G, Augustin H G. Blood vessel maturation in a 3-dimensional spheroidal coculture model: direct contact with smooth muscle cells regulates endothelial cell quiescence and abrogates VEGF responsiveness. *FASEB J* 2001; **15**(2): 447–57.
57. Baal N, Widmer-Teske R, McKinnon T, Preissner K T, Zygmunt M T. In vitro spheroid model of placental vasculogenesis: does it work? *Lab Invest* 2009; **89**: 152–63.
58. Cartwright J E, Kenny L C, Dash P R *et al.* Trophoblast invasion of spiral arteries: a novel in vitro model. *Placenta* 2002; **23**(2–3): 232–5.
59. Cartwright J E, Wareing M. An in vitro model of trophoblast invasion of spiral arteries. *Methods Mol Med* 2006; **122**: 59–74.
60. Crocker I P, Wareing M, Ferris G R *et al.* The effect of vascular origin, oxygen, and tumour necrosis factor alpha on trophoblast invasion of maternal arteries in vitro. *J Pathol* 2005; **206**(4): 476–85.
61. Dunk C, Petkovic L, Baczyk D *et al.* A novel in vitro model of trophoblast-mediated decidual blood vessel remodeling. *Lab Invest* 2003; **83**(12): 1821–8.
62. Red-Horse K, Rivera J, Schanz A *et al.* Cytotrophoblast induction of arterial apoptosis and lymphangiogenesis in an in vivo model of human placentation. *J Clin Invest* 2006; **116**(10): 2643–52.

Chapter 15

Long-term effects of uteroplacental insufficiency in animals

Robert H. Lane, Robert A. McKnight, and Qi Fu

Department of Pediatrics, University of Utah School of Medicine, Salt Lake City, USA

Intrauterine growth retardation (IUGR) complicates between 3 and 10% of all pregnancies. A common cause of IUGR is uteroplacental insufficiency (UPI), which is associated with many common complications of pregnancy, such as the pregnancy-induced hypertension (PIH) spectrum of diseases. For the clinician, IUGR predicts an increased risk for both perinatal and postnatal adult morbidities. The adult morbidities include pathophysiologies such as insulin resistance, insulin insufficiency, hypertension, dyslipidemia, and obesity. Because of the escalating burden that these morbidities place on societal health and healthcare systems of many countries, understanding the specific mechanisms through which uteroplacental insufficiency-induced IUGR (uIUGR) predisposes to these adult pathophysiologies is necessary if thoughtful and specific interventions are to be designed.

A true and testable understanding of the specific mechanisms necessarily encompasses physiology, cellular biology, and molecular biology. Human studies have obvious limitations in terms of tissue accessibility and lifespan. Furthermore, any model system of uIUGR must take into account interactions between tissues, cell types, metabolic systems, and molecular pathways, as well as the most important and yet most confounding issue, biological variability. Subsequently, it is clear that animal models of uIUGR are necessary to identify and test for key specific mechanisms of uIUGR pathophysiology because of the multidimensional nature of mammalian biology. This is true for the initiating events and the subsequent biological cascade induced by uIUGR that lead to the aforementioned adult pathophysiologies.

This chapter will review recent insights derived from animal models of uIUGR on a tissue-specific basis. Despite this approach, it will be important to recognize that the effects of uIUGR upon each tissue do not occur in isolation, but are a part of a whole body adaptation and response. This chapter will focus on observations of mechanisms relevant to the major postnatal pathophysiologies associated with uIUGR: (1) altered glucose homeostasis; (2) altered lipid homeostasis; and (3) hypertension; however, it should be noted that this is not an exclusive list. The chapter will then finish with a succinct discussion of relevant molecular mechanisms likely to be involved in the link between the intrauterine environment of uIUGR and these postnatal morbidities.

The majority of uIUGR models are characterized by hypoglycemia, decreased amino acid levels (particularly the branched chain amino acids leu, ile, and val), hypoxia, acidosis, and decreased availability of growth factors such as insulin and insulin-like growth factor-I (IGF-1). This is similar to the findings of periumbilical blood sampling studies comparing growth-retarded infants versus control. In contrast, IUGR models induced by maternal deprivation have been characterized by normal blood gas parameters and contrasting changes in fetal amino acid concentrations. Because of the wide continuum of the human genetics, conditions, and environmental context, both types of models are valid and necessary to further our understanding of IUGR biology and pathophysiology, so that human health can be improved in both the perinatal and postnatal periods.

Postnatal consequences of uIUGR

The recent surge in interest in uIUGR and IUGR in general has occurred secondary to the realization that these early life events impact upon adult health with worldwide implications. Though multiple human studies have demonstrated a link between IUGR and altered glucose homeostasis, three classic studies make this association very clearly. The first of these involved the Dutch famine of 1944–1945. The effect of the famine upon the Dutch population has been examined via multiple sources, including the Dutch famine cohort, as well as military induction records and self reports.

Interestingly, the timing of the maternal famine impacted the postnatal consequences to the offspring. Babies exposed to maternal famine in the first trimester suffered from an increased incidence of hypertension, dyslipidemia [1], and obesity [2]. In contrast, babies exposed to famine in the last trimester were more likely to exhibit impaired glucose tolerance, versus those babies who were born after the famine [3]. Other findings from the Dutch famine that have not received as much attention, though are likely to be just as relevant, are observed associations between experiencing the famine *in utero* and increased rates of schizophrenia and schizophrenia spectrum disorders, as well as antisocial personality disorders [4].

The second of the classic investigations involves the Barker Hertfordshire studies. Among the many salient findings was that men with impaired glucose sensitivity and non-insulin dependent diabetes were characterized by lower weight at birth and 1 year of age [5]. Interestingly, by 2005, a cohort from these studies demonstrated clear gender differences. Low birth weight in men increases the risk for cardiovascular disease, whereas low birth weight in women predisposes toward cardiovascular disease, diabetes, and pneumonia [6]. An astute and somewhat prophetic statement from this group is that 'poor nutrition early in life increases susceptibility to the affects of an affluent diet'.

The third investigation of major significance comes from the Nurses' Health Study which was established in 1976 and involved 122 000 married female registered nurses (aged 30–55) who responded to a questionnaire about their medical histories. This study added weight to the observations of the Barker group by noting significantly increased relative risk for cardiovascular disease and non-insulin dependent diabetes in women who were low birth weight versus women of median birth weight [7].

These large studies have provided important and seminal insight into the relationship between *in utero* growth restriction and altered postnatal glucose homeostasis. They have also provided the impetus to further studies that identify possible mechanisms.

Obviously, poor maternal nutrition played a causative role in the development of growth restriction, particularly within the Dutch famine cohort. However, uteroplacental insufficiency secondary to the pregnancy-induced hypertension spectrum of diseases is a leading cause of uIUGR in developed countries. Furthermore, with the insidious onslaught of Western dietary habits upon developing countries, uIUGR is becoming progressively more frequent and is associated with an increasing incidence of pregnancy-induced hypertensive diseases in developed and developing countries. This will greatly impact both immediate and future community health. The fact that it is occurring in the midst of a global epidemic of obesity is frightening and emphasizes the need to understand the mechanisms involved in translating early life events to postnatal disease (Tables 15.1, 15.2).

Liver

Glucose homeostasis

Hepatic glucose homeostasis plays a significant role in determining whole body glucose biology. This is because the liver is the major organ for glucose production via glycogenolysis and gluconeogenesis. Furthermore, unsuppressed hepatic glucose production is a component of pathological insulin resistance.

uIUGR alters hepatic glucose homeostasis. This consequence has been well established in the uIUGR rodent model of bilateral uterine artery ligation that has been characterized by multiple groups. In this model, investigators induce IUGR by ligating both uterine arteries at day 18 to 19 of gestation in the rat. Like the human infant suffering from uteroplacental insufficiency, the prenatal rat pups in the model experience moderate hypoxia, hypoglycemia, hypoinsulinemia, decreased levels of the branched

Table 15.1. Tissues affected by uIUGR

Liver
Skeletal muscle
Pancreas
Kidney
Other tissues
Heart
Lung
Adipose

chain amino acids, and decreased bioavailability of insulin-like growth factor 1 (IGF-1). Rat pups in this model are asymmetrically growth retarded and approximately 20% lighter than sham-operated controls. Birth weights are normally distributed within and between litters. Importantly, IUGR pups in this model develop early insulin resistance with hyperinsulinemia and progress toward diabetes in adulthood [8,9,10,11,12].

In this model of uIUGR, a significant focus of research has been on hepatic glycogenolysis and gluconeogenesis secondary to the direct physiological importance. The liver's role in these cellular processes is critical in both the perinatal and postnatal periods. In the perinatal period, these processes are critical because a common morbidity for IUGR infants is hypoglycemia. Early seminal studies by Ogata *et al.* suggested that uIUGR affects both processes. Specifically, uIUGR decreases hepatic glycogen content and delays activation of phosphoenolpyruvate carboxykinase (PEPCK), the rate limiting enzyme for gluconeogenesis when compared to livers from control pups or pups from sham-operated dams [13]. These studies are important to our understanding of the long-term consequences of uIUGR not only because of the possible postnatal pathological impact of perinatal hypoglycemia, but because they suggested that gene products associated with gluconeogenesis such as PEPCK may be targets of uIUGR.

A subsequent study of postnatal juvenile rats focused upon the gene product peroxisome proliferator-activated receptor-gamma coactivator-1 (PGC-1), which is a transcriptional coactivator that mediates hepatic glucose production by regulating mRNA levels of PEPCK (gluconeogenesis) and glucose-6-phosphatase (G6P) (glycogenolysis). The hypothesis of this study was that IUGR increases hepatic expression of PGC-1 as well as the PGC-1 downstream targets PEPCK and G6P. Indeed, IUGR did increase PGC-1 mRNA and protein levels to greater than 200% of control levels. Moreover, IUGR also increased mRNA levels of PEPCK and G6P. Within the context of the previous observations that insulin resistance occurs in this model, the findings suggest that a possible mechanism for this insulin resistance is through unsuppressed hepatic gluconeogenesis. These findings are conceptually important because they concretely demonstrate that an early life event such as uIUGR affects postnatal gene expression and phenotype.

Lipid homeostasis

Multiple postnatal diseases associated with aberrant lipid homeostasis threaten the IUGR infant. These diseases include obesity, cardiovascular disease, and dyslipidemia. Among the more relevant studies in the human literature is the follow up study by the Barker group that asked the question whether women are similarly at risk compared to men to the consequences of IUGR. Using a Hertfordshire cohort of 297 women, they found that waist to hip ratios and serum triglyceride levels fell with increasing birth weight, similar to glucose and insulin levels [14]. However, critics of these studies have questioned to what extent this data may be confounded by genetics.

In an attempt to address this genetic component, several groups have used discordant twin pairs to minimize the impact of genetics. These studies are particularly relevant within the context of uIUGR models because one of the causes of the discordance is a relative uteroplacental insufficiency to the smaller twin. Among the most interesting studies was that performed by Bo *et al.*, who used a cohort of 46 monozygotic and 32 dizygotic twins to evaluate the role of the intrauterine environment in predisposing affected individuals toward adult metabolic syndrome, with associated dyslipidemia. They found through logistic regression analysis that the relative risk of developing metabolic syndrome was increased when there was a greater discordance in birth weight between the twins [15]. These findings continue to emphasize the impact of environment on adult health.

During adulthood, the liver plays a significant role in regulating whole body lipid biology. Important functions of the liver in this context are oxidation of fatty acids and the synthesis of triglycerides. Because of the human studies discussed above, as well as the evidence of altered postnatal gene expression of enzymes involved in glucose homeostasis, it was hypothesized that uIUGR in the rat would affect hepatic mRNA levels of acetyl-CoA carboxylase (ACC) and carnitine palmitoyltransferase-1 (CPT1), hepatic malonyl-CoA levels, and serum triglyceride levels in juvenile and adult life. ACC and CPT1 are rate-limiting enzymes for fatty acid synthesis and fatty acid β-oxidation, respectively. Malonyl-CoA is the by-product of ACC function, and it inhibits CPT1 function.

An important finding of this study is that the effects of uIUGR are gender specific, at least for the targeted genes and metabolites of this study. More specifically, uIUGR significantly increased hepatic ACC mRNA levels and malonyl-CoA levels in adult male rats, while decreasing CPT1 mRNA levels in the same uIUGR males. Furthermore, uIUGR increased serum triglycerides in the adult uIUGR animals. In contrast, the uIUGR did not have a significant impact upon these same measures in the female animals [16]. The implication is that uIUGR leads to gender-specific altered expression and, probably, function of enzymes involved in hepatic fatty acid metabolism.

This concept of gender specificity is an important one to remember, and in both the human and animal literature, there are many examples that demonstrate the response to an early life stress is influenced by gender. The mechanisms behind these gender-specific responses are unknown. Questions that need to be answered include whether the differences are due to central regulation of the sex steroids, peripheral synthesis, degradation, and/or signaling.

Mitochondrial gene expression and function

The question of the influence of gender arose in the early studies of uIUGR, particularly as it related to mitochondria. This is due to the early observations that: (1) uIUGR crosses generations; (2) the fetus receives its mitochondria from its mother; and (3) many studies suggest that the gender effect is more likely to be transmitted through the mother. The latter point is controversial because studies exist that also demonstrate paternal transmission of IUGR both in human and rats. Regardless, these observations led to a nidus of interest in the effect of uIUGR on mitochondrial function.

The initial studies were performed by Ogata *et al.* who hypothesized that uIUGR in the rat would affect cellular energy and mitochondrial redox states. They found that the uIUGR rat fetus suffered from a diminished ATP/ADP ratio and mitochondrial NAD^+/NADH ratio, whereas the cytosolic NAD^+/NADH ratio was increased [17]. This demonstrates a disassociation between cytosolic and mitochondrial energy homeostasis. These changes were followed up with a study from the same group that used the technique of differential display RT-PCR to identify the gene mitochondrial protein NADH-ubiquinone oxireductase subunit 4L mRNA (ND-4L) as a possible target of uIUGR. Based on these findings, they hypothesized that uIUGR affects mRNA levels of multiple genes involved in ATP and NADH homeostasis. In the fetus, uIUGR increased ND-4L, adenine-nucleotide translocator-2 (ANT-2), mitochondrial malate dehydrogenase (MMD), and glucose-6-phosphate dehydrogenase (G6PD), whereas uIUGR decreased ornithine transcarbamylase (OTC) mRNA levels. In the juvenile rat, uIUGR increased mRNA levels of ND-4L, ANT-2, G6PD, OTC, MMD, and phosphofructokinase-2 (PFK-2) [18]. These findings are important because they demonstrate that uIUGR not only affects hepatic mitochondrial metabolic machinery while it is occurring, but it also continues to affect metabolism in the postnatal life, long after the time of the initial insult.

Finally, Peterside *et al.* isolated mitochondria from uIUGR and control juvenile animals to examine mitochondrial defects in oxidative metabolism. The most important and novel findings of this study were that oxidative phosphorylation of pyruvate, glutamate, succinate, and alpha ketoglutarate were significantly decreased in the juvenile uIUGR livers, when compared to control livers [19]. These studies from Ogata *et al.* and Peterside *et al.* demonstrate that the uIUGR significantly affects energy and substrate processing in the liver. The methodical and rigorous approach in these studies have demonstrated: (1) disassociation in energy states between the cytoplasm and the mitochondria; (2) altered expression of metabolic machinery; and (3) decreased mitochondrial function. Credit for this stepwise approach needs to be given to Edward S. Ogata, MD who initiated the interest in uIUGR and mitochondrial function, and guided his mentees toward subsequent studies.

Summary

Uteroplacental insufficiency-induced IUGR affects multiple processes in the postnatal liver. Using the model of bilateral uterine artery ligation, evidence exists that uIUGR alters the expression and function of genes involved in glucose, lipid, and energy homeostasis. This section has focused upon the aforementioned processes, however other systems have been assessed, though not as completely. One example involves branched chain amino acids. In studies by Kloesz *et al.* it was noted that uIUGR affects expression of enzymes involved in branched chain amino acid metabolism and transport [10]. All of the studies discussed above potentially affect whole body homeostasis, possibly leading to insulin resistance or dyslipidemia.

One of the more important findings, however, is the observation that the early life event of uIUGR leads to postnatal changes in hepatic gene expression. This is in spite of the fact that the uIUGR pups appear and act relatively normal. Breast milk from dams that underwent the bilateral uterine artery ligation is constitutionally similar to milk from control dams. The implication therefore of the postnatal changes in uIUGR rodent gene expression, and presumably the equivalent human homologs, is that significant early life events can program the expression of critical hepatic genes which can be carried over into postnatal life and thereby affect postnatal gene expression and subsequent phenotype. Considering the wide spectrum of events that potentially affect the human fetus, ranging from diseases of pregnancy-induced hypertension to maternal and early life malnutrition, the potential impact of this biological phenomenon upon community health and social resources could be significant.

Skeletal muscle

Mitochondrial gene expression and function

Evidence exists in humans and rats that IUGR alters peripheral metabolism, and this phenomenon may be causally linked to many of the morbidities associated with IUGR, such as insulin resistance and dyslipidemia. Several studies demonstrate that IUGR individuals modulate peripheral tissue energy homeostasis differently than appropriately sized individuals. For example, Chessex *et al.* demonstrated that IUGR increases lipid oxidation in 3–4-week-old infants [20]. Similarly, Bohler *et al.* found that IUGR decreases the respiratory quotient of infants through the first 8 weeks of life, suggesting an increase in lipid oxidation [21].

These early disorders of peripheral oxidation suggest that IUGR potentially affects skeletal muscle mitochondrial gene expression and function. Based upon the previous studies in the liver, it was hypothesized that IUGR would similarly affect mitochondrial NAD+/NADH ratios, as well as expression of ND-4L, adenine nucleotide translocator 1 (ANT1), and subunit C (SUC) of the F_1F_0-ATPase. ND-4L is a mitochondrial component of complex 1. ANT1 is the adenine nucleotide transporter isoform of skeletal muscle. SUC is necessary for the mitochondrial ATPase function, and previous studies suggest that SUC abundance is a rate-limiting step in the construction of the ATPase synthase complex.

Using the model of bilateral uterine artery ligation in the pregnant rat, uIUGR decreased the mitochondrial NAD^+/NADH ratio in postnatal skeletal muscle. Furthermore, uIUGR also decreased mRNA levels of ND-4L, SUC, and ANT1 in the same juvenile skeletal muscle [22,23]. These finding were among the first to suggest: (1) a mechanism for why uIUGR often retards postnatal growth; and (2) how uIUGR skeletal muscle intermediary metabolism may impact upon whole body glucose homeostasis. For the former, decreased expression of ND-4L, SUC, and ANT1 may limit ATP production, forcing the myocyte to minimize ATP expenditure. Because protein synthesis is one of the most costly users of ATP, this would limit growth. For the latter, a high NADH level can inhibit pyruvate dehydrogenase and thereby decrease the flux of glycolytic metabolites through the mitochondria. This would be particularly important in terms of whole body glucose homeostasis in that skeletal muscle metabolizes up to 70% of intravenous glucose. Consistent with these findings are those of Simoneau *et al.*, who observed that obese women with insulin resistance have a low aerobic–oxidative capacity in their skeletal muscle [24].

Finally, these studies in the uIUGR rat were supported by the follow up work of Peterside *et al.*, who described mitochondrial function and glucose uptake in skeletal muscle from uIUGR animals. In these studies, as predicted, uIUGR significantly decreased pyruvate dehydrogenase activity and impaired oxidative phosphorylation in postnatal skeletal muscle. For the latter, uIUGR specifically decreased pyruvate oxidation and ATP production in mitochondria. Moreover, these defects in mitochondrial function were associated with decreased glucose transporter recruitment and glucose transport response to insulin [25].

Two important concepts arise from these studies involving mitochondrial gene expression and function. The first is that as in the liver, uIUGR causes postnatal changes in mitochondrial gene expression. The second is that consequences of uIUGR are complex. There is unlikely to be one gene product that explains a specific defect secondary to uIUGR. Instead, the consequences of uIUGR are going to impact upon multiple pathways and systems. If the presumption is made that the response to uIUGR is an evolutionary adaptation because pregnancies have been suffering from uteroplacental insufficiency for as long as there have been pregnancies, then one of our goals for the future is an understanding of how the tissue-specific responses are coordinated. This could be through a central endocrine response, or it may be through a molecular response that allows for tissue specificity.

Lipid homeostasis

Considering the previously discussed effects of IUGR upon human lipid oxidation and the previously discussed findings in the uIUGR rat liver, a reasonable question is to ask whether skeletal muscle is similarly affected in terms of expression and function of fatty acid metabolizing enzymes. It was therefore hypothesized that gene expression and function of mitochondrial fatty acid β-oxidation enzymes would be altered in juvenile uIUGR muscle. It was further hypothesized that skeletal muscle triglyceride levels would be altered by uIUGR because altered intramuscular triglycerides have been associated with dysregulation of skeletal muscle metabolism.

The first of these hypotheses was tested by measuring mRNA levels of CPT-1 and trifunctional protein (TFP). CPT-1 catalyzes the exchange of acyl-carnitines across the mitochondrial outer membrane, and it is an important rate-determining step of fatty acid β-oxidation. TFP is an inner mitochondrial membrane protein that is involved in three of four reactions necessary for mitochondrial fatty acid β-oxidation, including the reduction of NAD^+ to NADH. TFP competes directly for NAD+ with Krebs cycle dehydrogenases. As a result, this intramitochondrial competition is another potential point of flux control connecting the Krebs cycle to β-oxidation. It was found that uIUGR increases mRNA levels of CPT-1 and TFP, while increasing TFP activity in isolated skeletal muscle mitochondria [23].

For the second hypothesis, it was found that uIUGR significantly increased skeletal muscle triglyceride levels nearly four-fold, despite increased CPT-1 and TFP gene expression and TFP function [23]. However, previous studies in other models have found that skeletal muscle triglycerides can positively correlate with fatty acid oxidation in both humans and rats [26,27]. The substrate fueling the increased lipid oxidation in these situations is likely derived from the diet or hepatic synthesis. As discussed in the liver portion of this chapter, uIUGR also increases expression of ACC, the rate-limiting step of hepatic fatty acid synthesis, and serum triglyceride levels. The accumulation of skeletal muscle triglycerides and increased β-oxidation machinery likely indicates a persistent deregulation between liver and skeletal muscle lipid metabolism that contributes to the altered metabolism seen on a whole body level in IUGR adults.

Three issues not well addressed to this point in the uIUGR skeletal muscle literature are: (1) the effects of uIUGR on skeletal muscle composition; (2) whether the effect of uIUGR varies based on skeletal muscle fiber type; and (3) whether these effects are gender specific. However, these issues were addressed in a study that measured skeletal muscle fiber types, as well as peroxisome proliferator-activated receptor γ coactivator-1 (PGC-1) expression in uIUGR and control juvenile skeletal muscle. PGC-1 is a transcriptional coactivator that induces expression of CPT-1. PGC-1 genotype polymorphisms have been linked to increased risk of type 2 diabetes.

The findings of this study were three-fold. First, uIUGR does not significantly alter skeletal muscle fiber distribution in the juvenile rat. Proportions of type 1, type 2A, and type 2B fibers were similar between control and IUGR animals. Second, the impact of uIUGR is muscle fiber specific, at least in terms of PGC-1 mRNA levels. Specifically, uIUGR significantly increased PGC-1 mRNA levels in extensor digitorum longus fibers (type 2) and decreased PGC-1 mRNA levels in soleus fibers (type 1). Finally, the response to uIUGR in terms of PGC-1 mRNA levels is gender specific, with male skeletal muscle being more robustly impacted than skeletal muscle from female uIUGR animals [28].

This study was among the first to note gender-specific differences in a rat model of uIUGR. Interestingly, humans also metabolize fat in a gender-specific manner. Sumner *et al.* found that only males were resistant to insulin's antilipolytic effects, whereas both genders were resistant to insulin glucoregulatory effects [29]. Because PGC-1 acts as a transcriptional coactivator with both estrogen and androgen receptors, the impact of uIUGR upon skeletal muscle PGC-1 expression and subsequent phenotype likely changes as the uIUGR individual progressively experiences sexual maturation, maturity, and senescence.

Summary

Uteroplacental insufficiency-induced IUGR affects expression and function of genes involved in energy and lipid homeostasis in skeletal muscle. Multiple genes and systems are impacted by uIUGR. This section focused upon mitochondrial and lipid metabolism because of the presence of integrative mutually supportive studies from separate institutions. However, evidence exists for other metabolic systems being affected, including branched chain amino acid homeostasis [10].

Regardless of the pathway, it is likely that uIUGR affects gene expression in a manner that is specific to muscle fiber type and gender. Further studies involving the impact of IUGR upon skeletal muscle need to assess these confounding effects. Moreover, the consequences of uIUGR on skeletal muscle phenotype from a study involving fetal muscle cannot be confidently applied to the adult phenotype, even if it is presumed that molecular biology stays relatively consistent, which by itself is an unlikely presumption. Not only is skeletal muscle relatively undifferentiated in the fetus, but regulation of gene expression is likely to vary over the lifetime of the individual as their endocrine and paracrine status evolves with age.

Pancreas

The pancreatic β-cell obviously plays a central role in glucose homeostasis. In general, with uIUGR insulin resistance has been observed in association with hyperinsulinemia in juvenile and young adult animals. As the uIUGR animal reaches senescence, there has been the finding of subsequent β-cell failure.

β-cells are found in pancreatic islets. Human islets are scattered throughout the pancreas. Islet cells can vary in size, but typically contain about 1000 cells of which nearly 80% are β-cells. β-cell production is initiated during fetal life and continues into neonatal life. Furthermore, β–cells respond to metabolic demands in juvenile and adult life with changes in cell size, number, and function [30]. Because of these characteristics, molecular mechanisms regulating β-cell biology must be considered with respect to the uIUGR phenotype.

Studies linking β-cell biology and uIUGR phenotype use both ovine models and rat models. Both of these animal models are vitally important in terms of describing the β-cell response to uIUGR. An intrinsic advantage of rodent models is the relatively short gestation and, similar to humans, postnatal dependence upon glucose as the primary carbohydrate for peripheral tissues. In contrast, adult sheep use fructose as their primary carbohydrate. However, a disadvantage of uIUGR rat models is that the pancreas is less developed in late gestation versus the human, whereas ovine *in utero* β-cell development closely parallels human β-cell ontogeny. As a result, this part of the chapter will be divided into sections involving ovine studies and rat studies, respectively.

Ovine studies and the β-cell

Ovine studies of uIUGR and its impact upon the β-cell clearly send two messages. The first is that uIUGR impacts β-cell number and mass at birth, as well as later in life. Using a model of uteroplacental insufficiency generated by removal of the endometrial caruncles from the non-pregnant uterus prior to conception, Gatford *et al.* observed that β-cell numbers correlated positively with fetal weight, but negatively with birth weight in adult male sheep [31].

The second is that uIUGR affects β-cell gene expression. Several families of genes have been studied. For example, using the aforementioned model of uIUGR involving endometrial caruncle removal, Gatford *et al.* were able to suggest that IGF-II and insulin receptor expression are important regulators of β-cell mass compensation, whereas voltage-gated calcium channel alpha 1D subunit expression is a determinant of β-cell function [31].

An important point as a follow-up to these two findings is whether the changes in β-cell number, mass, and gene expression affect overall β-cell function. In the uIUGR model of endometrial caruncle removal, Gatford *et al.* found that uIUGR does not impair insulin secretion, relative to glucose sensitivity before birth or in young offspring. However, with aging, β-cell insulin secretory capacity was markedly decreased in males. It appears that this defect was due to failure of the male adult sheep to increase β-cell mass needed to maintain appropriate insulin secretion relative to glucose-stimulated insulin secretion. Another interesting finding from this group is that uIUGR increased insulin sensitivity to free fatty acids in the postnatal sheep [31].

Rat studies and the β-cell

Similar to the ovine studies, studies of uIUGR and its impact upon the rat β-cell demonstrate that multiple aspects of β-cell biology are altered. Results vary slightly between groups, but the message is clear that uIUGR affects postnatal β-cell function in the uIUGR rat. For example, Styrud *et al.* performed bilateral uterine artery ligation at day 16 of gestation to induce uIUGR. This severe model of uIUGR decreased pancreatic β-cell mass and insulin content by 35–40% by as early as 1 day of age. By 3 months of age, β-cell mass was reduced by 40–45% in both genders. Interestingly, no difference in glucose tolerance was noted in the uIUGR animals at this age [32].

In contrast, using the model of bilateral uterine ligation at 19 days of gestation established by Ogata, Simmons *et al.* found that uIUGR does not affect β-cell mass, islet size, or pancreatic weight at 1 and 7 weeks of age, though at 7 weeks of age the uIUGR rats suffered from fasting hyperglycemia and hyperinsulinemia. However, at 15 weeks of age, uIUGR significantly decreased β-cell mass to 50% of control values. At 26 weeks of age, uIUGR further decreased β-cell mass to 33% of control values [11]. It should be noted there are considerable differences in the models based upon when the artery ligation is performed. For example, Styrud *et al.* found that bilateral uterine artery ligation at day 16 of gestation reduced litter size [32]. In contrast, bilateral uterine artery ligation at day 18 or 19 does not significantly affect litter size. Furthermore, it is not surprising that even moderate differences in similar models may produce different results. For example, Dumortier *et al.* demonstrated that in models of maternal malnutrition the cellular mechanisms are different depending on whether the model uses a low-energy diet or a low-protein diet [33].

In terms of β-cell function, Liao *et al.* found that adult male uIUGR rats generated from bilateral uterine artery ligation at 17 days' gestation were characterized by abnormal glucose tolerance tests. Specifically, they found that uIUGR resulted in hyperglycemia and peak serum insulin levels that were delayed, yet markedly higher than the control animals. Overall, the modified β-cell function index in the uIUGR adult males was only one half the values found in the control adult males [34].

Finally, in terms of how uIUGR affects β-cell energy homeostasis and molecular biology, Simmons *et al.* have proposed two separate mechanisms. The first involves uIUGR induction of mitochondrial dysfunction in the uIUGR β-cell, which leads to progressive production of free radicals and subsequent mitochondrial DNA damage [35]. The consequence is progressive deterioration of β-cell function. The second involves decreased expression of pancreatic and duodenal homeobox 1 transcription factor (Pdx-1), which is a critical factor for β-cell development and function [36].

Summary

Uteroplacental insufficiency-induced IUGR affects β-cell biology and gene expression. Issues not yet investigated in detail include: (1) the extent to which gender plays a role; and (2) the extent to which peripheral tissue metabolism contributes to β-cell deregulation considering the fact that some evidence supports that peripheral dysfunction appears to occur earlier than β-cell failure. More variability also appears to occur in the β-cell literature, though this is likely due to the extreme vulnerability of the β-cell and the complexity of β-cell homeostasis.

Kidney

Epidemiological evidence indicates that IUGR affects adult renal function and increases the risk for hypertension. Two recent epidemiological studies provide clear evidence of these phenomena. The first study is the HUNT 2 study from Hallan *et al.* They studied 7457 adults aged 20 to 30 years and found that intrauterine growth retardation was significantly associated with low normal kidney function; the more growth was retarded, the greater the risk. Furthermore, the impact of IUGR upon kidney function was more consistent and severe in men [37].

The second study came from four centers within the National Institute of Child Health and Human Developmental Neonatal Research Network. Over 1300 infants were followed through the first 6 years of life. IUGR was significantly associated with hypertension (relative risk of 1.8) when multivariate Poisson regression analysis was performed adjusting for: (1) maternal race and education; (2) maternal use of tobacco, alcohol, and cocaine; and (3) child's current body mass index [38]. The implications for adult health are obvious, and these implications have been a nidus for studies using models of uIUGR. Three messages are clear when reviewing the literature. The first is that uIUGR reduces nephron number. The second is that multiple pathways are altered, which underlines the complexity of the renal response to uIUGR. The third is that uIUGR does induce adult hypertension, at least in the rat.

In both the sheep and the rat, uIUGR decreases nephron number. Sheep complete nephrogenesis prior to term delivery, similar to the human. uIUGR can be induced in the sheep using microsphere injections into the fetal aorta, which disrupt oxygen and nutrient delivery. With this model, microsphere injection at

0.75 of gestation (144 days) negatively affects nephrogenesis, whereas microsphere injection at 0.8 of gestation does not affect nephron numbers, thereby establishing a critical time during gestation in the sheep when uteroplacental insufficiency affects nephron number [39]. In the rat, nephrogenesis begins on embryonic day 12 and is completed 7–10 days after birth. Therefore, the rat models employing late gestation insults can be used to study renal developmental issues analogous to mid and third trimester in humans [40]. Indeed, Pham *et al.* used the bilateral uterine ligation model of uIUGR to demonstrate that uteroplacental insufficiency decreases glomeruli number in the perinatal and juvenile uIUGR rat. Interestingly the decrease in glomeruli number was associated with an increase in renal apoptosis and caspase-3 activity in the uIUGR kidney, suggesting one possible mechanism [41]. However, several other mechanistic pathways have been found to be deregulated by uIUGR as well.

Three pathways appear to be particularly interesting: (1) those involved with renal glucocorticoid processing and cyclooxygenase-2 (COX2) expression; (2) those involved in vasculogenesis; and (3) those involved with the renin–angiotensin system. In terms of renal glucocorticoid processing, Baserga *et al.* observed that uIUGR rats generated from bilateral uterine artery ligation suffer from elevated corticosterone levels (the rat form of cortisol). In this aberrant endocrine environment, uIUGR decreases 11-β hydroxysteroid dehydrogenase (11HSD2) and COX2 expression in the perinatal kidney [42]. 11HSD2 converts active corticosterone to inert 11-dehydrocorticosterone. COX2 expression is responsive to glucocorticoid signaling and COX2 is necessary for normal nephrogenesis. COX2 knockout mice have marked renal pathology, including hypoplasia and tubular atrophy.

In juvenile animals, uIUGR continues to decrease renal 11HSD2 expression [42]. These findings are important because they demonstrate that deregulation of renal steroid homeostasis through 11HSD2 may have multiple consequences. First, decreased perinatal expression of 11HSD2 may lead to decreased COX2 expression and thereby less than optimal renal development during important periods of renal organogenesis. Second, decreased 11HSD2 may predispose the juvenile uIUGR to later hypertension secondary to increased sensitivity to either glucocorticoid or mineralocorticoid signaling. A human example of the latter occurs with excessive ingestion of licorice derivatives, such as glycyrrhetinic acid, which leads to sodium retention and increased blood pressure [43].

In terms of vasculogenesis, Baserga *et al.* hypothesized that uIUGR would decrease vascular endothelial growth factor (VEGF) and its receptors in juvenile and adult kidneys. This hypothesis was based upon the observation that VEGF is critical to renal development and modulated by steroid levels. They found that uIUGR decreased renal VEGF expression in perinatal and juvenile animals of both sexes. Surprisingly, they found that uIUGR increased VEGF levels in female adult kidneys, while not affecting VEGF levels in male adult kidneys. These findings were associated with relative glomerular hypertrophy in the male uIUGR animals versus female uIUGR animals, which is associated with hypertension [44]. The findings of decreased VEGF expression in the young uIUGR rats are important because they occur during a period of active nephrogenesis. The findings of increased VEGF renal expression in the adult female animals are intriguing, considering the more benign phenotype in the females. Interestingly, Alexander *et al.* have found that estrogen protects against hypertension in postpubertal female uIUGR offspring [45]. Furthermore, the same group has demonstrated that testosterone contributes to elevations in mean arterial blood pressure in uIUGR male adult animals [46].

In terms of the renin–angiotensin system, the Alexander group have clearly demonstrated that deregulation of this system is a common complication of uIUGR. Alexander *et al.* induce uIUGR by clipping the aorta above the iliac bifurcation, as well as the compensatory right and left ovarian arteries at day 14 of gestation. Pregnant rats used for the control group are not exposed to the surgical procedures. Their objective was to assess the renin–angiotensin system in this model. They found that uIUGR increased renal mRNA levels of renin and angiotensinogen in association with increased renal angiotensinogen converting enzyme (ACE) activity in old adult animals that were hypertensive. Interestingly, many of these changes were not present in the young adult hypertensive animals. Most importantly, renin–angiotensin system blockade or treatment with an ACE inhibitor administered from 2 to 4 weeks of age abolished subsequent hypertension [47]. Though there are some conflicting data from the sheep literature, where uIUGR did decrease nephron number without affecting renal renin–angiotensin system gene expression, this highlights the complexity of blood pressure regulation in terms of the kidney [39]. It also reinforces the importance of using multiple models to tease apart the many possible mechanisms through which uIUGR may affect the kidney, considering the wide continuum of human existence in terms of environment, heritage, and genetics.

A good example of the differences between the different models is the impact of uIUGR upon adult blood pressure. As mentioned above, Alexander *et al.* observed that reduced placental blood flow from day 14 of gestation increased systemic blood pressure in rats by day 120 of life [46]. Baserga *et al.* demonstrated that bilateral uterine artery ligation significantly increased blood pressure by day 140 of life [42]. In contrast, Louey *et al.* used umbilico-embolization to find that uIUGR decreases mean arterial pressures and relative hypotension through the first 8 weeks of life. In further contrast to the studies of Baserga *et al.* in the uIUGR rat, uIUGR did not significantly alter postnatal plasma concentrations of glucocorticoids [48].

Summary

Uteroplacental insufficiency-induced IUGR affects renal nephron number, gene expression, and systemic blood pressure. Different models of uIUGR identify different pathways and/or mechanisms that are likely to be relevant to the human condition. In a scientific environment that is often characterized by investigators looking for 'the answer', this is refreshing. It is also important, as more tools become available for meaningful translational research, to understand the many possible effects of uIUGR or any other perinatal insult. If we are going to move translational research beyond the field of looking for simple biomarkers of disease, we need as much information as possible on relevant biological mechanisms.

Other tissues

For liver, skeletal muscle, and kidney, linear stories are developing that deliver insight into how uIUGR impacts the molecular biology of these tissues and subsequent phenotype. Other tissues within the context of uIUGR have been studied, but the literature and subsequent story lines are less developed. A good example of this is the heart, which is particularly relevant considering the risk for cardiovascular morbidity in IUGR individuals. For example, Tsirka *et al.* have noted that uIUGR decreases cardiac glucose transporter expression and function in adult rats [49]. Morrison *et al.* observed that placental restriction in the sheep increases the relative proportion of mononucleated cardiomyocytes in the progeny [50]. However, little is known about the effect of uIUGR upon endothelial function.

Another good example of this is the lung, which is also relevant considering the association between IUGR and chronic lung disease of prematurity. Harding *et al.* (sheep) [51] in particular, as well as Lipsett *et al.* (sheep) [52] and O'Brien *et al.* (rat) [53] have made important contributions to the field. However, the connections between phenotype and molecular mechanisms for the lung and heart are not as well developed compared to liver, skeletal muscle, β-cell, and kidney. Even less is known about the impact of uIUGR upon adipocyte biology. In the latter arena, uIUGR studies have lagged significantly behind IUGR models involving maternal food restriction. We would suggest the reader refer to the works of Desai *et al.* for excellent references on the impact of maternal food restriction upon adipocyte biology in the IUGR rat [54,55,56,57].

Epigenetics

The central theme of this chapter is that uIUGR causes significant long-term changes in mRNA and subsequent phenotype. The potential phenotype of a cell, tissue, or organism is determined by the information contained within DNA: the genetics of that individual. However, the determination of the actual phenotype occurs through the transcription of that information. Long-term changes in transcriptional regulation occur through epigenetic regulation of gene expression.

Epigenetic regulation of gene expression is a fundamental feature of mammalian development that causes heritable and persistent changes in gene expression, without altering DNA sequence. Epigenetic regulation involves covalent modifications to DNA and histones. These modifications affect the three-dimensional structure of a cell's chromatin, the association of DNA and protein within the nucleus. DNA can be methylated at the C-5 position of cytosine within a CpG dinucleotide. Not all of the consequences of DNA methylation are known, but it is believed that DNA methylation affects transcription factor binding and may act as a marker or a tag for further modifications of chromatin. Generally, CpG methylation in a promoter region decreases expression, whereas CpG methylation in a downstream coding region is associated with increased expression [58].

Table 15.2. Genes affected by uIUGR

Liver	IGF-1 (insulin-like growth factor 1)
	PEPCK (phosphoenolpyruvate carboxykinase)
	PGC-1 (peroxisome proliferator-activated receptor γ coactivator-1)
	G6P (glucose-6-phosphatase)
	ACC (acetyl-CoA carboxylase)
	CPT1 (carnitine palmitoyltransferase-1)
	ND-4L (NADH-ubiquinone oxireductase subunit 4L)
	ANT-2 (adenine-nucleotide translocator-2)
	MMD (mitochondrial malate dehydrogenase)
	G6PD (glucose-6-phosphate dehydrogenase)
	OTC (ornithine transcarbamylase)
	PFK-2 (phosphofructokinase-2)
Skeletal muscle	ND-4L
	ANT1 (adenine nucleotide translocator 1)
	SUC (subunit C of the F_1F_0-ATPase)
	TFP (trifunctional protein)
	PGC-1
	ACC
	CPT-1
Pancreas	IGF-II (insulin-like growth factor II)
	Insulin receptor
	Voltage-gated calcium channel, alpha 1D subunit
	Pdx-1 (pancreatic and duodenal homeobox 1 transcription factor)
Kidney	11HSD2 (11-β hydroxysteroid dehydrogenase)
	COX2 (cyclooxygenase-2)
	VEGF (vascular endothelial growth factor)
	Renin
	Angiotensinogen
	ACE (angiotensinogen-converting enzyme)
Heart	Glucose transporters 1 and 4

A dynamic relationship exists between DNA methylation and covalent modifications of histones. Histones can be modified by multiple processes, including acetylation, methylation, and phosphorylation. These histone modifications can be read collectively as a 'histone code'. Considering that (1) each histone has multiple sites that can be modified by one or more processes, (2) eight histones make up each nucleosome which associates with one H1 linker protein, and (3) each nucleosome is associated with approximately 147 DNA base pairs within the nucleosome plus 30–40 bases within the linker region between each nucleosome for a total of approximately 30 million nucleosomes per diploid cell, the possible number of different histone codes is orders of magnitude greater than the total number of nucleosomes in each cell. It would be possible, for example, to uniquely mark all nucleosomes containing maternally vs paternally derived DNA. The important lesson is that the epigenetic information contained within the chromatin structure introduces a level of transcriptional regulation that is more complex than just the DNA sequence alone.

The first demonstration that uIUGR effects alter epigenetic information of a specific gene was published in 2003 by Pham *et al.* Because uIUGR affects renal p53 expression and p53 CpG methylation affects p53 expression, this group analyzed DNA methylation at multiple sites along the p53 gene. They found that uIUGR decreased CpG DNA methylation in the promoter and exons 5 through 8, as well as decreased expression of DNA methyltransferase 1 (DNMT1). DNMT1 performs both *de novo* and maintenance DNA methylation [41]. This study was particularly important in the field because it demonstrated that epigenetic modifications of specific genes occur in response to a late perinatal event, as opposed to the initial dogmatic view that epigenetic modifications are an embryonic event driven by gender-specific imprinting.

Since the original publication, the field has progressed considerably. Subsequent studies have demonstrated that uIUGR affects postnatal genome-wide epigenetic characteristics in both the liver and brain, as well as the epigenetic characteristics of specific genes previously discussed, such as hepatic PGC-1 [59,60]. Interestingly, these findings occur in association with modified tissue levels of one-carbon metabolites and zinc [61]. These associations are intriguing because one-carbon metabolism influences DNA methylation, and zinc is a cofactor for many chromatin-modifying enzymes. These findings are also important because they reveal possible nutritional interventions through which the impact of uIUGR may be modified.

Finally recent studies have demonstrated through more elaborate analyses involving DNA methylation and the histone code the impact of uIUGR on epigenetic modifications of chromatin. In 2006, Fu *et al.* published that uIUGR affects hepatic dual specificity phosphate 5 (DUSP5) expression and epigenetic characteristics into adulthood. In this study, the authors speculate that the perinatal changes of DUSP5 are likely to be protective, maximizing the hepatic stress response, whereas the same changes in DUSP5 expression are likely to lead to hepatic insulin resistance later in life [62]. In 2008, Simmons *et al.* described that uIUGR and the subsequent changes in the whole body milieu caused a progression of changes in β-cell PDX-1 expression from birth to adulthood [36].

Some important observations can be gleaned from the aforementioned studies of uIUGR and epigenetic 'programming' which differentiate the phenomena from epigenetics as a mechanism of embryonic 'imprinting'. The first is that epigenetic programming modulates the threshold for transcription, acting as a rheostat while epigenetic imprinting is an 'on or off' mechanism. Epigenetic programming occurs in a gene-, tissue-, and gender-specific manner in response to a stress such as uIUGR. Finally, epigenetic programming affects epigenetic modification across the whole gene, whereas epigenetic imprinting primarily affects promoter regions.

These differences make sense, if one presumes that epigenetic programming in response to uIUGR is an adaptive response that improves chances for survival and reproduction. This is particularly true for the observation that uIUGR often does not significantly affect promoters that have a high-density region of CpGs. DNA methylation of these regions causes gross 'on or off' consequences in terms of transcriptional regulation. In contrast, epigenetic modifications within a gene allow for a more graded response that results in a true fine tuning of transcriptional expression (Table 15.3). As a result, studies that focus solely on small regions of the promoter are quite limited in the statements they can make about how uIUGR is affecting epigenetic modifications and subsequent transcriptional regulation.

Table 15.3. Differences between epigenetic programming and imprinting

Epigenetic programming	Epigenetic imprinting
Modulating the threshold for transcription, acting as rheostat	An 'on or off' mechanism
Affecting epigenetic modification across the whole gene	Primarily affecting promoter regions

Summary

Uteroplacental insufficiency-induced IUGR affects the epigenetic characteristics of many genes. Mammalian epigenetics is complex, and the impact of altering epigenetic determinants may not be obvious or immediate. Concern exists about proposals and investigations that 'treat' epigenetic modifications in a non-specific manner. Shot gun genome-wide epigenetic modifications induced by an *in utero* intervention could subsequently modify expression of critical gene(s) that leads to an alternative morbidity. For example, in an attempt to reduce the risk for insulin resistance, one may turn on a gene that leads to an adult cancer. This may be more likely true when a pharmacological agent is used, for example one capable of altering chromatin structure such as the histone deacetylase inhibitor valproic acid, than when nutrition is used. This is because the latter may have evolved to allow intrinsic homeostatic mechanisms to dampen or self-regulate the consequences, whereas pharmacological intervention is immediate and can be extreme.

uIUGR affects epigenetics along the entire gene. The regulation of epigenetic modifications in response to uIUGR is specific to the tissue, gender, environment, genetics, and likely multiple other factors. We are at this time only at the earliest understanding of how epigenetic determinants define our immediate and long-term phenotypes and how *in utero* insults alter their roles.

References

1. Roseboom T J, van der Meulen J H, Osmond C *et al.* Plasma lipid profiles in adults after prenatal exposure to the Dutch famine. *Am J Clin Nutr* 2000; **72**(5): 1101–6.
2. Ravelli A C, van Der Meulen J H, Osmond C, Barker D J, Bleker O P. Obesity at the age of 50 y in men and women exposed to famine prenatally. *Am J Clin Nutr* 1999 ; **70**(5): 811–6.
3. Ravelli A C, van der Meulen J H, Michels R P *et al.* Glucose tolerance in adults after prenatal exposure to famine. *Lancet* 1998; **351**(9097): 173–7.

4. Hoek H W, Brown A S, Susser E. The Dutch famine and schizophrenia spectrum disorders. *Soc Psychiatry Psychiatr Epidemiol* 1998; **33**(8): 373–9.
5. Barker D J, Hales C N, Fall C H *et al.* Type 2 (non-insulin-dependent) diabetes mellitus, hypertension and hyperlipidaemia (syndrome X): relation to reduced fetal growth. *Diabetologia* 1993; **36**(1): 62–7.
6. Syddall H E, Sayer A A, Simmonds S J *et al.* Birth weight, infant weight gain, and cause-specific mortality: the Hertfordshire Cohort Study. *Am J Epidemiol* 2005; **161** (11): 1074–80.
7. Rich-Edwards J W, Colditz G A, Stampfer M J *et al.* Birthweight and the risk for type 2 diabetes mellitus in adult women. *Ann Int Med* 1999; **130**(4 Pt 1): 278–84.
8. Ogata E S, Bussey M E, LaBarbera A, Finley S. Altered growth, hypoglycemia, hypoalaninemia, and ketonemia in the young rat: postnatal consequences of intrauterine growth retardation. *Pediatr Res* 1985; **19**(1): 32–7.
9. Ogata E S, Bussey M E, Finley S. Altered gas exchange, limited glucose and branched chain amino acids, and hypoinsulinism retard fetal growth in the rat. *Metabolism: Clin Exp* 1986; **35**(10): 970–7.
10. Kloesz J L, Serdikoff C M, Maclennan N K, Adibi S A, Lane R H. Uteroplacental insufficiency alters liver and skeletal muscle branched-chain amino acid metabolism in intrauterine growth-restricted fetal rats. *Pediatr Res* 2001; **50**(5): 604–10.
11. Simmons R A, Templeton L J, Gertz S J. Intrauterine growth retardation leads to the development of type 2 diabetes in the rat. *Diabetes* 2001; **50**(10): 2279–86.
12. Unterman T G, Simmons R A, Glick R P, Ogata E S. Circulating levels of insulin, insulin-like growth factor-I (IGF-I), IGF-II, and IGF-binding proteins in the small for gestational age fetal rat. *Endocrinology* 1993; **132**(1): 327–36.
13. Lane R H, MacLennan N K, Hsu J L, Janke S M, Pham T D. Increased hepatic peroxisome proliferator-activated receptor-gamma coactivator-1 gene expression in a rat model of intrauterine growth retardation and subsequent insulin resistance. *Endocrinology* 2002; **143** (7): 2486–90.
14. Fall C H, Osmond C, Barker D J *et al.* Fetal and infant growth and cardiovascular risk factors in women. *BMJ (Clinical Research Ed)* 1995; **310**(6977): 428–32.
15. Bo S, Cavallo-Perin P, Scaglione L, Ciccone G, Pagano G. Low birthweight and metabolic abnormalities in twins with increased susceptibility to Type 2 diabetes mellitus. *Diabet Med* 2000; **17**(5): 365–70.
16. Lane R H, Kelley D E, Gruetzmacher E M, Devaskar S U. Uteroplacental insufficiency alters hepatic fatty acid-metabolizing enzymes in juvenile and adult rats. *Am J Physiol* 2001; **280**(1): R183–90.
17. Ogata E S, Swanson S L, Collins J W Jr, Finley S L. Intrauterine growth retardation: altered hepatic energy and redox states in the fetal rat. *Pediatr Res* 1990; **27**(1): 56–63.
18. Lane R H, Flozak A S, Ogata E S, Bell G I, Simmons R A. Altered hepatic gene expression of enzymes involved in energy metabolism in the growth-retarded fetal rat. *Pediatr Res* 1996; **39**(3): 390–4.
19. Peterside I E, Selak M A, Simmons R A. Impaired oxidative phosphorylation in hepatic mitochondria in growth-retarded rats. *Am J Physiol Endocrinol Metab* 2003; **285**(6): E1258–66.
20. Chessex P, Reichman B, Verellen G *et al.* Metabolic consequences of intrauterine growth retardation in very low birthweight infants. *Pediatr Res* 1984; **18**(8): 709–13.
21. Bohler T, Kramer T, Janecke A R, Hoffmann G F, Linderkamp O. Increased energy expenditure and fecal fat excretion do not impair weight gain in small-for-gestational-age preterm infants. *Early Human Dev* 1999; **54**(3): 223–34.
22. Lane R H, Chandorkar A K, Flozak A S, Simmons R A. Intrauterine growth retardation alters mitochondrial gene expression and function in fetal and juvenile rat skeletal muscle. *Pediatr Res* 1998; **43**(5): 563–70.
23. Lane R H, Kelley D E, Ritov V H, Tsirka A E, Gruetzmacher E M. Altered expression and function of mitochondrial beta-oxidation enzymes in juvenile intrauterine-growth-retarded rat skeletal muscle. *Pediatr Res* 2001; **50**(1): 83–90.
24. Simoneau J A, Colberg S R, Thaete F L, Kelley D E. Skeletal muscle glycolytic and oxidative enzyme capacities are determinants of insulin sensitivity and muscle composition in obese women. *FASEB J* 1995; **9** (2): 273–8.
25. Selak M A, Storey B T, Peterside I, Simmons R A. Impaired oxidative phosphorylation in skeletal muscle of intrauterine growth-retarded rats. *Am J Physiol Endocrinol Metab* 2003; **285**(1): E130–7.
26. Dyck D J, Miskovic D, Code L, Luiken J J, Bonen A. Endurance training increases FFA oxidation and reduces triacylglycerol utilization in contracting rat soleus. *Am J Physiol Endocrinol Metab* 2000; **278**(5): E778–85.
27. Schrauwen P, Wagenmakers A J, van Marken Lichtenbelt W D, Saris W H, Westerterp K R. Increase in fat oxidation on a high-fat diet is accompanied by an increase in triglyceride-derived fatty acid oxidation. *Diabetes* 2000; **49**(4): 640–6.
28. Lane R H, Maclennan N K, Daood M J *et al.* IUGR alters postnatal rat skeletal muscle peroxisome proliferator-activated receptor-gamma coactivator-1 gene expression

in a fiber specific manner. *Pediatric Res* 2003; **53**(6): 994–1000.

29. Sumner A E, Kushner H, Lakota C A, Falkner B, Marsh J B. Gender differences in insulin-induced free fatty acid suppression: studies in an African American population. *Lipids* 1996; **31** (Suppl): S275–8.

30. Bonner-Weir S, Deery D, Leahy J L, Weir G C. Compensatory growth of pancreatic beta-cells in adult rats after short-term glucose infusion. *Diabetes* 1989; **38** (1): 49–53.

31. Gatford K L, Mohammad S N, Harland M L *et al.* Impaired beta-cell function and inadequate compensatory increases in beta-cell mass after intrauterine growth restriction in sheep. *Endocrinology* 2008; **149**(10): 5118–27.

32. Styrud J, Eriksson U J, Grill V, Swenne I. Experimental intrauterine growth retardation in the rat causes a reduction of pancreatic B-cell mass, which persists into adulthood. *Biol Neonate* 2005; **88**(2): 122–8.

33. Dumortier O, Blondeau B, Duvillie B *et al.* Different mechanisms operating during different critical time-windows reduce rat fetal beta cell mass due to a maternal low-protein or low-energy diet. *Diabetologia* 2007; **50** (12): 2495–503.

34. Liao Y, Li H Q. [Impaired islet beta-cell function and insulin resistance in adult male rats born with intrauterine growth retardation.] *Beijing da xue xue bao Yi xue ban (Journal of Peking University)* 2005; **37**(4): 351–4.

35. Simmons R A, Suponitsky-Kroyter I, Selak M A. Progressive accumulation of mitochondrial DNA mutations and decline in mitochondrial function lead to beta-cell failure. *J Biol Chem* 2005; **280**(31): 28785–91.

36. Park J H, Stoffers D A, Nicholls R D, Simmons R A. Development of type 2 diabetes following intrauterine growth retardation in rats is associated with progressive epigenetic silencing of Pdx1. *J Clin Invest* 2008; **118**(6): 2316–24.

37. Hallan S, Euser A M, Irgens L M *et al.* Effect of intrauterine growth restriction on kidney function at young adult age: the Nord Trondelag Health (HUNT 2) Study. *Am J Kidney Dis* 2008; **51**(1): 10–20.

38. Shankaran S, Das A, Bauer C R *et al.* Fetal origin of childhood disease: intrauterine growth restriction in term infants and risk for hypertension at 6 years of age. *Arch Pediatr Adolesc Med* 2006; **160**(9): 977–81.

39. Zohdi V, Moritz K M, Bubb K J *et al.* Nephrogenesis and the renal renin-angiotensin system in fetal sheep: effects of intrauterine growth restriction during late gestation. *Am J Physiol* 2007; **293**(3): R1267–73.

40. Guron G, Friberg P. An intact renin-angiotensin system is a prerequisite for normal renal development. *J Hypertension* 2000; **18**(2): 123–37.

41. Pham T D, MacLennan N K, Chiu C T *et al.* Uteroplacental insufficiency increases apoptosis and alters p53 gene methylation in the full-term IUGR rat kidney. *Am J Physiol* 2003; **285**(5): R962–70.

42. Baserga M, Hale M A, Wang Z M *et al.* Uteroplacental insufficiency alters nephrogenesis and downregulates cyclooxygenase-2 expression in a model of IUGR with adult-onset hypertension. *Am J Physiol* 2007; **292**(5): R1943–55.

43. Lindsay R S, Lindsay R M, Edwards C R, Seckl J R. Inhibition of 11-beta-hydroxysteroid dehydrogenase in pregnant rats and the programming of blood pressure in the offspring. *Hypertension* 1996; **27**(6): 1200–4.

44. Baserga M, Bares A L, Hale M A *et al.* Uteroplacental insufficiency affects kidney VEGF expression in a model of IUGR with compensatory glomerular hypertrophy and hypertension. *Early Hum Dev* 2009; **85**(6): 361–7.

45. Ojeda N B, Grigore D, Robertson E B, Alexander B T. Estrogen protects against increased blood pressure in postpubertal female growth restricted offspring. *Hypertension* 2007; **50**(4): 679–85.

46. Ojeda N B, Grigore D, Yanes L L *et al.* Testosterone contributes to marked elevations in mean arterial pressure in adult male intrauterine growth restricted offspring. *Am J Physiol* 2007; **292**(2): R758–63.

47. Grigore D, Ojeda N B, Robertson E B *et al.* Placental insufficiency results in temporal alterations in the renin angiotensin system in male hypertensive growth restricted offspring. *Am J Physiol* 2007; **293**(2): R804–11.

48. Louey S, Cock M L, Stevenson K M, Harding R. Placental insufficiency and fetal growth restriction lead to postnatal hypotension and altered postnatal growth in sheep. *Pediatr Res* 2000; **48**(6): 808–14.

49. Tsirka A E, Gruetzmacher E M, Kelley D E *et al.* Myocardial gene expression of glucose transporter 1 and glucose transporter 4 in response to uteroplacental insufficiency in the rat. *J Endocrinol* 2001; **169**(2): 373–80.

50. Morrison J L, Botting K J, Dyer J L *et al.* Restriction of placental function alters heart development in the sheep fetus. *Am J Physiol* 2007; **293**(1): R306–13.

51. Harding R, Tester M L, Moss T J *et al.* Effects of intra-uterine growth restriction on the control of breathing and lung development after birth. *Clin Exp Pharmacol Physiol* 2000; **27**(1–2): 114–9.

52. Lipsett J, Tamblyn M, Madigan K *et al.* Restricted fetal growth and lung development: a morphometric analysis of pulmonary structure. *Pediatr Pulmonol* 2006; **41**(12): 1138–45.

53. O'Brien E A, Barnes V, Zhao L *et al.* Uteroplacental insufficiency decreases p53 serine-15 phosphorylation in term IUGR rat lungs. *Am J Physiol* 2007; **293**(1): R314–22.

54. Desai M, Gayle D, Babu J, Ross M G. Programmed obesity in intrauterine growth-restricted newborns: modulation by newborn nutrition. *Am J Physiol* 2005; **288**(1): R91–6.

55. Desai M, Gayle D, Han G, Ross M G. Programmed hyperphagia due to reduced anorexigenic mechanisms in intrauterine growth-restricted offspring. *Reproductive Sciences (Thousand Oaks, Calif)* 2007; **14**(4): 329–37.

56. Desai M, Babu J, Ross M G. Programmed metabolic syndrome: prenatal undernutrition and postweaning overnutrition. *Am J Physiol* 2007; **293**(6): R2306–14.

57. Desai M, Guang H, Ferelli M, Kallichanda N, Lane R H. Programmed upregulation of adipogenic transcription factors in intrauterine growth-restricted offspring. *Reproductive Sciences (Thousand Oaks, Calif)* 2008; **15** (8): 785–96.

58. Jones P L, Wolffe A P. Relationships between chromatin organization and DNA methylation in determining gene expression. *Semin Cancer Biol* 1999; **9**(5): 339–47.

59. Fu Q, McKnight R A, Yu X *et al.* Uteroplacental insufficiency induces site-specific changes in histone H3 covalent modifications and affects DNA-histone H3 positioning in day 0 IUGR rat liver. *Physiol Genom* 2004; **20**(1): 108–16.

60. Ke X, Lei Q, James S J *et al.* Uteroplacental insufficiency affects epigenetic determinants of chromatin structure in brains of neonatal and juvenile IUGR rats. *Physiol Genom* 2006; **25**(1): 16–28.

61. MacLennan N K, James S J, Melnyk S *et al.* Uteroplacental insufficiency alters DNA methylation, one-carbon metabolism, and histone acetylation in IUGR rats. *Physiol Genom* 2004; **18**(1): 43–50.

62. Fu Q, McKnight R A, Yu X, Callaway C W, Lane R H. Growth retardation alters the epigenetic characteristics of hepatic dual specificity phosphatase 5. *FASEB J* 2006; **20**(12): 2127–9.

Section 6 Chapter 16

Genetics

Fertile soil or no man's land: cooperation and conflict in the placental bed

David Haig

Department of Organismic and Evolutionary Biology, Harvard University, Cambridge, MA, USA

Introduction

In 1910, Gräfenberg wrote that ideas about relations between the human ovum and ovum bed [*Eibett*] had undergone a dramatic change during the previous decade. The ovum was no longer viewed as a passive object around which maternal tissues spread a protective cover. Far from being a helpless germ in need of protection, the ovum was a cheeky intruder [*ein frecher Eindringling*] that eats its way deep into the uterine mucosa. A popular comparison had been of the villi sinking into the endometrium as the roots of a tree sink into the earth, but Gräfenberg saw a hint of antagonism between the roots of the ovum and the surrounding soil. In his opinion, various structural and enzymatic features of the decidua were defensive reactions against the destructive ovum [1]. (I have translated the German *Ei* (egg) as ovum, the term used in the contemporary English literature. We would now call the 'ovum' an embryo.)

Grosser took a contrary view. Gräfenberg should not have taken Roux's 'struggle of parts within the organism' quite so literally. The primary function of the decidua was obvious; to act as a fertile soil [*Nährboden*] for supporting growth of the ovum. Toward this end, trophoblast and decidua formed an effective mutually coordinated, or better preservational, system in which one partner could not attack the other, nor the other defend itself, in opposition to what was imperative for the survival of the species [2: 289–290]. (*Nährboden* can be translated as fertile soil or as culture medium.)

My subject is the tension between hostile and amicable accounts of maternal–embryo relations; between a cooperative view, in which mother and embryo engage in mutual action in pursuit of common goals, and a conflictual view, in which mother and embryo have antagonistic goals and act at cross-purposes. This chapter has three parts. In the first part, I present a *partial* history of ideas about the maternal–fetal boundary of the gravid human uterus. It is a partial history in the dual sense of not complete and not impartial. A complete history would require a book-length exposition and fluency in multiple European languages but, in the space allotted, I can achieve no more than a sketch. My time span is from the late eighteenth century to the period between the World Wars. My exposition is not impartial because I discuss an idiosyncratic set of papers that appeal to me because of the images and metaphors employed to describe maternal–fetal relations. In the second part, I discuss the modern theoretical understanding of parent–offspring relations and how this predicts a complex interplay of cooperation and conflict. In the final part, I consider how this interplay is expressed in relations between the endometrium and early human embryos.

Mixed metaphors: historical interpretations of the maternal–fetal interface

Fundamental progress in understanding the maternal–fetal interface occurred in the brief 5-year period from 1895 to 1899. Before this period, there was considerable confusion about which cell types were fetal and which were maternal. Strange theories, from a modern perspective, were expounded (e.g. the chorion was a maternal tissue deposited around the ovum as it traversed the Fallopian tube, analogous to the white of a hen egg [3]). After this period, descriptions of the maternal–fetal interface are readily intelligible to a modern reader, although many details still remained to be elucidated. My account will race through the nineteenth century, outline the discoveries that caused this change in perspective, and then discuss early reactions to the realization that human embryos 'invaded' maternal tissues.

About the month of May 1754, John Hunter was called in to examine the uterus, with placenta *in situ*, of a woman who had died undelivered at full term. A colleague had previously injected red wax into the uterine arteries and yellow wax into the uterine veins. 'Upon cutting into the placenta [Hunter] discovered in many places of its substance, yellow injection; in others red, and in many others these two colours intermixed. This substance of the placenta, now filled with injection, had nothing of the vascular appearance, nor that of extravasation, but had a regularity in its form which showed it to be a natural cellular structure, fitted to be a reservoir for blood' [4]. ('Cellular structure' refers to the cavernous spaces of the placenta; beware of changes in meaning!)

The fetus, by contrast, had: 'a communication with the placenta of another kind. The arteries from the fœtus pass out to a considerable length, under the name of the umbilical chord, and when they arrive at the placenta, ramify upon its surface, sending into its substance branches which pass through it, and divide into smaller and smaller, till at last they terminate in veins; these uniting, become larger and larger, and end in one, which at last terminates in the proper circulation of the fœtus'[4].

Thus, Hunter had arrived at an essentially correct view of the maternal and fetal circulations in the term placenta: maternal blood passed out of the mother's circulation into the spongy substance of the placenta – a structure Hunter viewed as of solely fetal origin – before returning to the general maternal circulation. At no time was there admixture of maternal and fetal blood. Much of the nineteenth century involved controversy between Hunterians who accepted this view of placental blood flow and non-Hunterians who believed that maternal blood did not enter the placenta and that the Hunterian theory was based on experimental artifacts [5,6]. By the end of the century, the Hunterian view was predominant.

The precise nature of the covering of the tufts (villi) that projected into the cellular structure of the placenta was also controversial. Reid proposed an influential, but incorrect, resolution of this problem: 'when the blood of the mother flows into the placenta through the curling arteries of the uterus, it passes into a large sac formed by the inner coat of the vascular system of the mother, which is intersected in many thousands of different directions, by the placental tufts projecting into it like fringes, and pushing its thin wall before them in the form of sheaths, which closely envelope both the trunk and each individual branch composing these tufts. From this sac the maternal blood is returned by the utero-placental veins without having been extravasated, or without having left her own system of vessels' [7].

By the 1880s, advances in microscopical techniques had enabled a more accurate view of the villous sheath. Villi were now seen as covered by two layers: an outer syncytial layer and an inner cellular layer (Langhans' cells) adjacent to the mesenchymal core of the villus. There was great confusion, however, about the nature and origin of these layers (a review of the many hypotheses is beyond the scope of this chapter). Marchand made a crucial advance in 1895 when he recognized that 'decidual' tumors (choriocarcinomas of modern parlance) were composed of the same cellular elements as the villous sheath. At first, Marchand interpreted the sheath as a symbiosis between the syncytium, derived from the uterine (or tubal) epithelium, and ectodermal cells of fetal origin, but he soon recognized that both layers were fetal [8,9]. He now suggested that chorionepithelioma was the most appropriate name for these tumors.

In June 1897, Hubert Peters presented a very early human embryo at the Congress of the German Gynecological Society in Leipzig. This embryo had been found at autopsy of a young woman who had killed herself 3 days after a missed menstrual period. Peters' subsequent monograph described the embryo in detail, together with observations of the *Umlagerungszone*, a confusing region in which maternal and fetal cells were jumbled together amidst cellular debris. Peters' preparations made clear that the embryo had sunk into, and embedded itself within, the uterine mucosa (previous hypotheses had viewed the decidua as growing up and enveloping the embryo) and that the syncytium was of fetal origin [10]. (The original meaning of *Umlagerungszone* seems to have been a zone of transformation, see discussion by Grosser who preferred instead *Durchdringungszone* (penetration-zone) [2: 306–307].)

Prior to the late 1890s, the human embryo was not generally perceived as *invading* maternal tissues. The concept of trophoblastic invasion developed from an appreciation of the great destructive power of chorionepitheliomas; from the description of Peters' ovum embedded within the uterine mucosa; and from comparative studies of implantation in hedgehogs, rodents, and rabbits. After this change in outlook, the search for the maternal–fetal boundary shifted outward (to adopt the fetal perspective) from the lining of the chorionic villi into the *Umlagerungszone*. By the time that Teacher reviewed the literature on chorionepitheliomas in 1903, there was an emerging consensus that the syncytium was derived from fetal Langhans' cells and that the human embryo digested its way into the uterine lining (although some continued to defend older interpretations) [11].

Once trophoblast was recognized as invading maternal tissues, it was a small step (taken by several authors) to view the process of implantation as a conflict between maternal and fetal tissues, with the decidua functioning as a protective bulwark against intrusion by trophoblast [12,13,14,15,16]. Polano wrote of an antagonism between maternal tissues and the motherforeign tissues of the child, and described the latter as establishing outposts in enemy territory [*Vorposten in Feindesland*] [14]. In an authoritative review, published in 1910, Grosser claimed that most authors saw the formation of the decidua as 'a provision against the too intensive penetration of the ovum into the mucous membrane', but himself favored the alternative hypothesis that decidual cells functioned as a store of nutrients for use by the embryo [17: 139–140].

Gräfenberg applied bacteriological methods to investigate the respective roles of ovum and decidua in nidation. He prepared homogenates from first-trimester human placentas and showed that these contained a proteolytic activity that eroded protein-containing culture media. This activity was absent in placental homogenates from the second half of pregnancy. The proteolytic activity, however, was attenuated when placental homogenates were mixed with decidual homogenates, especially those prepared from first-trimester decidua. Therefore, Gräfenberg concluded the decidua produced antitryptic ferments (protease inhibitors) to act as a defense against the tryptic ferments (proteases) of the chorion. He suggested that Nitabuch's fibrinoid provided additional resistance, both mechanical and biochemical, to penetration by trophoblast [1]. For Linzenmeier, the ferments and antiferments described by Gräfenberg were the weapons [*Waffen*] used by fetal and maternal cells in their struggle [*Kampf*] in the contact zone [18].

On the eve of the conflagration that was to engulf Europe, Johnstone used eerily prescient language: 'The border zone . . . is not a sharp line, for it is in truth the fighting line where the conflict between the maternal cells and the invading trophoderm takes place, and it is strewn with such of the dead on both sides as have not already been carried off the field'. Despite these images, Johnstone concluded that the decidual reaction was 'in all probability indirectly but equally protective to the embryo, in that, by supporting and strengthening the maternal capillaries, it prevents a too sudden and too extensive opening up of the vessels. . . . The formation of the decidua is therefore to the mutual advantage of both mother and child' [19]. One could ascribe a defensive function to the decidua, employ militaristic metaphors, and yet view maternal–fetal relations as fundamentally harmonious.

Caffier extended Gräfenberg's experimental work on placental ferments after the Great War which provided him with a new metaphor for the maternal–fetal boundary: the fibrinoid layer of the border zone was a no man's land [*Niemandsland*] created by the reciprocal proteolytic actions of ovum and ovum bed. He suggested that abortion resulted from a preponderance of the proteolytic activity of the mother-soil [*Mutterboden*] whereas placenta accreta resulted from excess proteolytic activity of the embryo [20,21].

Kleine advanced similar views in his systematic pathology of the penetration zone, based on the modern perception that pregnancy was a biological struggle between maternal and fetal organisms. The decidua showed a defensive reaction against the attacks [*Angriffe*] of the trophoblast. Developmental abnormalities resulted from a mismatch between the aggressiveness of the fetal epithelium and the defensive powers of maternal tissues. Thus, overly strong defenses could result in an early abortion (by shutting off the embryo from the maternal blood supply) whereas weak defenses could result in the destructive infiltration of a chorionepithelioma. Kleine observed that a decidual reaction occurs exclusively in those mammals in which the trophoblast destroys the uterine mucosa, and interpreted this correlation as indirect evidence for antagonism between the decidua and trophoblast [22].

Where some saw 'a ruthless attack and an equally vigorous defense' others saw 'a nicely worked out co-operation to produce a definite harmonious end' [23]. For Mossman, the idea that the decidua functioned as a defensive bulwark was 'quite unsubstantiated'. It seemed more logical 'to assume that decidual tissue develops as a glycogen-storing tissue . . . partly at least for the purpose of being invaded and absorbed by trophoblast, rather than to prevent such invasion' [24: 168]. Here, Mossman referred to the principal hypothesis of those who viewed implantation as a cooperative process: decidual cells were provided by the mother as pabulum for nourishment of the embryo [25,26]. Bonnet saw the migration of leukocytes to the maternal–fetal border and their subsequent disintegration as a mechanism whereby the mother transported nutrients to the embryo [25]. (By contrast, Frassi interpreted the leukocytes as a means of halting the parasitic penetration of the ovum [13].)

None of the authors who described the maternal–fetal boundary as a battleground offered well-articulated reasons for why mother and offspring should be at war. Their use of military metaphors did not reflect strong theoretical preconceptions but was rather an attempt to make sense of what they saw through their microscopes. Undoubtedly, the images they chose to describe what they saw were shaped by the militaristic ethos of their age, but there were other strongly competing images of nurturing love of mothers for infants that could have been used if the histology had been different. After World War II, occasional descriptions can be found of the placental bed as a battleground or a no man's land but these passages lack the ferocity of the earlier period.

Evolutionary conflict in parent–offspring relations

Decidual reactions occur only in mammals with invasive placentation. This observation has been used to support different theories. McLaren interpreted the decidual reaction as evidence that the decidua functions as a barrier to trophoblast. 'If the decidual reaction were acting as a protective device, one would expect it to be more highly developed in those forms where mother and fetus are more intimately fused. The distribution of decidual development would thus seem to favor a protective rather than a nutritional role' [27]. But Robertson & Warner used the same correlation to make the opposite inference: 'There must be significance in the fact that only in hemochorial placentation is there development of a true decidua ... It may therefore be concluded that decidua is essential for the success of hemochorial placentation and it seems illogical to regard it as an impediment to the invasiveness of trophoblast when invasiveness is a *sine qua non*' [28]. McLaren implicitly assumed a conflictual relationship – borders are fortified where the threat of invasion is greatest – whereas Robertson & Warner implicitly assumed a cooperative partnership. Such differences of interpretation cannot be resolved or reconciled without an explicit theory of how maternal–fetal relations evolve. No such theory existed until the work of Robert Trivers [29,30].

Trivers defined parental investment as '*any investment by the parent in an individual offspring that increases the offspring's chances of surviving (and hence reproductive success) at the cost of the parent's ability to invest in other offspring*'. His definition was carefully worded. Parental investment provided a benefit (B) to the offspring at a cost (C) to the parent's fitness from other offspring. If a parental expenditure did not involve such a trade-off, then the expenditure did not qualify as investment [29]. He recognized that parental investment, defined this way, implied an evolutionary conflict between parents and offspring. From a parent's perspective, further investment was favored as long as $B > C$ but, from an offspring's perspective, further investment was favored as long as $B > rC$, where r was a measure of the probability that the parent's other offspring carried a copy of a randomly chosen gene in the offspring. Trivers concluded that genes in offspring are selected to obtain more investment from parents than genes in parents are selected to supply (because $r \leq 0.5$) [30]. I will attempt to give an intuitive idea of the interplay between cooperation and conflict in maternal–fetal relations with a simple graphical model that elides many theoretical complications.

Consider a plane with two axes (Fig. 16.1). One axis represents the effect of a new genetic variant on maternal residual fitness (ΔM, measured as changes in a mother's expected number of surviving offspring not including the fetus). The other axis represents the effect on fetal fitness (F, measured as changes in the fetus' probability of survival). The zero-point, where the axes cross, represents the evolutionary *status quo*. Points in the upper-right quadrant represent variants that enhance both fetal fitness and maternal residual fitness whereas points in the lower-left quadrant represent variants that reduce both measures. The other two quadrants represent variants that 'rebalance' maternal investment between the two asset classes. In the upper-left quadrant, maternal investment is shifted from the fetus to other offspring, whereas, in the lower-right quadrant, maternal investment is shifted from other offspring to the fetus. (In terms of Trivers' model negative values of ΔM correspond to a cost to the parent's fitness (C) whereas positive values of F correspond to a benefit to offspring fitness B.)

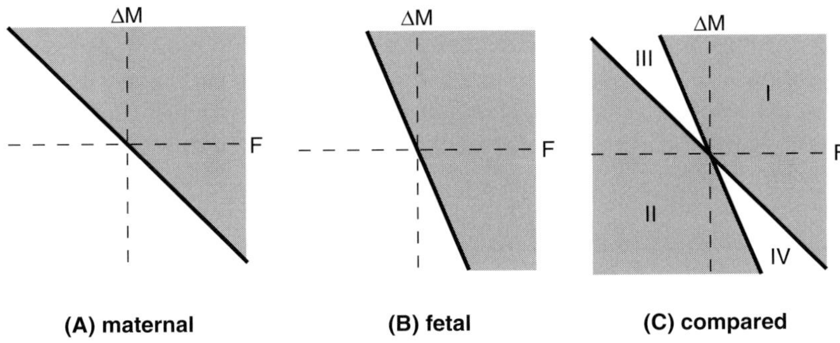

Fig. 16.1 Cooperation and conflict between maternal and fetal genes. *F* is the change in fetal fitness and ΔM the change in maternal residual fitness. (A) Maternal inclusive fitness is increased if $F + \Delta M > 0$ (shaded area). (B) Fetal inclusive fitness is increased if $F + r\Delta M > 0$ (shaded area) where *r* is the relatedness between two of a mother's offspring. (C) Figures A and B are compared. Maternal and fetal inclusive fitness both benefit in region I and both are reduced in region II. In region III, the mother benefits at the expense of the fetus. In region IV, the fetus benefits at the expense of the mother. These figures were drawn choosing $r = 0.5$ to maximize the area of mutual interest (regions I and II). The region of conflict (regions III and IV) expands for smaller *r* (i.e. lower relatedness among a mother's offspring).

For genes expressed in mothers, natural selection favors changes that satisfy $F + \Delta M > 0$ (shaded area of Fig. 16.1A). By contrast, for genes expressed in a fetus, natural selection favors changes that satisfy $F + r\Delta M > 0$ (shaded area of Fig. 16.1B). The zones of mutual and conflicting interests are visualized in Fig. 16.1C (obtained by combining Fig. 16.1A and Fig. 16.1B). The plane is divided into four regions. In region I, changes are favored independent of whether they are caused by a gene expressed in mothers or fetuses. In region II, changes are disfavored independent of where the gene is expressed. In region III, changes are favored if they are caused by a gene expressed in mothers but not if they are caused by a gene expressed in fetuses (and the reverse in region IV). Thus, regions I and II comprise the zone of *maternal–fetal cooperation* whereas regions III and IV comprise the zone of *maternal–fetal conflict*.

There are four points that I wish to make about the foregoing analysis. First, the evolution of maternal–fetal relations is complex because a mother and her fetus share some genes, but not all. The genes that are unshared create the opportunity for conflict whereas the genes that are shared restrain the escalation of conflict. Second, there is broad overlap between the interests of maternal and fetal genes. Genetic variants that enhance fetal fitness and maternal residual fitness (upper-right quadrant) will be favored by natural selection regardless of whether they are expressed in the mother or the fetus. Similarly, genetic variants that diminish both fitness measures (lower-left quadrant) will be purged by natural selection regardless of where they are expressed. The interests of maternal and fetal genes may even coincide when a fetus benefits at the cost of other offspring or vice versa (regions I and II extend into the upper-left and lower-right quadrants; Fig. 16.1C). Third, a successful genetic variant establishes a new status quo, around which new genetic variants are selected. Therefore, there will have been a mixture of 'cooperative' and 'antagonistic' gene substitutions in the evolution of any complex feature of maternal–fetal relations. There is no contradiction in the decidua having evolved *both* as a defensive barrier *and* as a nurturing environment for the young embryo. Fourth, much of the 'evolutionary action' may take place in the regions of conflict because fetal adaptations to acquire a little bit extra create the selective force for maternal adaptations to supply a little bit less, and so on *ad infinitum*. This may help to explain the rapid divergence of maternal–fetal relations among taxa, relative to the greater conservatism of physiological relations within individual organisms.

Implantation: a testing time

'If it is done then when tis done twer better it were done quickly.' –*Macbeth*

Trivers mentioned the possibility of prenatal conflict between mothers and offspring, but emphasized postnatal conflict [30]. Haigh [31] provided the first substantial attempt to apply the theory of parent–offspring conflict to understanding the details of maternal–fetal relations, and I have developed these ideas in a series of subsequent papers [32,33,34,35,36,37]. An interplay of cooperation and conflict is predicted to permeate all aspects of maternal–fetal relations, but in the remainder of this chapter I will focus on interactions in the first few weeks after conception.

Many human embryos abort early, often before a woman is aware she has conceived [38]. Moreover, frequent early losses have also been reported in other primates [39,40,41]. Most maternal investment occurs after the first weeks of gestation. Therefore, an early loss can usually be quickly replaced with little cost to a mother's lifetime reproduction. By contrast, continuation of a pregnancy with the birth of a sickly infant can substantially depress a mother's fitness as the child consumes maternal time and resources that could otherwise have been invested in higher-quality sibs. For these reasons, primate mothers are expected to 'test' embryos before commitment of major resources and to be physiologically 'risk-averse' about which embryos are allowed to establish a sustained pregnancy [42,43]. The maternal–embryo dialogue may resemble a job interview.

Earlier pregnancy losses have smaller costs for maternal fitness if resources can be redirected to other offspring (reproductive compensation). Natural selection favors the *amelioration* of deleterious effects in the absence of reproductive compensation but may favor their *accentuation* if resources can be reallocated. Maternal genes will benefit from the conversion of a small decrement in offspring fitness into a lethal difference if early death is associated with a sufficiently large increase in the fitness of other offspring. For these reasons, reproductive compensation is predicted to favor rigorous testing of early embryos and earlier expression of harmful effects [44,45].

If this were the whole story, one would expect embryonic screening to become ever more effective at increasing offspring quality. However, natural selection acting on genes expressed in embryos will tend to undermine the efficiency of screening because genes of lower-quality embryos have only a chance of their copies being present in higher-quality siblings. Such genes therefore must balance the certainty of a sure bet (investment in their own low-quality offspring) against the chance of a higher return (investment in a high-quality sib). For this reason, natural selection will favor embryos that create a more favorable impression at interview than reflects their true quality.

The complex relations between an examiner (mother) and an examinee (prospective offspring) cannot be pigeon-holed as purely cooperative or purely conflictual. An examiner's aim is to design tests that provide useful information about a candidate as cheaply as possible. The examinee wishes to pass. If the examinee is indeed of high quality, both parties benefit when this information is conveyed accurately, but, if the examinee is of poor quality, her best interest may be to dissemble. The challenge of test design is to ensure a tight correlation between attributes measured and qualities desired. Genes and pathways that are essential for cell survival are automatically, and reliably, tested at the earliest stages of development. But some functions are difficult to test: a mother cannot directly assess neural function in an embryo without neurons; poor visual acuity entails no disadvantage in the darkness of the womb [46: 247].

Any task that an embryo is required to perform tests all genes that are essential for completion of the task. Thus, the necessity for a small embryo to produce large quantities of chorionic gonadotropin (CG) tests not only the genes that encode the hormone's α- and β-subunits (the latter of little importance in postnatal life) but also the efficient functioning of the machinery of transcription, translation, glycosylation, and cellular secretion. Placental production of a luteinizing hormone (LH), the future CG, may have originated as a form of cheating that allowed embryos to evade maternal mechanisms of pregnancy termination (i.e. withdrawal of pituitary LH). But, the quantity of the placental hormone provided mothers with useable information about embryo quality and was incorporated into the testing procedure as a new requirement for embryos to exceed some threshold level of CG to block regression of the corpus luteum [31,35]. Although the original targets of CG were presumably maternal LH receptors of the ovary, CG appears to have acquired additional functions during implantation [47] allowing earlier, less costly, rejection of a subset of embryos.

Examinations select for individuals who are good at passing tests, and discriminate against otherwise equivalent individuals with poorer test performance. For this reason, the correlation between test performance and offspring quality will tend to degrade over evolutionary time as genes that enhance test-taking ability spread through the population. Examiners must add additional tasks or adjust expectations to maintain the usefulness of the testing procedure. For example, the acquisition of extra copies of CG genes and the prolongation of the hormone's half-life [48] would have enhanced an embryo's test performance without changing the resulting offspring's competence on tasks that really matter. Mothers are predicted to have responded evolutionarily by increasing the threshold of CG required to maintain pregnancy.

Early human embryos embed themselves within the endometrial stroma (as do the embryos of other apes). By contrast, monkey blastocysts attach to the endometrial surface but remain located within the uterine cavity [49,50]. Mossman considered the reasons for the evolution of interstitial implantation to be obscure. Platyrrhine and catarrhine monkeys develop perfectly adequate hemochorial placentae despite superficial implantation of their blastocysts. Therefore, interstitial implantation is not a *sine qua non* of hemochorial placentation [50: 152–154]. Embedded embryos experience an environment very different from that experienced by superficially attached embryos. It is an open question whether this novel environment created new opportunities for more thorough vetting of offspring.

A typical early pregnancy loss in ancestral primates probably took the form of an attached embryo being flushed out as the uterine lining was shed at the end of the estrous cycle. A superficially attached embryo would be eliminated by sloughing the outermost layer of the endometrium whereas a more deeply embedded embryo would survive. Therefore, interstitial implantation may have originated as an adaptation of embryos to evade this ancestral mechanism of pregnancy termination. Deeper shedding of the endometrium may then have evolved as a maternal countermeasure to re-establish effective testing. Thus, a history of facultative abortion, embryonic evasion of quality control, and maternal responses may help to explain the origin of interstitial implantation and copious menstruation.

The above scenario could be dismissed as no more than a just-so story, incapable of test, because it posits a unique series of unfossilizable events that occurred in an ancestral ape. However, some insight may be obtained from comparative studies of implantation, pregnancy loss, and menstruation in primates. The quantity of maternal tissue shed at menstruation varies markedly among monkeys and apes [51]. Does the depth of menstrual shedding correlate with the depth of implantation? How frequently is menstruation accompanied by an early pregnancy loss?

Schlusskoagulum

The evolutionary relations between a mother and a fetus are fundamentally similar to the relations between the same two genetic individuals after the birth of the fetus. Mothers care for and nurture their infants but do not accede to each and every demand [52]. And infants have evolved multiple stratagems – from charm to blackmail – for eliciting more maternal care. Maternal–fetal relations likewise involve an intricate admixture of cooperation and conflict. Prenatal relations do, however, differ in a couple of important respects from postnatal relations. In the earliest stages of pregnancy, there is little difference between the expected cost to a mother of raising the current embryo or trying again with another embryo. Therefore, mothers abandon early embryos much more readily than they would abandon a child. After an embryo is securely ensconced within the uterus, however, the offspring probably has far greater power to control the delivery of maternal investment than it has at any postnatal stage. The secretion of placental hormones and other factors into maternal blood allows the fetus to treat its mother's body as if it were a direct extension of the fetus's own soma.

Acknowledgments

Omer Bartov, Richard Bondi, Reimar Brüning, Jan Engelstädter, Karin Michels, Judith Ryan, and Claus Wedekind all provided help with translation from German. The paper has benefited from the insightful comments of Robert Pijnenborg.

References

1. Gräfenberg E. Beiträge zur Physiologie der Eieinbettung. *Z Geburtsh Gynäk* 1910; **65**: 1–35.
2. Grosser O. *Frühentwicklung Eihautbildung und Placentation des Menschen und der Säugetiere*. München: JF Bergmann; 1927.
3. Smith W T. The decidua, chorion, placenta, and umbilical cord. *Lancet* 1856; **1**: 171–5.
4. Hunter J. *Observations on certain parts of the animal oeconomy*. London; 1786.
5. Madge H M. On the anatomical relations between the mother and fœtus. *Trans Obstet Soc London* 1867; **8**: 348–60.
6. Hicks J B. The anatomy of the human placenta. *Trans Obstet Soc London* 1873; **14**: 149–207.
7. Reid J. On the anatomical relations of the blood-vessels of the mother to those of the fœtus in the human species. *Edinburgh Med Surg J* 1841; **55**: 1–12.
8. Marchand F. Ueber die sogenannten "decidualen" Geschwülste im Anschluss an normale Geburt, Abort, Blasenmole und Extrauterinschwangerschaft. *Monatsschr Gerburtsh Gynäk* 1895; **1**: 419–438, 513–561.

9. Marchand F. Ueber das maligne Chorion-Epitheliom, nebst Mittheilung von 2 neuen Fällen. *Z Geburtsh Gynäk* 1898; **49**: 173–258.
10. Peters H. *Ueber die Einbettung des menschlichen Eies und das früheste bisher bekannte menschliche Placentationsstadium*. Leipzig: F Deutike; 1899.
11. Teacher J H. On chorionepithelioma and the occurrence of chorionepitheliomatous and hydatidiform mole-like structures in teratomata. *J Obstet Gynæcol Brit Emp* 1903; **4**: 1–64, 145–199.
12. Fothergill W E. The function of the decidual cell. *Edinburgh Med J* 1899; **5**: 265–73.
13. Frassi L. Ueber ein junges menschliches Ei in situ. *Arch mikroskop Anat Entwicklungsg* 1907; **70**: 492–505.
14. Polano O. Ueber Verschwinden einer Schwangerschaft. Ein Beitrag zur Lehre von der Blasenmole. *Z Geburtsh Gynäk* 1907; **59**: 453–66.
15. Bryce T H, Teacher J H, Kerr J M M. *Contributions to the study of the early development and imbedding of the human ovum. II. An early ovarian pregnancy*. Glasgow: J MacLehose; 1908.
16. Ulezko-Stroganova K. Zur Frage von dem feinsten Bau des Deciduagewebes, seiner Histogenese, Bedeutung und dem Orte seiner Entwickelung im Genitalapparat der Frau. *Arch Gynaek* 1908; **86**: 542–63.
17. Grosser O. The development of the egg membranes and the placenta; menstruation. In: Keibel F, Mall F P, eds. *Manual of human embryology, Volume 1*. Philadelphia: JB Lippincott; 1910; pp. 91–179.
18. Linzenmeier G. Ein junges menschliches Ei in situ. *Arch Gynäk* 1914; **102**: 1–17.
19. Johnstone R W. Contribution to the study of the early human ovum. *J Obstet Gynaecol Brit Emp* 1914; **25**: 231–76.
20. Caffier P. Die proteolytische Fähigkeit von Ei und Eibett. (Experimentelle Studien mit Chorion und Decidua). *Zentralb Gynäk* 1929; **53**: 2410–25.
21. Caffier P. Zur Biologie von Ei und Eibett. *Klin Wochenschr* 1932; **11**: 1089–92.
22. Kleine H O. Zur Systematik der Pathologie der sog. Durchdringungszone. *Arch Gynäk* 1931; **145**: 459–73.
23. Arey L B. Placentation, fetal membranes and deciduae. In: Curtis A H, ed. *Obstetrics and gynecology*. Philadelphia: WB Saunders; 1933: pp. 442–76.
24. Mossman H W. Comparative morphogenesis of the fetal membranes and accessory uterine structures. *Contrib Embryol* 1937; **26**: 129–246.
25. Bonnet M. Ueber Syncytien, Plasmodien und Symplasma in der Placenta der Säugetiere und des Menschen. *Monatsschr Gerburtsh Gynäk* 1903; **18**: 1–51.
26. Ritter F. Ueber Deciduazellen und ihre Bedeutung. *Beitr Geburtsh Gynäk* 1910; **15**: 226–41.
27. McLaren A. Maternal factors in nidation. In: Park W W, ed. *The early conceptus, normal and abnormal*. St. Andrews: University of St. Andrews; 1965: pp. 27–33.
28. Robertson W B, Warner B. The ultrastructure of the human placental bed. *J Pathol* 1974; **112**: 203–11.
29. Trivers R L. Parental investment and sexual selection. In: Campbell B, ed. *Sexual selection and the descent of man, 1871–1971*. Chicago: Aldine Publishing; 1972: pp. 136–79.
30. Trivers R L. Parent-offspring conflict. *Amer Zool* 1974; **14**: 249–64.
31. Haig D. Genetic conflicts in human pregnancy. *Q Rev Biol* 1993; **68**: 495–532.
32. Haig D. Gestational drive and the green-bearded placenta. *Proc Natl Acad Sci USA* 1996; **93**: 6547–51.
33. Haig D. Placental hormones, genomic imprinting, and maternal-fetal communication. *J Evol Biol* 1996; **9**: 357–80.
34. Haig D. Altercation of generations: genetic conflicts of pregnancy. *Amer J Reprod Immunol* 1996; **35**: 226–32.
35. Haig D. Genetic conflicts of pregnancy and childhood. In: Stearns S C, ed. *Evolution in health and disease*. Oxford: Oxford University Press; 1999: pp. 77–90.
36. Haig D. Evolutionary conflicts in pregnancy and calcium metabolism: a review. *Placenta* 2004; **25** (Suppl A): S10-S15.
37. Haig D. Putting up resistance: maternal-fetal conflict over the control of uteroplacental blood flow. In: Aird W C, ed. *Endothelial biomedicine*. Cambridge: Cambridge University Press; 2007: pp. 135–41.
38. Wilcox A J, Weinberg C R, O'Connor J F *et al.* Incidence of early loss of pregnancy. *New Engl J Med* 1988; **319**: 189–94.
39. Small M F. Reproductive failure in macaques. *Amer J Primatol* 1982; **2**: 137–47.
40. Kuehl T J, Kang I S, Siler-Khodr T M. Pregnancy and early reproductive failure in the baboon. *Amer J Primatol* 1992; **28**: 41–8.
41. Hobson W C, Graham C E, Rowell T J. National Chimpanzee Breeding Program: Primate Research Institute. *Amer J Primatol* 1991; **24**: 257–63.
42. Kozlowski J, Stearns S C. Hypotheses for the production of excess zygotes: models of bet-hedging and selective abortion. *Evolution* 1989; **43**: 1369–77.
43. Haig D. Brood reduction and optimal parental investment when offspring differ in quality. *Amer Nat* 1990; **136**: 550–6.

44. Hamilton W D. The moulding of senescence by natural selection. *J Theor Biol* 1966; **12**: 12–45.

45. Hastings I M. Models of human genetic disease: how biased are the standard formulae? *Genet Res* 2000; **75**: 107–114.

46. Ridley M. *Mendel's demon*. London: Weidenfeld & Nicolson; 2000.

47. Licht P, Fluhr H, Neuwinger J *et al.* Is human chorionic gonadotropin directly involved in the regulation of human implantation? *Mol Cell Endocrinol* 2007; **269**: 85–92.

48. Henke A, Gromoll J. New insights into the evolution of chorionic gonadotropin. *Mol Cell Endocrinol* 2008; **291**: 11–19.

49. Wislocki G B. On the placentation of primates, with a consideration of the phylogeny of the placenta. *Contrib Embryol* 1929; **20**: 51–80.

50. Mossman H W. *Vertebrate fetal membranes*. New Brunswick: Rutgers University Press; 1987.

51. Strassmann B I. The evolution of endometrial cycles and menstruation. *Q Rev Biol* 1996; **71**: 181–220.

52. Hrdy S B. *Mother nature*. New York: Pantheon; 1999.

Chapter 17

The search for susceptibility genes

Linda Morgan

Institute of Genetics, University of Nottingham, Nottingham, UK

Introduction

The last decade has seen increasing evidence of the power of molecular genetics to generate novel hypotheses of disease etiology. Clinical observation suggests that there is a familial predisposition to a number of disorders associated with impaired placentation, including preeclampsia, fetal growth restriction, recurrent miscarriage, and preterm labor [1,2,3]. From this spectrum of disorders, preeclampsia is the condition which has attracted most attention from geneticists, and will be the focus of this chapter. The identification of susceptibility genes offers unique insights into the pathophysiology of disease. In many patients, perhaps the majority, preeclampsia has its origins in the early stages of pregnancy prior to the onset of symptoms, at a time when basic research into its etiology is impossible for practical and ethical reasons. Once the disease is established, pathophysiological research is hampered by the transient phenotype of the condition, and confounded by secondary responses to the widespread maternal endothelial damage. Genetic research is an attractive option, as the patient's genotype is unaffected by time or disease severity.

The evidence for inheritance

First-degree relatives of women affected by preeclampsia have a two- to three-fold increase in risk of the disorder compared with the rest of the pregnant population [4,5,6]. In genetic terminology, this is known as the relative risk ratio, λ_R, and is calculated as the ratio of the incidence of disease in first-degree relatives to its incidence in the population. A λ_R of 2 to 3 is typical of many complex disorders, including type 2 diabetes, Alzheimer's disease, and coronary artery disease. Susceptibility genes for these conditions have been identified, encouraging optimism that the search for genetic variants associated with preeclampsia will lead to similar successes.

A tendency for a disease to run in families may be due to shared genes or shared environmental influences such as diet and exposure to toxins and infections. Partitioning the contribution of genetic and environmental factors to disease has classically relied on twin studies. The underlying principle is intuitive: monozygotic twins share 100% of genes, whilst dizygotic twins share on average 50% of genes. If disease susceptibility is highly dependent on genetic factors, monozygotic twins will show significantly higher concordance rates than dizygotic twins. The proportion of variation in susceptibility to a disease which can be attributed to genetic variation is known as its heritability, h^2, which can take a value between 0 and 1. High values of h^2 justify attempts to identify causal genes.

Initial attempts to define the heritability of preeclampsia through twin studies were discouraging; discordance for preeclampsia amongst parous monozygotic twin sisters is common, and in some series no monozygotic twin pairs concordant for preeclampsia were identified [7]. The problem appears to have been one of sample power; even large twin registries contain limited numbers of parous twin sisters. The largest twin study to date made use of the Swedish Twin Registry, analyzing data from over 900 parous monozygotic twin sisters and almost 1200 dizygotic twins [8]. They included 8 pairs of monozygotic twins concordant for preeclampsia, and 47 pairs in whom only one sister developed preeclampsia. The corresponding figures for dizygotic twins were 2 concordant and 59 discordant pairs. Heritability for preeclampsia was estimated as 0.54, but even with this large sample 95% confidence intervals included 0 (0 to 0.71). Inclusion of non-proteinuric gestational hypertension with preeclampsia as a single category of pregnancy-induced hypertension yielded a heritability of 0.47 (95% C.I. 0.13–0.61).

A subsequent study analyzed data from over 700 000 pregnancies on the Swedish Birth Registry [9].

Text Box 17.1 Identification of susceptibility genes

- For many complex disorders of pregnancy, a family history in a first-degree relative is associated with a two- to three-fold increase in risk
- 35% of the variation in susceptibility to preeclampsia is attributed to maternal genes, and 20% to fetal genes
- Candidate gene studies in preeclampsia have failed to identify a universally accepted susceptibility gene
- Genome-wide screening is an unbiased approach to susceptibility gene discovery
- Genotyping 500 000 to 1 million selected single nucleotide polymorphisms captures over 80% of variation in the human genome

The incorporation of data from sibs (50% of genes shared on average) and half-sibs (25% gene sharing on average) generated a powerful study of the inheritance of preeclampsia. Heritability was estimated as 0.35 (95% C.I. 0.33–0.36) due to maternal genes, and 0.20 (95% C.I. 0.11–0.24) for fetal genes. This highlights an important challenge which must be addressed in studying the genetic basis of complex disorders of pregnancy: two genomes are involved, maternal and fetal, and the search for susceptibility genes should include both.

A number of approaches to gene discovery in complex disorders are possible (Text Box 17.1). The most extensively used strategy has been to study candidate genes suggested by pathophysiological considerations. An alternative approach is to screen the entire genome for evidence of susceptibility loci. For many years this could be achieved only by focusing on families with more than one affected subject using linkage analysis. Recent developments in genotyping technology and bioinformatics now make it possible to screen the genome for association with disease using a case–control design. The successes and challenges of each of these approaches as they apply to preeclampsia will be considered in turn.

Candidate gene studies

Our understanding of the pathophysiology of preeclampsia suggests that a number of biological mechanisms are involved. Many affected pregnancies demonstrate impaired trophoblastic invasion of maternal tissues, and this is understood to be an etiological factor in possibly the majority of cases. The process of trophoblast invasion requires the expression of proteinases, adhesion molecules, cytokines and their receptors, triggered in turn by the spatial and temporal coordination of transcription factor expression. It is clear that both maternal and fetal genes are involved in this process. The spectrum of maternal response to impaired placentation ranges from minimal, in uncomplicated fetal growth restriction, to fulminant preeclampsia with widespread endothelial activation and multisystem involvement. The nature and extent of the maternal pathology may also be genetically determined, most evidently in the response to oxidative stress, vascular reactivity, and thrombophilic tendency.

Candidate gene studies have focused primarily on maternal genes, including those encoding proteins involved in blood pressure regulation and sodium homeostasis, factors affecting endothelial reactivity, coagulation factors, cytokines and their receptors. Comprehensive reviews of these studies are available [2,10,11]. Most have adopted a case–control design, comparing the frequency of a genetic variant in affected women and in healthy pregnant controls. Disappointingly no universally accepted susceptibility gene has emerged from over a decade of research, and the field has been beset by inconsistent and conflicting results. This is typical of the experience in candidate gene studies of other complex disorders, and is the consequence of inadequately powered studies. With the near-completion and annotation of the human genome map, it is now known that there are approximately 25 000 human genes, many still of unknown function. The prior probability that any one of these genes is associated with preeclampsia is small; the likelihood of association with one of many polymorphisms within a specific gene is even lower. Whilst it has been argued that the biological candidacy of a particular gene increases its prior probability of association, the truth is that a more or less convincing case can be made for involvement of any gene. It is now widely accepted that evidence for genetic association requires more stringent levels of statistical significance to reduce the false-positive signals to an acceptable level. This is achievable only with large studies, and no candidate gene studies in preeclampsia have been published which achieve the statistical power that meets current consensus requirements.

A number of attempts have been made to improve the statistical power of candidate gene studies by combining reported results in a meta-analysis. This is fraught with the usual hazards associated with meta-analysis, including publication bias and heterogeneity between studies. Thrombophilia genes have attracted particular attention, and a number of meta-analyses have reported an association between the coagulation Factor V Leiden variant and preeclampsia [12,13,14]. One group has addressed the problem of selection bias in case–control studies by restricting meta-analysis to six cohort studies, including a total of 2085 cases and almost 20 000 controls [15]. These studies were statistically homogeneous, and provided evidence for an association between preeclampsia and possession of one or two copies of the Factor V Leiden variant (pooled OR 1.49; 95% CI 1.13–1.96, P = 0.003).

This interesting result, although it falls short of the significance threshold required for genome-wide significance, illustrates that the major benefit of genetic research does not lie in the identification of individuals who are genetically at high risk. The Factor V Leiden variant is carried by only about 5% of the population in Northern and Western Europe. It is therefore unlikely that, with currently available resources, antenatal testing of women for the Leiden variant to identify those at increased risk would be a worthwhile exercise. The importance of this finding, if verified, would be the incrimination of a thrombotic mechanism in susceptibility to preeclampsia. In an individual woman this may or may not be due to genetic factors, but preventative strategies aimed at reducing the risk of thrombotic events in all pregnancies would merit further investigation.

Linkage analysis

The lack of success in studies of candidate genes in complex disorders has encouraged researchers to turn to screening the entire genome, an unbiased approach which seeks to highlight regions of the genome (loci) which may harbor susceptibility genes. Until recently this could only be achieved by linkage analysis, which involves tracking the inheritance of genetic markers in multicase families.

Scattered throughout the human genome are highly polymorphic regions known as microsatellites or variable numbers of tandem repeats (VNTR). The latter name is more informative, as it describes the distinguishing feature of DNA sequence in these regions: multiple repeats of short sequences of 2, 3, or more nucleotide bases. The number of repeats at each VNTR is variable in the population, giving rise to multiple alleles. Amplification of the region containing the VNTR using the polymerase chain reaction generates fragments which differ in size according to the number of nucleotide repeats. These can be distinguished by electrophoresis, and used as markers to track the inheritance of specific alleles through families. A VNTR marker and a nearby (unknown) disease gene are likely to co-segregate within a family, as their proximity reduces the chance that they will be separated by meiotic recombination. Extensive experience of gene mapping in Mendelian disorders has resulted in the production of panels of VNTRs spread evenly throughout the genome. Approximately 500 VNTR markers provide sufficient coverage for an initial linkage screen of the entire genome. Linked regions may be many millions of bases in length, and include numerous genes, and loci highlighted in a first-pass genome-wide screen are usually fine-mapped by the addition of further markers.

The success of genome-wide linkage studies in identifying genes responsible for Mendelian disorders can hardly be overstated, but with few exceptions this approach has been disappointing in complex disorders. Early successes predating the molecular genetic era included the identification of linkage of type 1 diabetes to the HLA cluster [16]; subsequent molecular approaches have demonstrated linkage of Alzheimer's disease to the apolipoprotein E locus [17]. The common factor in these success stories has been the large effect size of the linked locus; for example, inheritance of a single copy of the apolipoprotein E4 allele confers a three-fold risk of developing Alzheimer's disease. The majority of genes underlying complex disorders appear to increase risk by less than 50%, and linkage analysis lacks the power to detect genes with such small effects.

Nevertheless, there have been some tantalizing results of genome-wide linkage studies of preeclamptic pedigrees. Genome-wide linkage studies have been undertaken by groups from Iceland, Australasia, Holland, and Finland [18,19,20,21]. The affected sib-pair approach has generally been used, or a modification to allow the use of more distantly related family members in affected pedigree analysis. The principle is based on Mendelian laws of inheritance; on average, 25% of sibs share 2 alleles, 50% share 1 allele, and 25% share neither allele. A statistically significant increase in sharing of a marker allele between two affected sibs suggests the presence of a nearby susceptibility gene. Recruiting an adequate number of affected sib-pairs with preeclampsia presents challenges, as the disease classification can only be applied to parous sisters – there is no phenotype which identifies carrier males or non-parous women.

Two loci, on the short and long arms of chromosome 2, were initially reported in a study of 124 Icelandic pedigrees [18]. The linked region on 2p was almost entirely due to two large multicase pedigrees, raising the possibility that in a small number of families preeclampsia is inherited as a monogenic disorder. This would be consistent with observations in other complex disorders. Examples include the Mendelian forms of type 2 diabetes presenting as MODY (maturity onset diabetes of the young) and of early onset Alzheimer's disease due to mutations in the presenilin genes [22,23]. The second linked locus in the Icelandic scan was on chromosome 2q, and this or a nearby locus was subsequently identified in a screen of 34 Australian/New Zealand pedigrees [19]. The linked region contains 120 genes, including the *ACVR2* gene which encodes an activin receptor. This gene was prioritized for further study, and a single nucleotide polymorphism (SNP) within *ACVR2* was associated with preeclampsia in the Australian/New Zealand pedigrees ($P = 0.007$) [24]. A subsequent study of 1138 preeclamptic women and 2270 normotensive pregnant controls from Norway provided modest support ($P = 0.01$) for an association with *ACVR2* [25]. Further replication studies are required to confirm and quantify the effect of this gene in preeclampsia.

A genomewide linkage scan of Dutch pedigrees identified a suggestive locus on chromosome 10q [20]. Re-analysis of the data under a model of genetic imprinting pointed to excess sharing of maternally inherited alleles between affected sisters [26]. Genetic imprinting describes the phenomenon of silencing of one copy of a gene, depending on its parent of origin. In the Dutch model, the susceptibility gene is paternally imprinted; in consequence, the paternally inherited copy of the gene is transcriptionally silent, and the variant inherited from the mother is the only active copy of the gene. Interestingly, a model of genetic imprinting in preeclampsia was suggested several years earlier based on epidemiological observations [27]. The *STOX1* gene, encoding a putative DNA-binding protein involved in the transition of invasive trophoblast to multinucleated cells, was suggested by the Dutch group as a likely susceptibility gene [28]. The model originally suggested has been modified to take account of subsequent studies which suggest that *STOX1* is not in fact imprinted in placenta [29]. Adequately powered replication studies are required to resolve the controversy surrounding the role of this gene in preeclampsia.

The most recent genome-wide linkage screen analyszed data from 15 Finnish pedigrees [21]. They also reported a linked locus on chromosome 2p, but at some distance from that identified by the Icelandic and Australasian groups. Evidence of linkage to chromosome 9 also reported by the Finnish group is of particular interest, as this locus includes a region which has been associated with type 2 diabetes and coronary artery disease in non-pregnant individuals [30,31]. Women with a history of preeclampsia are at increased risk of developing both of these conditions later in life, raising the possibility of a common genetic basis for these observations.

Genome-wide association screening

Genetic association studies comparing the frequency of genetic variants in cases and controls provide a more powerful strategy than linkage analysis for the identification of susceptibility loci in complex disorders [32]. When the Human Genome Map became available to researchers the pace of discovery of variation within the genome accelerated. The most extensively documented variants are those which result in a single base change, single nucleotide polymorphisms (SNPs). Over 10 million SNPs with a population frequency of at least 1% have now been described, an average density of 1 per 300 bases [33]. Most lie in non-coding regions of the genome, and therefore do not affect the amino acid sequence of encoded proteins. The functional effects of the majority of SNPs are unknown, but experimental evidence indicates that many affect gene regulation, and may therefore influence cell biology and susceptibility to disease.

The concept that common genetic variants might confer susceptibility to common diseases raised the daunting prospect of testing 10 million SNPs for association with disease. This is not impossible, but would be an expensive and time-consuming enterprise.

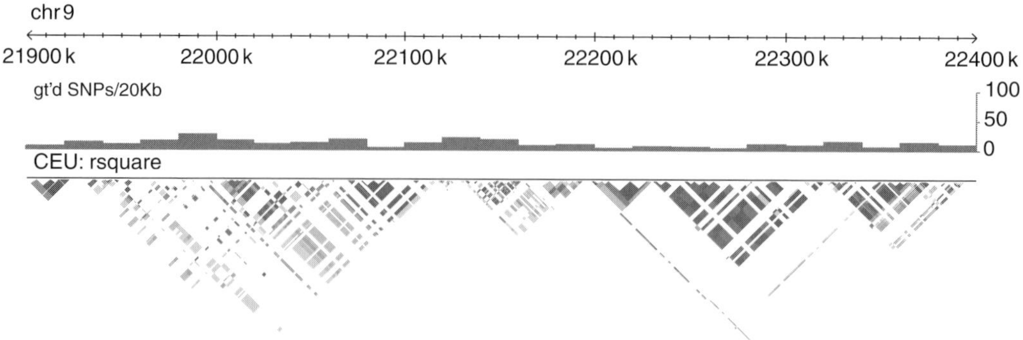

Fig. 17.1 Haplotype blocks in a segment of chromosome 9. Image generated from the HapMap website showing a 500 kilobase region of chromosome 9 in the CEU panel of subjects of north and west European ancestry. The upper horizontal line provides the coordinates of this segment on the human genome map. Below this, a histogram depicts the number of SNPs/20 kilobases genotyped by the HapMap project. The grid represents the linkage disequilibrium between each pair of SNPs; deeper intensities of color indicate greater correlation. Recombination hotspots separating haplotype blocks are clearly evident, with minimal linkage disequilibrium between blocks. This region of chromosome 9 harbors susceptibility genes for type 2 diabetes and coronary artery disease, and has been linked to preeclampsia in a study of Finnish pedigrees.

Fortunately it is not necessary to genotype all SNPs due to the correlation between nearby alleles. This arises because each SNP is the result of a single mutational event on an ancestral chromosome, bearing its own repertoire of SNP alleles. This genetic barcode is inherited as a block, unless either a further new mutation arises (a relatively rare event) or meiotic recombination leads to reshuffling of the ancestral alleles. Recombination does not occur evenly throughout the genome; recombination hotspots occur at an average spacing of 10–20 kilobases, and separate stretches of DNA known as haplotype blocks. SNP alleles within a haplotype block are not inherited independently in the population; in genetic parlance they are said to be in linkage disequilibrium (Fig. 17.1). Due to this correlation genotyping one SNP predicts the genotype at other nearby SNPs. This element of redundancy reduces the number of SNPs which must be physically genotyped to capture the variation in the human genome.

Our understanding of the architecture of human genetic variation owes much to the International HapMap Project, which was established with the aim of providing a map of genetic variation in a total of 270 individuals from four geographically diverse ethnic groups: 30 mother–father–offspring trios of northern and western European ancestry from Utah, USA (CEU) and 30 trios from the Yoruba in Ibadan, Nigeria (YRI); 45 unrelated Han Chinese individuals in Beijing (CHB) and 45 unrelated Japanese individuals in Tokyo (JPT). In the first and second phases of HapMap, over 3 million SNPs were genotyped, providing a mapping density of 1 SNP per kilobase [34,35]. The third phase of HapMap has extended the project to additional populations. This remarkable resource is freely available to researchers via the HapMap website [36]. Commercial providers have incorporated HapMap data into the design of the latest generation of genome-wide screening arrays, which use 500 000 to 1 million SNPs to capture over 80% of the variation in the genome.

Proof of principle has been provided by the success of a number of high-profile studies. An example is the Wellcome Trust Case Control Consortium (WTCCC) which utilized an array of 500 000 SNPs to screen 2000 affected individuals for each of seven common disorders, including coronary artery disease, type 1 and type 2 diabetes, and chronic hypertension [30]. Genotype frequencies were compared with those of a common control panel of 3000 UK subjects. Between 1 and 9 strong SNP association signals ($P < 5 \times 10^{-7}$) were detected for 6 of the 7 disorders, and a further 58 SNPs with moderate associations with disease were identified ($P < 1 \times 10^{-5}$). Some hits confirmed previously reported genetic associations, but the majority were novel, and many lie within regions of the genome which had not previously been considered as candidates for susceptibility loci.

The first wave of genome-wide association studies has established some important principles. First, the effect size of individual SNPs is small, typically conferring an odds ratio for disease of less than 1.5. Only large, well-powered studies are adequately powered to detect such small effects, and a sample of 2000 cases is now regarded as a minimum for genome-wide screening [30]. Second, consideration must be given to the impact of the multiple statistical comparisons entailed in genome-wide screening on the probability of generating false positive results. Applying a stringent level of statistical significance can help to reduce the false discovery rate, and a P value of 5×10^{-7} has been widely quoted – although a case could be made for increasing or decreasing this figure by an order of magnitude. Equally important is the replication of positive findings in an adequately powered, independent study, requiring as a minimum an equal number of cases and controls to the original study. The attrition in odds ratios commonly observed in replication studies argues for larger sample sizes for retesting the original findings of genome-wide association (GWA) screens.

A number of groups involved in genetic research in preeclampsia are now poised to undertake genome-wide association screening. Achieving the sample sizes required for informative genome-wide association screens and replication studies in preeclampsia will be possible only through national and international collaboration. This is particularly true if phenotypic subgroups are to be studied. As an example, two overlapping clinical presentations of preeclampsia are recognized: early onset preeclampsia, often severe and associated with fetal growth restriction; and preeclampsia presenting later in pregnancy, often following a milder clinical course for both mother and baby. Resolving whether these two extremes represent differing molecular subtypes of preeclampsia requires the analysis of large numbers of subjects with each phenotype, achievable only by sharing existing resources. A further advantage of cooperation between research groups is the prospect of pooling results from multiple genome-wide screens to maximize the power to detect variants with small effects. This has been demonstrated convincingly by the Diabetes Genetics Replication and Meta-analysis (DIAGRAM) consortium [37]. By combining the results of three genome-wide screens in a meta-analysis, and conducting replication studies on SNPs giving the strongest signals in over 24 000 cases and 30 000 controls, this international consortium identified 6 novel susceptibility loci for type 2 diabetes with odds ratios for disease of 1.15 or less. The small effect size of these loci accounts for the failure to detect them in individual GWA studies, and demonstrates the power of meta-analysis in gene-discovery efforts.

The fetal genotype

Fetal genotyping has been largely neglected in reported genetic studies of preeclampsia, although it is clear from epidemiological research that fetal genes have a part to play [9]. Differentiating between susceptibility genes active in the mother and those active in the fetus, though essential if genetic research is to provide insights into disease mechanisms, is not a straightforward challenge. Susceptibility variants which are over-represented in women affected by preeclampsia will inevitably be over-represented in their babies. Conversely, a variant gene which is active in the fetus is inherited from its mother 50% of the time on average, and consequently will be over-represented in maternal genes. One study design which distinguishes between maternal and fetal susceptibility genes is known as transmission disequilibrium testing [38]. This requires that the baby and both parents are genotyped in a large number of affected pregnancies. The principle is that parents who are heterozygous at a polymorphic site will transmit either allele to their offspring with an expected frequency of 50%. If one allele confers susceptibility to disease in the offspring, it will be transmitted at a higher than expected frequency from heterozygous parents. It is not necessary to genotype a control group in this design, as the non-transmitted allele acts as a paired control. The results are independent of the frequency of the fetal susceptibility allele in the parents (other than the effects on statistical power of low-frequency alleles) and therefore any distortion in the frequency of allele transmission to affected babies can be attributed to a gene active in the fetus. A further advantage of this approach is that it enables the identification of parent-of-origin effects, which might suggest a mechanism involving genetic imprinting. The transmission disequilibrium testing approach has been used in candidate gene studies [39], and a number of existing or on-going DNA collections have incorporated this option (e.g. the UK GOPEC Consortium; the Norwegian Mother and Child Study [39,40]).

A more challenging problem arises from the theoretical consideration that preeclampsia may be the result of interaction between maternal and fetal genes. The importance of impaired trophoblast invasion in the pathogenesis of preeclampsia suggests an almost endless number of mechanisms involving the interaction between adhesion molecules, proteinases, cytokines and their receptors, either maternally or fetally encoded. The role of paternal genes suggests the possibility of an immune mechanism, with maternal genes responding to paternally encoded fetal antigens. One approach to this challenge is to test a well-founded candidate pathway; an example is the studies of the maternal KIR genes and fetal HLA-C genotype described in Chapter 6 [41]. An alternative is to adopt an agnostic strategy of genome-wide screening of both maternal and fetal genomes. This immediately raises the problem of the vast number of statistical tests required if all possible interactions between maternal and fetal genetic variants are to be examined. This statistical dilemma is avoided if the fetal genome is viewed as one of many factors which affect the penetrance of maternal susceptibility genes, and vice versa. A genome-wide screen of the maternal or fetal genome would be expected to identify a gene of low penetrance due to maternal–fetal gene interactions, providing it were adequately powered. This would trigger the functional studies which would point to its accomplice in the other genome. The answers to this conundrum are not yet clear, but it is apparent that sample sizes beyond those currently available will be needed.

An interesting result arising from a candidate gene study arose from the observation that levels of the placental soluble receptor, sFlt-1, are elevated in women with preeclampsia [42]. This may contribute to maternal endothelial damage by binding circulating placental growth factor (PlGF), and suggests the involvement of fetally encoded placental genes. This has been explored in a study of pregnancies affected by the chromosomal abnormality trisomy 13. An increased incidence of preeclampsia in trisomy 13 pregnancies which progress to the second or third trimester has long been recognized, but the mechanism of this association was unclear [43]. The gene encoding sFlt-1 is located on chromosome 13, and therefore a trisomy 13 fetus has three copies of this gene. A retrospective comparison of sFlt-1 levels in first and second trimester plasma collected for antenatal screening demonstrated a significantly increased ratio of sFlt-1 to PlGF in trisomy 13 pregnancies, suggesting a possible mechanism for the increased incidence of preeclampsia, and illustrating the importance of giving due consideration to fetal genetic factors [44].

The benefits of genetic studies

In the early years of molecular genetic studies it was hoped that the identification of susceptibility genes for complex disorders would lead to the development of diagnostic tests which could be used to identify at-risk individuals (Text Box 17.2). For disorders of pregnancy this would have far-reaching implications for the delivery of antenatal care; scarce resources could be targeted at those women at highest risk. This optimism

Text Box 17.2 Translational benefits of gene discovery

- Elucidation of novel pathophysiological pathways may:
  - Inform strategies for disease prevention
  - Identify novel targets for therapeutic interventions
  - Encourage development of *in vitro* diagnostic tests
- Genetic testing to identify individuals at high risk:
  - Not currently applicable at an individual level
  - May prove useful in intervention studies for the selection of a group at increased risk

has been tempered by observations in other complex disorders; the effect size of individual genes is often too small to justify the expense of predictive genotyping at current costs. Type 2 diabetes, for which multiple susceptibility genes have been discovered in the last few years, provides a good example. In a prospective study of over 18 000 individuals from Sweden and Finland with a mean follow-up time of 23.5 years, 2201 participants developed type 2 diabetes [45]. The predictive values of clinical measurements, including BMI and family history, and genotyping at 16 SNPs in confirmed susceptibility genes for type 2 diabetes, were compared. Whilst the genotypes were significantly associated with the development of type 2 diabetes, their effect on the predictive value of clinical data alone was marginal. Assessment of the efficiency of genotyping in the prediction of disorders of placentation awaits the unequivocal identification of susceptibility genes.

The chief benefit of genetic studies in complex disorders is in providing clues to underlying molecular mechanisms. Indeed, the naming of susceptibility genes is the prelude to extensive research into their functional effects. The potential rewards are commensurate with the effort involved. A clear understanding of the molecular pathogenesis of a disease can provide a rational basis for the development of novel strategies for its prevention and cure. For disorders of placentation, genetics can provide unique insights into the molecular metier at the maternal–fetal interface in early pregnancy. It is important to bear in mind that a gene with a very small effect can nevertheless provide important clues to disease mechanisms. The detection of genes with very low odds ratios for disease is limited only by the size of the study. It is clear that extensive national and international collaboration between clinicians, geneticists, and bioinformaticians is vital to ensure that the advances in molecular genetics are translated into better outcomes for pregnancies at risk from disorders of placentation.

References

1. Ward K, Argyle V, Meade M, Nelson L. The heritability of preterm delivery. *Obstet Gynecol* 2005; **106**: 1235–9.
2. Chappell S, Morgan L. Searching for genetic clues to the causes of pre-eclampsia. *Clin Sci* 2006; **110**: 443–58.
3. Clausson B, Lichtenstein P, Cnattingius S. Genetic influence on birthweight and gestational length determined by studies in offspring of twins. *Br J Obstet Gynaecol* 2000; **107**: 375–81.
4. Lie R T, Rasmussen S, Brunborg H *et al.* Fetal and maternal contributions to risk of pre-eclampsia: population based study. *Brit Med J* 1998; **316**: 1343–7.
5. Chesley L C, Annitto J E, Cosgrove R A. The familial factor in toxemia of pregnancy. *Obstet Gynecol* 1968; **32**: 303–11.
6. Cincotta R B, Brennecke S P. Family history of pre-eclampsia as a predictor for pre-eclampsia in primigravidas. *Int J Gynaecol Obstet* 1998; **60**: 23–7.
7. Thornton J G, Macdonald A M. Twin mothers, pregnancy hypertension and pre-eclampsia. *Br J Obstet Gynaecol* 1999; **106**: 570–5.
8. Salonen Ros H, Lichtenstein P, Lipworth L, Cnattingius S. Genetic effects on the liability of developing pre-eclampsia and gestational hypertension. *Am J Med Genet* 2000; **91**: 256–60.
9. Cnattingius S, Reilly M, Pawitan Y, Lichtenstein P. Maternal and fetal genetic factors account for most of familial aggregation of preeclampsia: a population-based Swedish cohort study. *Am J Med Genet* 2004; **A130**: 365–71.
10. Lachmeijer A M A, Dekker G A, Pals G *et al.* Searching for preeclampsia genes: the current position. *Eur J Obstet Gyn R B* 2002; **105**: 94–113.
11. Wilson M L, Goodwin T M, Pan V L, Ingles S A. Molecular epidemiology of preeclampsia. *Obstet Gynecol Surv* 2003; **58**: 39–66.
12. Lin J, August P. Genetic thrombophilias and preeclampsia: a meta-analysis. *Obstet Gynecol* 2005; **105**: 182–92.
13. Dudding T E, Attia J. The association between adverse pregnancy outcomes and maternal factor V Leiden genotype: a meta-analysis. *Thromb Haemost* 2004; **91**: 700–11.
14. Kosmas I P, Tatsioni A, Ioannidis J P A. Association of Leiden mutation in Factor V gene with hypertension in pregnancy and pre-eclampsia: a meta-analysis. *J Hypertens* 2003; **21**: 1221–8.
15. Dudding T, Heron J, Thakkinstian A *et al.* Factor V Leiden is associated with pre-eclampsia but not with fetal growth restriction: a genetic association study and meta-analysis. *J Thromb Haemost* 2008; **6**: 1868–75.
16. Cudworth A G, Woodrow J C. Evidence for HL-A-linked genes in "juvenile" diabetes mellitus. *Br Med J* 1975; **3**(5976): 133–5.
17. Yu C-E, Payami H, Olson J M *et al.* The apolipoprotein E/CI/CII gene cluster and late-onset Alzheimer disease. *Am J Hum Genet* 1994; **54**: 631–42.
18. Arngrimsson R, Sigurardottir S, Frigge M L *et al.* A genome-wide scan reveals a maternal susceptibility locus for pre-eclampsia on chromosome 2p13. *Hum Mol Genet* 1999; **8**: 1799–805.
19. Moses E K, Lade J A, Guo G *et al.* A genome scan in families from Australia and New Zealand confirms the presence of a maternal susceptibility locus for pre-eclampsia, on chromosome 2. *Am J Hum Genet* 2000; **67**: 1581–5.
20. Lachmeijer A M A, Arngrimsson R, Bastiaans E J *et al.* A genome-wide scan for preeclampsia in the Netherlands. *Eur J Hum Genet* 2001; **9**: 758–64.
21. Laivuori H, Lahermo P, Ollikainen V *et al.* Susceptibility loci for preeclampsia on chromosomes 2p25 and 9p13 in Finnish families. *Am J Hum Gene* 2003; **72**: 168–77.
22. Malecki M T. Genetics of type 2 diabetes mellitus. *Diabetes Res Clin Pract* 2005; **68** (Suppl 1): S10–21.
23. Bird T D. Genetic aspects of Alzheimer disease. *Genet Med* 2008; **10**: 231–9.
24. Moses E K, Fitzpatrick E, Freed K A *et al.* Objective prioritization of positional candidate genes at a quantitative trait locus for pre-eclampsia on 2q22. *Mol Hum Reprod* 2006; **12**: 505–12.
25. Roten L T, Johnson M, Forsmo S *et al.* Association between the candidate susceptibility gene ACVR2A on chromosome 2q22 and pre-eclampsia in a large Norwegian population-based study (the HUNT study). *Eur J Hum Genet* 2009; **17**(2): 250–7.
26. Oudejans C B, Mulders J, Lachmeijer A M *et al.* The parent-of-origin effect of 10q22 in pre-eclamptic females coincides with two regions clustered for genes with down-regulated expression in androgenetic placentas. *Mol Hum Reprod* 2004; **10**: 589–98.
27. Graves J A M. Genomic imprinting, development and disease – is pre-eclampsia caused by a maternally imprinted gene? *Reprod Fert Develop* 1998; **10**: 23–9.

28. van Dijk M, Mulders J, Poutsma A *et al.* Maternal segregation of the Dutch preeclampsia locus at 10q22 with a new member of the winged helix gene family. *Nat Genet* 2005; **37**: 514–9.
29. Iglesias-Platas I, Monk D, Jebbink J *et al.* *STOX1* is not imprinted and is not likely to be involved in pre-eclampsia. *Nat Genet* 2007; **39**: 279–80.
30. The Wellcome Trust Case Control Consortium. Genome-wide association study of seven common diseases and 3000 shared controls. *Nature* 2007; **447**: 661–78.
31. Zeggini E, Weedon M N, Lindgren C M *et al.* Replication of genome-wide association signals in UK samples reveals risk loci for type 2 diabetes. *Science* 2007; **316**: 1336–41.
32. Risch N, Merikangas K. The future of genetic studies of complex human diseases. *Science* 1996; **273**: 1516–7.
33. http://www.ncbi.nlm.nih.gov/projects/SNP
34. The International HapMap Consortium. A haplotype map of the human genome. *Nature* 2005; **437**: 1299–319.
35. The International HapMap Consortium. A second generation human haplotype map of over 3.1 million SNPs. *Nature* 2007; **449**: 851–62.
36. http://www.hapmap.org
37. Zeggini E, Scott L J, Saxena R, Voight B F. Meta-analysis of genome-wide association data and large-scale replication identifies additional susceptibility loci for type 2 diabetes. *Nat Genet* 2008; **40**: 638–45.
38. Spielman R S, McGinnis R E, Ewens W J. Transmission test for linkage disequilibrium: the insulin gene region and insulin-dependent diabetes mellitus (IDDM). *Am J Hum Genet* 1993; **52**: 506–16.
39. The GOPEC Consortium. Disentangling fetal and maternal susceptibility for pre-eclampsia: a British multicenter candidate-gene study. *Am J Hum Genet* 2005; **77**: 127–31.
40. Magnus P, Irgens L, Haug K *et al.* Cohort profile: the Norwegian Mother and Child Cohort Study (MoBa). *Int J Epidemiol* 2006; **35**: 1146–50.
41. Hiby S, Walker J, O'Shaughnessy K *et al.* Combinations of maternal KIR and fetal HLA-C genes influence the risk of preeclampsia and reproductive success. *J Exp Med* 2004; **200**: 957–65.
42. Maynard S E, Min J Y, Merchan J *et al.* Excess placental soluble fms-like tyrosine kinase 1 (sFlt1) may contribute to endothelial dysfunction, hypertension, and proteinuria in preeclampsia. *J Clin Invest* 2003; **111**: 649–58.
43. Boyd P A, Lindenbaum R H, Redman C. Pre-eclampsia and trisomy 13: a possible association. *Lancet* 1987; **2** (8556): 425–7.
44. Bdolah Y, Palomaki G E, Yaron Y *et al.* Circulating angiogenic proteins in trisomy 13. *Am J Obstet Gynecol* 2006; **194**: 239–45.
45. Lyssenko V, Jonsson A, Almgren P *et al.* Clinical risk factors, DNA variants, and the development of type 2 diabetes. *N Engl J Med* 2008; **359**: 2220–32.

Chapter 18

Imprinting

Sayeda Abu-Amero and Gudrun E. Moore

Clinical and Molecular Genetics, Institute of Child Health, University College London, London, UK

Introduction

The placenta is the bridge between the mother and fetus and its importance for normal, robust fetal survival is documented in great detail in this book. The placenta permits oxygen and nutrients from maternal blood to pass through the walls of the villi and enter the fetal capillaries to feed the growing and developing fetus. Apart from the physiological means by which the placenta contributes to fetal growth and development, there is a recognized and definitive contribution from placental active genes. Of particular interest are those that can affect fetal growth via healthy effective placental development and function. These genes have been intensively studied and from these a set of genes have been identified which have parent-of-origin expression, termed imprinted genes.

Imprinting was first demonstrated by a set of elegant experiments in the 1980s where pronuclear transplantation in mice gave rise to completely maternal (gynogenetic) or paternal (androgenetic) conceptuses [1]. Neither genetically modified conceptuses developed into normal pregnancies and it was observed that gynogenotes had identifiable embryonic tissue but poor placental tissue compared to androgenotes, where embryonic development was poor but trophoblastic tissue was clearly evident [1,2]. In humans naturally occurring gynogenotes and androgenotes are clinically recognized as ovarian teratomas and hydatidiform moles respectively and are also non-viable.

Translational message: imprinting errors can have severe consequences on fetal development and in some non-viable pregnancies can lead to choriocarcinomas or ovarian teratomas

These observations showed an unequal contribution of maternal and paternal genomes to fetal development and suggested maternal genes were critical for embryonic growth and paternal genes for placental growth. This differential parental contribution to some specific genes is defined as genomic imprinting. Neither the whole maternal nor whole paternal genome displays this effect. This was shown by further experiments where heterozygous mice with Robertsonian and reciprocal translocations were interbred, resulting in mice with subchromosomal regions of uniparental disomy (UPD), i.e. two copies of either maternal (m) or paternal (p) genes for that region alone. Certain chromosomes/chromosomal regions showed no parent-of-origin effects whereas others had clear phenotypic effects [3]. These experiments have given rise to the construction of the mouse imprinted gene map (http://www.mgu.har.mrc.ac.uk/research/imprinted/imprin.html; WAMIDEX: https://atlas.genetics.kcl.ac.uk).

Imprinted genes are effectively hemizygous, compared to the biallelic expression of most other Mendelian genes. Either the maternal or paternal allele is expressed with the corresponding paternal or maternal allele said to be silenced or imprinted, respectively. The website, http://igc.otago.ac.nz, is regularly updated with pertinent information on the status of imprinted genes in man and mouse. Of these only 55 are known to be imprinted in humans compared to 85 in mice. Of the 55 known imprinted genes in humans, 26 are imprinted in the placenta and 13 of these have documented growth related effects (Table 18.1). There is an approximate 50:50 distribution of maternally and paternally expressed (paternally and maternally imprinted or silenced) genes. The trend for a smaller number of imprinted genes in humans may be related to why imprinting evolved in the first place. The most favored is the conflict or kinship hypotheses [4].

The conflict hypothesis proposes that successful selection of the paternal genome needs to create larger and fitter offspring which have a better

Table 18.1. Imprinted genes in human placenta

Location	Imprinted genes in human placenta	Acronym	Expressed allele	Human phenotype
6q24	**Pleiomorphic adenoma gene-like 1**	***PLAGL1* (*ZAC1*, *LOT1*)**	**P**	**TNDM**
7p12	**Growth factor receptor-bound protein 10**	***GRB10***	**P/M**	**SRS**
7q21.3	Sarcoglycan, epsilon	*SGCE*	P	Myoclonus dystonia
7q21.3	Paternally expressed gene 10	*PEG10*	P	NO DATA IN PLACENTA[a]
7q21.3	Protein phosphatase 1, regulatory (inhibitor) subunit 9A	*PPP1R9A*	M	Synapse formation in neural tissue
7q32.2	Carboxypeptidase A4	*CPA4*	M	Carboxypeptidase
7q32.2	**Mesoderm specific transcript**	***MEST***	**P**	**SRS/TNDM**
7q32.2	***MEST* intronic transcript 1**	***MESTIT1***	**P**	**GROWTH RELATED**
7q32.2	Kruppel-like factor 14	*KLF14*	M	NO DATA IN PLACENTA
11p15	**H19 (transcription factor)**	***H19***	**M**	**SRS/BWS**
11p15	**Insulin-like growth factor 2**	***IGF2***	**P**	**SRS/BWS**
11p15	Insulin-like growth factor 2 antisense	*IGF2AS*	P	NO DATA IN PLACENTA
11p15	**Potassium voltage gated channel KQT-like subfamily member 1**	***KCNQ1* (temporal)**	**M**	**BWS/LQT1/JLNS1**
11p15	***KCNQ1* overlapping transcript**	***KCNQ1OT1* (temporal)**	**P**	**BWS**
11p15	**Cyclin-dependent kinase inhibitor 1C**	***CDKN1C***	**M**	**BWS**
11p15	Solute carrier family 22, member 18	*SLC22A18*	M	NO DATA IN PLACENTA
11p15	**Pleckstrin homology-like domain family A member 2**	***PHLDA2***	**M**	**GROWTH RELATED**
11p15	Oxysterol binding protein-like 5	*OSBPL5*	M	NO DATA IN PLACENTA
14q32	**Delta-like 1 homolog**	***DLK1***	**P**	**GROWTH RELATED**
14q32	**Gene trap locus 2**	***GTL2***	**M**	**GROWTH RELATED**
15q11-q12	**Small nuclear ribonucleoprotein polypeptide N**	***SNRPN***	**P**	**PWS**
16p13	Zinc finger protein 597	*ZNF597*	M	NO DATA IN PLACENTA
19q13.41	Zinc finger protein 331	*ZNF331*	M	NO DATA IN PLACENTA
19q13.43	Paternally expressed gene 3	*PEG3*	P	NO DATA IN PLACENTA[a]
19q13.43	Zinc finger, imprinted 2	*ZIM2*	P(M)	NO DATA IN PLACENTA
20q13	Guanine nucleotide binding protein (alpha stimulating) complex locus	*GNAS (NESP55)*	M	AHO

26 genes are known to be imprinted in the human placenta, of which 13 have been shown to have growth-related effects (**bold**). These genes are detailed at http://igc.otago.ac.nz.

[a] PEG3 and *PEG10* are expressed in human placenta and are being investigated for growth-related effects (Ishida *et al.*, unpublished data).
TNDM, transient neonatal diabetes mellitus; SRS, Silver–Russell syndrome; BWS, Beckwith–Wiedemann syndrome; LQT1, long QT syndrome 1; JLNS1, Jervell and Lange–Nielsen syndrome 1; PWS, Prader–Willi syndrome; AHO, Albright hereditary osteodystrophy.

survival chance compared to weaker peers. The maternal genome carrying the offspring has a different need. In addition to producing fit offspring, she herself must survive for that pregnancy and also others to follow. Therefore the father promotes growth through expression of growth-promoting imprinted genes and the mother restricts growth through her growth-limiting imprinted genes. This hypothesis makes most sense when referring to polygamous species where many offspring in one litter are normal but may not be as valid in humans where polygamy is not common and singleton pregnancies are normal.

Translational message: imprinting may have occurred as a consequence of conflict between the two parental genomes with the paternal genome promoting growth and the maternal genome suppressing it

Much of what we know about imprinted genes has been understood from murine experiments involving targeted mutations and knockouts of imprinted genes. In humans, data have been obtained from clinically identified imprinting disorders such as Beckwith-Wiedemann syndrome (BWS - OMIM 130650) and Silver Russell syndrome (SRS - OMIM 180860). In mice the pathological effects of imprinted genes have also been studied in the placenta whereas this has been extremely limited in humans as most imprinted disorders are identified after birth such as BWS or in early childhood such as SRS [5,6].

Mechanism of imprinting

The mechanism controlling imprinting must ensure functional monoallelic expression of a gene which has two putatively functional alleles. The successful silencing of either the maternal or paternal copy of the allele is essential for correct dosage of the gene to be expressed.

DNA methylation is a general mechanism for controlling gene transcription and therefore protein translation. Methylation of DNA is typically seen at CpG sites where cytosine is converted to 5-methylcytosine (Me-CpG) by DNA methyltransferase. CpG sites are scattered throughout the genome but are clustered near promoters of genes and are often referred to as CpG islands. Differentially methylated regions (DMRs) are hallmarks of imprinted genes as the methylation of CpG islands here is dependent on which parental allele is being expressed, with methylation in most cases associated with silencing. Mouse knockouts of specific DMRs result in inappropriate imprinted gene expression, testifying to the role of DMRs in epigenetic gene regulation (http://www.informatics.jax.org). Regulation is extremely complex, with imprinted genes showing tissue-, developmental stage-, and isoform-specific monoallelic expression governed by methylation, trans-chromosomal interactions, histone modification, and numerous noncoding RNA species [7]. Allele-specific DNA methylation is established in the gamete during epigenetic reprograming which acts to suppress or activate gene expression.

Translational message: methylation is a key mechanism behind imprinting regulation

In this chapter specific imprinted genes or imprinted regions known to be imprinted in the human placenta with an effect on fetal growth and development are discussed in detail.

Imprinted genes on 11p15.5

The human 11p15.5 region is the most intensively studied imprinted region. One of the characteristics of imprinted genes is that they tend to occur in clusters which groups regulation of monoallelic expression. The 11p15.5 region comprises two recognized clusters of imprinted genes: the telomeric imprinting control region 1 (ICR1) and the centromeric imprinting control region 2 (ICR2).

ICR1: *H19* and *IGF2* (Insulin-like growth factor 2)

ICR1 includes the maternally expressed transcription factor *H19* and paternally expressed Insulin-like growth factor 2 (*IGF2*) and is controlled by the *H19* Differentially Methylated Domain (*H19* DMD) or ICR1. IGFII is a growth-promoting protein active during gestation and was the first imprinted gene to be described which is common to mouse and man [8]. IGFII mediates its growth-promoting functions via the Insulin-like growth factor I receptor (IGFIR) and is indirectly regulated via the Insulin-like growth factor II receptor (IGFRII) which acts as a signaling antagonist by sequestering IGFII. *IGF2* is expressed in most fetal tissues and five isoforms have been identified, generated by alternative splicing of its nine exons via different promoters [9].

H19 is a 2.3 kb non-coding RNA as evidenced by no recognizable open reading frame and is conserved at the RNA level. It localizes to cytoplasmic ribonucleoprotein particles suggesting it may be a riboregulator. The exact function of *H19* in the cell is unknown but it has been found highly expressed in a number of cancers.

H19 shows temporal regulation of imprinting with biallelic expression in placenta up to 10 weeks gestation after which expression is exclusively maternal, suggesting strict control of *H19* dosage is essential for placental and embryonic growth [10]. Postnatally, there is little expression of *H19* in any tissues except skeletal muscle, and in pubertal and pregnant females there is expression in the mammary glands and the uterus during pregnancy [11,12].

H19 contains a germline DMR which acts as an ICR regulating its expression as well as imprinted genes in the cluster. Both *IGF2* and *H19* possess additional DMRs known as the *IGF2* DMR2 and *H19* promoter, respectively, and are hypomethylated at all stages of placental development [13,14]. The 3' portion of the *H19* promoter shows progressive methylation of the paternal allele in placenta as pregnancy progresses demonstrating that the correct functional imprint is established at the onset of gestation by the *H19* DMD/ICR1.

The level of *H19* expression is negatively correlated with methylation of the somatic *H19* promoter DMR and as the promoter methylation increases, *H19* expression decreases with concomitant increase in *IGF2* expression and vice versa [15]. Cells grown in the presence of the cytosine methylation inhibitor, 5-aza-2'-deoxycytidine, have high levels of *H19*, low levels of *IGF2*, and grow more slowly compared to untreated cells due to the low levels of *IGF2* [15].

Due to the differential parental expression, inheritance of maternal deletion of *H19* in mice results in overgrown mice while paternal deletion of *Igf2* results in growth-restricted mice [16]. Paternal deletion of *H19* and maternal deletion of *Igf2* are phenotypically normal as these parental alleles are normally silenced. More interestingly, mice inheriting both a maternal deletion of *H19* and a paternal deletion of *Igf2* show no aberration in growth parameters at birth or postnatally [16]. The data together suggests that *H19* loss is not lethal in itself although it obviously controls *Igf2* expression which has potent growth-related functions.

Translational message: *IGF2* and *H19* methylation status could be used as indicators of tumorigenesis

In mice, a placental-specific transcript called *Igf2*P0 exists which is exclusively expressed in the labyrinthine layer [17]. *Igf2*P0 knockouts result in placental growth restriction followed by fetal growth restriction, unlike complete *Igf2* knockouts where there is simultaneous fetal and placental growth restriction [17]. The *Igf2*P0 knockout placenta shows morphological changes with proportionate reduction in cellular compartments and diffusional capabilities [17,18]. There is an equivalent P0 transcript in humans which is highly expressed in fetal skeletal muscle and much less in other adult tissues and term placenta suggesting it does not have the same role in humans as in mouse [9].

IGF2 has been studied by a number of investigators in human growth and development and its role has not yet been conclusively established. In a study by McMinn *et al.* [19] there was downregulation of *IGF2* in 38 intrauterine growth restricted (IUGR) placentae compared to 75 non-IUGR placentae, but no significant correlation of *IGF2* expression with birth weight [19]. In a similar study of 24 small-for-gestational age (SGA) placentae compared to 20 normal term placentae, downregulation of *IGF2* mRNA in all SGA placentae was demonstrated [14]. However, only one of the SGA placentae had concomitant biallelic expression of *H19* caused by hypomethylation of the *H19* DMD, which could explain the observed downregulation of *IGF2* mRNA. [14]. Hypomethylation of both the *H19* DMD and *H19* promoter in growth-restricted placentae has also been reported [14,20].

Apostolidou *et al.* [21] found no correlation for birth weight, placental weight, or head circumference with *IGF2* mRNA expression in 200 term placentae in a homogenous white European population. The same population was studied for methylation at the *H19* DMD but no relationship was found between methylation status and birth weight, head circumference, or placental weight as might have been expected if the *H19* DMD regulated these growth parameters through the effect of *H19* and/or *IGF2*.

Disruption of *H19* and *IGF2* imprinting has been well documented in BWS and more recently SRS. In 10% of BWS patients there is hypermethylation of *H19* resulting in loss of expression of *H19*, biallelic and hence overexpression of *IGF2* and overgrowth. In approximately 50% of SRS patients there is hypomethylation of *H19* and reduction of *IGF2* expression and growth restriction of placenta and consequently the fetus [20,22,23].

Translational message: methylation of ICR1 and ICR2 can be used as indicators of imprinting disorders such as SRS and BWS

ICR2: *KvDMR1*

ICR2 or *KvDMR1* regulates the paternally expressed *KCNQ1* overlapping transcript (*KCNQ1OT1*) and maternally expressed Potassium voltage gated channel KQT-like subfamily member 1 (*KCNQ1*) and Cyclin-dependent kinase inhibitor 1C (*CDKN1C/P57/KIP2*). All three genes are expressed in human placenta and have growth-related effects, most notably being implicated in BWS. *KvDMR1* is an intronic CpG island within the *KCNQ1* gene and loss of methylation of the *KvDMR1* is the most frequent alteration associated with BWS [24].

In the *Kcnq1* domain in mice there are 14 imprinted genes, eight of which are maternally expressed. Six of the orthologous genes retain their imprinting status in humans (*CDKN1C, KCNQ1, KCNQ1OT1*, Plekstrin homology-like domain family A member 2 (*PHLDA2*), solute carrier family 22 (organic cation transporter), member 18 (*SLC22A18*) and *SLC22AILS*) which are identified as being placenta-specific in their imprinting status [25].

The *p57* (*Kip2*) mouse model of preeclampsia clearly demonstrates the critical function of *Cdkn1c* as these mice demonstrate the full spectrum of preeclampsia. Pregnant females expressing normal levels of *p57(Kip2)* carry fetuses with no p57(Kip2) but still exhibit preeclampsia demonstrating that the condition is driven by fetal/placental transcripts [26]. In humans, *CDKN1C* transcripts have been found to be increased in IUGR placenta compared to normal placenta, though not significantly [19].

ICR2: *PHLDA2* (Plekstrin homology-like domain family A member 2)

ICR2 also regulates expression of *PHLDA2*, which is a tumor suppressor gene demonstrating sequence similarity to T cell death-associated gene 51 (*TDAG51*), a gene implicated in apoptosis, making *PHLDA2* the first apoptosis-related imprinted gene to be described in any species [27]. *PHLDA2* is most highly expressed in the trophoblast of placenta and additionally in bronchial epithelium cells, liver, and prostate. It has recently been shown to be expressed statistically significantly higher in term placenta of low birth weight babies compared to normal birth weight babies, which fits in well with its role as a growth suppressor [21]. The same study found no relationship with Mesoderm specific transcript (*MEST*), *IGF2R* or *IGF2*, and birth weight. In a study of 38 human IUGR placentae and 75 normal placentae, *PHLDA2* expression was significantly increased compared to *MEST* with appropriate *PHLDA2* protein tissue distribution as shown by immunocytochemistry [28]. However neither study found any relationship with *PHLDA2* expression and term placenta weight itself. The effects of *PHLDA2* on placental growth may be more obvious during the first and second trimester of pregnancy which would contribute toward our understanding of *PHLDA2* during development.

In mice *Phlda2* is located on chromosome 7, and is expressed quite specifically in the visceral endoderm of yolk sac and labyrinthine trophoblast of placenta, tissues critical for maternal/fetal material exchange [29]. Its expression and imprinting is controlled by *Kcnq1* as disruption of *Kcnq1* by targeted chromosomal translocations in mice resulted in loss of imprinting of *Phlda2* as well as *Cdkn1c* and *Slc22a1l*, which are located in the same imprinting cluster [30]. In viable mice created null for *Phlda2* there was expansion of spongiotrophoblast and overgrowth of placenta with little effect on the fetus [31]. The role of *Phlda2* in placental growth was further delineated by breeding *Phlda2* null mice into mutant *Igf2* background where placental phenotype, but not fetal phenotype, was partly rescued. Salas *et al.* [32] saw that *Phlda2*(+/+); *Kvdmr1*(+/-) fetuses had both fetal and placental growth restriction, while loss of *Phlda2* on a wild-type background resulted in placentomegaly.

In mice, *Phlda2* expression phases out in mid to late gestation as placental growth ceases contrasting with humans where placenta grows throughout gestation with persistent *PHLDA2* mRNA and protein expression. Exposure of human trophoblasts *in vitro* to hypoxic conditions reduced *PHLDA2* mRNA expression and protein production and together with the evidence of murine *Phlda2* restricting placental growth, this suggests that downregulation of *PHLDA2* expression counteracts the effect of hypoxia on fetal growth [33]. *PHLDA2* is the only imprinted gene studied to date in the placenta to show a significant effect on birth weight in humans [21]. Given its obvious role in fetal growth restriction it has potential as a biomarker, which has profound clinical implications.

Translational message: *PHLDA2* could potentially be used as a diagnostic tool for IUGR in humans

Imprinted genes on chromosome 15

Angelman's (AS – OMIM 105830) and Prader–Willi syndromes (PWS – OMIM 176270) are two syndromes with different clinical presentations but caused by opposite genetic abnormalities in the same chromosomal region and were the first imprinting disorders described in man. AS infants often present with feeding problems and are characterized by cognitive and developmental delay, seizures, and inappropriate smiling and laughter. It is caused by loss of maternal gene(s) on 15q11–13 which includes ubiquitin-protein ligase E3A (*UBE3A*) as well as pUPD15. *UBE3A* is maternally expressed in the hippocampus and cerebellum and codes for an E6-AP ubiquitin ligase.

PWS babies present with hypotonia, feeding difficulties leading to hyperphagia, and excessive weight gain in childhood. They also show delayed puberty in adolescence, short stature, and obesity, which persists into adulthood, and behavioral and cognitive problems. PWS is caused by deletion of the paternally expressed genes, small nuclear ribonucleoprotein polypeptide N (*SNRPN*) and *NECDIN* on 15q11–13, which is generally sporadic but can be caused by mUPD15. The role of the placenta in PWS or AS has not been clearly demonstrated although cases of mUPD 15 in mosaic trisomy 15 chorion villus sampling (CVS) have been described [34,35].

Translational message: important to diagnose PWS correctly as it is often confused with Down's syndrome: management of condition can benefit patient

Imprinted genes on chromosome 7: *MEST* (Mesoderm specific transcript) and *GRB10* (Growth factor receptor-bound protein 1)

Mesoderm-specific transcript (*MEST*)

MEST localizes to human chromosome 7q32 and was the first imprinted gene identified on chromosome 7, and is expressed in all major fetal tissues including placental trophoblast and endothelium [36]. It is abundantly expressed in androgenotes and essentially absent in gynogenotes attesting to its exclusive paternal parent-of-origin. It has 98% amino acid similarity to mouse *Mest*. There are two isoforms of *MEST*; *MEST*-isoform 1 is paternally expressed whereas *MEST*-isoform 2 is generally biallelically expressed as seen in adult lymphocytes, i.e. human *MEST* is imprinted in an isoform-specific manner [37]. Recently, *MEST*-isoform 2 was shown to be imprinted in a subset of placentae with imprinting status being regulated by the level of methylation [28]. As well as two isoforms of *MEST*, a non-coding antisense RNA transcript called *MEST* intronic transcript 1 (*MESTIT1*) is derived from intron 1, and transcribed in the opposite direction to *MEST*. Like most other non-coding RNAs, it has been proposed that *MESTIT1* is involved in regulation of *MEST* expression [38].

Mest localizes to mouse chromosome 6, and was originally discovered during a systematic screen in mice for imprinted genes, using subtraction hybridization, and was designated Paternally expressed gene 1 (*Peg 1*) [39]. Lefebvre *et al.* [40] identified a CpG island in exon 1 of *Mest* with an unmethylated paternal allele and methylated maternal allele. By targeted mutations of this gene, they demonstrated that the effect was reversibly silenced through the maternal germline compared to paternal transmission where the mutated gene was expressed, resulting in growth restriction and poor postnatal growth. *Mest* was the first imprinted gene to be described with behavioral effects and is found in the hypothalamus, preoptic area, and septum of the brain [41,42]. Female mice deficient for *Mest* exhibit impaired placentophagia and abnormal maternal behavior.

Growth factor receptor-bound protein 10 (*GRB10*)

The Growth factor receptor-bound protein 10 (*GRB10*) is one of a group of small adaptor proteins, i.e. they have no intrinsic effect themselves but possess protein-binding motifs which permit interactions with other proteins such as the insulin receptor (IR) and IGFIIR. There are multiple isoforms from alternatively spliced transcripts showing isoform- and tissue-specific imprinting. *GRB10* is a maternally expressed growth suppressor gene in fetal skeletal muscle and placental villous trophoblast but paternally expressed in fetal brain and is expressed from both parental alleles in all other tissues investigated including term placenta [43,44,45,46,47]. It is located on human 7p11.2-p12 and is still considered a strong candidate gene for SRS despite no reported cases of SRS being caused by mutations in *GRB10* [46,48,49,50].

In mice, *Grb10* localizes to 11p and is maternally expressed in all tissues except the brain, making it the first gene to be described showing opposite imprinting in man and mouse. Disruption of the maternal allele resulted in mice which are approximately 30% larger than wild-type with equally growth-enhanced placentae; however, the liver showed disproportionate overgrowth compared with relative sparing of the brain [51]. Arnaud *et al.* [44] investigated upstream regions and methylation profiles of man and mouse to understand the contrary imprinting patterns of *GRB10*/*Grb10*. Both genes displayed well-conserved sequences upstream and similar methylation patterns suggesting that the differences are due to the way the imprinting mark is read. Coan *et al.* [52] studied the natural intra-litter variation in placental nutrient efficiency in normal pregnant mice by examining the morphology, nutrient transfer, and expression of genes involved in growth, including *Grb10*, among day 16 and 19 gestation of the lightest and heaviest placentae. The lightest placenta showed evidence of morphological and physical changes which supported increased nutrient transfer. This permits the placenta to maximize fetal growth late in pregnancy in the face of adverse placental conditions, i.e. smaller placentae work harder to support fetal growth [52].

The growth-related phenotype associated with *Grb10* in mice suggested it would be a good candidate for SRS where mUPD 7 is associated with IUGR and postnatal growth restriction, although pUPD7 is not always associated with overgrowth in the few cases documented [53,54]. *GRB10* has been shown to be biallelic in term placenta [43,46]. However it may have potent effects during early pregnancy when it is monoallelically expressed in villous trophoblast, the placental tissue involved in nutrient transfer (Monk *et al.*, unpublished observations). Additionally, imprinting of *GRB10* in the brain may be associated with feeding behavior as mUPD 7 patients are known to have feeding problems [5].

ZAC1 on chromosome 6

Transient neonatal diabetes mellitus (TNDM) is defined as diabetes in a term infant occurring in the first 6 weeks of life and recovery by 18 months of age, accompanied by IUGR [55]. A substantial proportion of these infants go on to develop diabetes later in life. The first genetic clue to the cause of TNDM was found in patients with pUPD for chromosome 6 presenting with TNDM and later this region was observed in paternal duplications of 6q24 also presenting with TNDM, thereby delineating the region of interest [56,57]. The parent-specific origin of the phenotype suggested that imprinted genes may be localized to this region and Zinc finger protein 1/pleiomorphic adenoma gene-like 1/Lost On Transformation 1 (*ZAC1*/*PLAGL1*/*LOT1*) associated with apoptosis and cell cycle arrest, and Hydatidiform mole-associated and imprinted transcript (*HYMAI*) were found in the relevant region.

ZAC1/*PLAGL1*/*LOT1* is zinc finger transcription factor of the PLAG family and localizes to human chromosome 6q24–25 and is a growth suppressor. It is a transcriptional regulator for the pituary adenylate cyclase-activating polypeptide type 1 receptor which is recognized as the most potent insulin secretagog and controls insulin secretion in the pancreatic islet in an autocrine manner [58]. It is maternally imprinted or silenced and paternally expressed which is contrary to the conflict hypothesis. Loss of *ZAC1* in humans is also associated with cancers. *HYMAI* is also paternally expressed and is an untranslated mRNA with unknown function.

The *Zac1* mouse homolog is located on chromosome 10 and is also imprinted but the phenotypic features seen in humans are not mirrored in mice with the corresponding chromosome anomalies [59]. It has been shown that inactivation of *Zac1* results in IUGR, altered bone formation, and neonatal lethality [60]. Transgenic mice carrying the human paternal TNDM locus exhibit the classical human phenotype of hyperglycemia in neonates and impaired glucose tolerance in adults [61]. More interestingly, *Zac1* has been shown to alter the expression of other imprinted genes such as *Igf2*, *H19*, *Cdkn1c*, and *Dlk1* which are located on different chromosomes, pointing to the existence of additional trans-acting regulation of imprinted genes [60,62].

The role of *ZAC1* in human placenta is not clear and expression levels in term placenta do not correlate with birth weight, placental weight, or head circumference (Iglesias *et al.*, unpublished observations). It has been shown that in mice it has minimal effect on growth when the paternal allele is selectively deleted from the placenta, and does not significantly alter placental histology or the transport capacity of nutrients across the placental membranes [60].

Zinc finger protein 57 (*ZFP57*) is a Kruppel-associated box (KRAB) zinc finger protein recently shown to mediate methylation imprinting at several ICRs in the genome [63]. *ZFP57* mutations have been shown in TNDM patients, all of whom were hypomethylated for the *PEG3* and *GRB10* DMRs as well as the TNDM locus attesting to its role in methylation at multiple sites [64]. In mice, it has been shown that *Zfp57* is involved in establishment and maintenance of imprinting of several loci in the genome [65].

Translational message: mutations in *ZFP57* may be responsible for disorders caused by different imprinted genes in the genome

Imprinted genes on chromosome 14

Distinct phenotypes are seen in mUPD14 and pUPD14 cases. Earlier work by Sutton and Shaffer [66] focused on the search for imprinted gene(s), localization(s), and function(s) by comparing mUPD14 and pUPD14 cases with paternal and maternal chromosome 14 deletions, respectively. Their work suggested 14q23-q32 was the most likely region to contain imprinted gene(s). In fact, this region harbors a cluster of imprinted genes: paternally expressed Delta-like 1 homolog (*DLK1*) and Retrotransposon-like 1 (*RTL1*) and maternally expressed Gene trap locus 2 (*GTL2/MEG3*), RNA imprinted and accumulated in the nucleus (*RIAN/MEG8*), and *RTL1* antisense (*RTL1as*). *DLK1* is a paternally expressing growth promoter and *GTL2* is an untranslated mRNA.

In man, mUPD14 is characterized by pre- and postnatal growth restriction, early onset of puberty, scoliosis, and muscle hypotonia [67,68]. For the rarer pUPD14 cases, polyhydraminos, edema, and skeletal deformities have been described [69,70]. Recently it has been suggested that the associated DMR, *DLK-GTL2* IG-DMR, regulates the maternally inherited imprinted region, and phenotypes seen in the mUPD14 and pUPD14 cases are caused by disturbances in *RTL1* and *DLK1* expression [71]. Their role in human placenta and growth has not been determined although *DLK1* is strongly expressed and *GTL2* is moderately expressed; *RTL1* is not expressed in the human placenta.

The syntenic region on mouse chromosome 12 with *Dlk1* and *Gtl2* shows appropriate growth disturbances in UPD conceptuses – with mUPD12 resulting in late embryonic or early neonatal lethality accompanied by IUGR and pUPD12 mice similarly resulting in embryonic lethality but an overgrowth phenotype including placentomegaly [72]. In heterozygous mice with paternal loss of *RTL*, inadequate placental development results in neonatal lethality as opposed to heterozygous mice with maternal loss of *RTL* which are also neonatally lethal but have overdevelopment of the placenta [73]. *Dlk1* in mice is involved in somite formation and segmentation and skeletal muscle maturation defects seen in mice are comparable to the scoliosis seen in humans [74]. In mice, *Dlk1* and *Gtl2* have been shown to be coexpressed and their expression is reciprocally controlled in a manner similar to *H19* and *IGF2* [75].

Conclusion

Imprinted genes are most highly expressed during fetal development and growth with some involved in early postnatal growth. Recently it has been shown that there is downregulation of mRNA of 11 imprinted genes in multiple organs as ageing occurs which included *Igf2*, *H19*, *Zac1*, *Mest*, *Peg3*, *Dlk1*, *Gtl2*, *Grb10*, *Ndn*, *Cdkn1c*, and *SLC38a4* [76]. The downregulation of these genes was due to changes in promoter methylation except for *Mest*, *Peg3*, and *Zac1* [76].

The complexity of the human placenta has not been underestimated but with the added influence of imprinted genes, its complete function has adopted another evolutionary dimension. Imprinted genes are found in clusters throughout the genome exhibiting coordinated expression although many have specific independent expression pathways. Imprinting is different in man and mouse as is clear from studies showing tissue and gestation expression differences as well as imprinting status. A concerted effort is required to investigate known imprinted genes in the human placenta to elucidate the individual contribution of each gene in fetal and placental growth and development. Interestingly with the data as described above very few imprinted genes in man are placental specific and only a few have an obvious specialized role in human growth. However, the ones that do, such as *PHLDA2*, are potentially very important.

References

1. Barton S C, Surani M A, Norris M L. Role of paternal and maternal genomes in mouse development. *Nature* 1984; **311**: 374–6.
2. McGrath J, Solter D. Completion of mouse embryogenesis requires both maternal and paternal genomes. *Cell* 1984; **37**: 179–83.
3. Cattanach B M, Kirk M. Differential activity of maternally and paternally derived chromosome regions in mice. *Nature* 1985; **315**: 496–8.
4. Moore T, Haig D. Genomic imprinting in mammalian development: a parental tug-of-war. *Trends Genet* 1991; 7(2): 45–9.
5. Abu-Amero S, Monk D, Frost J *et al.* The genetic aetiology of Silver-Russell syndrome. *J Med Genet* 2008; **45**(4): 193–9.
6. Weksberg R, Shuman C, Smith A C. Beckwith-Wiedemann syndrome. *Am J Med Genet C Semin Med Genet* 2005; **137C**(1): 12–23.
7. Ideraabdullah F Y, Vigneau S, Bartolomei M S. Genomic imprinting mechanisms in mammals. *Mutat Res* 2008; **647**(1–2): 77–85.
8. DeChiara T M, Robertson E J, Efstratiadis A. Parental imprinting of the mouse insulin-like growth factor II gene. *Cell* 1991; **64**: 849–59.
9. Monk D, Sanches R, Arnaud P *et al.* Imprinting of *IGF2* P0 transcript and novel alternatively spliced INS-IGF2 isoforms show differences between mouse and human. *Hum Mol Genet* 2006; **15**(8): 1259–69.
10. Arima T, Matsuda T, Takagi N *et al.* Association of *IGF2* and *H19* imprinting with choriocarcinoma development. *Cancer Genet Cytogenet* 1997; **93**(1): 39–47.
11. Brunkow M E, Tilghman S M. Ectopic expression of the *H19* gene in mice causes prenatal lethality. *Genes Dev* 1991; **5**(6): 1092–101.
12. Adriaenssens E, Lottin S, Dugimont T *et al.* Steroid hormones modulate *H19* gene expression in both mammary gland and uterus. *Oncogene* 1999; **18**(31): 4460–73.
13. Jinno Y, Ikeda Y, Yun K *et al.* Establishment of functional imprinting of the *H19* gene in human developing placentae. *Nat Genet* 1995; **10**(3): 318–24.
14. Guo L, Choufani S, Ferreira J *et al.* Altered gene expression and methylation of the human chromosome 11 imprinted region in small for gestational age (SGA) placentae. *Dev Biol* 2008; **320**(1): 79–91.
15. Gao Z H, Suppola S, Liu J *et al.* Association of *H19* promoter methylation with the expression of *H19* and IGF-II genes in adrenocortical tumors. *J Clin Endocrinol Metab* 2002; **87**(3): 1170–6.
16. Leighton P A, Ingram R S, Eggenschwiler J *et al.* Disruption of imprinting caused by deletion of the *H19* gene region in mice. *Nature* 1995; **375**(6526): 34–9.
17. Constância M, Hemberger M, Hughes J *et al.* Placental-specific IGF-II is a major modulator of placental and fetal growth. *Nature* 2002; **417**(6892): 945–8.
18. Coan P M, Fowden A L, Constancia M *et al.* Disproportional effects of *Igf2* knockout on placental morphology and diffusional exchange characteristics in the mouse. *J Physiol* 2008; **586**(Pt 20): 5023–32.
19. McMinn J, Wei M, Schupf N *et al.* Unbalanced placental expression of imprinted genes in human intrauterine growth restriction. *Placenta* 2006; **27**(6–7): 540–9.
20. Abu-Amero S, Wakeling E L, Preece M *et al.* Commentary: epigenetic signatures of Silver-Russell syndrome. *J Med Genet*, in press.
21. Apostolidou S, Abu-Amero S, O'Donoghue K *et al.* Elevated maternal expression of the imprinted *PHLDA2* gene is associated with low birth weight. *J Mol Med* 2007; **85**(4): 379–87.
22. Gicquel C, Rossignol S, Cabrol S *et al.* Epimutations of the telomeric imprinting control region on chromosome 11p15 in Silver-Russell syndrome. *Nat Genet* 2005; **37** (9): 1003–7.
23. Yamazawa K, Kagami M, Nagai T. Molecular and clinical findings and their correlations in Silver-Russell syndrome: implications for a positive role of *IGF2* in growth determination and differential imprinting regulation of the IGF2-H19 domain in bodies and placentas. *J Mol Med* 2008; **86**(10): 1171–81.
24. Du M, Zhou W, Beatty L G *et al.* The *KCNQ1OT1* promoter, a key regulator of genomic imprinting in human chromosome 11p15.5. *Genomics* 2004; **84**(2): 288–300.

25. Monk D, Arnaud P, Apostolidou S *et al.* Limited evolutionary conservation of imprinting in the human placenta. *PNAS USA* 2006; **103**(17): 6623–8.

26. Knox K S, Baker J C. Genome-wide expression profiling of placentas in the *p57/Kip2* model of preeclampsia. *Mol Hum Reprod* 2007; **13**(4): 251–63.

27. Lee M P, Feinberg A P. Genomic imprinting of a human apoptosis gene homologue, *TSSC3. Cancer Res* 1998; **58** (5): 1052–6.

28. McMinn J, Wei M, Sadovsky Y *et al.* Imprinting of *PEG1/MEST* isoform 2 in human placenta. *Placenta* 2006; **27**(2–3): 119–26.

29. Frank D, Mendelsohn C L, Ciccone E *et al.* A novel pleckstrin homology-related gene family defined by *Ipl/Tssc3*, *TDAG51*, and *Tih1*: tissue-specific expression, chromosomal location, and parental imprinting. *Mamm Genome* 1999; **10**(12): 1150–9.

30. Cleary M A, van Raamsdonk C D, Levorse J *et al.* Disruption of an imprinted gene cluster by a targeted chromosomal translocation in mice. *Nat Genet* 2001; **29** (1): 78–82.

31. Frank D, Fortino W, Clark L *et al.* Placental overgrowth in mice lacking the imprinted gene *Ipl. PNAS USA* 2002; **99**(11): 7490–5.

32. Salas M, John R, Saxena A *et al.* Placental growth retardation due to loss of imprinting of *Phlda2*. *Mech Dev* 2004; **121**(10): 1199–210.

33. Kim H S, Roh C R, Chen B *et al.* Hypoxia regulates the expression of *PHLDA2* in primary term human trophoblasts. *Placenta* 2007; **28**(2–3): 77–84.

34. Cassidy S B, Lai L-W, Erickson R P *et al.* Trisomy 15 with loss of the paternal 15 as a cause of Prader-Willi syndrome due to maternal disomy. *Am J Hum Genet* 1992; **51**: 701–8.

35. Purvis-Smith S G, Saville T, Manass S *et al.* Uniparental disomy 15 resulting from ‘correction’ of an initial trisomy 15 (Letter). *Am J Hum Genet* 1992; **50**: 1348–50.

36. Kobayashi S, Kohda T, Miyoshi N *et al.* Human *PEG1/MEST*, an imprinted gene on chromosome 7. *Hum Molec Genet* 1997; **6**(5): 781–6.

37. Kosaki K, Kosaki R, Craigen W J *et al.* Isoform-specific imprinting of the human *PEG1/MEST* gene. *Am J Hum Genet* 2000; **66**(1): 309–12.

38. Nakabayashi K, Bentley L, Hitchins M P *et al.* Identification and characterization of an imprinted antisense RNA (*MESTIT1*) in the human *MEST* locus on chromosome 7q32. *Hum Molec Genet* 2002; **11**: 1743–56.

39. Kaneko-Ishino T, Kuroiwa Y, Miyoshi N *et al.* Peg1/Mest imprinted gene on chromosome 6 identified by cDNA subtraction hybridization. *Nat Genet* 1995; **11**: 52–9.

40. Lefebvre L, Viville S, Barton S C *et al.* Genomic structure and parent-of-origin-specific methylation of *Peg1*. *Hum Molec Genet* 1997; **6**: 1907–15.

41. Lefebvre L, Viville S, Barton S C *et al.* Abnormal maternal behaviour and growth retardation associated with loss of the imprinted gene *Mest. Nat Genet* 1998; **20**: 163–9.

42. Keverne E B. Genomic imprinting and the maternal brain. *Prog Brain Res* 2001; **133**: 279–85.

43. Blagitko N, Mergenthaler S, Schulz U *et al.* Human *GRB10* is imprinted and expressed from the paternal and maternal allele in a highly tissue- and isoform-specific fashion. *Hum Molec Genet* 2000; **9**: 1587–95.

44. Arnaud P, Monk D, Hitchins M *et al.* Conserved methylation imprints in the human and mouse *GRB10* genes with divergent allelic expression suggests differential reading of the same mark. *Hum Mol Genet* 2003; **12**(9): 1005–19.

45. Hikichi T, Kohda T, Kaneko-Ishino T *et al.* Imprinting regulation of the murine *Meg1/Grb10* and human *GRB10* genes; roles of brain-specific promoters and mouse-specific CTCF-binding sites. *Nucleic Acids Res* 2003; **31**: 1398–406.

46. Hitchins M P, Monk D, Bell G M *et al.* Maternal repression of the human *GRB10* gene in the developing central nervous system; evaluation of the role for *GRB10* in Silver-Russell syndrome. *Eur J Hum Genet* 2001; **9**: 82–90.

47. Monk D, Arnaud P, Frost J *et al.* Reciprocal imprinting of human GRB10 in placental trophoblast and brain: evolutionary conservation of reversed allelic expression. *Hum Mol Genet* 2009; **18**: 3066–74.

48. Mergenthaler S, Hitchins M P, Blagitko-Dorfs N *et al.* Conflicting reports of imprinting status of human *GRB10* in developing brain: how reliable are somatic cell hybrids for predicting allelic origin of expression? *Am J Hum Genet* 2001; **68**(2): 543–5.

49. Monk D, Wakeling E L, Proud V *et al.* Duplication of 7p11.2-p13, including *GRB10*, in Silver-Russell syndrome. *Am J Hum Genet* 2000; **66**(1): 36–46.

50. Monk D, Smith R, Arnaud P *et al.* Imprinted methylation profiles for proximal mouse chromosomes 11 and 7 as revealed by methylation-sensitive representational difference analysis. *Mamm Genome* 2003; **14**(12): 805–16.

51. Charalambous M, Smith F M, Bennett W R *et al.* Disruption of the imprinted *Grb10* gene leads to disproportionate overgrowth by an Igf2-independent mechanism. *PNAS USA* 2003; **100**(14): 8292–7.

52. Coan P M, Angiolini E, Sandovici I *et al.* Adaptations in placental nutrient transfer capacity to meet fetal growth demands depend on placental size in mice. *J Physiol* 2008; **586**(Pt 18): 4567–76.

53. Hoglund P, Holmberg C, de la Chapelle A *et al.* Paternal isodisomy for chromosome 7 is compatible with normal growth and development in a patient with congenital chloride diarrhea. *Am J Hum Genet* 1994; **55**: 747–52.

54. Pan Y, McCaskill C D, Harrisom G M *et al.* Paternal uniparental disomy of chromosome 7 associated with complete situs inversus and immotile cilia. *Am J Hum Genet* 1998; **62**(6): 1551–5.

55. Temple I K, Shield J P. Transient neonatal diabetes, a disorder of imprinting. *J Med Genet* 2002; **39**(12): 872–5.

56. Temple I K, James R S, Crolla J A *et al.* An imprinted gene(s) for diabetes? *Nat Genet* 1995; **9**(2): 110–2.

57. Temple I K, Gardner R J, Robinson D O *et al.* Further evidence for an imprinted gene for neonatal diabetes localized to chromosome 6q22-q23. *Hum Mol Genet* 1996; **5**(8): 1117–21.

58. Kamiya M, Judson H, Okazaki Y *et al.* The cell cycle control gene *ZAC*/PLAGL1 is imprinted: a strong candidate gene for transient neonatal diabetes. *Hum Molec Genet* 2000; **9**: 453–60.

59. Smith R J, Arnaud P, Konfortova G *et al.* The mouse *Zac1* locus: basis for imprinting and comparison with human *ZAC*. *Gene* 2002; **292**(1–2): 101–12.

60. Varrault A, Gueydan C, Delalbre A *et al.* *Zac1* regulates an imprinted gene network critically involved in the control of embryonic growth. *Dev Cell* 2006; **11**(5): 711–22.

61. Ma D, Shield J P, Dean W *et al.* Impaired glucose homeostasis in transgenic mice expressing the human transient neonatal diabetes mellitus locus, *TNDM*. *J Clin Invest* 2004; **114**(3): 339–48.

62. Arima T, Kamikihara T, Hayashida T *et al.* *ZAC*, *LIT1* (*KCNQ1OT1*) and *p57KIP2* (*CDKN1C*) are in an imprinted gene network that may play a role in Beckwith-Wiedemann syndrome. *Nucleic Acids Res* 2005; **33**(8): 2650–60.

63. Hirasawa R, Feil R. A KRAB domain zinc finger protein in imprinting and disease. *Dev Cell* 2008; **15**(4): 487–8.

64. Mackay D J, Callaway J L, Marks S M *et al.* Hypomethylation of multiple imprinted loci in individuals with transient neonatal diabetes is associated with mutations in*ZFP57*. *Nat Genet* 2008; **40**(8): 949–51.

65. Li X, Ito M, Zhou F *et al.* A maternal-zygotic effect gene, *Zfp57*, maintains both maternal and paternal imprints. *Dev Cell* 2008; **15**(4): 547–57.

66. Sutton V R, Shaffer L G. Search for imprinted regions on chromosome 14: comparison of maternal and paternal UPD cases with cases of chromosome 14 deletion. *Am J Med Genet* 2000; **93**(5): 381–7.

67. Kotzot D. Maternal uniparental disomy 14 dissection of the phenotype with respect to rare autosomal recessively inherited traits, trisomy mosaicism, and genomic imprinting. *Ann Genet* 2004; **47**(3): 251–60.

68. Ruggeri A, Dulcetti F, Miozzo M *et al.* Prenatal search for UPD 14 and UPD 15 in 83 cases of familial and de novo heterologous Robertsonian translocations. *Prenat Diagn* 2004; **24**(12): 997–1000.

69. Cotter P D, Kaffe S, McCurdy L D *et al.* Paternal uniparental disomy for chromosome 14: a case report and review. *Am J Med Genet* 1997; **70**(1): 74–9.

70. Kurosawa K, Sasaki H, Sato Y *et al.* Paternal UPD14 is responsible for a distinctive malformation complex. *Am J Med Genet* 2002; **110**(3): 268–72.

71. Ogata T, Kagami M, Ferguson-Smith A C. Molecular mechanisms regulating phenotypic outcome in paternal and maternal uniparental disomy for chromosome 14. *Epigenetics* 2008; **3**(4): 181–7.

72. Georgiades P, Watkins M, Surani M A *et al.* Parental origin-specific developmental defects in mice with uniparental disomy for chromosome 12. *Development* 2000; **127**(21): 4719–28.

73. Sekita Y, Wagatsuma H, Nakamura K *et al.* Role of retrotransposon-derived imprinted gene, *Rtl1*, in the feto-maternal interface of mouse placenta. *Nat Genet* 2008; **40**(2): 243–8.

74. Sutton V R, McAlister W H, Bertin T K *et al.* Skeletal defects in paternal uniparental disomy for chromosome 14 are re-capitulated in the mouse model (paternal uniparental disomy 12). *Hum Genet* 2003; **113**(5): 447–51.

75. Schmidt J V, Matteson P G, Jones B K *et al.* The *Dlk1* and *Gtl2* genes are linked and reciprocally imprinted. *Genes Dev* 2000; **14**(16): 1997–2002.

76. Lui J C, Finkielstain G P, Barnes K M *et al.* An imprinted gene network that controls mammalian somatic growth is down-regulated during postnatal growth deceleration in multiple organs. *Am J Physiol Regul Integr Comp Physiol* 2008; **295**(1): R189–96.

Section 7 Chapter 19

Risk factors, predictors, and future management

The epidemiology of preeclampsia with focus on family data

Rolv Skjaerven[1,2], Kari K. Melve[1,2], and Lars J. Vatten[3]

[1]Department of Public Health and Primary Health Care, University of Bergen, Bergen, Norway
[2]Medical Birth Registry of Norway, National Institute of Public Health, Bergen, Norway
[3]Department of Public Health, Norwegian University of Science and Technology, Trondheim, Norway

Introduction

In this review of epidemiological aspects of preeclampsia we focus on family data, with particular emphasis on the recurrence of preeclampsia within sibships and between generations. We also include effects related to change of partner and effects related to time interval between births, and we explain how effects related to change of partner can be confounded by other factors. To a large extent we have relied on data from the Medical Birth Registry of Norway (MBRN), since this review reflects the contents of a presentation given at the 'Placental Bed' Symposium in Leuven in 2007.

Family data in Norway are unique in that they cover all births that have taken place over a period of more than 40 years, starting in 1967. These data can be organized according to sibships, i.e. by linking all births of a particular mother, including children that she might have with different fathers. Also, the life course reproduction of all women and men born in 1967 or later can be followed, and linked back to their own birth records. Thus, it is possible to study variation in reproduction by pregnancy conditions at birth, and the recurrence of pregnancy outcomes from one generation to the next. The data cover a period of approximately 40 years, and we therefore start this review by analyzing time trends. Although most of the results have been previously published, we also include some new analyses using extended data, 1967–2006.

Trends in occurrence and shift in the distribution of length of gestation

In Norway the occurrence of preeclampsia, as captured by MBRN, has almost doubled from 1967 to 2006, from a total of 3.0% in first pregnancies at the beginning of the period to almost 6.0% for the last 5 years, and from 1.4% to 2.7% in second (and higher) pregnancies. Various factors may explain this development. The general increase in the prevalence of obesity and type 2 diabetes in women, and the lower prevalence of smoking in pregnancy, may account for some of the increase, but the higher incidence may also be due to improved ascertainment of the diagnosis. Demographic factors, including lower parity and higher maternal age, have also contributed. The increase has been relatively stronger for preeclampsia with preterm delivery (from 0.4% to 1.3% for first pregnancies, and 0.2% to 0.6% for second and higher pregnancies), which to a large extent is due to early delivery of infants to women with severe preeclampsia.

Trends in survival

Preeclampsia has been a major cause of stillbirth and infant mortality. For the period 1967–1978, stillbirth associated with preeclampsia was more than four-fold higher compared to stillbirth in pregnancies not afflicted by preeclampsia [1]. This excess risk has been dramatically reduced, and for the period 1991–2003, excess risk was only about 30% (odds ratio, 1.34, 95% confidence interval (CI) 1.07–1.68). However, neonatal mortality associated with preeclampsia did not improve throughout this period. The large improvement in stillbirths is caused by better clinical management, whereas the lack of improvement in neonatal mortality is a prevailing challenge.

For recurrent preeclampsia during the period 1967–1978 we found that perinatal mortality in second pregnancies was four-fold higher compared to women with preeclampsia in the first but not in the second pregnancy, and five-fold higher compared to women

Table 19.1. Recurrence of total and preterm preeclampsia by period of birth, Norway 1967–2006

	Total preeclampsia			Preeclampsia, delivered preterm		
Period of birth	Recurrence risk (%)	Baseline risk (%)	RR (95% CI)	Recurrence risk (%)	Baseline risk (%)	RR (95% CI)
1967–78	10.9	1.1	11 (10–12)	4.9	0.11	47 (32–71)
1979–88	15.7	1.5	12 (11–13)	9.5	0.21	50 (39–66)
1989–98	16.8	1.5	13 (12–14)	9.5	0.31	34 (28–41)
1999–06	16.6	1.6	12 (11–13)	12.6	0.5	29 (24–34)
Total[a]	15.2	1.4	11.7 (11.2–12.1)	9.9	0.27	34.1 (30.5–38.2)

[a] Total RR is adjusted for maternal age (5 categories: <20, 20–24, 25–29, 30–34, 35+) and period (4 levels), categorized.

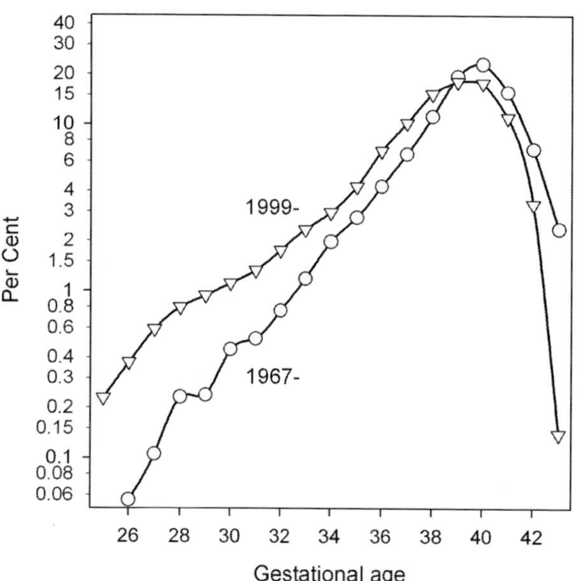

Fig. 19.1 Gestational age distributions (log scale) for all preeclampsia cases, singleton pregnancies for two periods in Norway, 1967–78 and 1999–2006. Restricted to pregnancies with gestational age between 25 and 43 weeks.

without preeclampsia in either the first or second pregnancy. For the period 1999–2006, there was no such excess risk in perinatal mortality.

The great improvement related to stillbirth is clearly the result of induced early delivery of the most severe cases of preeclampsia. The higher tendency in recent years to induce births has substantially increased the proportion of preterm cases of preeclampsia. For instance, the proportion of preeclampsia in gestational weeks 30–33 has increased four- to six-fold from 1967–78 to 1999–2006 (see Fig. 19.1).

Recurrence of preeclampsia

Women with a history of preeclampsia are at increased risk of preeclampsia and other adverse pregnancy outcomes in subsequent pregnancies. According to a recent review by Barton and Sibai, 'no single biomarker can be used in the prediction of recurrent preeclampsia, and various potentially preventive agents, such as supplementation with fish oil, calcium, vitamin C and E, or the use of antihypertensive medication, have shown no clear effects' [2].

There are few other outcomes of pregnancy where recurrence is as high as for preeclampsia, and preterm preeclampsia holds the highest recurrence risk. In Norway, recurrence, measured as relative risk for total preeclampsia, has remained nearly unchanged over 40 years, although the absolute risk at baseline and the absolute risk of recurrence have gradually increased over time (Table 19.1). The increase in the risk of recurrent preterm preeclampsia is less pronounced than the increase in the baseline risk, and over time the relative risk of recurrence, compared to women without preeclampsia in their first pregnancy, has decreased from almost 50 to 29. Technically, this reduction in relative risk corresponds to a significant interaction between preeclampsia in the first pregnancy and period (P for interaction 0.0002). Again, the increase in risk for preterm preeclampsia is most likely a consequence of the clinical practice of early delivery of severe preeclampsia, ending in preterm birth.

Selective fertility and recurrence of preeclampsia within sibships

Usually, recurrence of preeclampsia is studied using data from two successive pregnancies, preferably the first and second pregnancy. Preeclampsia is related to increased risk of a perinatal death, and it is well documented that fertility subsequent to a perinatal death is increased [3]. The likelihood that a woman will continue to another pregnancy following a perinatal death is about 10% higher than expected, and more than one loss strengthens this tendency. Thus, one might expect that preeclampsia would also be associated with a similar increase in fertility, but we found the opposite [4]. For instance, following two preeclamptic pregnancies, fertility was reduced by 20%, and if these preeclamptic pregnancies were preterm, subsequent fertility was 40% lower than would be expected in women without a history of preeclampsia.

Figure 19.2 illustrates the recurrence risk of preeclampsia in families (all sibships in Norway, 1967–2006). This 'risk-tree' shows the branching of preeclampsia risk at each category of parity, given preeclampsia in the previous pregnancy. For instance, there was 16% risk of preeclampsia in the second pregnancy among women who had preeclampsia in the first (solid line), compared to 1.5% in the second pregnancy among women without preeclampsia in the first (broken line). This figure shows some important aspects of the recurrence pattern. First, among women with at least one preeclamptic pregnancy, the risk of preeclampsia is never reduced to the baseline level. Second, the relative risk of preeclampsia in women with one or two previous pregnancies with preeclampsia is practically independent of parity. The risk following one preeclamptic pregnancy is around 15% in second, third or fourth pregnancy, and is at least 30% following two preeclamptic pregnancies (regardless of these being first and second, second and third, or first and third pregnancies).

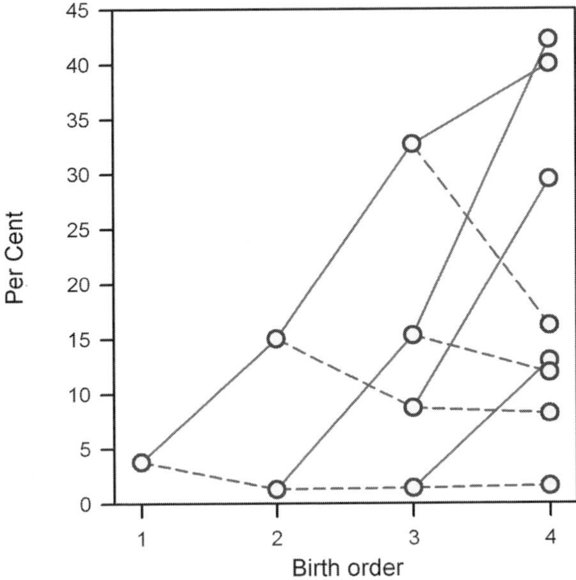

Fig. 19.2 Preeclampsia by history of preeclampsia in previous pregnancies. At each node, a solid line indicates the increased risk due to preeclampsia in the previous pregnancy; a broken line indicates the risk without preeclampsia. All singleton pregnancies in Norway, 1967–2006. Confined to women with same partners in all pregnancies.

Change of partner, interval between pregnancies and immunology

Several studies have found that change of partner between pregnancies is associated with increased risk of preeclampsia [5,6,7,8]. The higher risk of preeclampsia in a pregnancy following change of partner has stimulated research aiming to identify possible underlying mechanisms. This observation has been particularly important for immunological studies of preeclampsia. It has been suggested that the protective effect of multiparity is lost with change of partner, and that 'genuine preeclampsia' is a disease of first pregnancies [9]. Also, it has been reported that exposure to semen provides protection against developing preeclampsia, and that artificial donor insemination and oocyte donation may result in a substantial increase in the risk of preeclampsia [10]. Thus, epidemiologial studies suggest that immune maladaptation is involved in the etiology of preeclampsia .

However, three papers from Scandinavia [11,12,13], based on very large population data, have shown that change of partner is not likely to be associated with increased risk of preeclampsia; on the contrary, the results of these studies suggest that change of partner is associated with reduced risk. All these studies showed that the effect of partner change was heavily confounded by time interval between pregnancies. Thus, there was a longer time interval between pregnancies among women who had experienced a change of partner, and after taking this difference into account, the higher risk was completely attenuated, and showed a slightly reduced risk associated with change of partner. Nonetheless, this issue remains controversial, and the 'primipaternity' hypothesis still receives considerable attention [14,15,16,17].

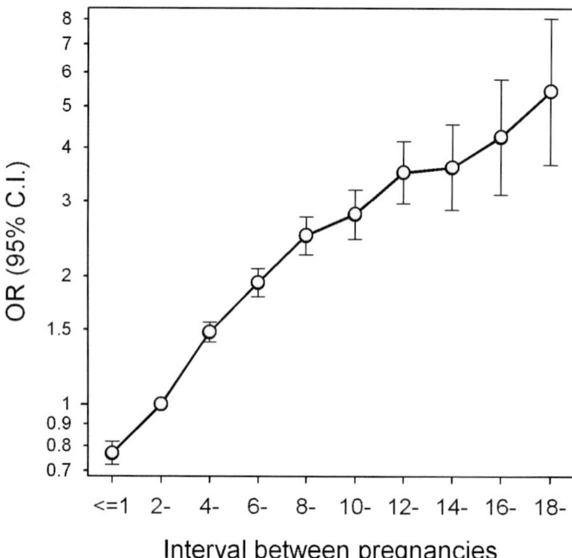

Fig. 19.3 Preeclampsia in second pregnancy by interval between pregnancies. All singleton pregnancies in Norway, 1967–2006 for women without preeclampsia in first pregnancy. OR values were adjusted for period of birth, maternal age (first birth), and change of partner.

In Fig. 19.3, we have reanalyzed the data of the original study, extended the study period to 2006, and included approximately 700 000 women, as compared to the 550 000 women in the original analysis [12]. By restricting time intervals between births from 1 to 18 years, and restricting the analysis to women without preeclampsia in the first pregnancy, the risk increase per year between pregnancies corresponds to an OR of 1.12 (95% CI 1.11–1.13), which again corresponds to more than five times higher risk between the longest and the shortest time interval between pregnancies. In the analyses we adjusted for period and maternal age of first birth, and for change of partner.

The crude relative risk of preeclampsia for women who had a new partner corresponds to an OR of 1.24 (95% CI 1.17–1.30), but the time interval between births is substantially different for women with a new partner (mean = 7.2 years, SD = 3.8) and women with the same partner in the second pregnancy (mean = 3.3 years, SD = 1.9). In our data, approximately 10% of the women had a new partner. After adjustment for differences in time interval between pregnancies, the effect of having a new partner was not only attenuated, it was reversed to the opposite, yielding an odds ratio of 0.80 (95% CI 0.75–0.85). This suggests that a change of partner is associated with a reduced risk of preeclampsia in a subsequent pregnancy.

Another factor that also could contribute to this effect is the prevalence of smoking, since smoking is associated with reduced risk of preeclampsia [18]. For smoking to play a role in these estimates, change of partner should be associated with higher prevalence of smoking. In Norway, change of partner between pregnancies is more likely to occur among women with relatively low level of education (19%) compared to women with high (6%) level of education [19], and given the higher prevalence of smoking in the former group, this may suggest that adjustment for smoking could also be relevant for the association of change of partner with risk of preeclampsia.

Previous studies have been unclear as to whether *recurrence risk* also increases by interval between pregnancies, and whether there is an effect of change of partner related to recurrence [11,13]. Using the extended data (1967–2006), the effects of interval between pregnancies and partner change were similar to those reported above also for women who had preeclampsia in the first pregnancy. The unadjusted effect of change of partner corresponds to an OR of 0.98 (95% CI 0.88–1.10), after adjustment for time period and maternal age the OR was 0.93 (95% CI 0.82–1.04), and after adding time interval between births the OR was 0.86 (95% CI 0.76–0.99).

Thus, after adjustment for time interval between births, there is a reduced risk of preeclampsia associated with change of partner, both for first occurrence of preeclampsia in the second pregnancy, and related to recurrence of preeclampsia from the first to the second pregnancy.

Women (and men) who have changed partner from one pregnancy to the next are more common in current data. For the first period (1967–1978), only 6% had a new partner, whereas in the most recent period (1999–2006), 14% have changed partner between the first and second pregnancy. Mean age at the second pregnancy and the time interval between pregnancies have also increased over time. In the most recent period, mean interval between births was 8.2 years for women who had changed partner, and 3.2 years for women with the same partner. Thus, given the strong effect on preeclampsia by time interval between pregnancies, studies that fail to adjust for this factor in the assessment of partner change and subsequent risk of preeclampsia are prone to bias.

In a recent review [20] entitled 'Is the immune maladaptation hypothesis still standing?', Dekker and Robillard find support for the immunological

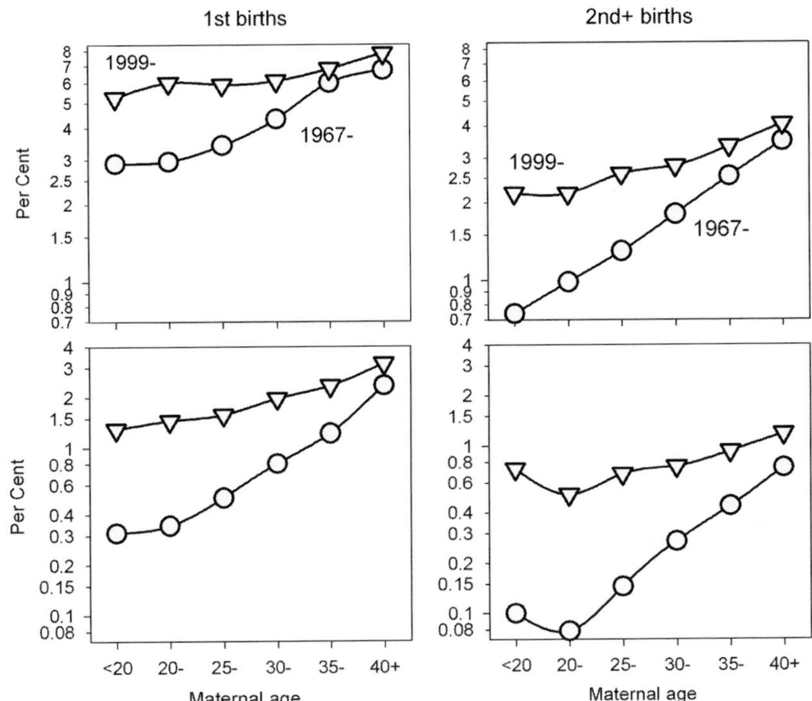

Fig. 19.4 Proportions of preeclampsia by maternal age categories in first and second pregnancies by two periods in Norway, 1967–78 and 1999–2006. Upper two panels: total preeclampsia; lower two panels: preterm preeclampsia.

mechanisms in the studies of Li and Wi [21] and Lie *et al.* [22] and claim that 'these studies indicate that changing paternity plays a different role in women with or without a history of preeclampsia, and that analyses must be stratified by history of disease'. However, the results from our extended analysis (see above), with adjustment for interval between births, suggest that the effects related to change of partner are independent of whether the preeclampsia is a recurrence or a first occurrence. It is a weakness of the study by Li and Wi that the effect of a new partner is assessed within data that only allow a 3-year time interval between births. Since the time interval related to change of partner is typically longer, a 3-year window between two successive pregnancies will by itself introduce bias. The forces of selective fertility will also introduce bias [3,4].

Maternal age and parity

First birth and high maternal age are well known risk factors for preeclampsia. In Fig. 19.4 we present the risk of preterm preeclampsia by maternal age, stratified by parity, and compare trends for the first (1967–1978) and the most recent period (1999–2006). The figure shows the secular increase in preeclampsia by maternal age at childbearing; it is noteworthy that the increase was higher in younger than in older age groups, and that the increase is relatively stronger for preterm than for term preeclampsia.

One explanation for these trends may be the current increase in overweight and obesity [23,24,25], since obesity is known to increase the risk of pregnancy-related hypertension and preeclampsia. The work by Villamor and Cnattingius [26] shows that 10% increase in BMI from the first to the second pregnancy may result in more than 50% higher risk of preeclampsia in the second pregnancy. Given this increase in BMI between pregnancies, they observed similar excess risks for gestational hypertension, gestational diabetes, and LGA (large-for-gestation age), and they also reported higher risks for stillbirths and cesarean delivery associated with BMI increase between pregnancies.

In their recent review, Barton and Sibai [2] reported that women 40 years of age or older have 10–20% risk of preeclampsia. The risk for these women, as reported to the MBRN, is 8% during the most recent period (1999–2006); however, the risk is only 4% for second and higher parities.

For second and higher parity, previous preeclampsia will dramatically increase the risk regardless of maternal age (see Table 19.1). Also, high maternal age will increase the likelihood of a new partner, and a new partner is in turn related to longer time interval between pregnancies. While a new partner will be rare if the mother is young at her second birth, for instance 20–24 years (9%), it is more likely that a 40-year-old mother will have a new partner (21%) and, therefore, these demographic factors will substantially influence the risk of preeclampsia at the age of 40 years.

Due to the effect of interval between pregnancies, the risk for preeclampsia in the second pregnancy for women at the age of 40 will vary depending on age at first pregnancy. The risk of women who were 20–24 years at first pregnancy was 3.5 times higher (OR = 3.5, 95% CI 1.9–6.5) compared to women who were 35–39 years. The risk for the latter group of women was 2.4% for the years 1999–2006.

Thus, the age effect for preeclampsia varies greatly, and depends on parity, partner-change, and time interval since a previous pregnancy, in addition to the higher risk conferred by a previous pregnancy with preeclampsia.

Smoking and recurrence of preeclampsia

The lower risk of preeclampsia associated with smoking is well documented [18], as is the higher risk of perinatal death associated with preeclampsia among mothers who smoke. However, it is not clear if smoking is associated with the risk of recurrence of preeclampsia. In our material, among non-smoking women with the same partner in both pregnancies, the recurrence risk was 15.4% compared to the baseline risk of 1.6% in women without previous preeclampsia, yielding an odds ratio of 11.4 (95% CI 9.9–13.1). Among smoking women, the recurrence risk was 14.9%, compared to a baseline risk of 0.85%, yielding an odds ratio in smoking women of 20.5 (95% CI 10.1–41.5). Thus, the recurrence risk in smoking and non-smoking women appears to be comparable, but the odds ratio is higher for women who smoke, due to the lower baseline risk, that is nearly half that of non-smoking women.

Recurrence between generations

Genetic factors are important causes of preeclampsia [27,28], and it was recently estimated that 35% of the variance in liability is attributable to maternal genetic effects, 20% to genes of the fetus, and 13% to combined genetic effects [29]. We have shown [30] that preeclampsia tends to repeat in the second generation, i.e. if a mother experienced preeclampsia, her female offspring's risk of preeclampsia was twice as high as in other women (OR = 2.2; 95% CI 2.0–2.4). Surprisingly, a sister who was born after a pregnancy without preeclampsia was also at increased risk (OR = 2.0; 95% CI 1.7–2.3). Moreover, if a brother was born after preeclampsia, his partner's risk was also increased (OR = 1.5; 95% CI 1.3–1.7), suggesting that fetal genes transmitted from the father could be important. The conclusions from that study were as follows: 'It seems reasonable to attribute the observed patterns of familial predisposition to genetic inheritance. Daughters born after a preeclamptic pregnancy may carry their mothers' susceptibility genes, as well as genes from either parent that operate through the fetus. Their sisters who were born after pregnancies not complicated by preeclampsia would be at lower risk as they are less likely to be carrying the genes that operate through the fetus. Still they are just as likely to be carrying their mothers' susceptibility genes. Thus, sisters of affected men and women have about twice the risk of women with no family history of preeclampsia'.

Also, 'For men who were born after preeclampsia, the higher risk of fathering a preeclamptic pregnancy can solely be attributed to paternal factors. Brothers who were born after a pregnancy without preeclampsia would have a low probability of carrying fetal risk genes, which is confirmed by the near baseline risk of preeclampsia among pregnancies they father' [30].

An effect of the father's influence has also been demonstrated by Lie *et al.* [22]. They showed that men who father a preeclamptic pregnancy have almost twice the risk of fathering a preeclamptic pregnancy in another woman. They conclude that both the mother and the fetus contribute to the risk of preeclampsia, and that the fetal contribution partly comes from paternal genes.

Fetal growth restriction and preeclampsia

The relation between preeclampsia and fetal growth restriction is well established [31,32,33]. It has been shown that the association of preeclampsia with small-for-gestational age (SGA) offspring is stronger for the second than for the first pregnancy [31]. In this study the odds ratio for SGA in multiparous women was estimated to be 29 (95% CI 5.2–167.5), compared to 4.1 (CI 1.2–14.1) for nulliparous women. As indicated by the confidence interval limits, these estimates are uncertain due to small samples.

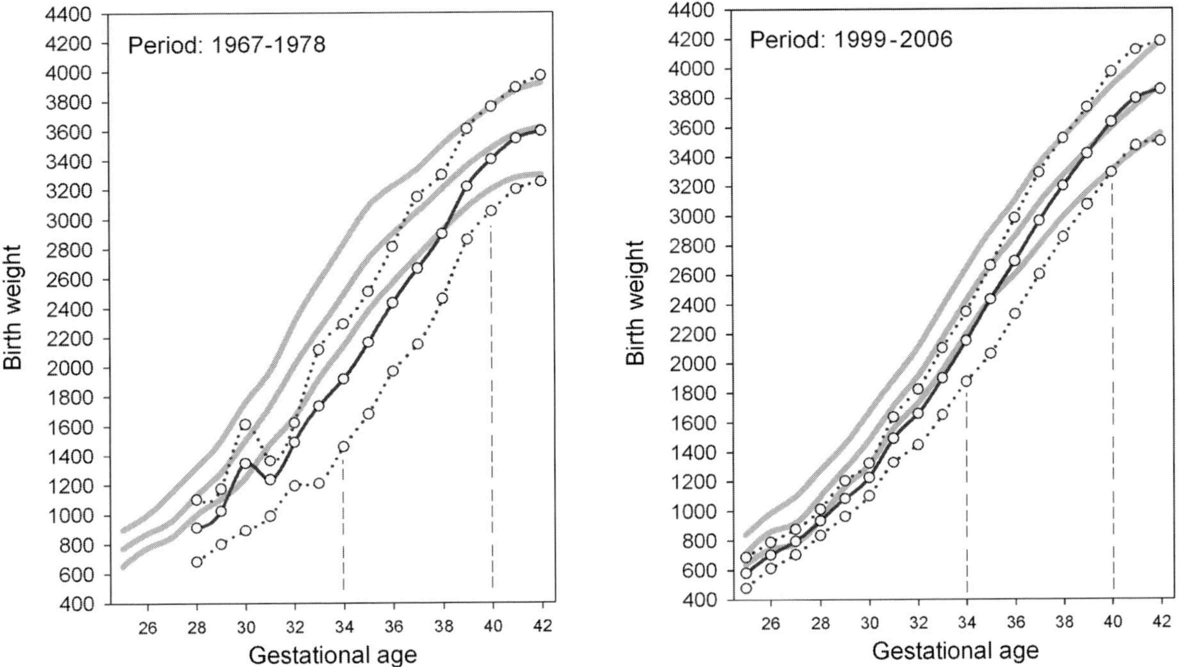

Fig. 19.5 Percentiles for birth weight by gestational age (25th, 50th, and 75th percentiles) for singleton first pregnancies affected by preeclampsia (marked with open circles and lines) and normotensive pregnancies (no markers) in two periods in Norway, 1967–78 and 1999–2006.

Using data from the Medical Birth Registry of Norway (1999–2006), we re-estimated these relations. In pregnancies delivered to term, the relation between SGA and preeclampsia was stronger in second than in first pregnancies (OR = 2.6; CI 2.4–2.8 and 1.9; CI 1.8–2.0, respectively), while in preterm pregnancies there was no difference (OR = 4.0; CI 3.7–4.3, adjusted for parity). In these evaluations we used 'growth standards' that were not stratified by parity [34].

Also, pregnancies with large babies (or large-for-gestational age, LGA) are afflicted by preeclampsia [33,35]. In pregnancies delivered to term, the association with LGA was similar for first and second pregnancies (OR=1.3; CI 1.3–1.4, adjusted for parity). In pregnancies delivered preterm, we observed no association between preeclampsia and LGA offspring.

In studies of siblings it has been suggested that small infants are associated with higher risk of preeclampsia in a subsequent pregnancy. Rasmussen and Irgens [36] showed that the risk of preeclampsia in the second pregnancy was three-fold higher among women with a small child (< third percentile of birth weight by gestational age) in the first pregnancy, compared to women who delivered infants at or above this percentile. Similar results have been shown by Zhang *et al.* [37]. Two Scandinavian studies have recently shown that this relation holds between generations, i.e. women who themselves were small at birth have higher risk (50–70% increase) of preeclampsia compared to other women [38,39].

In Fig. 19.5 we compare the 75th, 50th, and 25th percentiles for singleton newborns affected by preeclampsia (marked lines) compared to singletons of normotensive pregnancies (non-marked lines) for two time periods, 1967–78 and 1999–2006. The figure shows some distinct differences between the two periods. For preeclampsia, there was much more variation in the first period, and preterm birth weights were lower in the first than in the second period. However, there was no difference in birth weight by preeclampsia status at 40 weeks of gestation.

Vatten and Skjaerven [33] concluded in their study that 'For preeclampsia diagnosed around term, there was a U-shaped association with birth weight. Compared with appropriate birth weights for gestation, the risk of term preeclampsia was more than fourfold higher (relative risk (RR) 4.5, 95% CI 4.3 to 4.7) if the baby's birth weight was lower than two

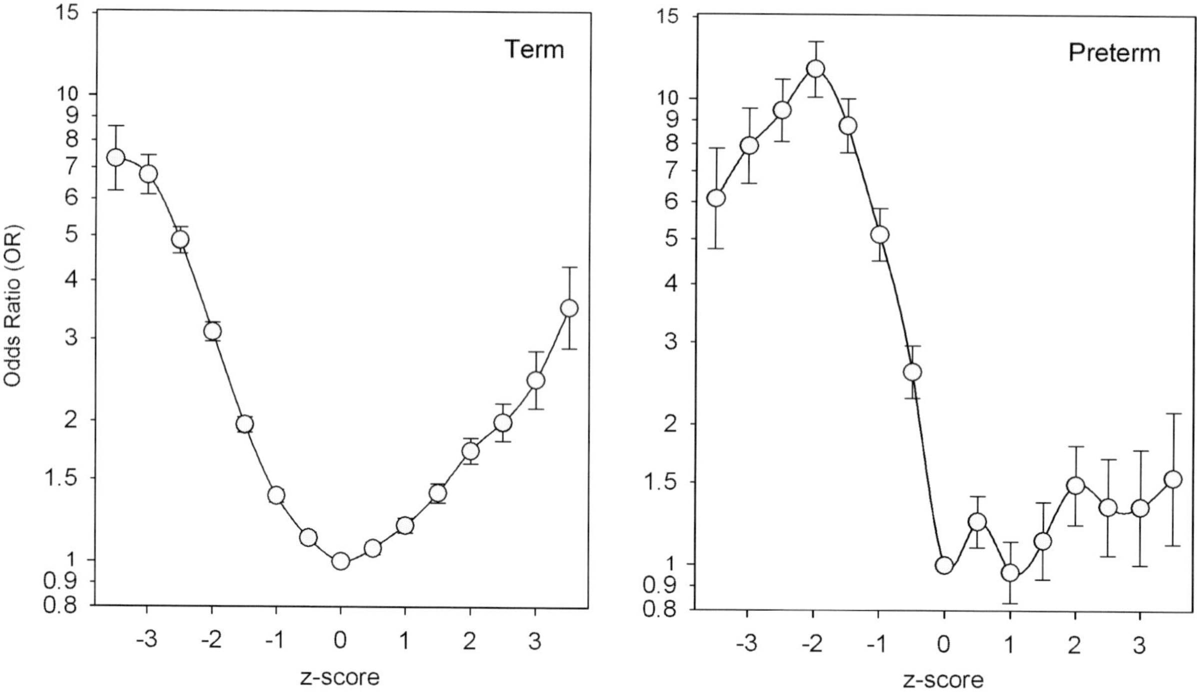

Fig. 19.6 Preeclampsia by z-scores of birth weight by gestational age in singleton, term, and preterm pregnancies. OR values relative to z-score = 0 as reference, adjusted for period (4 categories), maternal age (5 categories), parity (2 categories). Norway, 1967–2006.

standard deviations under the mean. For birth weights three standard deviations or higher than the mean, preeclampsia was more than twice as likely (RR 2.6, 95% CI 2.2–2.9). In contrast, the risk of preterm preeclampsia displayed an L-shaped association with birth weight. Low birth weight (less than 2 standard deviations) was associated with greatly increased risk (RR 9.9, 95% CI 9.1–10.9), but for high birth weights (3 standard deviations or above), there was no association with the risk of preterm preeclampsia (RR 1.2, 95% CI 0.7–2.1)'. Further: 'Whereas preeclampsia with preterm delivery associated with low birth weight may be caused by underlying placental abnormality, preeclampsia delivered at term may represent a mixture of conditions, ranging from mild preeclampsia with moderate placental affection to hypertensive conditions in pregnancy without placental dysfunction'.

Preeclampsia – more than one disease

Several authors have suggested that the definition of preeclampsia may include more than one disease [33,40,41,42]. It has become a convention to distinguish between preeclampsia with term or preterm delivery. However, within the term category, there may also be two distinct subtypes: those associated with fetal growth restriction, and those pregnancies with large-for-gestational age offspring as demonstrated by our earlier work [33]. In Fig. 19.6 we have reassessed the main results from this paper, presented as OR-values, adjusted for period, parity, and maternal age categories.

In the study that related high birth weight for age with preeclampsia, Xiong *et al.* conclude 'This study challenges the currently held belief that reduced utero-placental perfusion is the unique pathophysiologic process in preeclampsia' [35]. The processes leading to preeclampsia are probably very different for those cases where the baby is severely growth restricted and those where the baby is large. The maternal condition causes growth restriction in the former situation, whereas preeclampsia in the latter situation is due to the excess fetal growth. The very strong dose–response relation for term pregnancies may illustrate a genetic conflict between the mother and the baby [43], although it is intriguing that a large baby in the preterm period does not trigger the same responses in the mother.

Strong heterogeneity is also seen in the effects related to preeclampsia and later maternal mortality. Women with a history of preeclampsia have very different risks of cardiovascular disease depending on the severity of the preeclamptic condition. Whereas the risk of cardiovascular death among women with preterm preeclampsia is eight-fold higher (hazard ratio (HR) = 8.1; 95% CI 4.3–15.3) than in women with no history of preeclampsia, women with term delivery have only a moderately increased (HR = 1.7; 95% CI 1.0–2.7) risk [44]. Recent work by Funai *et al.* [45] seems to indicate that women who in a subsequent pregnancy are normotensive are protected from early death. However, after 20 years the hazard is similar to other women with preeclampsia. Vikse *et al.* [46] showed that the relation between preeclampsia and later development of renal disease is stronger in women with only one pregnancy, than in women with more than one pregnancy, and women with severe preeclampsia in a first pregnancy are less likely to continue with subsequent pregnancies. Also, among women who had preeclampsia in only one of two pregnancies, the risk of renal disease was higher if preeclampsia occurred in the second pregnancy than if it occurred in the first pregnancy. The same trend was seen for women with three pregnancies.

Another aspect related to the possibility of preeclampsia being more than one disease may be derived from the recurrence of preeclampsia following a twin pregnancy affected by preeclampsia. Trogstad *et al.* [47] showed that a history of preeclampsia in a previous twin pregnancy may be associated with reduced risk of recurrence in a subsequent pregnancy compared to having preeclampsia in a previous singleton pregnancy. The authors conclude that 'although the maternal organism is likely to be heavily burdened by a preeclamptic twin pregnancy, our results implicate that no permanent changes in the mother are likely to take place that would increase her risk of recurrent preeclampsia'. The authors did not show many details related to the risk of recurrence, and we therefore reanalyzed the data using the complete material from 1967 to 2006. The baseline risk in the second pregnancy following a singleton with preeclampsia was similar to the risk following a twin in the first pregnancy. As shown earlier (see Table 19.1), there was a tendency for the baseline risk to increase by period, but the recurrence risk also increased. Thus, for women with two singleton pregnancies, the recurrence risk was remarkably stable (11.7; 95% CI 11.2–12.1). Given preeclampsia in a twin first pregnancy, there was a lower risk of recurrence to a subsequent singleton pregnancy (OR = 7.9; 95% CI 4.2–15.0 for the period 1967–1986, and OR = 4.5; 95% CI 2.5–8.0 for the period 1987–2006). The lower odds ratios were due to the higher baseline risk, and to a lower risk of recurrence in the last period. Still, the main impression of these analyses was that the recurrence risk of preeclampsia after a twin pregnancy is much lower than after a singleton pregnancy.

Sibships and the relevance of other adverse outcomes

A history of small-for-gestational age or low birth weight offspring is related to an increased risk of preeclampsia in a subsequent pregnancy [36]. Smith *et al.* [48] have also shown that a history of preeclampsia, preterm delivery, and delivery of a small-for-gestational age infant increased the risk of unexplained stillbirth in the second pregnancy. Their risk for a stillbirth in the next pregnancy was two-fold (OR = 2.1; 95% CI 1.5–3.0).

In Table 19.2 we have summarized the relation between some basic risk factors and preeclampsia between first and second pregnancies. The relations between preeclampsia and low birth weight (LBW), preterm birth, and small-for-gestational age (both 10th and 2.5th percentiles: SGA10 and SGA2.5) are strong, and tend to be even stronger in the most recent period (1999–2006). Also, the effects of the risk factors in first pregnancy on preeclampsia in the second pregnancy tend to be stronger than the reverse effect: the effect of preeclampsia on LBW, preterm birth, and SGA in the second pregnancy. Finally, preterm preeclampsia provides the stronger link.

Conclusions

Family data provide valuable insight into the epidemiology of preeclampsia, both for prediction purposes and to improve our understanding of the etiology. Preeclampsia is a maternal disease, with a pattern of repetition within sibships. The condition may also be triggered by the fetus itself and the increased risk may be genetically transmitted from the father. Given that patterns of preterm and term preeclampsia differ so much, it seems reasonable to suggest that preeclampsia

Table 19.2. Recurrence between preeclampsia and selected adverse outcomes measured as odds rations (OR) with 95% confidence intervals, first to second singleton pregnancies, Norway 1967–2006

Total material	**Outcome of second pregnancy**				
Exposure, first pregnancy	LBW	Stillbirth	SGA10	SGA2.5	Preterm
Preeclampsia	1.5 (1.4–1.6)	1.5 (1.4–1.7)	1.2 (1.1–1.2)	1.5 (1.4–1.6)	1.3 (1.3–1.4)
Preterm preeclampsia	4.0 (3.6–4.5)	3.4 (2.7–4.3)	2.2 (2.0–2.4)	3.1 (2.7–3.6)	3.3 (3.0–3.7)
Restricted to first birth in 1999–2006					
Preeclampsia	1.7 (1.5–1.9)	1.4 (1.1–1.9)	1.4 (1.3–1.5)	1.8 (1.5–2.1)	1.5 (1.3–1.6)
Preterm preeclampsia	4.1 (3.3–5.1)	3.0 (1.8–4.8)	2.4 (2.0–2.9)	3.3 (2.5–4.4)	3.4 (2.8–4.1)
Total material	***Exposure, condition in first pregnancy***				
Outcome of second pregnancy	LBW	Stillbirth	SGA10	SGA2.5	Preterm
Preeclampsia	2.4 (2.3–2.6)	2.6 (2.3–3.0)	1.4 (1.3–1.5)	1.9 (1.7–2.0)	2.1 (2.0–2.3)
Preterm preeclampsia	5.9 (5.2–6.8)	5.9 (4.7–7.4)	2.5 (2.2–2.8)	3.8 (3.3–4.5)	4.4 (3.8–5.0)
Restricted to first birth in 1999–2006					
Preeclampsia	3.0 (2.7–3.4)	3.0 (2.2–3.9)	1.5 (1.3–1.7)	2.2 (1.9–2.6)	2.6 (2.3–3.0)
Preterm preeclampsia	7.9 (6.3–9.7)	7.4 (4.9–11.2)	2.7 (2.1–3.3)	4.3 (3.2–5.7)	4.8 (3.9–6.1)

Women with recurrent preeclampsia were excluded.
For abbreviations, see text.

may cover more than one biological entity, and differences between preeclampsia in the first and subsequent pregnancies contribute to the impression that different causes may be involved. In recent years the proportion of preeclampsia with preterm delivery has increased due to early induction of pregnancy. This clinical practice has also changed important epidemiological features of preeclampsia.

References

1. Basso O, Rasmussen S, Weinberg C R *et al.* Trends in fetal and infant survival following preeclampsia. *Jama* 2006; **296**(11): 1357–62.
2. Barton J R, Sibai B M. Prediction and prevention of recurrent preeclampsia. *Obstet Gynecol* 2008; **112**(2 Pt 1): 359–72.
3. Skjaerven R, Wilcox A J, Lie R T, Irgens L M. Selective fertility and the distortion of perinatal mortality. *Am J Epidemiol* 1988; **128**(6): 1352–63.
4. Skjaerven R, Melve K K. Selective fertility: the examples of perinatal death and preeclampsia. *Norsk Epidemiologi* 2007; **17**(2): 175–80.
5. Need J A. Pre-eclampsia in pregnancies by different fathers: immunological studies. *BMJ* 1975; **1**(5957): 548–9.
6. Robillard P Y, Dekker G A, Hulsey T C. Revisiting the epidemiological standard of preeclampsia: primigravidity or primipaternity? *Eur J Obstet Gynecol Reprod Biol* 1999; **84**(1): 37–41.
7. Robillard P Y, Hulsey T C, Alexander G R *et al.* Paternity patterns and risk of preeclampsia in the last pregnancy in multiparae. *J Reprod Immunol* 1993; **24**(1): 1–12.
8. Trupin L S, Simon L P, Eskenazi B. Change in paternity: a risk factor for preeclampsia in multiparas. *Epidemiology* 1996; **7**(3): 240–4.
9. Dekker G A, Sibai B M. Etiology and pathogenesis of preeclampsia: current concepts [see comments]. *Am J Obstet Gynecol* 1998; **179**(5): 1359–75.
10. Dekker G A, Robillard P Y, Hulsey T C. Immune maladaptation in the etiology of preeclampsia: a review of corroborative epidemiologic studies. *Obstet Gynecol Surv* 1998; **53**(6): 377–82.
11. Basso O, Christensen K, Olsen J. Higher risk of pre-eclampsia after change of partner: an effect of longer

interpregnancy intervals? *Epidemiology* 2001; **12**(6): 624–9.

12. Skjaerven R, Wilcox A J, Lie R T. The interval between pregnancies and the risk of preeclampsia. *N Engl J Med* 2002; **346**(1): 33–8.
13. Trogstad L I, Eskild A, Magnus P, Samuelsen S O, Nesheim B I. Changing paternity and time since last pregnancy; the impact on pre-eclampsia risk. A study of 547 238 women with and without previous pre-eclampsia. *Int J Epidemiol* 2001; **30**(6): 1317–22.
14. Deen M E, Ruurda L G, Wang J, Dekker G A. Risk factors for preeclampsia in multiparous women: primipaternity versus the birth interval hypothesis. *J Matern Fetal Neonatal Med* 2006; **19**(2): 79–84.
15. Dekker G, Robillard P Y. The birth interval hypothesis: does it really indicate the end of the primipaternity hypothesis? *J Reprod Immunol* 2003; **59**(2): 245–51.
16. Hjartardottir S, Leifsson B G, Geirsson R T, Steinthorsdottir V. Paternity change and the recurrence risk in familial hypertensive disorder in pregnancy. *Hypertens Pregnancy* 2004; **23**(2): 219–25.
17. Zhang J, Patel G. Partner change and perinatal outcomes: a systematic review. *Paediatr Perinat Epidemiol* 2007; **21** (Suppl 1): 46–57.
18. Cnattingius S, Mills J L, Yuen J, Eriksson O, Salonen H. The paradoxical effect of smoking in preeclamptic pregnancies: smoking reduces the incidence but increases the rates of perinatal mortality, abruptio placentae, and intrauterine growth restriction. *Am J Obstet Gynecol* 1997; **177**(1): 156–61.
19. Vatten L J, Skjaerven R. Effects on pregnancy outcome of changing partner between first two births: prospective population study. *BMJ* 2003; **327**(7424): 1138.
20. Dekker G, Robillard P Y. Pre-eclampsia: is the immune maladaptation hypothesis still standing? An epidemiological update. *J Reprod Immunol* 2007; **76**(1–2): 8–16.
21. Li D K, Wi S. Changing paternity and the risk of preeclampsia/eclampsia in the subsequent pregnancy. *Am J Epidemiol* 2000; **151**(1): 57–62.
22. Lie R T, Rasmussen S, Brunborg H *et al.* Fetal and maternal contributions to risk of pre-eclampsia: population based study. *BMJ* 1998; **316**(7141): 1343–7.
23. Guelinckx I, Devlieger R, Beckers K, Vansant G. Maternal obesity: pregnancy complications, gestational weight gain and nutrition. *Obes Rev* 2008; **9**(2): 140–50.
24. Catalano P M. Increasing maternal obesity and weight gain during pregnancy: the obstetric problems of plentitude. *Obstet Gynecol* 2007; **110**(4): 743–4.
25. Catalano P M. Management of obesity in pregnancy. *Obstet Gynecol* 2007; **109**(2 Pt 1): 419–33.
26. Villamor E, Cnattingius S. Interpregnancy weight change and risk of adverse pregnancy outcomes: a population-based study. *Lancet* 2006; **368**(9542): 1164–70.
27. Esplin M S, Fausett M B, Fraser A *et al.* Paternal and maternal components of the predisposition to preeclampsia. *N Engl J Med* 2001; **344**(12): 867–72.
28. Salonen Ros H, Lichtenstein P, Lipworth L, Cnattingius S. Genetic effects on the liability of developing pre-eclampsia and gestational hypertension. *Am J Med Genet* 2000; **91**(4): 256–60.
29. Cnattingius S, Reilly M, Pawitan Y, Lichtenstein P. Maternal and fetal genetic factors account for most of familial aggregation of preeclampsia: a population-based Swedish cohort study. *Am J Med Genet A* 2004; **130A**(4): 365–71.
30. Skjaerven R, Vatten L J, Wilcox A J *et al.* Recurrence of pre-eclampsia across generations: exploring fetal and maternal genetic components in a population based cohort. *BMJ* 2005; **331**(7521): 877.
31. Eskenazi B, Fenster L, Sidney S, Elkin E P. Fetal growth retardation in infants of multiparous and nulliparous women with preeclampsia. *Am J Obstet Gynecol* 1993; **169**(5): 1112–8.
32. Xiong X, Mayes D, Demianczuk N *et al.* Impact of pregnancy-induced hypertension on fetal growth. *Am J Obstet Gynecol* 1999; **180**(1 Pt 1): 207–13.
33. Vatten L J, Skjaerven R. Is pre-eclampsia more than one disease? *BJOG* 2004; **111**(4): 298–302.
34. Skjaerven R, Gjessing H K, Bakketeig L S. Birthweight by gestational age in Norway. *Acta Obstet Gynecol Scand* 2000; **79**(6): 440–9.
35. Xiong X, Demianczuk N N, Buekens P, Saunders L D. Association of preeclampsia with high birth weight for age. *Am J Obstet Gynecol* 2000; **183**(1): 148–55.
36. Rasmussen S, Irgens L M, Albrechtsen S, Dalaker K. Predicting preeclampsia in the second pregnancy from low birth weight in the first pregnancy. *Obstet Gynecol* 2000; **96**(5 Pt 1): 696–700.
37. Zhang J, Troendle J F, Levine R J. Risks of hypertensive disorders in the second pregnancy. *Paediatr Perinat Epidemiol* 2001; **15**(3): 226–31.
38. Zetterstrom K, Lindeberg S, Haglund B, Magnuson A, Hanson U. Being born small for gestational age increases the risk of severe pre-eclampsia. *BJOG* 2007; **114**(3): 319–24.
39. Rasmussen S, Irgens L M. Pregnancy-induced hypertension in women who were born small. *Hypertension* 2007; **49**(4): 806–12.

40. Ness R B, Roberts J M. Heterogeneous causes constituting the single syndrome of preeclampsia: a hypothesis and its implications. *Am J Obstet Gynecol* 1996; **175**(5): 1365–70.

41. Roberts J M, Redman C W. Pre-eclampsia: more than pregnancy-induced hypertension. *Lancet* 1993; **341** (8858): 1447–51.

42. Roberts J M, Catov J M. Preeclampsia more than 1 disease: or is it? *Hypertension* 2008; **51**(4): 989–90.

43. Haig D. Genetic conflicts in human pregnancy. *Q Rev Biol* 1993; **68**(4): 495–532.

44. Irgens H U, Reisaeter L, Irgens L M, Lie R T. Long term mortality of mothers and fathers after pre-eclampsia: population based cohort study. *BMJ* 2001; **323**(7323): 1213–7.

45. Funai E F, Friedlander Y, Paltiel O *et al.* Long-term mortality after preeclampsia. *Epidemiology* 2005; **16**(2): 206–15.

46. Vikse B E, Irgens L M, Leivestad T, Skjaerven R, Iversen B M. Preeclampsia and the risk of end-stage renal disease. *N Engl J Med* 2008; **359**(8): 800–9.

47. Trogstad L, Skrondal A, Stoltenberg C *et al.* Recurrence risk of preeclampsia in twin and singleton pregnancies. *Am J Med Genet A* 2004; **126**(1): 41–5.

48. Smith G C, Shah I, White I R, Pell J P, Dobbie R. Previous preeclampsia, preterm delivery, and delivery of a small for gestational age infant and the risk of unexplained stillbirth in the second pregnancy: a retrospective cohort study, Scotland, 1992–2001. *Am J Epidemiol* 2007; **165**(2): 194–202.

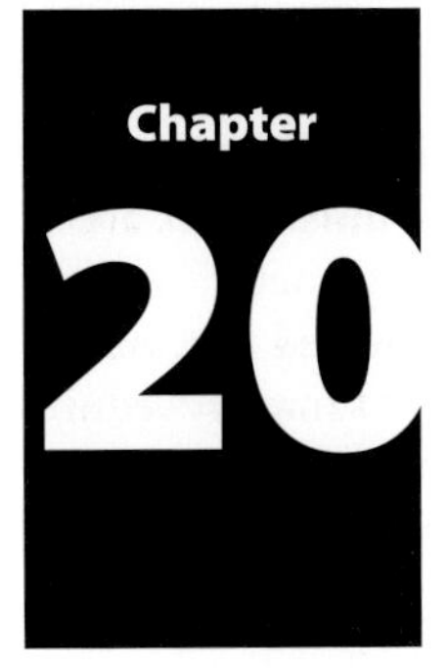

Assisted reproductive technology and the risk of poor pregnancy outcome

Marc J. N. C. Keirse[1] and Frans M. Helmerhorst[2]

[1]Department of Obstetrics, Gynaecology and Reproductive Medicine, Flinders University, Adelaide, South Australia, Australia
[2]Department of Gynaecology & Reproductive Medicine and Department of Clinical Epidemiology, Leiden University Medical Center, Leiden, The Netherlands

Introduction

As the very purpose of assisted reproductive technology (ART) is to assist infertile people in creating a healthy baby, anything short of this is basically a poor outcome. The majority of such poor outcomes are failure to achieve pregnancy and early pregnancy loss, but these are not dealt with in this chapter. Neither are the rare life-threatening situations, such as ovarian hyperstimulation syndrome, or other maternal morbidity that is more common after assisted than after natural conceptions [1].

This chapter will deal with perinatal outcomes, i.e. outcomes of pregnancies that have surpassed the early hurdles and have evolved far enough to result in a birth, internationally defined as the separation from its mother of a fetus weighing 500 g or more [2]. Although fetal weights vary widely, especially among pregnancies that end too early for one reason or another [3], this almost invariably implies a gestational age of at least 20 weeks. In Australia, where every fetus with a gestational age of 20 weeks or more is registered as a birth, fetuses of 500 g or more at 20 weeks account for less than 1 in 100 000 births [4]. Also, most studies on perinatal outcome after ART apply a 500 g, if not a 1000 g, cut-off point, with some using or adding gestational age limits ranging between 20 and 28 weeks. This can create considerable variation among studies particularly for an outcome such as perinatal death [5]. While this limits the generalizability of comparisons across studies, it would not affect within study comparisons provided the same criteria and definitions are applied to both ART and control groups.

It has been argued, however, that meta-analyses of published comparative studies grossly overestimate the risk of poor outcome after ART in comparison to population-based data [6]. In part, this may be due to differences in definitions as to what constitutes ART and what does not, with population-based studies more likely to ignore low-technology fertility-enhancing treatments and include these among the natural conceptions.

Whatever the explanation may be, it emphasizes the need for clear definitions of both the outcomes studied, and the exposures that are alleged to lead to these outcomes, not to mention due consideration of the limitations of the data that are available

Definitions and limitations of the data

Definitions of assisted reproductive technology (ART)

ART involves a whole gamut of interventions, used either as a single intervention or in combination, to address alleged dysfunction of one or more of the four crucial elements needed to achieve a successful pregnancy. These are: the presence of (1) a suitable oocyte and (2) a suitable sperm cell; (3) an opportunity for these two to meet and join; and (4) a suitable environment for the resulting zygote to develop. In about a third of all infertile couples it is either not known where the primary problem is or it is not confined to only one of these four elements. Thence, a whole diversity of treatments has evolved that, along with their acronyms, tend to confuse the non-initiated just as much as they confuse those who wish to explore what causes the difference in outcome between assisted and natural conceptions.

The European Society of Human Reproduction and Embryology (ESHRE) [7], in its position paper 'Good Clinical Treatment in Assisted Reproduction', tabulated the following treatments as assisted reproductive technology (ART): 'ovarian induction'[1], intrauterine insemination (IUI), *in vitro* fertilization (IVF), intracytoplasmic sperm injection (ICSI), and cryopreservation of embryos. The American Society of Reproductive Medicine (ASRM) [8], in its guide for patients on 'Assisted reproductive technologies', refers to several phases and variations of IVF: ovarian stimulation, ICSI, cryopreservation of embryos, gamete intrafallopian transfer (GIFT), zygote intrafallopian transfer (ZIFT), donor sperm, donor eggs, and donor embryos, as well as surrogacy/gestational carrier. Other definitions refer to ART as treatments in which both oocytes and sperm are handled outside the body [9].

In this chapter, we will consider any of the following as a form of ART when assessing the effect of ART on pregnancy outcome. Thereafter, we shall try to elucidate whether some of these variations or specific elements of ART carry greater or smaller risks of poor outcome than others.

- Controlled ovarian hyperstimulation (COHS) intended to enhance follicle maturation up to the point of ovulation. It is usually achieved with either clomiphene citrate, a non-steroidal antiestrogen that occupies the nuclear estrogen receptor in the hypothalamus and pituitary, thereby reducing the inhibiting action of estradiol and stimulating the release of follicle-stimulating hormone (FSH), or directly by administration of the gonadotropin FSH. The FSH glycoprotein that is administered can be derived either from the urine of postmenopausal women or from recombinant technology.
- Ovulation induction generally with human chorionic gonadotropin (hCG) (derived from the urine of pregnant women), which has a similar action on the dominant follicle(s) as the endogenous luteinizing hormone (LH) or, more recently, with a recombinant LH.
- Intrauterine insemination (IUI). This is commonly conducted after mild COHS (with clomiphene citrate or with gonadotropins) to obtain maturation of a maximum of two or three follicles. Selected spermatozoa are inseminated in the uterus, generally also after ovulation induction with hCG.
- *In vitro* fertilization (IVF): a procedure that consists of COHS, ovulation induction, oocyte retrieval, *in vitro* fertilization of the oocyte, embryo culture, and embryo transfer (ET).
- Gamete intrafallopian transfer (GIFT). After COHS and ovulation induction, the oocytes are retrieved by laparoscopy and the gametes (oocytes and spermatozoa) are then transferred together to the woman's fallopian tubes in the same procedure; fertilization takes place in the fallopian tube rather than in the laboratory.
- Zygote intrafallopian transfer (ZIFT) is similar to an IVF procedure, except that the fertilized oocyte is transferred to the fallopian tube by laparoscopy rather than to the uterus.
- Intracytoplasmic sperm injection (ICSI) is an IVF procedure with the addition of a single sperm being injected directly into each mature egg.
- *In vitro* maturation (IVM) of oocytes is a relatively new ART technique in which relatively immature oocytes are harvested without prior ovarian stimulation. Maturation occurs in the laboratory before fertilization using either IVF or ICSI.
- Cryopreservation of either sperm, oocytes, or embryos.
- Embryo transfer (ET) after 'donation' of either sperm, oocytes, or embryo.
- Surrogacy carrier, which implies that the oocyte is derived from one woman while the pregnancy is carried by another.

Definitions of perinatal outcome

The most direct and most relevant measure of perinatal outcome is the live birth of a healthy neonate. Defining a healthy neonate may seem easy enough, but it is not. A preterm infant born at 35 weeks' gestation may seem perfectly healthy, but by virtue of being born too early is still likely to experience significant health problems both in the short and in the long term [10,11]. Birth defects, a major concern of new ART procedures that has received considerable attention in the past, are a case in point. Extreme variability among studies in both definition and ascertainment of congenital malformations has been noted [12,13]. A large proportion of malformations is not detected at birth and, whether detected or not, some, including some cardiac malformations, are of little consequence throughout infancy. A systematic review by Hansen *et al.* [13] showed several methodological limitations of the available data, including inadequate or absent definition of a birth defect, inadequate information on how, when, and by whom birth defects had been ascertained, different methods of assessing birth

[1] We assume that this does not imply that ovaries are 'induced', but refers to ovarian stimulation and ovulation induction.

defects in ART and comparison groups, lack of suitable comparison data, and greater surveillance of the ART group than applied after natural conceptions.

We have chosen to address primarily perinatal death, defined as either stillbirth or death within the first week of life (early neonatal death), as an outcome that is entirely unambiguous. Considering the rarity of this outcome, ranging from 4.7 to 10.9 per 1000 births among 24 member states of the European Union (EU) in 2004 [14], we have added (very) low birth weight and (very) preterm birth as the most commonly used surrogate measures of poor pregnancy outcome and infant health.

In accordance with international definitions [2], low birth weight (LBW) is defined as a weight of < 2500 g, very low birth weight (VLBW) as < 1500 g, and extremely low birth weight (ELBW) as < 1000 g. Preterm birth is defined as birth before 37 completed weeks of gestation, very preterm as less than 32 weeks, and severely preterm as less than 28 weeks.

A large number of studies of pregnancy outcome after ART also provide data on small for gestational age (SGA), usually defined as a birth weight below the 10th centile of weight for gestation. The underlying assumption is that this parameter can provide some information on the (in)adequacy of fetal growth. However, this also assumes that intrauterine growth restriction occurs with the same frequency (i.e. 10%) at all gestational ages, which is a clear fallacy [3]. There is a good deal of evidence which suggests that factors which influence gestational age at birth also influence weight for gestation [3]. From the available studies, it is not always clear what birth weight for gestational age standards were used [15]. Thus, is it often not clear either whether parity-specific standards were used, although parity generally differs substantially between ART and natural conceptions and greatly influences birth weight [3]. We, therefore, chose not to incorporate such data to avoid comparisons that may not stand up to scrutiny. Nonetheless, there are clear indications that small for gestational age is significantly more common after ART than after natural conceptions [12,15,16], but controlling for differences in gestational age and the frequency of preterm birth in such data remains problematic.

Limitations of the available data

It is clear that, in comparison with natural conceptions, outcomes of ART are influenced by three main factors: first, the background characteristics of people relying on ART to achieve pregnancy, the most common being higher maternal age, nulliparity, and a history of infertility, all of which are known contributors to a less than average perinatal outcome [17,18, 19,20]; second, the ART techniques themselves, which may influence gametes, zygotes, and implantation in a number of ways that are not fully understood [21]; and third, the propensity of ART specialists to aim for a pregnancy of whatever nature, thereby overcoming what thousands of years of evolution have tended to ensure: singleton instead of multiple pregnancies [22]. Only a few decades ago, multifetal pregnancies were heralded in the media as major achievements of ART. Whilst such outcomes are now generally considered as irresponsible, it may take a few more decades before rates of twin pregnancies that exceed those of natural conceptions are viewed in the same way [23,24].

Without doubt multiple pregnancies are the main culprit of poor pregnancy outcome after ART versus natural conceptions. It was neatly established more than 50 years ago, well before the advent of ART, that every additional fetus in human pregnancy curtails both fetal weight and length of gestation [25], which are powerful predictors of infant health and survival. Where policies of single ET (SET) have not yet been instituted, there usually is a more than 20-fold difference in the frequency of twin pregnancies between ART and natural conceptions. The need to differentiate multiple pregnancies from singleton pregnancies when assessing the effect of ART seems to be well recognized. It must also be considered, though, that the large excess of twin pregnancies among ART compared with natural pregnancies is almost entirely due to dizygotic twins [26,27], which are well known to have better perinatal outcomes than monozygotic twins [28]. Unless chorionicity or zygosity is taken into account, any comparison of outcomes between ART and natural conceptions is likely to be seriously biased [15].

Controlling for all other elements, let alone adjusting for the many confounders that are not known, is an exercise that is doomed to fail and responsible for a great deal of contradictory information in the literature. Controlled studies of pregnancy outcome after ART, whether population based or comparative cohort studies (often erroneously referred to as case–control studies) [16,29,30,31], usually derive their controls from birth registrations. These are not necessarily accurate with respect to important birth outcomes, even perinatal death [32,33], let alone in registering the mode of conception [34]. Poor registration of the mode of conception does not apply only to low-technology fertility-enhancing treatments. Several countries have registers for *in vitro* fertilization (IVF) [35] and all industrialized nations have birth registrations, but joining these is not an exercise that has received a great deal of attention. IVF registers may register pregnancies with little concern for their outcome [36]. At the other end, mode of conception is usually of little concern when registering a birth. Among 15 member states of the European Union (EU), for example, only Flanders in Belgium, Finland, Germany, and Sweden collected information about infertility management as part of their medical registration of births in 2000 [37]. By 2004, only half of the then 24 EU members could provide some data on births after ART and only six regions or nations (Flanders, France, Italy, the Netherlands, Slovenia, and Finland) could provide data by type of ART [14].

In this context it must be realized that birth, in addition to anything else, is also a public event, whereas conception rarely is. It is fallacious to assume that absence of information on the mode of conception in birth registrations implies natural conception. Flanders, in Belgium, which has been registering mode of conception as part of its birth registry for many years, provides an excellent example of this. Of 8.1% of births with missing data on mode of conception between 1991 and 2002 more than 95% were due to deliberate omissions for privacy reasons [38]. These women were more likely to be nulliparous and less likely to have twins or preterm infants than women with recorded mode of conception [38]. Noteworthy too is that the percentage of births with unregistered mode of conception decreased significantly over time from 11.9% in 1992–93 to 6.1% in 2002–03, suggesting that the increase in ART has also removed some of the secrecy surrounding it. An earlier comparison between medical birth and IVF registrations in Finland showed that about 20% of IVF births were not reported as such in the medical birth register [34]. Whether and to what extent such observations are responsible for two- to three-fold differences in the percentage of ART among women giving birth in neighboring countries (e.g. 4.5% in Flanders versus 2.6% in the Netherlands and 4.9% in France versus 1.7% in Italy) [14] is impossible to determine. Yet, they need to be taken into account when interpreting the results of so-named population-based studies.

It would be wrong to assume that the above is of no importance in the interpretation of data from comparative cohort studies. These usually attempt to correct for a number of influential confounders, such as plurality, parity, infant gender, maternal age, and occasionally others, such as smoking or socioeconomic status, that might be known. However, the way in which so-named matching or controlling for various characteristics is achieved can have a major influence on the comparisons. For example, a large comparative study between assisted and natural conceptions reported a perinatal mortality rate of 5.2 per 1000 among natural conceptions when matching ART and natural conceptions for maternal age and infant sex [30]. Yet, the perinatal mortality increased more than two-fold, to 12.1 per 1000, among natural conceptions, when parity and gestational age were added to the matching criteria [30]. It is not always known either whether matching between cases and controls was done individually, on a one to one basis, or by group, creating groups with similar proportions of the known predictor values.

A further complicating factor in assessing published data is an apparent tendency among ART specialists to insert too many eggs not only in the uterus, but also into the literature [23]. Several publications dealing with the same cohort or with partially overlapping cohorts is a regrettably common phenomenon in the literature dealing with perinatal outcome after ART. Often it is impossible to disassemble such data into unique nominators or denominators.

The above indicates that published data on perinatal outcome after ART, including systematic reviews of such data, need to be interpreted with a great deal of caution. Clearly, the most satisfactory way to assess differences in outcome between ART and natural conceptions would be a controlled trial with randomized assignment to either receive or not receive a particular form of ART [39]. However, none large enough to address perinatal outcome has been conducted and it is questionable whether any ever should be.

Perinatal outcome in singleton pregnancies

The first indication that the perinatal outcome of singleton pregnancies is worse after ART than after

Table 20.1. Meta-analysis summary data with 95% confidence intervals for selected birth outcomes in singleton pregnancies after ART versus natural conception as reported by Helmerhorst *et al.* [15] and Jackson *et al.* [12]

Outcome	Relative risk[a] (Helmerhorst *et al.* [12])		
	Matched studies[b]	Unmatched studies	Odds ratio[a] (Jackson *et al.* [12])
Birth < 32 weeks	3.27 (2.03–5.28)	no data	3.10 (2.00–4.80)
Birth < 37 weeks	2.04 (1.80–2.32)	1.94 (1.31–2.88)	1.95 (1.73–2.20)
Birth weight < 1500 g	3.00 (2.07–4.36)	1.57 (0.21–11.7)	2.70 (2.31–3.14)
Birth weight < 2500 g	1.70 (1.50–1.92)	2.58 (1.80–3.60)	1.77 (1.40–2.22)
Cesarean section	1.54 (1.44–1.66)	2.33 (1.95–2.79)	2.13 (1.72–2.63)
Neonatal intensive care	1.27 (1.16–1.40)	1.38 (0.67–2.86)	1.60 (1.30–1.96)
Perinatal death	1.68 (1.11–2.55)	3.77 (1.15–12.4)	2.19 (1.61–2.98)

[a] With 95% confidence intervals between brackets.
[b] Matched refers to studies in which cases and comparison groups were matched for a number of important predictors of outcome, mostly including maternal age, parity, and infant gender.

natural conception dates back nearly 25 years [40]. In the years thereafter, several comparative studies confirmed that association [30,41,42,43,44,45], while others did not [29,31,46]. It took nearly 20 years, though, before any attempt was made to systematically review the available evidence using the technique of meta-analysis that had become popularized in the meantime. Two such reviews were published in 2004 [12,15]. Although they differed in several respects, both reviews only considered studies with a comparison group of natural conceptions. So, case reports, case series, registry reports, and studies without a comparison group were all excluded.

The first review, by Helmerhorst *et al.* [15], incorporated all forms of ART, consisting predominantly of IVF, but also IUI, while the review of Jackson *et al.* [12] attempted to address specifically IVF pregnancies. Jackson *et al.* [12] required studies to be adjusted for maternal age and parity and, therefore, excluded some studies that were included in the review of Helmerhorst *et al.* [15]. On the other hand, Jackson *et al.* [12] included three studies that were excluded by Helmerhorst *et al.* [15] because of inadequate data. Despite these differences, the conclusions, summarized in Table 20.1, were remarkably similar.

Virtually all of the studies included in both reviews originated from Europe, but in the same year Schieve *et al.* [9] reported on singleton live births from ART in the USA in 1996–2000 registered by the Centers for Disease Control and Prevention. ART was defined as treatments in which both oocytes and sperm are handled outside the body, and outcomes studied were preterm birth, term and preterm low birth weight, and very low birth weight. All of these occurred significantly more frequently after ART than in the general population [9]. Another review of singleton IVF and ICSI pregnancies versus natural singleton conception was published the following year [16]. It too differed in a number of respects, but basically confirmed the conclusions of the two previous reviews.

Perinatal mortality

Systematic reviews of the various studies (Table 20.1) indicate an approximately two-fold increase in perinatal mortality in ART compared with naturally conceived singletons. Given the uncertainty as to what contributes to this marked increase in mortality other than the higher frequency of preterm and very preterm birth, we conducted a further analysis on more than 450 000 singleton births in Flanders, Belgium, registered by the Study Center for Perinatal Epidemiology (SPE) in the years 2000 to 2007. The SPE registration covers all births in Flanders (Northern Belgium), with a population of about 6 million. Excluding births with unknown mode of conception, we calculated the risk for a singleton fetus that had reached a weight of 500 g either to be stillborn or to die in the first week of life at any time thereafter. The method for doing so was pioneered and described by Yudkin *et al.* in 1987 [47].

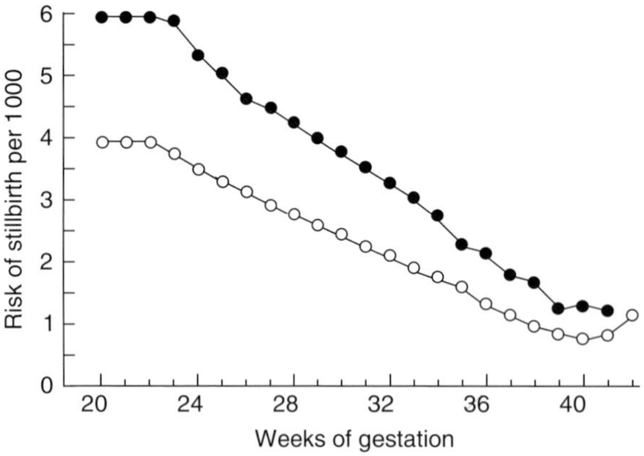

Fig. 20.1 Risk of subsequent stillbirth per 1000 unborn singleton fetuses at each week of gestation in ART (closed symbols) and naturally conceived (open symbols) pregnancies. Based on >450 000 singleton births with known mode of conception (4.2% after ART) registered by the Study Center for Perinatal Epidemiology in Flanders, Belgium, in 2000–2007.

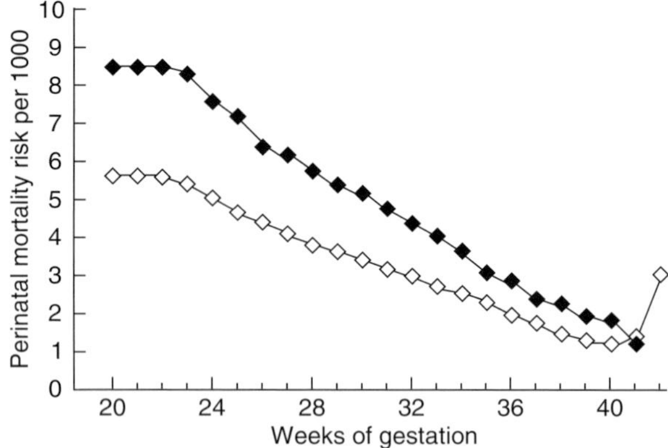

Fig. 20.3 Risk of perinatal death (stillbirth and early neonatal death) per 1000 unborn singleton fetuses at each week of gestation in ART (closed symbols) and naturally conceived (open symbols) pregnancies. Based on > 450 000 singleton births with known mode of conception (4.2% after ART) registered by the Study Center for Perinatal Epidemiology in Flanders, Belgium, in 2000–2007.

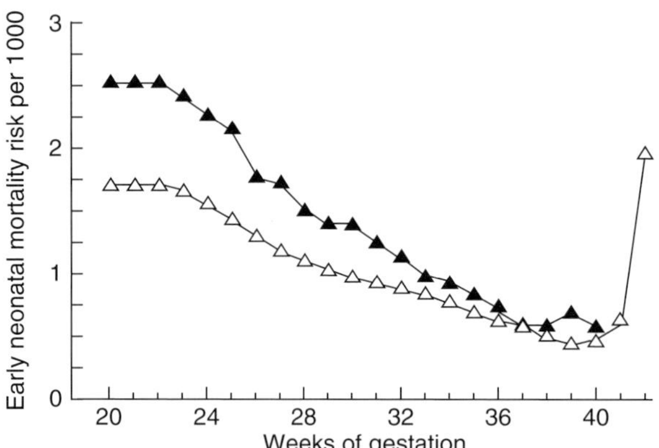

Fig. 20.2 Risk of death in the first week of life expressed per 1000 unborn singleton fetuses at each week of gestation in ART (closed symbols) and naturally conceived (open symbols) pregnancies. Based on > 450 000 singleton births with known mode of conception (4.2% after ART) registered by the Study Center for Perinatal Epidemiology in Flanders, Belgium, in 2000–2007.

The data show that the difference in the risk of stillbirth in particular (Fig. 20.1), but to a lesser extent also the risk of early neonatal death (Fig. 20.2), between ART and natural conceptions is sustained throughout gestation. Consistent with what has been argued previously [6], the data seem to confirm that the difference in risk in population-based studies tends to be smaller than systematic reviews of controlled studies would suggest, especially as the current data have not been corrected for confounders, such as maternal age, parity, and many others that may influence the difference between ART and natural conceptions. Nevertheless, they clearly indicate that the increased risk of perinatal death cannot be explained entirely by an increase in preterm birth as it is sustained up to 40 weeks of gestation, leveling off only thereafter as very few ART pregnancies are allowed to proceed postterm (Fig. 20.3). The conclusions were similar when the analyses were confined to normally formed infants.

Preterm and very preterm birth

Frequencies of preterm birth have been on the increase in most industrialized nations since the end of the last century, but rates, let alone the factors that contribute to them [38,48,49,50,51,52,53,54], are not always easy to interpret. For example, in the United States, preterm births increased from 7.3% to 8.4% between 1990 and 2000 in Whites, but decreased from 17.0% to 15.3% in Blacks [55]. In Flanders, preterm births in singleton pregnancies rose from 4.9% to 6.3% and very preterm births from 0.72% to 0.87% between 1991–93 and 2000–02 [38]. Rates of preterm among live born singletons varied from 4.4% in Ireland to 9.4% in Austria among 24 member states of the European Union in 2004 [14].

There is no doubt that some of the increase in preterm birth rates in singleton pregnancies is due to ART, an effect that was first reported nearly 25 years ago [40] and has been well demonstrated in systematic reviews since (Table 20.1). Using population-based data of more than 675 000 singleton births in

Table 20.2. Crude and adjusted odds ratios for the effect of ART versus natural conception on the frequency of preterm birth and low birth weight among 675 422 singleton pregnancies in Flanders, Belgium, from 1991 to 2002

Outcome	Odds ratio (95% confidence interval)		
	Unadjusted	Adjusted[a]	Preterm adjusted[b]
Birth < 28 weeks	2.22 (1.84–2.67)	1.99 (1.65–2.39)	Not applicable
Birth < 32 weeks	2.05 (1.82–2.30)	1.81 (1.61–2.03)	Not applicable
Birth < 37 weeks	1.72 (1.64–1.81)	1.57 (1.50–1.65)	Not applicable
Birth weight < 1000 g	2.46 (2.08–2.90)	2.07 (1.76–2.44)	1.38 (1.16–1.63)
Birth weight < 1500 g	2.25 (2.01–2.51)	1.91 (1.70–2.13)	1.21 (1.14–1.46)
Birth weight < 2500 g	1.66 (1.57–1.75)	1.45 (1.38–1.53)	1.17 (1.09–1.25)

[a] Adjusted for maternal age, parity, year of conception, induction of labor, and elective cesarean section.
[b] Adjusted for maternal age, parity, year of conception, induction of labor, elective cesarean section, and gestational age categories.
Based on data from Keirse *et al.* [38].

Flanders, it was shown that this effect is not limited to late preterm births, but is also seen for very (< 32 weeks) and severely (< 28 weeks) preterm births [38]. Indeed, the effect appears to be larger for the very early preterm births (Table 20.2), which is consistent with data of the systematic reviews [12,15].

The effect remains when adjustment is made for maternal age, parity, year of conception, and also for obstetric intervention to end pregnancy whether by induction of labor or by elective cesarean section (Table 20.2). The latter is an important observation given that obstetric intervention both at term and preterm is far more common in ART than in naturally conceived pregnancies [12,15,38]. The frequency of obstetric intervention to end pregnancy was 38.2% (95% CI 38.1–38.3) in singleton pregnancies from natural conceptions, compared with 43.0% (95% CI 42.3–43.7) for singleton pregnancies after ART in that Flemish cohort [38]. In preterm pregnancies, however, the difference was from 34.3% (95% CI 33.8–34.8) to 41.2% (95% CI 39.0–43.5), virtually all of it related to a higher rate of elective preterm cesarean sections before the onset of labor [38].

Low birth weight and very low birth weight

The frequency of low birth weight after ART obviously relates to differences in parity but also to differences in the gestational age distribution compared with natural conceptions. One would expect, therefore, that low birth weight will be more common in ART singletons. The systematic reviews confirm this in that the frequency of both low birth weight and very low birth weight is significantly higher after ART than after natural conceptions (see Table 20.1) [12,15]. Interestingly and similar to what is seen with preterm birth, the differential effect appears to be larger for very low birth weight than for all low birth weight infants (see Table 20.1).

We assessed this in a multivariable analysis on the same 1991 to 2002 Flemish cohort mentioned above [38], both with and without correcting for known confounders including differences in gestational age. The data, shown in Table 20.2, indicate a clear gradient with the frequency of birth weights < 1000 g being significantly more affected than those < 2500 g. The gradient becomes substantially less, with overlapping 95% confidence intervals, when differences in gestational age are taken into account, but it does not disappear entirely. The difference with natural conceptions, however, remains statistically significant for all low birth weight categories, indicating that there are independent influences of ART on both gestational age and weight at birth.

Perinatal outcome in twin pregnancies

There can be no doubt that the practice of inserting multiple embryos in the uterus to have at least one healthy infant has been counterproductive in terms of

Table 20.3. Meta-analysis summary data with 95% confidence intervals for selected birth outcomes in twin pregnancies after ART versus natural conception as reported by Helmerhorst *et al.* [15]

Outcome	Relative risk (95% confidence interval)[a]	
	Matched studies[b]	Unmatched studies
Birth < 32 weeks	0.95 (0.78–1.15)	1.20 (0.82–1.78)
Birth < 37 weeks	1.07 (1.02–1.13)	0.99 (0.80–1.23)
Birth weight < 1500 g	0.89 (0.74–1.07)	1.46 (1.01–2.11)
Birth weight < 2500 g	1.03 (0.99–1.08)	1.12 (1.06–1.19)
Cesarean section	1.21 (1.11–1.32)	1.17 (1.06–1.29)
Neonatal intensive care	1.05 (1.01–1.09)	1.26 (1.16–1.36)
Perinatal death	0.58 (0.44–0.77)	0.84 (0.53–1.32)

[a] Only 3 of 17 studies included in the meta-analysis controlled for zygosity [15].
[b] Matched refers to studies in which cases and comparison groups were matched for a number of important predictors of outcome, mostly including maternal age, parity, and infant gender.

perinatal outcome and hardship inflicted on families and society [22]. While we [22,23] and others [24], have argued this for many years, most responsible ART centers nowadays have either adopted SET (single embryo transfer) policies or vacillate between SET and DET (dual embryo transfer; often wrongly referred to as 'double' embryo transfer [24,56,57], as if the embryos are duplicates of each other). Some countries have made reimbursement of IVF procedures dependent on the implementation of such policies [58,59].

Contrary to the attention devoted to embryo reduction and the 'vanishing twin syndrome', remarkably little attention has been devoted to differences in outcome between naturally and ART conceived twin pregnancies. This is not surprising given that the potential for bias in such comparisons by far exceeds that of comparisons among singleton pregnancies. Chorionicity, which is the main confounder in such comparisons [26], is rarely available in birth registers or other data sets from which comparison groups tend to be drawn.

One systematic review is available, though [15]. Its results, based on 10 matched and 7 non-matched comparative studies, are summarized in Table 20.3. While these need to be interpreted with caution, it would seem that people have taken an excessively great deal of comfort from the fact that twin pregnancies from ART generally seem to do equally well or, in terms of perinatal mortality, even somewhat better than naturally conceived twins. To assess the validity of that assumption in the broadest of terms, we conducted logistic regression analyses uncorrected for zygosity on all twin births registered by the Study Center for Perinatal Epidemiology in Flanders, Belgium, from 1991 to 2002 (Table 20.4). The results are, therefore, heavily biased in favor of ART given that only a small proportion of these twins would be monozygotic compared with approximately 30% of the naturally conceived twin pregnancies [26,27]. This is notwithstanding that monozygotic twinning is more common with ART than with natural conceptions for reasons that are not entirely elucidated [27,59].

Contrary to what might have been expected from the systematic review (see Table 20.3) [15], there was no difference in perinatal mortality between ART and naturally conceived twins, despite their zygosity advantage and a marked increase in the rate of obstetric intervention, both induction of labor and cesarean section (see Table 20.4). Preterm birth and low birth weight were more common in ART twins than in naturally conceived twins. The difference in low birth weight disappeared after controlling for maternal confounders and for elective delivery in particular. Nonetheless, given that 36% of twin pregnancies are the result of ART compared with only 3% of singleton pregnancies [38], little comfort with regard to perinatal health can be derived from these data (Table 20.4).

Elements contributing to poor perinatal outcome in singletons after ART

Infertility or its treatment

It is reasonably well established that a history of failure to conceive is associated with poorer than average perinatal outcome, including perinatal death [19], irrespective of whether infertility treatment is instituted or not. The issue, therefore, is not whether infertility itself rather than its treatment contributes to the poorer outcomes of ART, but how large the contribution of each is likely to be. Unfortunately, there is no clear answer to it.

Romundstad *et al.* [20] recently reported on more than a million singleton births using data from the

Table 20.4. Crude and adjusted odds ratios for the effect of ART versus natural conception on perinatal outcome in 8016 naturally conceived and 4538 ART twin pregnancies in Flanders, Belgium, from 1991 to 2002

Outcome	Odds ratio (95% confidence interval)		
	Unadjusted	Adjusted	P value[a]
Birth < 28 weeks	1.10 (0.94–1.30)		n.s.
Birth < 32 weeks	1.04 (0.95–1.15)		n.s.
Birth < 37 weeks	1.18 (1. 12–1.25)	1.09 (1.04–1.16) [b]	0.002
Birth weight < 1000 g	1.10 (0.95–1.28)		n.s.
Birth weight < 1500 g	0.99 (0.90–1.09)		n.s.
Birth weight < 2500 g	1.13 (1.08–1.19)	0.99 (0.96–1.06) [b]	n.s.
Cesarean section	1.28 (1.21–1.34)	1.16 (1.10–1.22) [c]	< 0.001
Induction of labor	1.09 (1.03–1.16)	1.13 (1.06–1.20)[c]	< 0.001
Elective delivery	1.21 (1.15–1.28)	1.20 (1.14–1.27)[c]	< 0.001
Perinatal death	0.97 (0.83–1.13)	0.95 (0.81–1.11)[b]	n.s.

[a] n.s. = not statistically significant.
[b] Adjusted for maternal age, parity, year of conception, induction of labor, and elective cesarean section, but not for zygosity.
[c] Adjusted for maternal age, parity, and year of conception, but not for zygosity.
Based on data from Keirse *et al.* [38].

Medical Birth Registry of Norway from 1984 to 2006. Among these were 2546 assisted conceptions with a sibling born after natural conception. In 56% of these the ART birth preceded the natural conception birth. Whilst they confirmed higher rates of adverse outcomes among assisted conceptions, there was little difference in either low birth weight, preterm birth, or perinatal mortality between the ART and natural conception siblings, suggesting that the effect of infertility per se may be larger than it is commonly thought to be.

Kapiteijn *et al.* [21], on the other hand, used a Dutch population-based cohort to compare the perinatal outcome of 2239 IVF singletons with that of 6343 infertile women, defined as failure to conceive within 1 year of regular coitus, who eventually conceived naturally. The odds ratios for very preterm (< 32 weeks) and mildly preterm (32–36 weeks) birth in the IVF group versus the control group were respectively 2.0 (95% CI 1.4–2.9) and 1.5 (95% CI 1.3–1.8). Similarly, the odds ratio was 2.8 (95% CI 1.9–3.9) for very low birth weight (< 1500 g) and 1.6 (95% CI 1.2–1.8) for birth weights between 1500 and 2499 g. Adjustment for maternal age and primiparity did not materially affect these risk estimates [21].

Controlled ovarian (hyper)stimulation (COHS)

Recently, awareness has arisen that COHS, as a crucial element of many ART techniques, might be a major contributor to the poor perinatal outcome [60]. However, perinatal outcome data of singletons conceived after IVF in a natural cycle, for instance, have not been published. Recently some data have been gathered on outcomes after IVF in a modified natural cycle, i.e. after or during administration of a gonadotropin-releasing hormone (GnRH) analogue, a low dose of FSH is administered for a short period of time, followed by hCG ovulation induction. In a single-center retrospective study, the rate of (very) low birth weight and (very) preterm birth among 84 singletons resulting from IVF with such a modified ovarian stimulation did not differ from that among 106 singletons from IVF with the usual COHS treatment [61], but only very large differences would be detected with this sample size.

Adverse perinatal outcomes were observed more frequently in 263 singletons born to women who received only COHS compared with 5096 naturally conceived controls born in the same French hospital over the same period of time, while there was no difference in outcome between these COHS births and 162 IVF singletons (Table 20.5) [62]. After stratification for the number of years of involuntary childlessness, a Swedish group [63] still found a significantly increased risk of preterm birth and low birth weight in singletons conceived after just COHS in comparison with naturally conceived singletons [63]. Ombelet *et al.* [64] used data of the Flemish Study Center for Perinatal Epidemiology (SPE) to select women with COHS and constitute a matched group with natural conceptions. However, the COHS group contained women with and without IUI and with and without timed intercourse,

Table 20.5. Perinatal outcomes after controlled ovarian hyperstimulation (with or without timed intercourse) and/or intrauterine insemination (IUI)

Study type[a]	Author	COHS procedure			Controls[b]			RR	95% CI
		Cases	*N*	%	Cases	*N*	%		
Preterm birth < 37 weeks									
Controlled ovarian hyperstimulation – IUI									
Matched	Nuojua-Huttunen [65]	8	92	8.7	14	276	5.1	1.71	0.74–3.96
	Nuojua-Huttunen [65]	8	92	8.7	21	276	7.6	1.14	0.52–2.49 †
	Ombelet [64]	938	12 021	7.8	514	12 021	4.2	**1.82**	**1.64–2.03**
Unmatched	Gaudoin [66]	17	132	12.9	7541	109 288	6.9	**1.87**	**1.20–2.91**
Controlled ovarian hyperstimulation alone									
Unmatched	Olivennes [62]	16	263	6.1	224	5096	4.4	1.38	0.85–2.26
Very preterm birth < 32 weeks									
Controlled ovarian hyperstimulation – IUI									
Matched	Ombelet [64]	152	12 021	1.3	47	12 021	0.4	**3.23**	**2.33–4.48**
Controlled ovarian hyperstimulation alone									
Unmatched	Olivennes [62]	6	263	2.3	20	5096	0.4	**5.01**	**2.35–14.4**
Low birth weight < 2500 g									
Controlled ovarian hyperstimulation – IUI									
Matched	Nuojua-Huttunen [65]	8	92	8.7	17	276	6.2	1.41	0.63–3.16
	Nuojua-Huttunen [65]	8	92	8.7	19	276	6.9	1.26	0.28–1.14 †
	Ombelet [64]	794	12 021	6.6	441	12 021	3.7	**1.80**	**1.61–2.02**

Table 20.5. (cont.)

Study type[a]	Author	COHS procedure			Controls[b]			RR	95% CI
		Cases	*N*	%	Cases	*N*	%		
Unmatched	Gaudoin [66]	26	132	19.7	7760	109 302	7.1	**2.77**	**1.96–3.92**
Controlled ovarian hyperstimulation alone									
Unmatched	Olivennes [62]	18	263	6.8	183	5096	3.6	**1.91**	**1.19–3.04**
Very low birth weight < 1500 g									
Controlled ovarian hyperstimulation – IUI									
Matched	Ombelet [64]	159	12 021	1.3	50	12 021	0.4	**3.18**	**2.32–4.37**
Controlled ovarian hyperstimulation alone									
Unmatched	Olivennes [62]	6	263	2.3	20	5096	6.4	**5.01**	**2.35–14.4**

[a] See footnote to Table 20.1 for definition of study type.
[b] Controls are natural conceptions except for the data of Nuojua-Huttunen *et al.* [65] indicated by † which are IVF controls.
[c] Relative risk and 95% confidence interval (bold values indicate statistical significance).

making it difficult to interpret the contribution of each to the differences observed (see Table 20.5) [64].

Although the clinical heterogeneity both within and among the studies does not permit one to combine them in order to reach a firm conclusion, they seem to indicate that the risk differential between COHS conceptions and naturally conceived singletons is roughly similar to that between IVF and naturally conceived singletons (Table 20.5).

Intrauterine insemination (IUI)

Six studies, including the study of Ombelet *et al.* [64] mentioned above, have examined the perinatal outcome after IUI, but the studies show a great diversity and most of the women undergoing IUI also had ovarian stimulation and/or ovulation induction. Because of this, the data have, as far as possible, been incorporated in Table 20.5. Because of their diversity, these studies need to be considered individually rather than being combined, as none of them actually provides clear evidence on the effects of IUI per se.

A Finnish group [65] compared the outcome of 92 singleton pregnancies after controlled ovarian hyperstimulation and IUI in 1991–96 with two control groups. One consisted of 276 singleton IVF pregnancies and the other of 276 naturally conceived singletons, derived from the Finnish Medical Birth register and matched for year of delivery, age, parity, socioeconomic variables, and smoking.

Gaudoin *et al.* [66] compared outcomes of 132 singleton pregnancies after treatment with COHS (GnRH agonist, FSH, hCG) and IUI (97 with partner and 35 with donor sperm) with data of about 109 000 singletons contained in a Scottish database.

In a Belgian study, De Sutter and coworkers [67] compared the outcome of 112 singletons, conceived by IUI after ovulation was induced by hCG with or without prior clomiphene stimulation, with 112 IVF singletons matched for maternal age, parity, and plurality. Not surprisingly, given the numbers involved, no differences in outcome were detected [67].

De Geyter *et al.* [68] in Switzerland compared a mere 37 singletons, born after COHS and IUI, with 56 IVF singletons, 147 ICSI singletons and 443 singletons naturally conceived by infertile people. Data on preterm birth and low birth weight were not provided, but the authors concluded that pregnancy duration and infant weight were significantly reduced after IVF and ICSI but not after COHS and IUI [68].

Table 20.6. Frequencies of preterm birth and low birth weight in singletons conceived by ICSI versus natural conceptions

Study type[a]	Author	ICSI			Natural conception			RR	95% CI[b]
		Cases	*N*	%	Cases	*N*	%		
Preterm birth < 37 weeks									
Matched	Sutcliffe [70]	18	208	8.6	14	221	6.3	1.37	0.70–2.68
	Ombelet [72]	152	1655	9.2	260	3278	7.9	1.16	0.99–1.42
	Knoester [71]	6	87	6.9	0	85	0.0	Undetermined	
Unmatched	Katalinic [73]	248	2055	12.1	524	7861	6.7	**1.81**	**1.57–2.09**
Very preterm birth < 32 weeks									
Matched	Ombelet [72]	27	1655	1.6	51	3278	1.5	1.13	0.92–1.39
Low birth weight < 2500 g									
Matched	Ombelet [72]	132	1655	7.9	231	3278	7.0	0.83	0.69–1.01
	Knoester [71]	7	87	8.0	1	85	1.2	6.84	0.86–54.5
Unmatched	Katalinic [73]	224	2055	10.9	417	7861	5.3	**2.05**	**1.76–2.40**
Very low birth weight < 1500 g									
Matched	Ombelet [72]	32	1655	1.9	51	3278	1.5	1.24	0.80–1.93
Unmatched	Katalinic [73]	66	2055	3.2	86	7861	1.1	**2.94**	**2.14–4.03**

[a] See footnote to Table 20.1 for definition of study type.
[b] Relative risk and 95% confidence interval (bold values indicate statistical significance).

An Australian group [69] compared the preterm birth rate of singletons conceived after so-named high-technology ART (IVF, ICSI, and GIFT) and low-technology ART (IUI, usually after COHS, and donor insemination, usually in a natural cycle) with naturally conceived singletons. Preterm birth rates were respectively 12.5%, 8.5%, and 5.5% [69].

In-vitro fertilization (IVF) with and without intracytoplasmic sperm injection (ICSI)

In the early phases after the introduction of ICSI, male infertility was the predominant indication for this type of ART. This might give additional clues on the extent to which female infertility per se or, alternatively, COHS contributes to poor outcome, but no studies strictly limited to male factor infertility have been conducted to specifically address this question. Some other data, which have involved comparisons of ICSI pregnancies with either naturally conceived pregnancies or IVF pregnancies, some designed to assess long-term outcomes of ICSI [70,71], are available (Table 20.6).

A British study [70] recruited 208 singletons conceived by ICSI and a control group of 221 naturally conceived singletons from 22 fertility centers and local nurseries throughout the UK [70]. Controls were selected to match cases as closely as possible for social class, maternal educational attainment, region, sex, and race. A Flemish (Belgian) retrospective study [72] identified 1655 singletons born after ICSI and compared these with 3278 naturally conceived singletons, matched for maternal age, parity, place of delivery, year of birth, and fetal sex, drawn from a cohort of 430 565 births (1997–2004) [72]. In yet another study, 2055 ICSI singletons from a prospective nationwide German cohort study (1998–2000) were compared with 7861 singletons, born in Magdeburg hospitals in 1993–2002 [73]. A smaller Dutch single center study compared ICSI singletons born between 1996 and 1999 with singletons born after conventional IVF and after natural conception, matched for several confounders [71]. The comparison concentrated on outcomes at 5 to 8 years of age and, contrary to the matching between ICSI and natural conceptions, matching between ICSI and IVF offspring was only achieved for infants born at term [71].

A further three Belgian studies compared outcomes after ICSI with those after conventional IVF (Table 20.7) [74,75,76]. One of these [74] incorporated the same ICSI singletons that were in a previous report [72]. The other two were single center studies reported from two different centers in Brussels [75,76].

In a Swedish register study on ART (1981–2001) children born after standard IVF and after ICSI were compared [77]. Two data sets were used: children born up to 1996 ($N = 4517$) with only 7.2% ICSI, and from 1996 to 2001 (N = 16 280) with 30% ICSI. The authors found no significant differences in preterm birth or low birth weight between singleton infants born after standard IVF or after ICSI, but separate data for IVF and ICSI singletons were not provided [77].

Cryopreservation of gametes

There is no evidence that insemination with cryopreserved sperm per se adversely affects perinatal outcome, but the available data are not necessarily easy to interpret. For example, Hoy *et al.* [78] compared the outcomes of donor insemination using cryopreserved semen with a ‘control group of 7717 normally conceived pregnancies from the general population’ in Victoria, Australia. There are no separate data for singletons and twins, but 24% of the donor insemination cycles had received ovarian stimulation resulting in a six-fold higher rate of multiple pregnancies with donor insemination. Lansac *et al.* [79] compared 8943 singletons from donor inseminations with cryopreserved sperm with 13 631 singletons from a French national register. Rates of preterm birth were respectively 4.8% versus 5.9% and rates of low birth weight 4.7% versus 6.2%, but the numbers involving also COHS are not known.

Cryopreservation of embryos

The ability to freeze embryos and thaw them for ET later on, when first introduced, added an entirely new

Table 20.7. Frequencies of preterm birth and low birth weight in singletons conceived by ICSI or by conventional IVF

Study type[a]	Author	ICSI			IVF			RR	95% CI[b]
		Cases	*N*	%	Cases	*N*	%		
Preterm birth < 37 weeks									
Unmatched	Bonduelle [75]	126	1500	8.4	140	1555	9.0	0.93	0.74–1.17
	Govaerts [76]	6	66	9.1	7	65	10.8	0.84	0.30–2.38
	Ombelet [74]	152	1655	9.2	491	3974	12.4	**0.74**	**0.63–0.88**
Very preterm birth < 32 weeks									
Unmatched	Govaerts [76]	1	66	1.5	1	65	1.5	0.98	0.06–15.4
	Ombelet [74]	27	1655	9.2	74	3974	1.9	0.88	0.57–1.36

Table 20.7. (cont.)

Study type[a]	Author	ICSI			IVF			RR	95% CI[b]
		Cases	*N*	%	Cases	*N*	%		
Low birth weight < 2500 g									
Unmatched	Govaerts [76]	2	61	3.3	3	63	4.8	0.69	0.12–3.98
	Bonduelle [75]	106	1493	7.1	121	1551	7.8	0.91	0.71–1.17
	Ombelet [74]	132	12 021	6.6	441	12 021	3.7	0.83	0.69–1.01
Very low birth weight < 1500 g									
Unmatched	Govaerts [76]	1	61	1.6	1	63	1.6	1.03	0.07–16.1
	Bonduelle [75]	22	1467	1.5	28	1555	1.8	0.83	0.48–1.45
	Ombelet [74]	32	1655	1.9	81	3974	2.0	0.95	0.63–1.42

[a] See footnote to Table 20.1 for definition of study type.
[b] Relative risk and 95% confidence interval (bold values indicate statistical significance).

dimension to ART techniques. On the one hand, there is the question of whether freezing and thawing might affect the outcome. On the other hand, this has enabled ET to be performed in natural cycles without prior COHS. It has also created another dimension in terms of what to do with so-named 'surplus' embryos, an issue that has evoked a great deal of discussion larded with emotional, ethical, legal, and religious arguments that are well beyond the scope of this chapter. Just as it is difficult to steer a path of scientific neutrality among these arguments, it is also difficult to assess the effects of frozen and fresh without taking the influences of ART with or without COHS and many other confounders into account.

Whilst we consider that this is an important issue that may help to unravel some of the unanswered questions regarding the effects of ART on perinatal outcome, our attempt to do so is only in its infancy. Therefore, Table 20.8 merely shows a brief summary of some of the published data. Readers will note that there are large differences in outcome among studies, even among those with substantial numbers of subjects. Some studies have dealt specifically with IVF or ICSI and others with ART which in these studies would involve both IVF and ICSI. In one of the studies [80], some infants appear to have only birth weights but no gestational age, for reasons that are not explained [80]. All of this should emphasize the need for caution when interpreting the results of the individual studies and for considering not only statistical, but also clinical heterogeneity when trying to combine them with meta-analysis techniques. Nonetheless, as ET of frozen and thawed embryos is frequently performed in a natural cycle, the apparent advantage for singletons originating from frozen embryos may well reflect a difference between natural and stimulated cycles.

Singleton outcomes from multiple, dual and single embryo transfer (Tables 20.9 and 20.10)

Many singletons were born over the decades in which ART techniques evolved from multiple embryo transfer (MET) to dual embryo (DET) and single (SET) embryo transfer. This should have allowed reasonable comparisons between these forms of ET, if only there had been as much interest in achieving a healthy infant as there was in achieving a pregnancy of whatever description [22]. Due to the emphasis on short-term successes rather than long-term outcomes, these opportunities were lost. Fortunately, they are not likely ever to return.

To test whether ET of more than one embryo could offer an implantation advantage or disadvantage for the

Table 20.8. Preterm birth and low birth weight rates in singletons after ART with frozen embryos versus fresh embryos

Study type[a]	Author	ART	Frozen embryo			Fresh embryo			RR	95% CI[b]
			Cases	*N*	%	Cases	*N*	%		
Preterm birth < 37 weeks										
Matched	Wennerholm [81]	IVF	9	160	5.6	18	160	11.3	0.50	0.23–1.08
Unmatched	Wada [80]	IVF	19	158	12.0	67	494	13.6	0.89	0.55–1.43
	Belva [82]	IVF	34	281	12.1	140	1523	9.2	1.32	0.93–1.87
	Belva [82]	ICSI	44	381	11.6	126	1476	8.5	1.35	0.98–1.87
	Schieve [9]	ART	1404	8533	16.5	6103	47 586	12.8	**1.28**	**1.22–1.35**
	Wang [83]	ART	437	3833	11.4	1008	7695	13.1	**0.87**	**0.78–0.97**
	Shih [84]	ART	220	2387	9.2	383	3110	12.3	**0.75**	**0.64–0.88**
Very preterm birth< 32 weeks										
Matched	Wennerholm [81]	IVF	2	160	1.3	0	160	0.0	undetermined	
Low birth weight < 2500 g										
Matched	Wennerholm [81]	IVF	8	160	5.0	12	160	7.5	0.67	0.28–1.59
Unmatched	Wada [80]	IVF	13	177	7.3	68	527	12.9	0.57	0.32–1.00
	Belva [82]	IVF	20	281	7.1	121	1523	7.9	0.90	0.57–1.41
	Belva [82]	ICSI	24	381	6.3	106	1476	7.2	0.88	0.57–1.35
	Schieve [9]	ART	921	8533	10.8	6400	47 586	13.5	**0.80**	**0.75–0.86**
	Wang [83]	ART	277	3847	7.2	829	7676	10.8	**0.67**	**0.59–0.76**
	Shih [84]	ART	220	2387	9.2	383	3110	12.3	**0.75**	**0.64–0.88**
Very low birth weight < 1500 g										
Unmatched	Belva [82]	IVF	17	281	6.1	167	1523	11.0	**0.55**	**0.34–0.89**
	Belva [82]	ICSI	13	381	3.4	125	1476	8.5	**0.40**	**0.23–0.71**
	Schieve [9]	ART	136	8533	1.6	1031	47 586	2.2	**0.74**	**0.62–0.88**

[a] See footnote to Table 20.1 for definition of study type.
[b] Relative risk and 95% confidence interval (bold values indicate statistical significance).

one developing embryo after ART, De Neubourg *et al.* [85] analyzed the perinatal outcome of IVF/ICSI singletons after SET over a 6-year period (1998–2003) during which they progressively introduced SET from 12.4% to 53.8% and compared these to naturally conceived singletons in the same period (Table 20.9). Another Belgian group compared SET and DET singletons [56]. Poikkeus *et al.* [86] compared a 7-year cohort of SET singletons (1997–2003) at Helsinki University Hospital with naturally conceived singletons from the Finnish Medical Birth Register, which may or may not have been accurate enough in determining whether conceptions were natural, [34] and also with DET singletons. In the absence of controlling for characteristics that may have had an affect on determining whether women received SET or DET, data may be summarized as in Table 20.10. It remains difficult, though, to reach firm conclusions from these data except for a marked

Table 20.9. Preterm birth and low birth weight rates in singletons after single embryo transfer (SET) ART versus natural singleton conceptions

Study type[a]	Author	SET singletons			Natural conceptions			RR	95% CI[b]
		Cases	*N*	%	Cases	*N*	%		
Preterm birth < 37 weeks									
Unmatched	De Neubourg [85]	25	251	10.0	3669	59 535	6.2	**1.62**	**1.11–2.35**
	Poikkeus [86]	33	269	12.3	666	15 037	4.4	**2.77**	**2.00–3.85**
Very preterm birth < 32 weeks									
Unmatched	De Neubourg [85]	2	251	0.8	468	59 535	0.8	1.01	0.25–4.04
	Poikkeus [86]	3	269	1.1	108	15 037	0.7	1.55	0.50–4.86
Low birth weight < 2500 g									
Unmatched	De Neubourg [85]	15	251	6.0	3050	59 535	5.1	1.17	0.71–1.91
	Poikkeus [86]	15	269	5.6	441	15 037	2.9	**1.90**	**1.15–3.14**
Very low birth weight < 1500 g									
Unmatched	De Neubourg [85]	2	251	0.8	466	59 535	0.8	1.19	0.70–2.03
	Poikkeus [86]	3	269	1.1	86	15 037	0.6	1.95	0.62–6.13

[a] See footnote to Table 20.1 for definition of study type.
[b] Relative risk and 95% confidence interval (bold values indicate statistical significance).

reduction in the frequency of twin pregnancies and their associated complications after SET compared with DET, which has been a constant and self-evident observation in several other studies.

Other studies, not reviewed here, have examined the effects of embryo reduction on perinatal outcome. Basically, they investigate whether adverse effects of technology can be counteracted by more technology, rather than addressing the root of the problem: 'too many eggs in the same basket' [22,23].

ART with COHS and multiple oocytes or ET of more than one embryo after IVF or ICSI not infrequently results in a singleton birth. Loss of one or more of the embryos has become known as the 'vanishing twin syndrome' and has led to the realization that this is a frequent occurrence in both naturally conceived and ART pregnancies, and can have a major impact on the outcome of the remaining 'singleton' [87]. Spontaneous reduction of one or more gestational sacs occurring before the 12th week of gestation has been reported in 36% of twin pregnancies [88] and so-named 'missed abortion' in the first trimester in 10.4% to 12.2% [89,90]. Regrettably, the literature on the effect of the 'vanishing twin syndrome' on the perinatal outcome of ART singletons is also compounded by non-vanished double publications [89,91].

Nonetheless, two main conclusions can be reached from the available data. First, there is an inverse relationship between pregnancy duration and birth weight on the one hand and the initial gestational sac number on the other hand, irrespective of the number of infants that is eventually born [88]. This would seem to extend the classical observations of McKeown and Record in 1952 [25], on the effect of fetal numbers at birth, back up to the number present at the time of implantation. Second, gestational age at the time of 'vanishing' is inversely related to poor outcome, i.e. the earlier in gestation the twin 'vanishes', the poorer the outcome [87][89].

When combining these data (Table 20.11), impossible as it seems to be, we can certainly conclude that the difference in perinatal outcome between ART and naturally conceived singletons cannot be explained entirely by multiple or dual embryo transfer.

Donor oocytes

Donor oocytes introduce a main difference in ART in that 100% rather than 50% of the resulting zygote is foreign to the woman. Schieve *et al.* [9] collected perinatal outcome data of singleton infants conceived with freshly fertilized donor oocytes (N = 6432) and with women's own freshly fertilized oocytes (N = 47 586) in the United States in the period 1996–2000. Preterm birth rates were

Table 20.10. Preterm birth and low birth weight rates in singletons after single embryo transfer (SET) versus dual embryo transfer (DET)

Study type[a]	Author	SET singletons			DET singletons			RR	95% CI[b]
		Cases	*N*	%	Cases	*N*	%		
Preterm birth < 37 weeks									
Unmatched	De Sutter [56]	25	404	6.2	45	431	10.4	0.59	0.37–1.14
	Poikkeus [86]	33	269	12.3	26	230	11.3	1.09	0.67–1.76
Very preterm birth < 32 weeks									
Unmatched	Poikkeus [86]	3	269	1.1	3	230	1.3	0.86	0.17–4.20
Low birth weight < 2500 g									
Unmatched	De Sutter [56]	17	404	4.2	50	431	11.6	**0.36**	**0.21–0.62**
	Poikkeus [86]	15	269	5.6	22	230	9.6	0.58	0.31–1.10
Very low birth weight < 1500 g									
Unmatched	Poikkeus [86]	3	269	1.1	2	230	0.9	1.28	0.22–7.61

[a] See footnote to Table 20.1 for definition of study type.
[b] Relative risk and 95% confidence interval (bold values indicate statistical significance).

Table 20.11. Preterm birth and low birth weight rates in singleton pregnancies with a vanishing twin versus natural singleton conceptions

Study type	Author	Left as singletons			Natural conceptions			RR	95% CI[a]
		Cases	*N*	%	Cases	*N*	%		
Preterm birth < 37 weeks									
Matched	Shebl [92]	9	46	19.6	8	92	8.7	2.25	0.93–5.45
Unmatched	La Sala [90]	14	84	16.7	96	602	15.9	**10.5**	**6.23–17.5**
Very preterm birth < 32 weeks									
Matched	Shebl [92]	2	46	4.3	2	92	2.2	2.00	0.29–13.7
Unmatched	La Sala [90]	2	84	2.4	15	602	2.5	0.96	0.22–4.10
Low birth weight < 2500 g									
Matched	Shebl [92]	12	46	26.1	11	92	12.0	**2.18**	**1.04–4.56**
Unmatched	La Sala[90]	9	84	10.7	78	602	13.0	0.83	0.43–1.59
	Pinborg [89]	24	642	3.7	120	5237	2.3	1.63	1.06–2.51
Very low birth weight < 1500 g									
Matched	Shebl [92]	2	46	4.3	2	92	2.2	2.00	0.29–13.7
Unmatched	La Sala [90]	1	84	1.2	19	602	3.2	0.38	0.05–2.78

[a] See footnote to Table 20.1 for definition of study type.
[b] Relative risk and 95% confidence interval (bold values indicate statistical significance).

higher among singletons conceived with donor oocytes (16.8% versus 12.8%), but rates of low birth weight, although roughly similar to the preterm birth rate, did not differ, being respectively 14.5% and 13.4%. Neither was there a significant difference in very low birth weight (2.5% versus 2.2%). Several elements, other than genetic difference, e.g. enhancement of endometrial sensitivity, presence or absence of ovarian stimulation, etc., may also differ and would need to be taken into account.

General conclusions

It has been estimated that abolition of all ART, although not a feasible proposition, would reduce preterm birth numbers by 13% and very preterm births by 14% [38], with major reductions in morbidity in infancy and childhood and major benefits for public health and health care expenditure [11,93].Undoubtedly, the highest potential for reducing the frequency of adverse perinatal outcome after ART is in the avoidance of multiple pregnancies. As ART procedures, such as IVF and ICSI, are potentially far more effective than natural conceptions at limiting the number of fetuses per pregnancy, the continuing excess of multiple pregnancies is poor testimony to the interest of ART specialists in perinatal and public health. Suggestions that ART conceived twins may not be worse off than naturally conceived twins [15] does not alter this, especially as such data are heavily biased in favor of ART by not controlling for chorionicity or zygosity.

It is undeniable that some of the poor perinatal outcome of ART relates to the characteristics of people relying on ART in order to achieve a pregnancy, but how large that contribution actually is remains difficult to determine. The preexisting characteristics are multiple, including among others age, parity, and a history of infertility, and they are further compounded by an obstetric tendency to intervene in such pregnancies before problems arise [38]. Singleton pregnancies from assisted reproduction have a significantly worse perinatal outcome in terms of mortality, birth weight, and delivery too early in pregnancy than non-assisted singleton pregnancies after adjustment for major confounders, such as maternal age, parity, and fetal sex. The difference seems to exist throughout gestation, with the most marked effects seen at the lower end of the distributions of gestational age and birth weight. There is a great deal of mainly circumstantial evidence that ovarian stimulation is at least partially responsible for these poor outcomes. Differences in outcome with natural conceptions seem to be similar for COHS and IVF, whereas pregnancies from ET of thawed embryos, which is usually performed in natural cycles, appear to do better.

Implications for clinical practice

The main goal of ART is or should be to achieve a healthy singleton infant born at term, which is achieved more often now than it was in the past. Greater emphasis on single rather than multiple embryo transfer has gone a long way in reducing unwarranted outcomes of ART. The data suggest, though, that among ART techniques, controlled ovarian hyperstimulation (COHS) is largely responsible for the worse perinatal outcome after ART than after natural conception, although the causal factors in female infertility play a role as well. Patients seeking ART need to be informed about this and about the likely effects, both beneficial and adverse, of the various treatment modalities. The likelihood of achieving pregnancy is important, but it is not the ultimate criterion by which success or failure should be measured. Moreover, before embarking on ART, doctors must discuss and address known risk factors of adverse outcome, such as smoking, alcohol use, and obesity.

Implications for research

There is an obvious need for better and more detailed information based on consistent, unambiguous, and uniform definitions that are comparable among studies. Many of the results available thus far will need confirmation, preferably in different populations. ART registers in general will need to give more attention to substantive outcomes other than treatments used or pregnancies achieved. We may also need to find better ways of controlling for various confounders.

Perhaps more essential than controlling for confounders is to find explanations for the observed associations and the means to address them. In the absence of random allocation, a prerequisite for translating association into causation would seem to be a biologically plausible mechanism linking the two phenomena. Indirect evidence suggests that COHS does not greatly affect the oocyte, but may have marked effects on uterine receptivity and subsequent implantation [94,95,96]. Rodents treated with urinary gonadotropins show an increase in pre- and postimplantation mortality, impaired implantation, and prolonged gestation [97]. Further exploration of the various components of ART may yet provide significant clues as to what causes the difference in outcome with natural conceptions and how to remedy this.

References

1. Källén B. Maternal morbidity and mortality in in-vitro fertilization. *Best Pract Res Clin Obstet Gynaecol* 2008; **22**: 549–58.
2. WHO. Standards and reporting requirements related to fetal, perinatal, neonatal and infant mortality. In: *International statistical classification of diseases and related health problems: instruction manual*, 10th revision, Vol 2. Geneva: World Health Organization; 1993.
3. Keirse M J N C. International variations in intrauterine growth. *Eur J Obstet Gynecol Reprod Biol* 2000; **92**: 21–8.
4. Roberts C L, Lancaster P A L. Australian national birthweight percentiles by gestational age. *Med J Aust* 1999; **170**: 114–18.
5. Graafmans W C, Richardus J H, Macfarlane A *et al.* Comparability of published perinatal mortality rates in Western Europe: the quantitative impact of differences in gestational age and birthweight criteria. *BJOG* 2001; **108**: 1237–45.
6. Blickstein I. Does assisted reproduction technology, per se, increase the risk of preterm birth? *BJOG* 2006; **113** (Suppl 3): 68–71
7. ESHRE. *Good clinical treatment in assisted reproduction: An ESHRE position paper.* http://www.eshre.com/binarydata.aspx?type=doc/Good_Clinical_treatment_in_Assisted_Reproduction_ENGLISH.pdf (accessed December 2008).
8. ASRM. *Assisted reproductive technologies.* http://www.asrm.org/Patients/patientbooklets/ART.pdf (accessed December 2008).
9. Schieve L A, Ferre C, Peterson H B *et al.* Perinatal outcome among singleton infants conceived through assisted reproductive technology in the United States. *Obstet Gynecol* 2004; **103**: 1144–53.
10. McIntire D D, Leveno K J. Neonatal mortality and morbidity rates in late preterm births compared with births at term. *Obstet Gynecol* 2008; **111**: 35–41.
11. McLaurin K K, Hall C B, Jackson A J *et al.* Persistence of morbidity and cost differences between late-preterm and term infants during the first year of life. *Pediatrics* 2009; **123**: 653–9.
12. Jackson R A, Gibson K A, Wu Y W *et al.* Perinatal outcomes in singletons following in vitro fertilization: a meta-analysis. *Obstet Gynecol* 2004; **103**: 551–63.
13. Hansen M, Bower C, Milne E *et al.* Assisted reproductive technologies and the risk of birth defects: a systematic review. *Hum Reprod* 2005; **20**: 328–38.
14. EURO-PERISTAT project with SCPE, EUROCAT and EURONEONET. European Perinatal Health Report 2008. http://www.europeristat.com/bm.doc/european-perinatal-health-report-2.pdf (accessed January 2009).
15. Helmerhorst F M, Perquin D A M, Donker D, Keirse M J N C. Perinatal outcome of singletons and twins after assisted conception: a systematic review of controlled studies. *BMJ* 2004; **328**: 261–5.
16. McDonald S D, Murphy K, Beyene J *et al.* Perinatal outcomes of singleton pregnancies achieved by in vitro fertilization: a systematic review and meta-analysis. *J Obstet Gynaecol Can* 2005; **27**: 449–59.
17. Montan S. Increased risk in the elderly parturient. *Curr Opin Obstet Gynecol* 2007; **19**: 110–2.
18. Luke B, Brown M B. Elevated risks of pregnancy complications and adverse outcomes with increasing maternal age. *Hum Reprod* 2007; **22**: 1264–72.
19. Draper E S, Kurinczuk J J, Abrams K R *et al.* Assessment of separate contributions to perinatal mortality of infertility history and treatment: a case-control analysis. *Lancet* 1999; **353**: 1746–9.
20. Romundstad L B, Romundstad P R, Sunde A *et al.* Effects of technology or maternal factors on perinatal outcome after assisted fertilisation: a population-based cohort study. *Lancet* 2008; **372**: 737–43.
21. Kapiteijn K, de Bruijn C S, de Boer E *et al.* Does subfertility explain the risk of poor perinatal outcome after IVF and ovarian hyperstimulation? *Hum Reprod* 2006; **21**: 3228–34.
22. Keirse M J N C, Helmerhorst F M. The impact of assisted reproduction on perinatal health care. *Soc Prev Med* 1995; **40**: 343–51.
23. Keirse M J N C, Helmerhorst F M. Too many eggs? Ideally one egg and one offspring. *BMJ* 2004; **328**: 302–3.
24. Gerris J, Van Royen E. Avoiding multiple pregnancies in ART. A plea for single embryo transfer. *Hum Reprod* 2000; **15**: 1884–8.
25. McKeown T, Record R G. Observations on foetal growth in multiple pregnancy in man. *J Endocrinol* 1952; **8**: 386–401.
26. Chow J S, Benson C B, Racowsky C *et al.* Frequency of a monochorionic pair in multiple gestations: relationship to mode of conception. *J Ultrasound Med* 2001; **20**: 757–60.
27. Aston K I, Peterson C M, Carrell D T. Monozygotic twinning associated with assisted reproductive technologies: a review. *Reproduction* 2008; **136**: 377–86.
28. Sherer D M. Adverse perinatal outcome of twin pregnancies according to chorionicity: review of the literature. *Am J Perinatol* 2001; **18**: 23–37.
29. Dhont M, De Neubourg F, Van der Elst J *et al.* Perinatal outcome of pregnancies after assisted reproduction: a case-control study. *J Assist Reprod Genet* 1997; **14**: 575–80.

30. Dhont M, De Sutter P, Ruyssinck G *et al.* Perinatal outcome of pregnancies after assisted reproduction: a case-control study. *Am J Obstet Gynecol* 1999; **181**: 688–95.

31. Isaksson R, Gissler M, Tiitinen A. Obstetric outcome among women with unexplained infertility after IVF: a matched case-control study. *Hum Reprod* 2002; **17**: 1755–61.

32. Keirse M J N C. Perinatal mortality rates do not contain what they purport to contain. *Lancet* 1984; **1**: 1166–9.

33. Anthony S, van der Pal-de Bruin K M, Graafmans W C *et al.* The reliability of perinatal and neonatal mortality rates: differential under-reporting in linked professional registers vs. Dutch civil registers. *Paediatr Perinat Epidemiol* 2001; **15**: 306–14.

34. Gissler M, Silverio M M, Hemminki E. In-vitro fertilisation pregnancies and perinatal health in Finland 1991–1993. *Hum Reprod* 1995; **10**: 1856–61.

35. Andersen A N, Gianaroli L, Felberbaum R *et al.* Assisted reproductive technology in Europe, 2002: results generated from European registers by ESHRE. *Hum Reprod* 2006; **21**: 1680–97.

36. Kremer J A M, Bots R S G M, Cohlen B *et al.* Tien jaar resultaten van in-vitrofertilisatie in Nederland. *Ned Tijdschr Geneeskd* 2008; **152**: 146–52.

37. Wildman K, Blondel B, Nijhuis J *et al.* European indicators of health care during pregnancy, delivery and the postpartum period. *Eur J Obstet Gynecol Reprod Biol* 2003; **111**: S53–65.

38. Keirse M J N C, Hanssens M, Devlieger H. Trends in preterm birth in Flanders, Belgium, from 1991 to 2002. *Paediatr Perinat Epidemiol* 2009; **23**: 522–32.

39. Buck Louis G M, Schisterman E F, Dukic V M *et al.* Research hurdles complicating the analysis of infertility treatment and child health. *Hum Reprod* 2005; **20**: 12–8.

40. Lancaster P A L, Johnston W I H, Wood C *et al.* Australian in vitro fertilisation collaborative group. High incidence of preterm births and early losses in pregnancy after in vitro fertilisation. *BMJ* 1985; **291**: 1160–3.

41. Tan S L, Doyle P, Campbell S *et al.* Obstetric outcome of in vitro fertilization pregnancies compared with normally conceived pregnancies. *Am J Obstet Gynecol* 1992; **167**: 778–84.

42. Verlaenen H, Cammu H, Derde M P *et al.* Singleton pregnancy after in vitro fertilization: expectations and outcome. *Obstet Gynecol* 1995; **86**: 906–10.

43. Tanbo T, Dale P O, Lunde O, Moe N, Abyholm T. Obstetric outcome in singleton pregnancies after assisted reproduction. *Obstet Gynecol* 1995; **86**: 188–92.

44. Reubinoff B E, Samueloff A, Ben Haim M *et al.* Is the obstetric outcome of in vitro fertilized singleton gestations different from natural ones? A controlled study. *Fertil Steril* 1997; **67**: 1077–83.

45. Koudstaal J, Braat D D, Bruinse H W *et al.* Obstetric outcome of singleton pregnancies after IVF: a matched control study in four Dutch university hospitals. *Hum Reprod* 2000; **15**: 1819–25.

46. Olivennes F, Rufat P, Andre B *et al.* The increased risk of complication observed in singleton pregnancies resulting from in-vitro fertilization (IVF) does not seem to be related to the IVF method itself. *Hum Reprod* 1993; **8**: 1297–300.

47. Yudkin P L, Wood L, Redman C W. Risk of unexplained stillbirth at different gestational ages. *Lancet* 1987; **1**: 1192–4.

48. Yang H, Kramer M S, Platt R W *et al.* How does early ultrasound scan estimation of gestational age lead to higher rates of preterm birth? *Am J Obstet Gynecol* 2002; **186**: 433–37.

49. Joseph K S, Kramer M S, Marcoux S *et al.* Determinants of preterm birth rates in Canada from 1981 through 1983 and from 1992 through 1994. *New Engl J Med* 1998; **339**: 1434–9.

50. Craig E D, Thompson J M D, Mitchell E A. Socioeconomic status and preterm birth: New Zealand trends, 1980 to 1999. *Arch Dis Child* 2002; **86**: F42–6.

51. Cnattingius S, Forman M R, Berendes H W *et al.* Effect of age, parity, and smoking on pregnancy outcome: a population-based study. *Am J Obstet Gynecol* 1993; **168**: 16–21.

52. Langhoff-Roos J, Kesmodel U, Jacobsson B *et al.* Spontaneous preterm delivery in primiparous women at low risk in Denmark: population based study. *BMJ* 2006; **332**: 937–9.

53. Tracy S K, Tracy M B, Dean J *et al.* Spontaneous preterm birth of liveborn infants in women at low risk in Australia over 10 years: a population-based study. *BJOG* 2007; **114**: 731–5.

54. Ancel P Y, Saurel-Cubizolles M J, Di Renzo G C *et al.* Very and moderate preterm births: are the risk factors different? *BJOG* 1999; **106**: 1162–70.

55. Schempf A H, Branum A M, Lukacs S L *et al.* The contribution of preterm birth to the Black-White infant mortality gap, 1990 and 2000. *Am J Public Health* 2007; **97**: 1255–60.

56. De Sutter P, Delbaere I, Gerris J *et al.* Birthweight of singletons after assisted reproduction is higher after single- than after double-embryo transfer. *Hum Reprod* 2006; **21**: 2633–7.

57. Pandian Z, Templeton A, Serour G *et al.* Number of embryos for transfer after IVF and ICSI: a Cochrane review. *Hum Reprod* 2005; **20**: 2681–7.

58. Gerris J. IVF and ICSI reimbursed in Belgium. *J Assist Reprod Genetics* 2004; **21**: 135.

59. Gerris J M R. Single embryo transfer and IVF/ICSI outcome: a balanced appraisal. *Hum Reprod Update* 2005; **2**: 105–121.

60. Ombelet W, De Sutter P, Van der Elst J *et al.* Multiple gestation and infertility treatment: registration, reflection and reaction: the Belgian project. *Hum Reprod Update* 2005; **11**: 3–14.

61. Pelinck M J, Keizer M H, Hoek A *et al. Eur J Obstet Gynecol Reprod Med*, in press.

62. Olivennes F, Rufat P, André B *et al.* The increased risk of complication observed in singleton pregnancies resulting from in-vitro fertilization (IVF) does not seem to be related to the IVF method itself. *Hum Reprod* 1993; **8**: 1297–300.

63. Källén B, Olausson P O, Nygren K G. Neonatal outcome in pregnancies from ovarian stimulation. *Obstet Gynecol* 2002; **100**: 414–9.

64. Ombelet W, Martens G, De Sutter P *et al.* Perinatal outcome of 12,021 singleton and 3108 twin births after non-IVF-assisted reproduction: a cohort study. *Hum Reprod* 2006; **21**: 1025–32.

65. Nuojua-Huttunen S, Gissler M, Martikainen H *et al.* Obstetric and perinatal outcome of pregnancies after intrauterine insemination. *Hum Reprod* 1999; **14**: 2110–5.

66. Gaudoin M, Dobbie R, Finlayson A *et al.* Ovulation induction/intrauterine insemination in infertile couples is associated with low-birth-weight infants. *Am J Obstet Gynecol* 2003; **188**: 611–6.

67. De Sutter P, Veldeman L, Kok P *et al.* Comparison of outcome of pregnancy after intra-uterine insemination (IUI) and IVF. *Hum Reprod* 2005; **20**: 1642–6.

68. de Geyter C, de Geyter M, Steimann S *et al.* Comparative birth weights of singletons born after assisted reproduction and natural conception in previously infertile women. *Hum Reprod* 2006; **21**: 705–12.

69. Wang J X, Norman R J, Kristiansson P. The effect of various infertility treatments on the risk of preterm birth. *Hum Reprod* 2002; **17**: 945–9.

70. Sutcliffe A G, Taylor B, Saunders K *et al.* Outcome in the second year of life after in-vitro fertilisation by intracytoplasmic sperm injection: a UK case-control study. *Lancet* 2001; **357**: 2080–4.

71. Knoester M, Helmerhorst F M, Vandenbroucke J P *et al.* Perinatal outcome, health, growth, and medical care utilization of 5- to 8-year-old intracytoplasmic sperm injection singletons. *Fertil Steril* 2008; **89**: 1133–46.

72. Ombelet W, Peeraer K, De Sutter P *et al.* Perinatal outcome of ICSI pregnancies compared with a matched group of natural conception pregnancies in Flanders (Belgium): a cohort study. *Reprod Biomed Online* 2005; **11**: 244–53.

73. Katalinic A, Rösch C, Ludwig M *et al.* Pregnancy course and outcome after intracytoplasmic sperm injection: a controlled, prospective cohort study. *Fertil Steril* 2004; **81**: 1604–16.

74. Ombelet W, Cadron I, Gerris J *et al.* Obstetric and perinatal outcome of 1655 ICSI and 3974 IVF singleton and 1102 ICSI and 2901 IVF twin births: a comparative analysis. *Reprod Biomed Online* 2005; **11**: 76–85.

75. Bonduelle M, Liebaers I, Deketelaere V *et al.* Neonatal data on a cohort of 2889 infants born after ICSI (1991–1999) and of 2995 infants born after IVF (1983–1999). *Hum Reprod* 2002; **17**: 671–94.

76. Govaerts I, Devreker F, Koenig I *et al.* Comparison of pregnancy outcome after intracytoplasmic sperm injection and in-vitro fertilization. *Hum Reprod* 1998; **13**: 1514–8.

77. Källén B, Finnström O, Nygren K G *et al.* In vitro fertilization (IVF) in Sweden: infant outcome after different IVF fertilization methods. *Fertil Steril* 2005; **84**: 611–7.

78. Hoy J, Venn A, Halliday J *et al.* Perinatal and obstetric outcomes of donor insemination using cryopreserved semen in Victoria, Australia. *Hum Reprod* 1999; **14**: 1760–4.

79. Lansac J, Thepot F, Mayaux M J *et al.* Pregnancy outcome after artificial insemination or IVF with frozen semen donor: a collaborative study of the French CECOS Federation on 21,597 pregnancies. *Eur J Obstet Gynecol Reprod Biol* 1997; **74**: 223–8.

80. Wada I, Macnamee M C, Wick K *et al.* Birth characteristics and perinatal outcome of babies conceived from cryopreserved embryos. *Hum Reprod* 1994; **9**: 543–6.

81. Wennerholm U B, Hamberger L, Nilsson L *et al.* Obstetric and perinatal outcome of children conceived from cryopreserved embryos. *Hum Reprod* 1997; **12**: 1819–25.

82. Belva F, Henriet S, Van den Abbeel E *et al.* Neonatal outcome of 937 children born after transfer of cryopreserved embryos obtained by ICSI and IVF and comparison with outcome data of fresh ICSI and IVF cycles. *Hum Reprod* 2008; **23**: 2227–38.

83. Wang Y A, Sullivan E A, Black D *et al.* Preterm birth and low birth weight after assisted reproductive technology-related pregnancy in Australia between 1996 and 2000. *Fertil Steril* 2005; **83**: 1650–8.

84. Shih W, Rushford D D, Bourne H *et al.* Factors affecting low birthweight after assisted reproduction technology: difference between transfer of fresh and cryopreserved embryos suggests an adverse effect of oocyte collection. *Hum Reprod* 2008; **23**: 1644–53.

85. De Neubourg D, Gerris J, Mangelschots K *et al.* The obstetrical and neonatal outcome of babies born after

single-embryo transfer in IVF/ICSI compares favourably to spontaneously conceived babies. *Hum Reprod* 2006; **21**: 1041–6.

86. Poikkeus P, Gissler M, Unkila-Kallio L *et al.* Obstetric and neonatal outcome after single embryo transfer. *Hum Reprod* 2007; **22**: 1073–9.
87. Johnson C D, Zhang J. Survival of other fetuses after a fetal death in twin or triplet pregnancies. *Obstet Gynecol* 2002; **99**: 698–703.
88. Dickey R P, Taylor S N, Lu P Y *et al.* Spontaneous reduction of multiple pregnancy: incidence and effect on outcome. *Am J Obstet Gynecol* 2002; **186**: 77–83.
89. Pinborg A, Lidegaard O, la Cour Freiesleben N *et al.* Consequences of vanishing twins in IVF/ICSI pregnancies. *Hum Reprod* 2005; **20**: 2821–9.
90. La Sala G B, Villani M T, Nicoli A *et al.* Effect of the mode of assisted reproductive technology conception on obstetric outcomes for survivors of the vanishing twin syndrome. *Fertil Steril* 2006; **86**: 247–9.
91. Pinborg A, Lidegaard O, La Cour Freiesleben N *et al.* Vanishing twins: a predictor of small-for-gestational age in IVF singletons. *Hum Reprod* 2007; **22**: 2702–14.
92. Shebl O, Ebner T, Sommergruber M *et al.* Birth weight is lower for survivors of the vanishing twin syndrome: a case-control study. *Fertil Steril* 2008; **90**: 310–4.
93. Mangham L J, Petrou S, Doyle L W *et al.* The cost of preterm birth throughout childhood in England and Wales. *Pediatrics* 2009; **123**: e312–27.
94. Horcajadas J A, Riesewijk A, Polman J *et al.* Effect of controlled ovarian hyperstimulation in IVF on endometrial gene expression profiles. *Mol Hum Reprod* 2005; **11**; 195–205.
95. Tavaniotou A, Albano C, Smitz J *et al.* Impact of ovarian stimulation on corpus luteum function and embryonic implantation. *J Reprod Immunol* 2002; **55**: 123–30.
96. Horcajadas J A, Mínguez P, Dopazo J *et al.* Controlled ovarian stimulation induces a functional genomic delay of the endometrium with potential clinical implications. *J Clin Endocrinol Metab* 2008; **93**: 4500–10.
97. Sibug R M, Datson N, Tijssen A M *et al.* Effects of urinary and recombinant gonadotrophins on gene expression profiles during the murine peri-implantation period. *Hum Reprod* 2007; **22**: 75–82.

Angiogenic factors and preeclampsia

May Lee Tjoa[1], Eliyahu V. Khankin[1], Sarosh Rana[2,3], and S. Ananth Karumanchi[1,2,3,4]

[1]Department of Medicine, Beth Israel Deaconess Medical Center and Harvard Medical School, Boston, MA, USA
[2]Obstetrics and Gynecology, Beth Israel Deaconess Medical Center and Harvard Medical School, Boston, MA, USA
[3]Maternal Fetal Medicine Division, Beth Israel Deaconess Medical Center and Harvard Medical School, Boston, MA, USA
[4]Howard Hughes Medical Institute, Chevy Chase, MD, USA

Introduction

Preeclampsia is a systemic syndrome of pregnancy, which is characterized by widespread maternal endothelial dysfunction [1]. It is a leading cause of maternal and neonatal morbidity and mortality, affecting between 3% and 5% of all pregnancies in the developed world [2]. Symptoms of preeclampsia include *de novo* hypertension and proteinuria usually after 20 weeks of gestation. Although the exact molecular pathogenesis of preeclampsia is largely unknown, it is widely accepted that placental dysfunction is a major factor in the development of preeclampsia.

The placenta plays a key pathogenic role in preeclampsia based on two observations. First, to date the only effective treatment of preeclampsia is removal of the placenta. Women suffering from preeclampsia often see their symptoms resolve within 24 to 48 hours of delivery. Second, women with a molar pregnancy, in which there is hyperplastic growth of the placenta in the absence of a fetus, may be affected by preeclampsia. These patients may develop severe early onset preeclampsia and the symptoms usually resolve when the molar tissue is removed [3,4]. More recently, studies have shown that an imbalance in the secretion of placenta-associated angiogenic proteins contributes to the pathogenesis of the disease. These proteins include the antiangiogenic factors soluble fms-like tyrosine kinase 1 (sFlt1) and soluble endoglin. This chapter will focus on the emerging role of angiogenic and antiangiogenic factors in the pathogenesis of preeclampsia and how these factors may play an important role in mediating the clinical features of the disease.

Clinical features and epidemiology of preeclampsia

Preeclampsia is characterized by new-onset hypertension and proteinuria usually after 20 weeks of gestation. Management of preeclampsia varies according to the severity of the symptoms [5]. Hypertension can vary among patients, with those experiencing mild blood pressure elevations often prescribed bed rest. Severe preeclampsia, in which usually large blood pressure elevations occur, is accompanied by headache and visual changes and often leads to preterm delivery and intrauterine growth restriction (IUGR). Edema has historically been considered a symptom of preeclampsia, although its use in the clinical diagnosis of the disorder has diminished in recent years. However, sudden and severe onset of edema in the facial area or hands can be useful in detecting the onset of preeclampsia.

Other complications of preeclampsia include seizures (eclampsia), acute renal failure, pulmonary edema, liver failure, hemolysis, and thrombocytopenia. The three later complications constitute the HELLP (hemolysis, elevated liver enzymes, low platelets) syndrome, a very severe complication of preeclampsia. The maternal and neonatal mortality rates are significantly higher when HELLP syndrome occurs. Eclampsia is less common in developed countries than in developing countries. Although eclampsia frequently occurs in the presence of hypertension and proteinuria, it is known to also affect healthy pregnant women without any warning signs. Approximately one-third of all eclampsia cases occur postpartum [6]. In total, preeclampsia and its more severe complications are responsible for 10–15% of maternal deaths worldwide per year [2]. In developed countries, where maternal symptoms can be managed in a highly technical environment and early delivery is instituted when the maternal condition deteriorates, most maternal deaths are avoided. However, the burden of morbidity and mortality often falls on the neonates, who require specialized care in the case of preterm birth and low birth weight.

Preeclampsia is a complex disorder, characterized by genetic, immunological, and environmental factors.

In general, the highest risk factors for preeclampsia are primiparity, high body mass index, prepregnancy hypertension, maternal diabetes, and multifetal gestation [7,8,9]. In an early genetic epidemiological study published several years ago, it was shown that the incidence of preeclampsia in first-time pregnancies was 26% in daughters, 25% in granddaughters, and 8% in daughters-in-law of women who had had preeclampsia themselves [10]. A more recent study indicated that women with preeclampsia were 2.3 times more likely to have a sister who had preeclampsia [11]. Epidemiological studies also suggest that paternal genetic contributions in addition to maternal genes may contribute susceptibility to preeclampsia [12]. Well-known features of preeclampsia can be explained by maternal immune maladaptation. Increased time between subsequent pregnancies, change of partner between subsequent pregnancies, prolonged barrier contraception use, and conception by intracellular sperm injection have all been indicated as risk factors for preeclampsia [13,14,15,16].

Early vascular development

Adequate feto-maternal exchange of oxygen, nutrients, and waste products via the circulation is vital to the successful maintenance of pregnancy and growth of the fetus. An intricate network of vessels must be established, linking the growing fetus to maternal blood supply. The processes of vasculogenesis (the formation of new types of blood vessels from angioblasts) and angiogenesis (process of neovascularization from existing blood vessels) are vital during early gestation.

A detailed description and overview of angiogenesis in normal placenta is presented in Chapter 7. A brief account of normal placental vascular development as it relates to angiogenic factors is presented here. Vasculogenesis starts around 21 days postconception [17]. As the primary villi cores begin to fill with mesenchymal cells, secondary villi are formed. The mesenchymal cells then differentiate into hemangiogenic precursor cells, which later will form the lining of the first blood vessels in the placenta, and into Hofbauer cells, macrophages that may play a role in vasculogenesis [18] and trophoblast differentiation [19].

Throughout early pregnancy, these primitive vessels continue to transform into an extensive network of blood vessels through branching and nonbranching angiogenesis. As the network of blood vessels grows in the placenta, there is simultaneous remodeling of the maternal uterine vessels. Throughout the first weeks of pregnancy, the cytotrophoblast cells located within the villi differentiate into extravillous trophoblast (EVT) cells. These EVT cells migrate into the maternal tissue, where they home towards the maternal spiral arteries. A complex physiological remodeling of these vessels ensues, which converts these low-caliber, high-resistance spiral arteries into very-high-caliber, low-resistance blood vessels.

The establishment of the placental vasculature and the vascular remodeling of maternal vessels are related processes. The rise in oxygen levels not only stimulates the growth of the fetus, but also causes an upregulation of a range of adhesion molecules by cytotrophoblast cells that facilitate trophoblast invasion [20]. The converted maternal spiral arteries in the endometrium ensure that a steady blood supply reaches the placenta, thereby increasing the number of new placental vessels. It is likely that angiogenic disturbances exist at the feto-maternal interface and in the placental bed as the establishment of the placental vasculature and the vascular remodeling of maternal vessels are interwined processes. Although angiogenic imbalance has been implicated in maternal endothelial dysfunction resulting in preeclampsia (see below) and much is known about the lack of spiral arteriolar remodeling, unfortunately no causal data are available for the role of these angiogenic factors in the pathogenesis of abnormal placentation noted in preeclampsia and IUGR.

Placental origin of maternal disease

Based on the observation that the only definite cure for preeclampsia is removal of the placenta, it stands to reason that the placenta plays an important role in the development of the disorder. In 1972, Brosens and colleagues were the first to note that physiological remodeling of the maternal spiral arteries was shallow or absent in cases of preeclampsia [21]. Indeed, it has been demonstrated in histological studies that the physiological remodeling of the spiral arteries is confined only to those vessels in the decidual portion of the endometrium [22,23]. Consequently, the spiral arteries in the myometrium retain their endothelial linings and muscular walls, thereby retaining their high-resistance phenotype. The failure of vascular remodeling is thought to be one of the first steps leading to preeclampsia. Trophoblast cells from preeclamptic pregnancies fail to switch the expression of epithelial cell-associated cell surface integrins to an endothelial phenotype, thereby limiting their invasive potential [24]. Defective trophoblast invasion and inadequate maternal spiral artery conversion has also been observed in IUGR without preeclampsia. Concerning the virtual absence of trophoblast invasion in spontaneous abortion, Ball *et al.* found in a large series of early spontaneous miscarriages (≤ 12 weeks) that trophoblast invasion was normal [25] while in late miscarriages (≥ 13 weeks) there was impaired invasion [26]. Therefore, the role of trophoblast invasion is crucial to successfully maintaining a pregnancy.

Hypoxia likely induces the expression of a number of factors that activate the maternal endothelium, which leads to the widespread maternal endothelial dysfunction seen in overt preeclampsia [27,28,29]. Oxidative stress activates leukocytes, platelets, and neutrophils in the intervillous space [30,31]. In turn, these activated cells are able to generate free oxygen radicals upon contact with the endothelium, which stimulates the expression of inflammatory cytokines such as interleukin-6 (IL-6) [27,32]. Levels of inflammatory cytokines, including IL-6 and tumor necrosis factor alpha (TNF-α), are significantly higher in preeclampsia patients than in women with healthy pregnancies [33,34,35]. While the levels of these inflammatory factors reflect endothelial dysfunction which is part of the clinical syndrome, they are most likely secondary effects as they are elevated after onset of clinical disease.

The factors that do regulate the vascular remodeling and facilitate the formation of vessels are just beginning to be understood. These factors include angiogenic growth factors such as vascular endothelial growth factor (VEGF), placental growth factor (PlGF), and their receptors Flt1 (VEGFR1) and KDR/Flk1 (VEGFR2). Angiogenic growth factors that have been implicated in placental vascularization are Tie-1, Tie-2, and endoglin. Hypoxia regulates the expression of these factors. In the case of preplacental hypoxia, due to high altitude or medical conditions such as asthma or chronic anemia, reduced maternal oxygen levels exist even before pregnancy. When the gene profiles from placentae from preplacental hypoxic pregnancies are investigated in comparison to preeclamptic placentae, the same expression patterns of hypoxia-inducible transcription factors are found [36,37]. Hypoxia inducible factor (HIF)-1 modulates the expression of Flt1 and KDR/FLK1 [38,39]. HIF-1 levels are increased in preeclampsia [39]. An HIF-1 target, TGF-β3, is also elevated in preeclamptic placentae and is thought to prevent trophoblast invasion [40,41].

Angiogenic growth factors

Vascular endothelial growth factor (VEGF)

VEGF represents a family of growth factors involved in both vasculogenesis and angiogenesis. This family consists of at least seven members: VEGF-A, VEGF-B, VEGF-C, VEGF-D, VEGF-E, PlGF, and snake venom-derived VEGFs (such as from *Trimeresurus flavoviridis*, designated usually as svVEGF) [42]. All members except VEGF-E and svVEGF are encoded by the mammalian genome. The VEGF family members are summarized briefly below. For a more extensive overview on the various angiogenic growth factors and their receptors, please refer to Chapter 7 of this book.

VEGF-A plays a central role in angiogenesis as well as in vasculogenesis. Studies demonstrate that homozygous and heterozygous knockouts of the *VEGF-A* gene (*VEGF-A* mice) die *in utero* due to a vast variety of defects in angiogenesis, indicating that basal levels of VEGF-A supplied by two alleles are absolutely essential for complete formation of mature and functioning vasculature [43,44]. VEGF-A serves as an effective ligand of VEGF receptor type 1 (VEGFR1) also known as Flt1 and VEGF receptor type 2 (VEGFR2) designated as KDR/Flk1.

VEGF-B binds to and activates only Flt1. The angiogenic activity of VEGF-B is almost 10-fold lower than that of VEGF-A. However, under some pathological conditions, for example cancer, VEGF-B could be a significant source of pathological angiogenesis [45].

VEGF-C/VEGF-D play crucial roles in the process of lymphangiogenesis. Both factors are initially created in premature forms which are processed by digestion with various endogenous protein convertases, by which they acquire high affinity to VEGFR3 [46].

VEGF-E (OrfVEGF) represents a group of proteins encoded by the genome of the Orf virus (sheep/goat parapox-virus) [47]. Unlike VEGF-A, VEGF-E family proteins bind and activate KDR/Flk1, but not Flt1. This leads to their ability to induce significant angiogenic effects, without the 'side effects' of edema or inflammation that are commonly observed during treatment with VEGF-A [48].

Placental growth factor (PlGF)

The structure of PlGF is highly homologous to VEGF-A as it contains a *PDGF*-domain which is 53% similar to the *PDGF*-domain in the *VEGF* gene. Despite this obvious similarity, its properties are somewhat different from those of VEGF. First cloned from a term placenta cDNA library and mapped to chromosome 14 [49], four isoforms of PlGF have since been identified. All isoforms bind tightly to Flt1 but not KDR/Flk1. It is thought that PlGF acts as a potent angiogenic growth factor by amplifying VEGF-signaling by displacing VEGF from Flt1, allowing it to bind to KDR/Flk1 instead [50,51].

Despite its name implicating solely placental origin, PlGF expression has been found in a variety of placenta-derived tissues such as choriocarcinoma and human umbilical vein endothelial cells. PlGF has also been shown to be strongly expressed by the villous trophoblast [52]. It is believed that secretion of PlGF by trophoblast cells regulates the vascularization process in both the decidua and in the placenta. The localization of PlGF to villous trophoblasts and VEGF to mesenchymal-derived cells and endothelial cells suggests that these two factors mediate angiogenesis separately [52,53]. More recently, it was discovered that uterine natural killer (uNK) cells also express PlGF. These cells are phenotypically distinct from their blood counterparts through their ability to produce angiogenic growth factors, including PlGF, to promote trophoblast invasion [54]. In mice lacking uNK cells, the spiral arteries feeding into the placenta are not physiologically transformed as in normal mice, thereby suggesting an angiogenic role for uNK cells during early pregnancy [55].

VEGF receptors

Currently, the family of VEGF receptors (VEGFR) consists of three members: VEGFR1, VEGFR2, and VEGFR3. VEGFR1 and VEGFR2 are ligands of VEGF-A. They play a pivotal role in regulation of angiogenesis, while VEGFR3, which has a high affinity to VEGF-C and VEGF-D, stimulates lymphangiogenesis [56,57].

VEGFR1/Flt1 (fms-like tyrosine kinase 1)

VEGFR1 exists as both a cell membrane-bound form as well as a soluble form (sFlt1). Both are derived from an alternatively spliced mRNA product of the complete tyrosine kinase (membrane-bound Flt1). Flt1 has a extremely high affinity for VEGF-A, especially when compared to VEGFR2, while PlGF binds to Flt1 but not to VEGFR2. Interestingly, the tyrosine kinase activity of Flt1 is relatively modest, approximately 10-fold lower than that of VEGFR2, which renders Flt1 only a mild stimulant of endothelial proliferation under normal physiological conditions. Flt1 expression is most prominent by vascular endothelial cells. It is also expressed by cells of monocyte/macrophage lineage, in which stimulation of Flt1 induces migration of these cells [58,59,60]. Flt1 protein has been immunolocalized to the syncytiotrophoblast layer as well as endothelial cells in the placental villi. VEGFR1 has a limiting role on angiogenesis during the early stages of embryogenesis. This is displayed by the fact that Flt1-knockout mice die at E8.5–9.0 due to an overgrowth and dysfunction of blood vessels [61].

VEGFR2

VEGFR2 (also referred to as KDR/Flk1) exhibits an extremely strong tyrosine kinase activity although its ability to bind VEGF-A is approximately one order of magnitude weaker than that of Flt1. Mice lacking both copies of Flk1 (*flk-1 (-/-)* mice) die at E8.5 due to a lack of blood vessel development, a finding that indicates that VEGFR2 signaling is essential for the functional vascular system evolution in the developing embryo [62]. VEGFR2 generates a variety of angiogenic signals, plays a pivotal role in endothelial proliferation and in cell migration/morphogenesis including tubular formation. KDR/Flk1 expression has been localized almost exclusively to the endothelial cells of the placental villi [63]. In patients with severe preeclampsia, expression of Flt1 was significantly higher in the placenta, but the expression of KDR/Flk1 remained unchanged [63].

Endoglin

More recently, an angiogenic factor, endoglin, has been implicated in preeclampsia [64]. Endoglin (Eng) is a cell-surface co-receptor of transforming growth factors (TGF)-β1 and TGF-β3 [65]. Both TGF-β1 and TGF-β3 belong to the TGF-β superfamily, which also includes activin, inhibin, bone morphogenetic proteins, and follistatins. TGF-β signaling regulates a diverse array of cellular functions such as cellular growth, differentiation, and development. It has been shown that TGF-β isoforms prevent trophoblast invasion and there is an overexpression of TGF-β3 in preeclamptic placentae [40,66,67].

Mutations in the *ENG* gene lead to a condition called hereditary hemorrhagic telangiectasia type 1 (HHT1), an autosomal dominant disorder characterized by arteriovenous malformations and focal loss of capillaries [68]. Endoglin-null mice die *in utero* due to defective angiogenesis and cardiovascular development, while endoglin-heterozygous mice develop characteristics reminiscent of HHT1 [69]. Haploinsufficient mice (Eng) demonstrate impaired vasodilation and decreased levels of eNOS in their kidneys and femoral arteries, showing that Eng is also an important regulator of vascular homeostasis [70].

Eng is expressed at high levels by the syncytiotrophoblast, as well as by cytotrophoblast cells undergoing differentiation to an invasive phenotype. Both TGF-β1 and TGF-β3 are potent inhibitors of trophoblast differentiation and migration [67]. Normally, TGF-β1 and TGF-β3 levels are downregulated during early pregnancy, but it has been shown that TGF-β3 expression is selectively upregulated in preeclamptic placentae [66]. It has been shown that the inhibitory effects of TGF-β1 and TGF-β3 require Eng binding [71]. Based on these data, it thought that Eng may play a role in mediating the effects of placental hypoxia through the TGF-β pathway.

Role of angiogenic factors in the maternal syndrome

Recent work has shown that circulating antiangiogenic factors play an important role in the pathogenesis of preeclampsia [72] (see Fig. 21.1). The clinical symptoms of preeclampsia can generally all be attributed to endothelial dysfunction, leading to end-organ damage and hypoperfusion. It has been hypothesized that the endothelial dysfunction of preeclampsia may represent an antiangiogenic state that is mediated by high circulating levels of soluble fms-like tyrosine kinase 1 (sFlt1) (antiangiogenic) and low levels of circulating PlGF and VEGF (both proangiogenic) [72]. sFlt1, a splice variant of the VEGF (vascular endothelial growth factor) receptor Flt1, which lacks the transmembrane and cytoplasmic domains, is made in large amounts by the placenta and is released into the maternal circulation [73]. sFlt1 acts as a potent VEGF and PlGF antagonist by binding these molecules in the circulation and in the target tissues such as the kidney. VEGF stabilizes endothelial cells in mature blood vessels and is particularly important in maintaining fenestrated endothelia in renal, liver, and brain tissue, all organs that are implicated in preeclampsia [74]. Increased sFlt1 levels in preeclampsia are accompanied by decreased levels of circulating free PlGF and VEGF, a finding noted by several groups [75]. Overexpression of sFlt1 by adenoviral transfer in pregnant and non-pregnant rats produces hypertension, proteinuria, and glomerular endotheliosis, characteristic of preeclampsia [76]. The presence of preeclampsia-like phenotype in non-pregnant animals exposed to sFlt1 suggests that it acts directly on the maternal vasculature. When a soluble form of KDR/Flk1 was administered to pregnant rats, they did not develop any symptoms reflective of preeclampsia [76]. This suggests that antagonism of both PlGF and VEGF is necessary to induce preeclampsia.

When adult mice are administered anti-VEGF therapies, the animals develop glomerular endothelial damage and proteinuria [77]. In a knockdown model in mice, a 50% reduction in renal VEGF resulted in substantial glomerular endotheliosis and proteinuria,

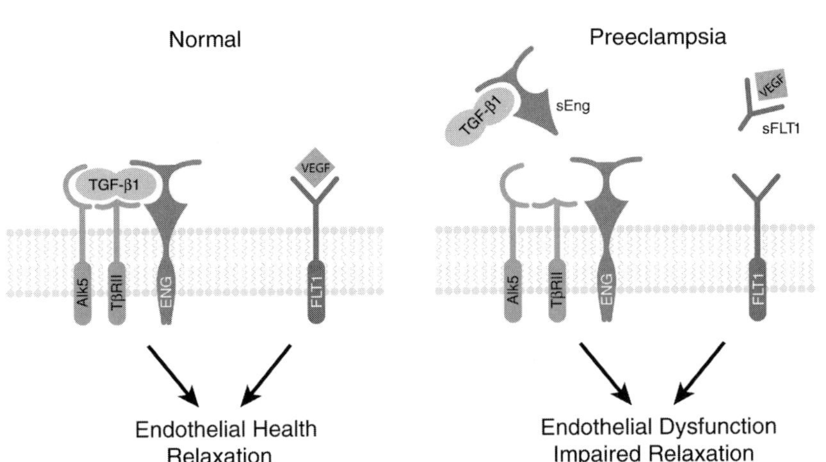

Fig. 21.1 sFlt1 and sEng cause endothelial dysfunction by antagonizing VEGF and TGF-β1 signaling. During normal pregnancy, vascular homeostasis is maintained by physiological levels of VEGF and TGF-β1 signaling in the vasculature. In preeclampsia, excess placental secretion of sFlt1 and sEng inhibits VEGF and TGF-β1 signaling, respectively, in the vasculature. This results in endothelial cell dysfunction, including decreased prostacyclin and nitric oxide production, and release of procoagulant proteins. Figure reproduced with permission from Karumanchi *et al.* [118].

similar to the kidney pathologies found in preeclamptic women [78]. In antiangiogenesis tumor therapy trials, cancer patients, who are given anti-VEGF antibodies in an attempt to limit tumor angiogenesis, develop hypertension, proteinuria, and loss of glomerular endothelial fenestrae [79,80]. Therefore, the early loss of VEGF function, as demonstrated by the decrease in circulating free VEGF and PlGF in presymptomatic preeclampsia patients [81], probably leads to the renal pathologies characteristic of preeclampsia.

Recently, several isoforms of sFlt1 have been demonstrated to be produced by the placenta [82]. One of these isoforms is referred to as sFlt1–14 and is expressed only in humans and in primates [83]. sFlt1–14 differs from sFlt1 by lacking the C-terminal 31 amino acids and containing intron 14 coded unique 28 amino acids in the C-terminus. Sela *et al.* identified sFlt1–14 as the primary isoform produced by the placenta in preeclamptic women. Interestingly, they identified placental syncytial knots as the major source of sFlt1–14. These structures are induced by placental hypoxia and are noted predominantly in preeclamptic placentae.

Soluble endoglin (sEng), a truncated form of endoglin, has been shown recently to be upregulated in preeclamptic placentae [64]. sEng is a cell surface coreceptor for TGF-β, which binds and antagonizes TGF-β in the extracellular milieu. It was demonstrated that sEng is upregulated in preeclampsia and that it disrupts formation of endothelial tubes *in vitro* and induces vascular permeability and hypertension *in vivo*. Furthermore, sEng in combination with sFlt1 was shown to amplify endothelial dysfunction and induce more severe clinical signs of preeclampsia including HELLP syndrome and cerebral edema that resembles eclampsia [64,84].

Hypoxia is known to influence the expression of angiogenic growth factors. Hypoxia decreases PlGF expression in placentae [85]. It has also been shown that hypoxia upregulates the expression of the soluble Flt1 protein in primary trophoblast cultures from first trimester placentae and increases its secretion into culture media [86]. Trophoblast cells isolated from preeclamptic placentae produce more sFlt1 and sEng and less PlGF than trophoblast cells from healthy placentae when cultured under normoxic and hypoxic conditions [87]. HIF-1, a key regulator of sFlt1 and sEng, is known to be expressed significantly higher in preeclampsia placentae, indicating a possible mechanism for the increase in sFlt1 and sEng secretion during preeclampsia [39]. Makris *et al.* demonstrated in a model of preeclampsia, based on uteroplacental perfusion insufficiency induced in pregnant non-human primates, that there was a significant elevation in the placental sFlt1 mRNA expression and an elevation in circulating sFlt1 levels [88]. Similar findings have been reported by Gilbert *et al.* in a rat model of preeclampsia [89]. Additional pathways such as deficient heme-oxygenase expression, autoantibodies against angiotensin type 1 receptor, and deficient catechol-*O*-methyl transferase have been proposed to play key roles in the regulation of sFlt1 production [90]. The exact role of these pathways in human preeclampsia is still being debated.

Angiogenic growth factors and IUGR

It has long been recognized that preeclampsia and IUGR share many common clinical and pathological features. IUGR is a common complication of preeclampsia, and abnormal uterine blood flow detected by Doppler ultrasound in early pregnancy is associated with an increased risk for both disorders. Babies that are growth-restricted *in utero* usually display asymmetry of growth, with their head circumference being disproportionately large compared to their body length. Genetic variation amongst different populations can lead to some ethnic groups having smaller babies at birth, for example amongst Asian populations, but these infants are not necessarily growth restricted *in utero*. In this chapter we focus on IUGR due to placental insufficiency. It is unknown why some women with placental insufficiency develop the systemic syndrome of preeclampsia, while some have small-for-gestational age (SGA) babies without these maternal symptoms. Variability in clinical phenotype is probably attributable to individual environmental and genetic differences that alter the maternal response to the placental disease.

With regard to angiogenic factors, studies have been performed measuring levels in placentae from normotensive pregnancies complicated by IUGR. There are some discrepancies in the study results. Using densitometric analysis of Western blots, Yinon and coworkers found that placentae from pregnancies complicated by IUGR had increased levels of endoglin and its soluble form, sEng [91]. A different study using the same approach did not find any alterations in endoglin levels in IUGR placentae, nor in circulating sEng levels [92]. Levels of Flt1 were found to be higher in IUGR placentae compared to normal placentae by immunostaining [63]. It was also shown that severe IUGR placentae have an increased expression of sFlt1 protein [93]. However, in the case of late onset IUGR, in which the extent of placental ischemia is often less pronounced than in early onset IUGR, levels of placental sFlt1 protein, as well as HIF-1α protein, were not altered compared to healthy placentae [94]. This study shows that in cases of IUGR, a distinction between early onset IUGR and late onset IUGR should be made in order to avoid discrepancies in data. However, given the pathological and clinical overlap between IUGR and preeclampsia, it is believed that the two conditions probably share common pathophysiological underpinnings, at least at the level of insufficient placental vascular development.

Clinical perspectives

Although currently there is not any definitive therapeutic or preventive strategy for preeclampsia, accumulating clinical data suggest that early detection, monitoring, and supportive care are beneficial to both the patient and the fetus. Reliable prediction of preeclampsia would allow prompt and close prenatal monitoring, leading to early diagnosis, which will enable timely intervention such as treatment with steroids to accelerate fetal lung maturation, intravenous magnesium therapy combined with bed rest and antihypertensive medications for seizure prophylaxis, and, when indicated, expeditious delivery. Furthermore, a reliable prognostic biomarker for preeclampsia would enable targeted studies of therapies and preventive strategies, including existing clinical standard treatments (e.g. aspirin for high-risk groups), further validation of somewhat controversial ones (i.e. calcium, L-arginine), as well as development of novel approaches to the therapy. However, no screening test has been proven to be accurate enough yet to become a standard for widespread clinical use.

Since the first report describing association between dysregulation of the above-mentioned angiogenic factors and preeclampsia, multiple studies have reproduced these findings. Levine and colleagues studied circulating angiogenic proteins in serum of women enrolled in the Calcium for Preeclampsia Prevention (CPEP) trial [95]. They found that concentrations of sFlt1, which were previously reported to be increased in women with established preeclampsia [96], begin to increase steeply approximately 5 weeks before the onset of the clinical maternal syndrome. In parallel with the increase in sFlt1 levels, decreases in the free PlGF and free VEGF levels are observed, suggesting that those levels could be the result of binding by sFlt1. In addition, association between sFlt1 and PlGF levels and severity of preeclampsia was evident: in general, women who developed severe and/or early onset preeclampsia had higher sFlt1 and lower PlGF levels at each time interval studied. Interestingly, this finding held true for women who simultaneously developed both preeclampsia and IUGR.

A similar study by Chaiworapongsa and coworkers compared levels of serum sFlt1 in normal pregnant women to those in patients with preeclampsia. This study determined that mean plasma sFlt1 concentration was significantly higher in preeclamptics compared to normal pregnancies up to 6–10 weeks before first clinical manifestation of the syndrome [119]. In line with these findings, in a nested case-control study by Rana *et al.* [97], levels of sFlt1 and sEng were already elevated at 17–20 weeks of gestation in those women who developed preeclampsia later during pregnancy. The sequential changes in sFlt1 and sEng levels between the second and third trimesters were greatest in those patients who developed early onset preeclampsia, a finding that has also been noted by other groups [98]. However, levels of sFlt1 and sEng did not differ significantly between the control and preeclampsia groups at 11–13 weeks of gestation [97].

In a prospective study by Stepan *et al.*, high sFlt1 levels and lower than normal PlGF levels during the second trimester preceded preeclampsia development, with the most pronounced differences seen in women who developed early onset preeclampsia [99]. Of interest to note is that normotensive women who were enrolled in this study and who delivered a growth-restricted newborn had higher sFlt1 and lower PlGF levels, compared to healthy pregnancies, but these differences were not statistically significant. Combining the measurements with uterine Doppler imaging analysis did not improve the prediction of adverse pregnancy outcomes in the case of sEng. However, when combining abnormal US Doppler findings with sFlt1 levels, sensitivity and specificity of Doppler to predict preeclampsia increased to 79% and 80%, respectively.

In contrast, Romero and coworkers found that alterations in PlGF and sEng levels were already evident as early as at 10 weeks of gestation in those pregnancies that later developed the IUGR pattern, while sFlt1 levels were predictive only for preeclampsia, but not IUGR [100]. Various studies have been able to reproduce the finding that both sFlt1 and sEng are elevated in preeclampsia [99,101,102,103]. Although there are some discrepancies in the data regarding the predictive values of circulating angiogenic growth factors for IUGR, it can be concluded that they are potentially very useful tools for predicting pregnancies at risk for preeclampsia, especially severe, early onset preeclampsia that is accompanied by IUGR.

Other studies have looked at alternative ways to develop biomarkers for clinical use. One study focused on measuring urinary PlGF levels in pregnant women participating in the CPEP trial. The authors were able to show that levels of urinary PlGF were significantly lower at 25–28 weeks of gestation in those women who went on to develop preeclampsia. Moreover, urinary PlGF levels were lowest in those women who developed early onset preeclampsia or who also delivered a growth restricted baby [104]. In a study performed by Purwosunu and colleagues, levels of circulating mRNA of Flt1 and endoglin were significantly increased in the plasma of preeclampsia patients compared to healthy pregnant women and levels of circulating mRNA levels of these angiogenic factors correlated with the severity of preeclampsia [105]. Although this study was performed using samples from women with overt preeclampsia, the results agree with the assumption that excessive placental secretion of sFlt1 and sEng is a primary feature of preeclampsia.

Currently, the only definitive treatment for preeclampsia is delivery of the fetus and placenta. In the late second and early third trimester, preeclampsia requiring delivery to preserve the health of the mother can result in significant neonatal morbidity and mortality due to prematurity and its complications. Both preeclampsia and IUGR have been shown to have long-term health consequences for both mother and child. Women who suffered from preeclampsia during pregnancy have a higher risk of developing cardiovascular disease [106,107], undergoing kidney biopsy [108], and end-stage renal disease [109] in later life. It has been observed that 40% of former preeclampsia patients had microalbuminuria 3–5 years postpregnancy [110]. Former preeclampsia patients also exhibit characteristics of metabolic syndrome [111,112] and increased insulin resistance [113] shortly after pregnancy, which may contribute to the overall long-term risks of developing cardiovascular disease. Although there is still controversy over whether IUGR is linked to cardiovascular disease and diabetes in later life (Barker hypothesis [114,115]), there has been support for this through an epidemiological study linking low birth weight to subsequent preeclampsia in adulthood [116].

Identification of sFlt1 and sEng as key plausible pathogenic links between placental pathology and maternal endothelial damage provides hope that these biomarkers may also be effective therapeutic targets. Potential therapies may be directed at restoring normal angiogenic balance in the maternal circulation – that is, the relative biological activity of proangiogenic factors such as VEGF and PlGF relative to antiangiogenic factors such as sFlt1 and sEng. One such potential therapy, VEGF-121, was recently shown to diminish hypertension and proteinuria in a rat model of sFlt1-induced preeclampsia, without apparent harm to the fetus [117]. Such therapies may transform the way preeclampsia is treated. Any intervention that allows clinicians to safely postpone delivery for even a few days to weeks could have a tremendous impact on overall neonatal morbidity and mortality. Taking into consideration the long-term health consequences of both preeclampsia and IUGR, it is justifiable to develop novel therapeutics that target the angiogenic imbalance present in women suffering from either or both pregnancy disorders. Although more molecular data and prospective clinical trails are warranted, we soon may see real improvements in the management of this ancient syndrome.

References

1. Redman C W, Sargent I L. Latest advances in understanding preeclampsia. *Science* 2005; **308**: 1592–4.

2. WHO. *World Health Report: Make every mother and child count*. Geneva: World Health Organization; 2005.

3. Page E W. The relation between hydatid moles, relative ischemia of the gravid uterus and the placental origin of eclampsia. *Am J Obstet Gynecol* 1939; **37**: 291–3.

4. Norwitz E R, Repke J T. Preeclampsia prevention and management. *J Soc Gynecol Investig* 2000; **7**: 21–36.

5. Sibai B, Dekker G, Kupferminc M. Pre-eclampsia. *Lancet* 2005; **365**: 785–99.

6. Sibai B. Diagnosis, prevention, and management of eclampsia. *Obstet Gynecol* 2005; **105**: 402–10.

7. Alderman B W, Sperling R S, Daling J R. An epidemiological study of the immunogenetic aetiology of pre-eclampsia. *Br Med J (Clin Res Ed)* 1986; **292**: 372–4.
8. Bhattacharya S, Campbell D M, Liston W A, Bhattacharya S. Effect of body mass index on pregnancy outcomes in nulliparous women delivering singleton babies. *BMC Public Health* 2007; **7**: 168.
9. Roman H, Robillard P Y, Hulsey T C, *et al.* Obstetrical and neonatal outcomes in obese women. *West Indian Med J* 2007; **56**: 421–6.
10. Chesley L C, Annitto J E, Cosgrove R A. The familial factor in toxemia of pregnancy. *Obstet Gynecol* 1968; **32**: 303–11.
11. Carr D B, Epplein M, Johnson C O, Easterling T R, Critchlow C W. A sister's risk: family history as a predictor of preeclampsia. *Am J Obstet Gynecol* 2005; **193**: 965–72.
12. Esplin M S, Fausett M B, Fraser A *et al.* Paternal and maternal components of the predisposition to preeclampsia. *N Engl J Med* 2001; **344**: 867–72.
13. Robillard P Y, Hulsey T C, Perianin J *et al.* Association of pregnancy-induced hypertension with duration of sexual cohabitation before conception. *Lancet* 1994; **344**: 973–5.
14. Skjaerven R, Wilcox A J, Lie R T. The interval between pregnancies and the risk of preeclampsia. *New Engl J Med* 2002; **346**: 33–8.
15. Trogstad L I, Eskild A, Magnus P, Samuelsen S O, Nesheim B I. Changing paternity and time since last pregnancy; the impact on pre-eclampsia risk. A study of 547 238 women with and without previous pre-eclampsia. *Int J Epidemiol* 2001; **30**: 1317–22.
16. Wang J X, Knottnerus A M, Schuit G *et al.* Surgically obtained sperm, and risk of gestational hypertension and pre-eclampsia. *Lancet* 2002; **359**: 673–4.
17. Demir R, Kaufmann P, Castellucci M, Erbengi T, Kotowski A. Fetal vasculogenesis and angiogenesis in human placental villi. *Acta Anat (Basel)* 1989; **136**: 190–203.
18. Seval Y, Korgun E T, Demir R. Hofbauer cells in early human placenta: possible implications in vasculogenesis and angiogenesis. *Placenta* 2007; **28**: 841–5.
19. Khan S, Katabuchi H, Araki M, Nishimura R, Okamura H. Human villous macrophage-conditioned media enhance human trophoblast growth and differentiation in vitro. *Biol Reprod* 2000; **62**: 1075–83.
20. Zhou Y, Fisher S J, Janatpour M *et al.* Human cytotrophoblasts adopt a vascular phenotype as they differentiate: a strategy for successful endovascular invasion? *J Clin Invest* 1997; **99**: 2139–51.
21. Brosens I A, Robertson W B, Dixon H G. The role of spiral arteries in the pathogenesis of pre-eclampsia. *Obstet Gynecol Annu* 1972; **1**: 177–91.
22. Gerretsen G, Huisjes H J, Elema J D. Morphological changes of the spiral arteries in the placental bed in relation to pre-eclampsia and fetal growth retardation. *Br J Obstet Gynaecol* 1981; **88**: 876–81.
23. Meekins J W, Pijnenborg R, Hanssens M, McFadyen I R, van Asshe A. A study of placental bed spiral arteries and trophoblast invasion in normal and severe pre-eclamptic pregnancies. *Br J Obstet Gynaecol* 1994; **101**: 669–74.
24. Zhou Y, Damsky C H, Fisher S J. Preeclampsia is associated with failure of human cytotrophoblasts to mimic a vascular adhesion phenotype: one cause of defective endovascular invasion in this syndrome? *J Clin Invest* 1997; **99**: 2152–64.
25. Ball E, Robson S C, Ayis S, Lyall F, Bulmer J N. Early embryonic demise: no evidence of abnormal spiral artery transformation or trophoblast invasion. *J Pathol* 2006; **208**: 528–34.
26. Ball E, Bulmer J N, Ayis S, Lyall F, Robson S C. Late sporadic miscarriage is associated with abnormalities in spiral artery transformation and trophoblast invasion. *J Pathol* 2006; **208**: 535–42.
27. Many A, Hubel C A, Fisher S J, Roberts J M, Zhou Y. Invasive cytotrophoblasts manifest evidence of oxidative stress in preeclampsia. *Am J Pathol* 2000; **156**: 321–31.
28. Vaughan J E, Walsh S W. Oxidative stress reproduces placental abnormalities of preeclampsia. *Hypertens Preg* 2002; **21**: 205–23.
29. Walsh S W. Maternal-placental interactions of oxidative stress and antioxidants in preeclampsia. *Semin Reprod Endocrinol* 1998; **16**: 93–104.
30. Redman C W, Sacks G P, Sargent I L. Preeclampsia: an excessive maternal inflammatory response to pregnancy. *Am J Obstet Gynecol* 1999; **180**: 499–506.
31. Sacks G P, Studena K, Sargent K, Redman C W. Normal pregnancy and preeclampsia both produce inflammatory changes in peripheral blood leukocytes akin to those of sepsis. *Am J Obstet Gynecol* 1998; **179**: 80–6.
32. Ala Y, Palluy O, Favero J *et al.* Hypoxia/reoxygenation stimulates endothelial cells to promote interleukin-1 and interleukin-6 production: effects of free radical scavengers. *Agents Actions* 1992; **37**: 134–9.
33. Kupferminc M J, Peaceman A M, Aderka D, Wallach D, Socol M L. Soluble tumor necrosis factor receptors and interleukin-6 levels in patients with severe preeclampsia. *Obstet Gynecol* 1996; **88**: 420–7.

34. Kupferminc M J, Peaceman A M, Wigton T R, Rehnberg K A, Socol M L. Tumor necrosis factor-alpha is elevated in plasma and amniotic fluid of patients with severe preeclampsia. *Am J Obstet Gynecol* 1994; **170**: 1752–7; discussion 1757–9.

35. Sharma A, Satyam A, Sharma J B. Leptin, IL-10 and inflammatory markers (TNF-alpha, IL-6 and IL-8) in pre-eclamptic, normotensive pregnant and healthy non-pregnant women. *Am J Reprod Immunol* 2007; **58**: 21–30.

36. Soleymanlou N, Jurisica I, Nevo O *et al.* Molecular evidence of placental hypoxia in preeclampsia. *J Clin Endocrinol Metab* 2005; **90**: 4299–308.

37. Zamudio S, Wu Y, Ietta F *et al.* Human placental hypoxia-inducible factor-1alpha expression correlates with clinical outcomes in chronic hypoxia in vivo. *Am J Pathol* 2007; **170**: 2171–9.

38. Nevo O, Soleymanlou N, Wu Y *et al.* Increased expression of sFlt-1 in in vivo and in vitro models of human placental hypoxia is mediated by HIF-1. *Am J Physiol Regul Integr Comp Physiol* 2006; **291**: R1085–93.

39. Rajakumar A, Brandon H M, Daftary A, Ness R, Conrad K P. Evidence for the functional activity of hypoxia-inducible transcription factors overexpressed in preeclamptic placentae. *Placenta* 2004; **25**: 763–9.

40. Caniggia I, Winter J L. Adriana and Luisa Castellucci Award lecture 2001. Hypoxia inducible factor-1: oxygen regulation of trophoblast differentiation in normal and pre-eclamptic pregnancies – a review. *Placenta* 2002; **23** (Suppl A): S47–57.

41. Nishi H, Nakada T, Hokamura M *et al.* Hypoxia-inducible factor-1 transactivates transforming growth factor-beta3 in trophoblast. *Endocrinology* 2004; **145**: 4113–8.

42. Shibuya M, Claesson-Welsh L. Signal transduction by VEGF receptors in regulation of angiogenesis and lymphangiogenesis. *Exp Cell Res* 2006; **312**: 549–60.

43. Carmeliet P, Ferreira V, Breier G *et al.* Abnormal blood vessel development and lethality in embryos lacking a single VEGF allele. *Nature* 1996; **380**: 435–9.

44. Ferrara N, Carver-Moore K, Chen H *et al.* Heterozygous embryonic lethality induced by targeted inactivation of the VEGF gene. *Nature* 1996; **380**: 439–42.

45. Kanda M, Nomoto S, Nishikawa Y *et al.* Correlations of the expression of vascular endothelial growth factor B and its isoforms in hepatocellular carcinoma with clinico-pathological parameters. *J Surg Oncol* 2008; **98**: 190–6.

46. McColl B K, Paavonen K, Karnezis T *et al.* Proprotein convertases promote processing of VEGF-D, a critical step for binding the angiogenic receptor VEGFR-2. *Faseb J* 2007; **21**: 1088–98.

47. Lyttle D J, Fraser K M, Fleming S B, Mercer A A, Robinson A J. Homologs of vascular endothelial growth factor are encoded by the poxvirus orf virus. *J Virol* 1994; **68**: 84–92.

48. Kiba A, Sagara H, Hara T, Shibuya M. VEGFR-2-specific ligand VEGF-E induces non-edematous hyper-vascularization in mice. *Biochem Biophys Res Comm* 2003; **301**: 371–7.

49. Maglione D, Guerriero V, Viglietto G, Delli-Bovi P, Persico M G. Isolation of a human placenta cDNA coding for a protein related to the vascular permeability factor. *Proc Natl Acad Sci U S A* 1991; **88**: 9267–71.

50. Autiero M, Waltenberger J, Communi D *et al.* Role of PlGF in the intra- and intermolecular cross talk between the VEGF receptors Flt1 and Flk1. *Nat Med* 2003; **9**: 936–43.

51. Carmeliet P, Moons L, Luttun A *et al.* Synergism between vascular endothelial growth factor and placental growth factor contributes to angiogenesis and plasma extravasation in pathological conditions. *Nat Med* 2001; **7**: 575–83.

52. Ahmed A, Dunk C, Ahmad S, Khaliq A. Regulation of placental vascular endothelial growth factor (VEGF) and placenta growth factor (PIGF) and soluble Flt-1 by oxygen – a review. *Placenta* 2000; **21** (Suppl A): S16–24.

53. Vuorela P, Hatva E, Lymboussaki A *et al.* Expression of vascular endothelial growth factor and placenta growth factor in human placenta. *Biol Reprod* 1997; **56**: 489–94.

54. Hanna J, Goldman-Wohl D, Hamani Y *et al.* Decidual NK cells regulate key developmental processes at the human fetal-maternal interface. *Nat Med* 2006; **12**: 1065–74.

55. Tayade C, Hilchie D, He H *et al.* Genetic deletion of placenta growth factor in mice alters uterine NK cells. *J Immunol* 2007; **178**: 4267–75.

56. Alitalo K, Carmeliet P. Molecular mechanisms of lymphangiogenesis in health and disease. *Cancer Cell* 2002; **1**: 219–27.

57. Veikkola T, Jussila L, Makinen T *et al.* Signalling via vascular endothelial growth factor receptor-3 is sufficient for lymphangiogenesis in transgenic mice. *Embo J* 2001; **20**: 1223–31.

58. Barleon B, Sozzani S, Zhou D *et al.* Migration of human monocytes in response to vascular endothelial growth factor (VEGF) is mediated via the VEGF receptor flt-1. *Blood* 1996; **87**: 3336–43.

59. Clauss M, Weich H, Breier G *et al.* The vascular endothelial growth factor receptor Flt-1 mediates biological activities: implications for a functional role of placenta growth factor in monocyte activation and chemotaxis. *J Biol Chem* 1996; **271**: 17629–34.

60. Sawano A, Iwai S, Sakurai Y *et al.* Flt-1, vascular endothelial growth factor receptor 1, is a novel cell surface marker for the lineage of monocyte-macrophages in humans. *Blood* 2001; **97**: 785–91.

61. Fong G, Rassant J, Gertenstein M M B. Role of Flt-1 receptor tyrosine kinase in regulation of assembly of vascular endothelium. *Nature* 1995; **376**: 66–7.

62. Shalaby F, Rossant J, Yamaguchi T P *et al.* Failure of blood-island formation and vasculogenesis in Flk-1-deficient mice. *Nature* 1995; **376**: 62–6.

63. Helske S, Vuorela P, Carpen O *et al.* Expression of vascular endothelial growth factor receptors 1, 2 and 3 in placentae from normal and complicated pregnancies. *Mol Hum Reprod* 2001; **7**: 205–10.

64. Venkatesha S, Toporsian M, Lam C *et al.* Soluble endoglin contributes to the pathogenesis of preeclampsia. *Nat Med* 2006; **12**: 642–9.

65. Barbara N P, Wrana J L, Letarte M. Endoglin is an accessory protein that interacts with the signaling receptor complex of multiple members of the transforming growth factor-beta superfamily. *J Biol Chem* 1999; **274**: 584–94.

66. Caniggia I, Grisaru-Gravnosky S, Kuliszewsky M, Post M, Lye S J. Inhibition of TGF-beta 3 restores the invasive capability of extravillous trophoblasts in preeclamptic pregnancies. *J Clin Invest* 1999; **103**: 1641–50.

67. Jones R L, Stoikos C, Findlay J K, Salamonsen L A. TGF-beta superfamily expression and actions in the endometrium and placenta. *Reproduction* 2006; **132**: 217–32.

68. McAllister K A, Grogg K M, Johnson D W *et al.* Endoglin, a TGF-beta binding protein of endothelial cells, is the gene for hereditary haemorrhagic telangiectasia type 1. *Nat Genet* 1994; **8**: 345–51.

69. Bourdeau A, Dumont D J, Letarte M. A murine model of hereditary hemorrhagic telangiectasia. *J Clin Invest* 1999; **104**: 1343–51.

70. Jerkic M, Rivas-Elena J V, Prieto M *et al.* Endoglin regulates nitric oxide-dependent vasodilatation. *Faseb J* 2004; **18**: 609–11.

71. St-Jacques S, Forte M, Lye S J, Letarte M. Localization of endoglin, a transforming growth factor-beta binding protein, and of CD44 and integrins in placenta during the first trimester of pregnancy. *Biol Reprod* 1994; **51**: 405–13.

72. Maynard S, Epstein F H, Karumanchi S A. Preeclampsia and angiogenic imbalance. *Ann Rev Med* 2008; **59**: 61–78.

73. Clark D E, Smith S K, He Y *et al.* A vascular endothelial growth factor antagonist is produced by the human placenta and released into the maternal circulation. *Biol Reprod* 1998; **59**: 1540–8.

74. Esser S, Wolburg K, Wolburg H *et al.* Vascular endothelial growth factor induces endothelial fenestrations in vitro. *J Cell Biol* 1998; **140**: 947–59.

75. Levine R J, Karumanchi S A. Circulating angiogenic factors in preeclampsia. *Clin Obst Gynecol* 2005; **48**: 372–86.

76. Maynard S E, Min J Y, Merchan J *et al.* Excess placental soluble fms-like tyrosine kinase 1 (sFlt1) may contribute to endothelial dysfunction, hypertension, and proteinuria in preeclampsia. *J Clin Invest* 2003; **111**: 649–58.

77. Sugimoto H, Hamano Y, Charytan D *et al.* Neutralization of circulating vascular endothelial growth factor (VEGF) by anti-VEGF antibodies and soluble VEGF receptor 1 (sFlt-1) induces proteinuria. *J Biol Chem* 2003; **278**: 12605–8.

78. Eremina V, Sood M, Haigh J *et al.* Glomerular-specific alterations of VEGF-A expression lead to distinct congenital and acquired renal diseases. *J Clin Invest* **111**: 707–716.

79. Eremina V, Jefferson J A, Kowalewska J *et al.* VEGF inhibition and renal thrombotic microangiopathy. *New Engl J Med* 2008; **358**: 1129–36.

80. Zhu X, Wu S, Dahut W L, Parikh C R. Risks of proteinuria and hypertension with bevacizumab, an antibody against vascular endothelial growth factor: systematic review and meta-analysis. *Am J Kidney Dis* 2007; **49**: 186–93.

81. Polliotti B M, Fry A G, Saller D N *et al.* Second-trimester maternal serum placental growth factor and vascular endothelial growth factor for predicting severe, early-onset preeclampsia. *Obstet Gynecol* 2003; **101**: 1266–74.

82. Thomas C P, Andrews J I, Liu K Z. Intronic polyadenylation signal sequences and alternate splicing generate human soluble Flt1 variants and regulate the abundance of soluble Flt1 in the placenta. *Faseb J* 2007; **21**: 3885–95.

83. Sela S, Itin A, Natanson-Yaron S *et al.* A novel human-specific soluble vascular endothelial growth factor receptor 1: cell-type-specific splicing and implications to vascular endothelial growth factor homeostasis and preeclampsia. *Circ Res* 2008; **102**: 1566–74.

84. Maharaj A S, Walshe T E, Saint-Geniez M *et al.* VEGF and TGF-beta are required for the maintenance of the choroid plexus and ependyma. *J Exp Med* 2008; **205**: 491–501.

85. Shore V H, Wang T H, Wang C L *et al.* Vascular endothelial growth factor, placenta growth factor and their receptors in isolated human trophoblast. *Placenta* 1997; **18**: 657–65.

86. Nagamatsu T, Fujii T, Kusumi M *et al.* Cytotrophoblasts up-regulate soluble fms-like tyrosine kinase-1

expression under reduced oxygen: an implication for the placental vascular development and the pathophysiology of preeclampsia. *Endocrinology* 2004; **145**: 4838–45.

87. Gu Y, Lewis D F, Wang Y. Placental productions and expressions of soluble endoglin, soluble fms-like tyrosine kinase receptor-1, and placental growth factor in normal and preeclamptic pregnancies. *J Clin Endocrinol Metab* 2008; **93**: 260–6.

88. Makris A, Thornton C, Thompson J *et al.* Uteroplacental ischemia results in proteinuric hypertension and elevated sFLT-1. *Kidney Int* 2007; **71**: 977–84.

89. Gilbert J S, Babcock S A, Granger J P. Hypertension produced by reduced uterine perfusion in pregnant rats is associated with increased soluble fms-like tyrosine kinase-1 expression. *Hypertension* 2007; **50**: 1142–7.

90. Parikh S M, Karumanchi S A. Putting pressure on pre-eclampsia. *Nat Med* 2008; **14**: 810–12.

91. Yinon Y, Nevo O, Xu J *et al.* Severe intrauterine growth restriction pregnancies have increased placental endoglin levels: hypoxic regulation via transforming growth factor-beta 3. *Am J Pathol* 2008; **172**: 77–85.

92. Jeyabalan A, McGonigal S, Gilmour C, Hubel C A, Rajakumar A. Circulating and placental endoglin concentrations in pregnancies complicated by intrauterine growth restriction and preeclampsia. *Placenta* 2008; **29**: 555–63.

93. Nevo O, Many A, Xu J *et al.* Placental expression of soluble fms-like tyrosine kinase 1 is increased in singletons and twin pregnancies with intrauterine growth restriction. *J Clin Endocrinol Metab* 2008; **93**: 285–92.

94. Rajakumar A, Jeyabalan A, Markovic N *et al.* Placental HIF-1 alpha, HIF-2 alpha, membrane and soluble VEGF receptor-1 proteins are not increased in normotensive pregnancies complicated by late-onset intrauterine growth restriction. *Am J Physiol Regul Integr Comp Physiol* 2007; **293**: R766–74.

95. Levine R J, Maynard S E, Qian C *et al.* Circulating angiogenic factors and the risk of preeclampsia. *New Engl J Med* 2004; **350**: 672–83.

96. Koga K, Osuga Y, Yoshino O *et al.* Elevated serum soluble vascular endothelial growth factor receptor 1 (sVEGFR-1) levels in women with preeclampsia. *J Clin Endocrinol Metab* 2003; **88**: 2348–51.

97. Rana S, Karumanchi S A, Levine R J *et al.* Sequential changes in antiangiogenic factors in early pregnancy and risk of developing preeclampsia. *Hypertension* 2007; **50**: 137–42.

98. Vatten L J, Eskild A, Nilsen T I *et al.* Changes in circulating level of angiogenic factors from the first to second trimester as predictors of preeclampsia. *Am J Obstet Gynecol* 2007; **196**:239. e231–236.

99. Stepan H, Unversucht A, Wessel N, Faber R. Predictive value of maternal angiogenic factors in second trimester pregnancies with abnormal uterine perfusion. *Hypertension* 2007; **49**: 818–24.

100. Romero R, Nien J K, Espinoza J *et al.* A longitudinal study of angiogenic (placental growth factor) and anti-angiogenic (soluble endoglin and soluble vascular endothelial growth factor receptor-1) factors in normal pregnancy and patients destined to develop preeclampsia and deliver a small for gestational age neonate. *J Matern Fetal Neonatal Med* 2008; **21**: 9–23.

101. Moore Simas T A, Crawford S L, Solitro M J *et al.* Angiogenic factors for the prediction of preeclampsia in high-risk women. *Am J Obstet Gynecol* 2007; **197**: e241–8.

102. Stepan H, Geipel A, Schwarz F *et al.* Circulatory soluble endoglin and its predictive value for preeclampsia in second-trimester pregnancies with abnormal uterine perfusion. *Am J Obstet Gynecol* 2008; **198**: e171–6.

103. Wikstrom A K, Larsson A, Eriksson U J *et al.* Placental growth factor and soluble FMS-like tyrosine kinase-1 in early-onset and late-onset preeclampsia. *Obstet Gynecol* 2007; **109**: 1368–74.

104. Levine R J, Thadhani R, Qian C *et al.* Urinary placental growth factor and risk of preeclampsia. *Jama* 2005; **293**: 77–85.

105. Purwosunu Y, Sekizawa A, Farina A *et al.* Evaluation of physiological alterations of the placenta through analysis of cell-free messenger ribonucleic acid concentrations of angiogenic factors. *Am J Obstet Gynecol* 2008; **198**: e121–7.

106. Smith G C, Pell J P, Walsh D. Pregnancy complications and maternal risk of ischaemic heart disease: a retrospective cohort study of 129 290 births. *Lancet* 2001; **357**: 2002–6.

107. Wilson B J, Watson M S, Prescott G J *et al.* Hypertensive diseases of pregnancy and risk of hypertension and stroke in later life: results from cohort study. *BMJ* 2003; **326**: 845.

108. Vikse B E, Irgens L M, Bostad L, Iversen B M. Adverse perinatal outcome and later kidney biopsy in the mother. *J Am Soc Nephrol* 2006; **17**: 837–45.

109. Vikse B E, Irgens L M, Leivestad T, Skjaerven R, Iversen B M. Preeclampsia and the risk of end-stage renal disease. *New Engl J Med* 2008; **359**: 800–9.

110. Bar J, Kaplan B, Wittenberg C *et al.* Microalbuminuria after pregnancy complicated by pre-eclampsia. *Nephrol Dial Transplant* 1999; **14**: 1129–32.

111. Pouta A, Hartikainen A L, Sovio U *et al.* Manifestations of metabolic syndrome after hypertensive pregnancy. *Hypertension* 2004; **43**: 825–31.

112. Forest J C, Girouard J, Masse J *et al.* Early occurrence of metabolic syndrome after hypertension in pregnancy. *Obstet Gynecol* 2005; **105**: 1373–80.

113. Wolf M, Hubel C A, Lam C *et al.* Preeclampsia and future cardiovascular disease: potential role of altered angiogenesis and insulin resistance. *J Clin Endocrinol Metab* 2004; **89**: 6239–43.

114. Barker D J, Gluckman P D, Godfrey K M *et al.* Fetal nutrition and cardiovascular disease in adult life. *Lancet* 1993; **341**: 938–41.

115. Hales C N, Barker D J, Clark P M *et al.* Fetal and infant growth and impaired glucose tolerance at age 64. *BMJ* 1991; **303**: 1019–22.

116. Klebanoff M A, Secher N J, Mednick B R, Schulsinger C. Maternal size at birth and the development of hypertension during pregnancy: a test of the Barker hypothesis. *Arch Intern Med* 1999; **159**: 1607–12.

117. Li Z, Zhang Y, Ying Ma J *et al.* Recombinant vascular endothelial growth factor 121 attenuates hypertension and improves kidney damage in a rat model of preeclampsia. *Hypertension* 2007; **50**: 686–92.

118. Karumanchi S A, Epstein F H. Placental ischemia and soluble fms-like tyrosine kinase 1: cause or consequence of preeclampsia? *Kidney Int* 2007; **71**: 959–61.

119. Chaiworapongsa T, Romero R, Kim Y M *et al.* Plasma soluble vascular endothelial growth factor receptor-1 concentration is elevated prior to the clinical diagnosis of pre-eclampsia. *J Matern Fetal Neonatal Med* 2005; **17**: 3–18.

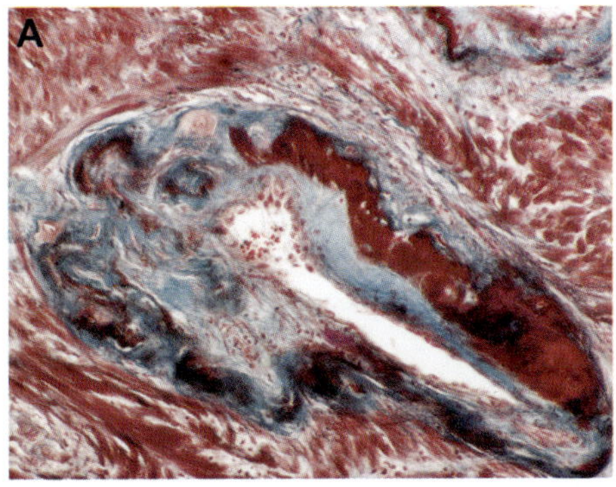

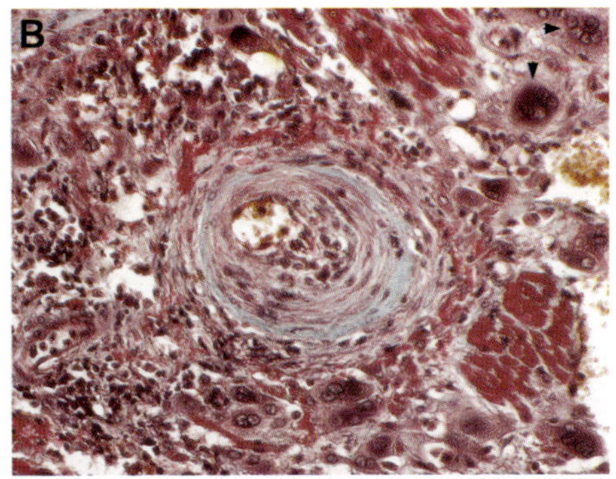

Fig. 3.1 (A) Uteroplacental artery showing marked distension and replacement of the muscular and elastic tissue in the wall by fibrinoid and invaded trophoblast. (B) A spiral artery in the junctional zone myometrium in severe preeclampsia showing absence of physiological changes and surrounded by interstitial trophoblast (Masson trichrome).

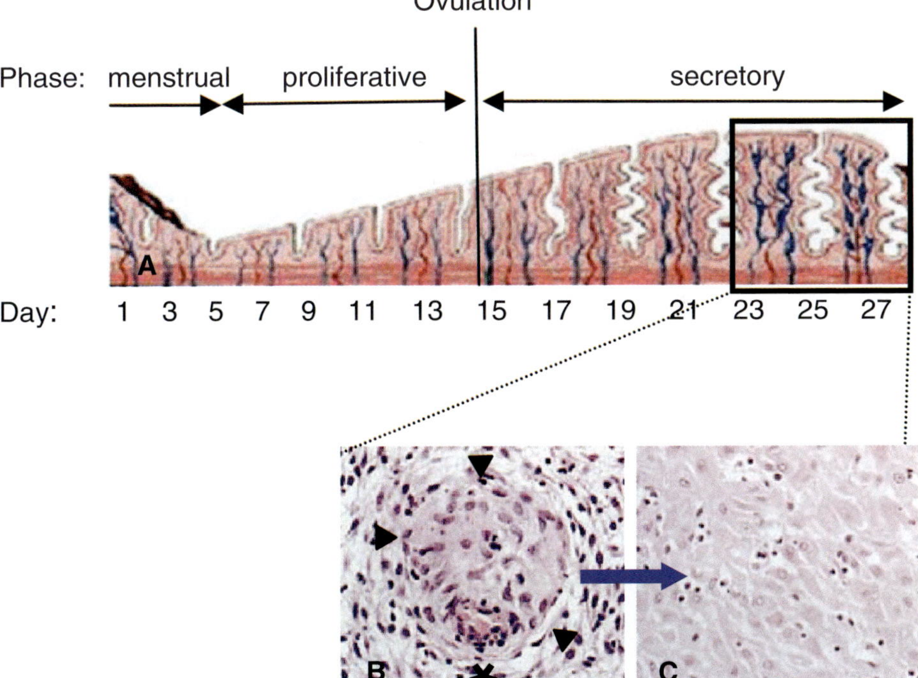

Fig. 5.1 Cyclic decidualization of the endometrial stromal compartment during the menstrual cycle. (A) The postovulatory rise in progesterone levels initiates endometrial differentiation in preparation for pregnancy. (B) As is the case in other menstruating species, the human endometrium exhibits spontaneous decidualization during the late secretory phase of the cycle, a process initiated around the terminal spiral arteries (*) and characterized by epithelioid transformation of stromal fibroblasts (arrowheads). (C) The decidual process continues to evolve and in pregnancy encompasses the entire stromal compartment.

Fig. 5.3 Morphological changes and functional reprogramming upon decidualization. (A) Cytoskeletal organization and stress fiber formation. Phalloidin staining (red) of filamentous-actin in undifferentiated endometrial stromal cells (left panel) and cells decidualized in culture for 72 hours (right panel). (B) In concert, endometrial stromal cells acquire unique functions essential for pregnancy.

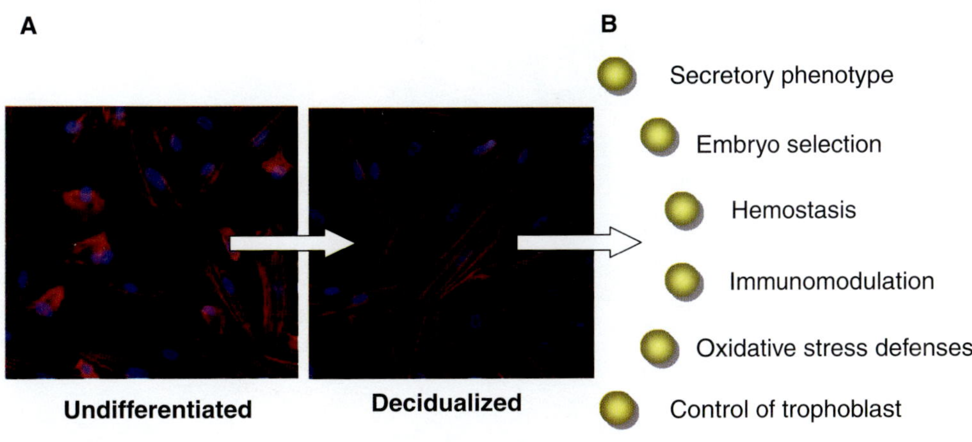

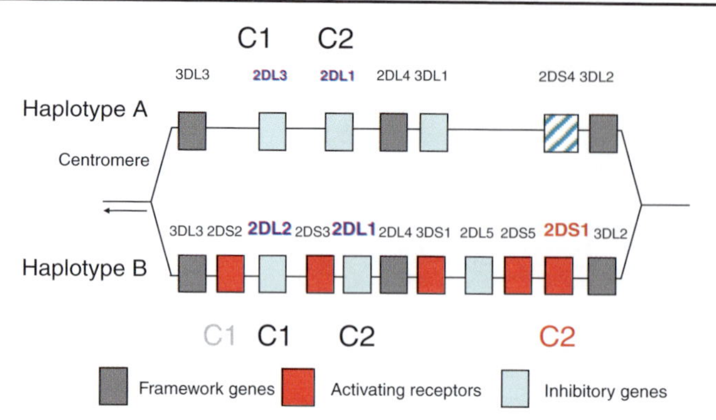

Fig. 6.1 Two representative KIR haplotypes of A and B type.

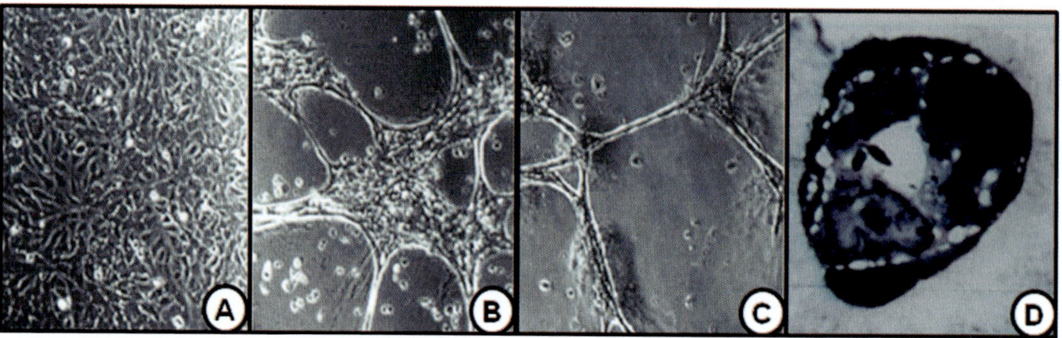

Fig. 7.1 (A) HUVEC grown for 48 hours on gelatin-coated plastic exhibit typical 'cobblestone' morphology. When the cells are cultured on Matrigel® for 8 hours (B) or 48 hours (C) they retract and form three-dimensional capillary-like bridges and tubules. (D) A high-power cross-section of the latter structure reveals a central lumen. Reproduced with permission from De Groot *et al.* 1995 [10].

Fig. 8.1 Color flow mapping of the utero and umbilico-placental circulations at 7 weeks of gestation.

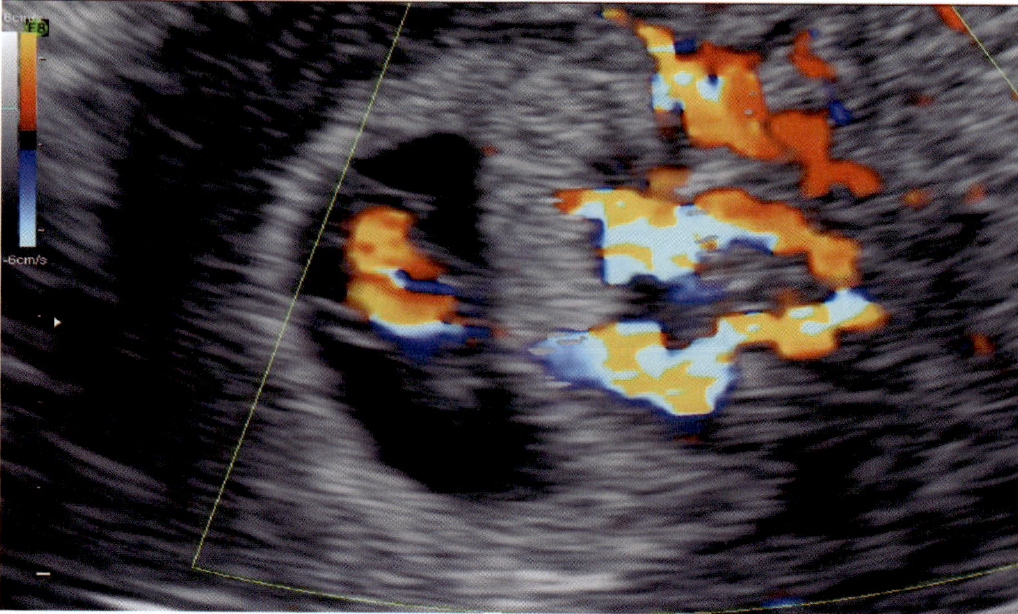

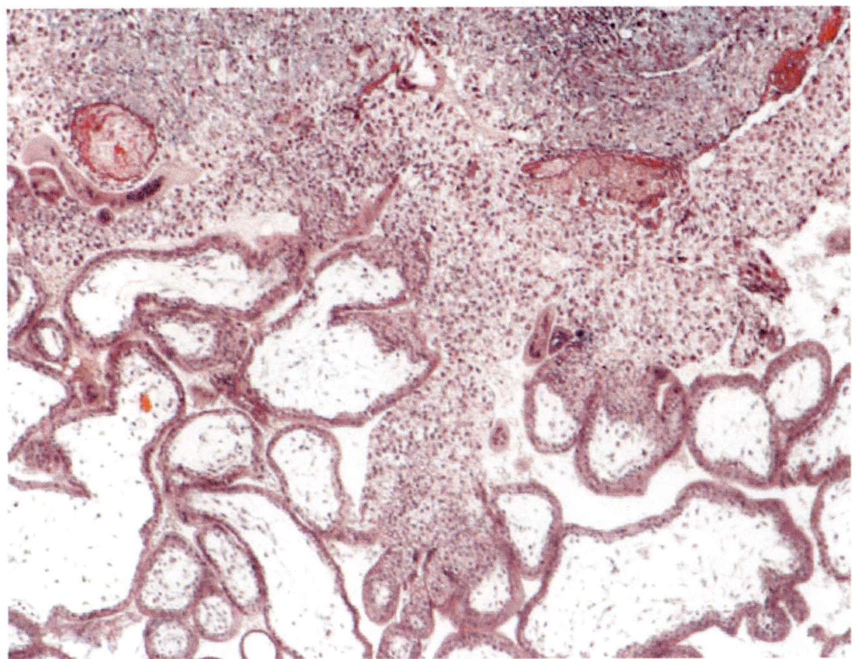

Fig. 8.2 Histological view of the materno-placental interface (deciduochorial) showing the cytotrophoblastic cell shell (hysterectomy specimen No H710: 4 mm embryo of 6 weeks of gestation, Boyd Collection, Department of Anatomy, University of Cambridge).

Fig. 11.5 Cytokeratin (red)/CD31 (blue) double immunostaining of a remodeled spiral artery, illustrating endothelial repair (*End*) after intramural incorporation of the trophoblast (*IMT*). The insert is a high-power picture showing a trophoblastic cell very close to the lumen, covered by a very thin layer of endothelium. Reproduced with permission from Pijnenborg *et al.* [7], Copyright Elsevier (2006).

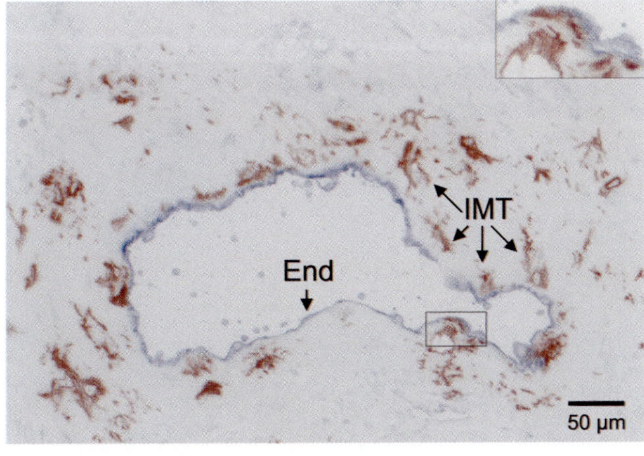

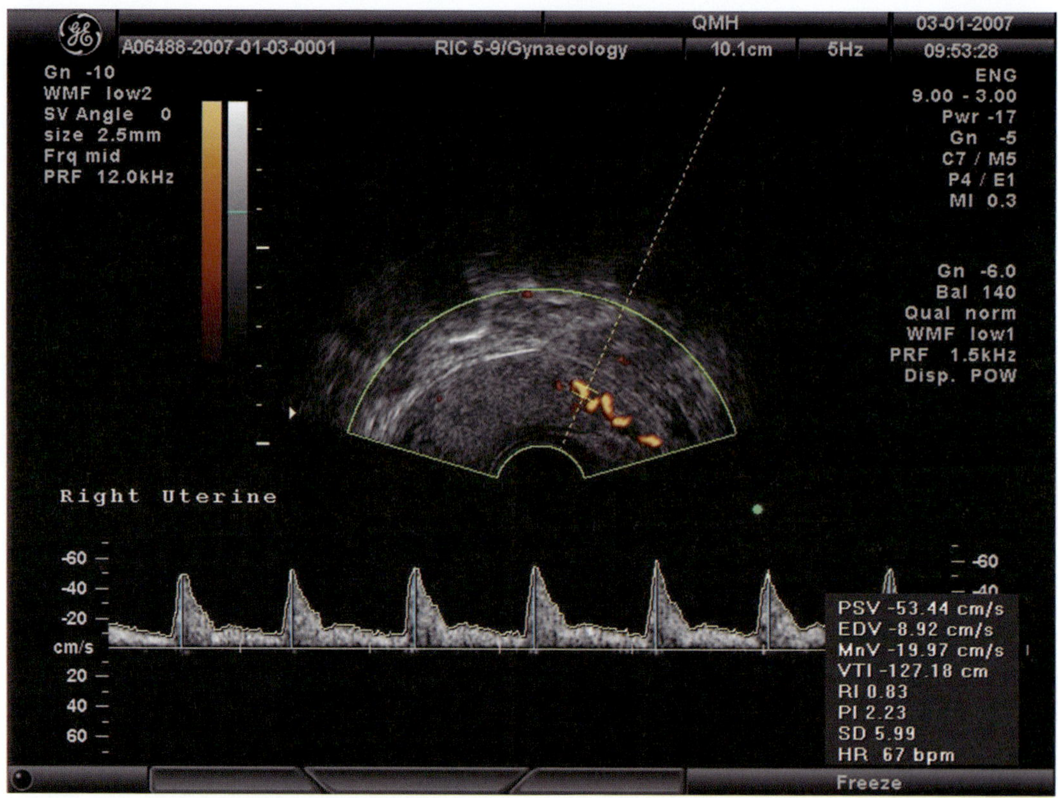

Fig. 10.1 Uterine blood flow measured by 2D Doppler ultrasound.

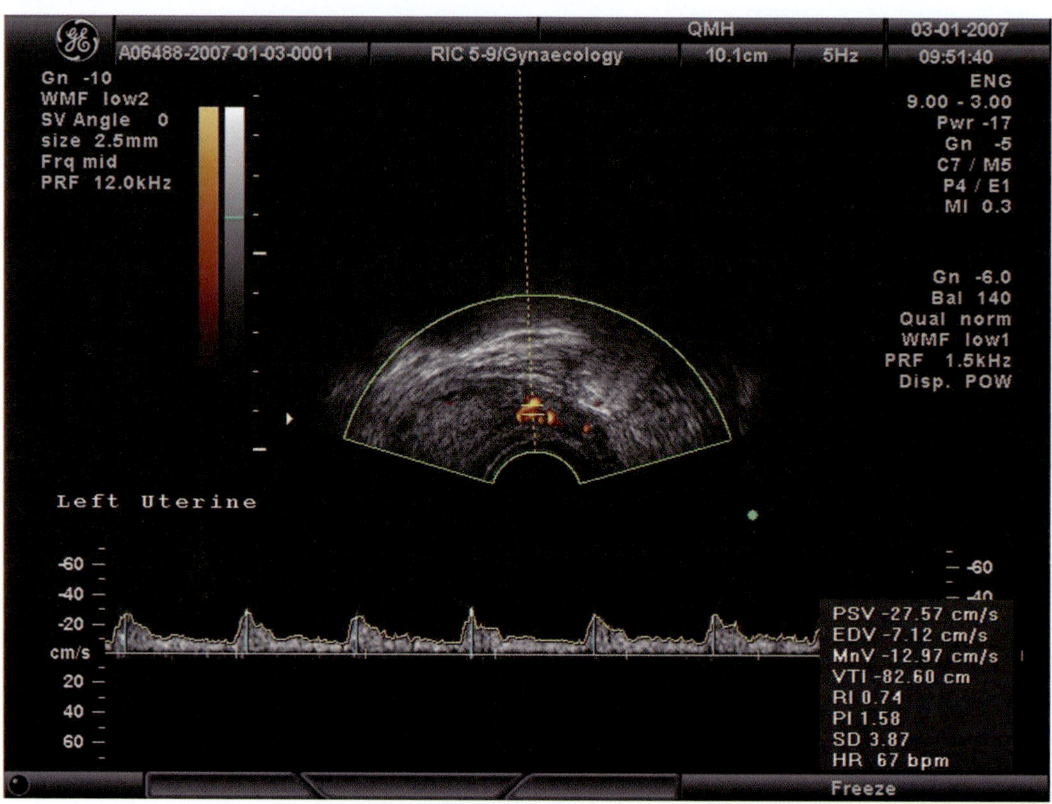

Fig. 10.1b

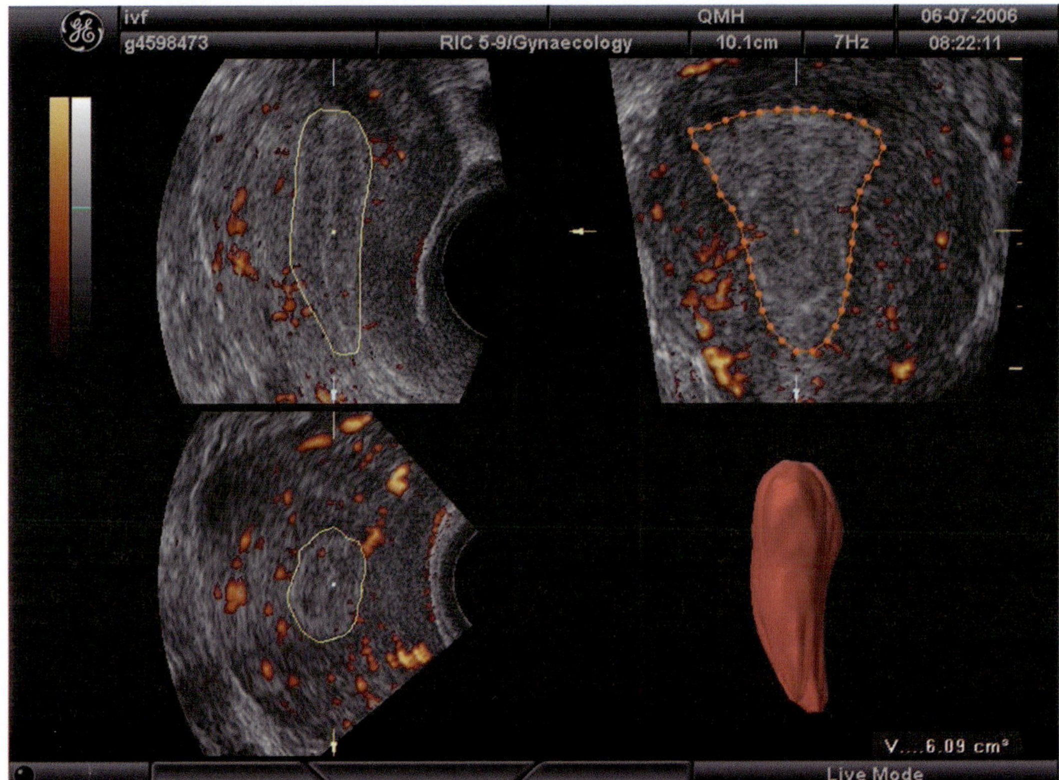

Fig. 10.2 Endometrial volume and blood flow measured by 3D Doppler ultrasound.

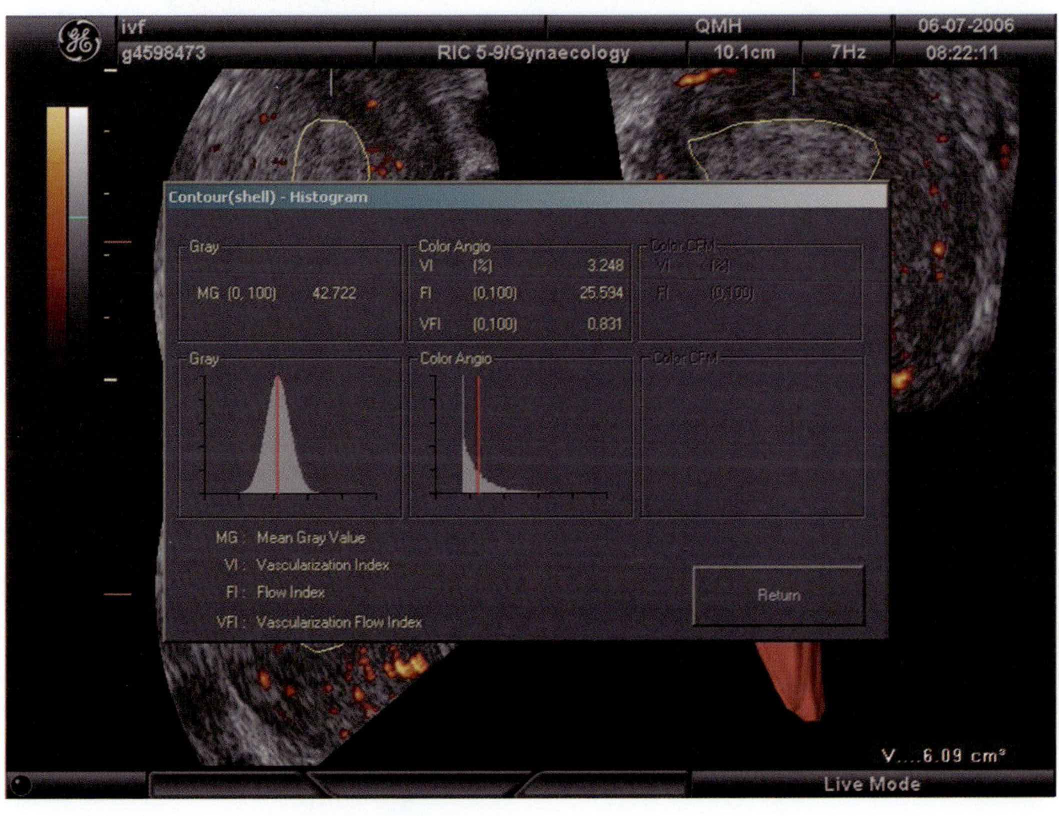

Fig. 10.2b

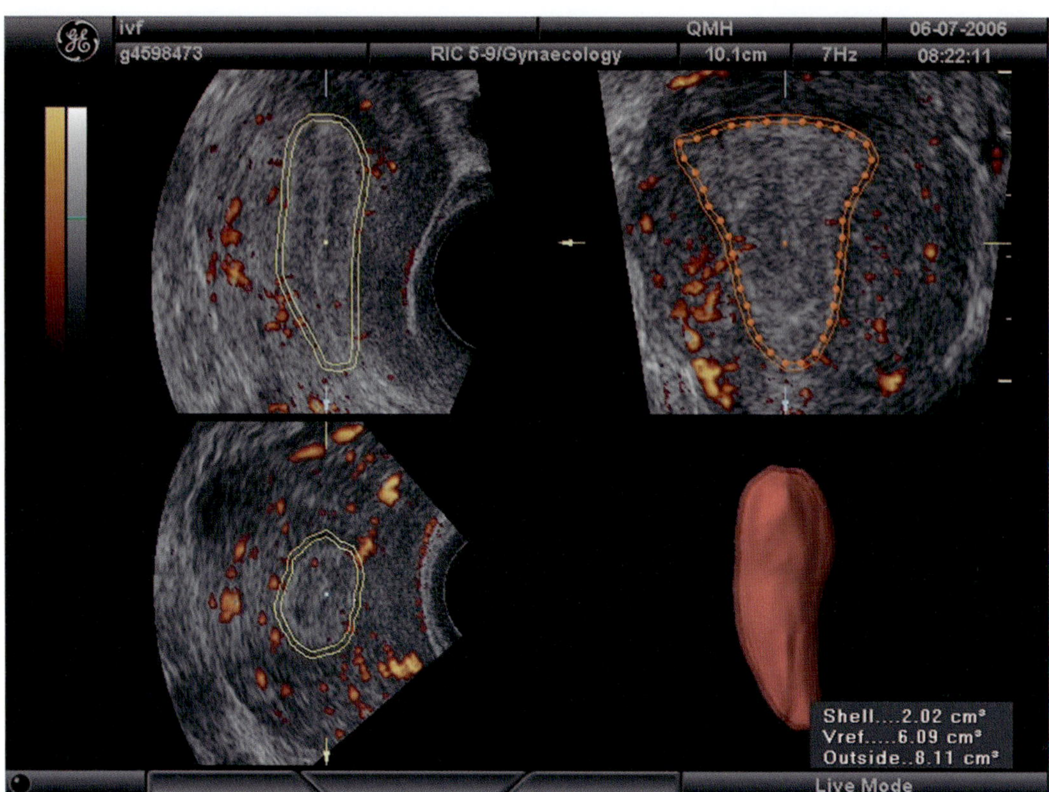

Fig. 10.3 Subendometrial volume and blood flow measured by 3D Doppler ultrasound.

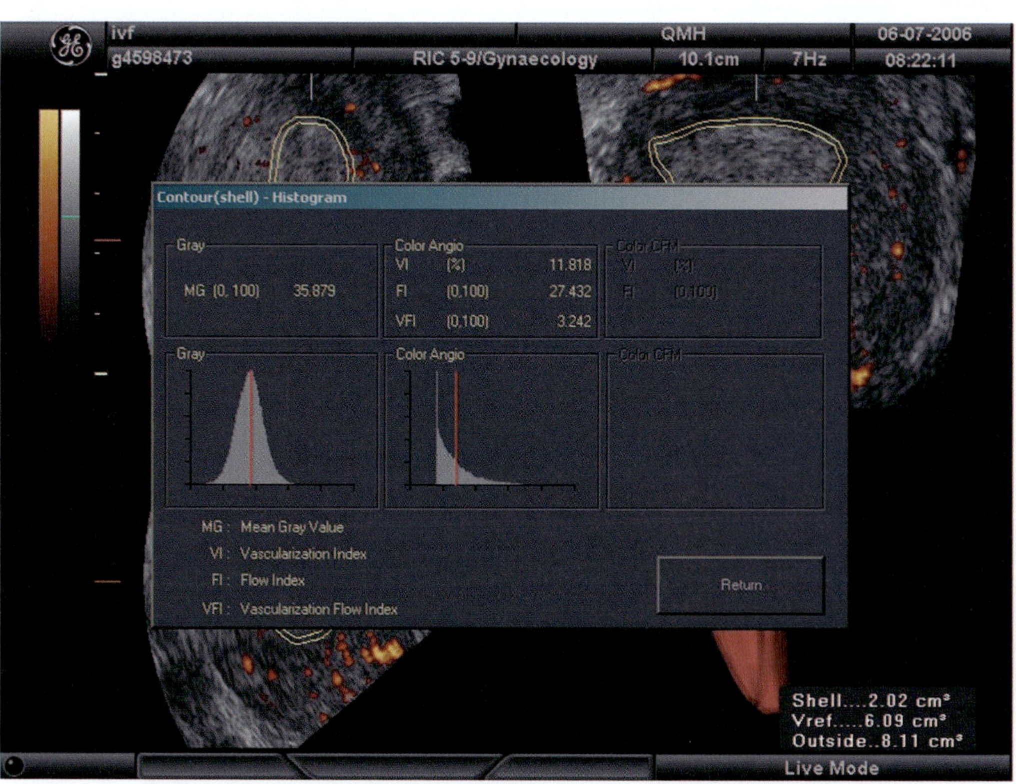

Fig. 10.3b

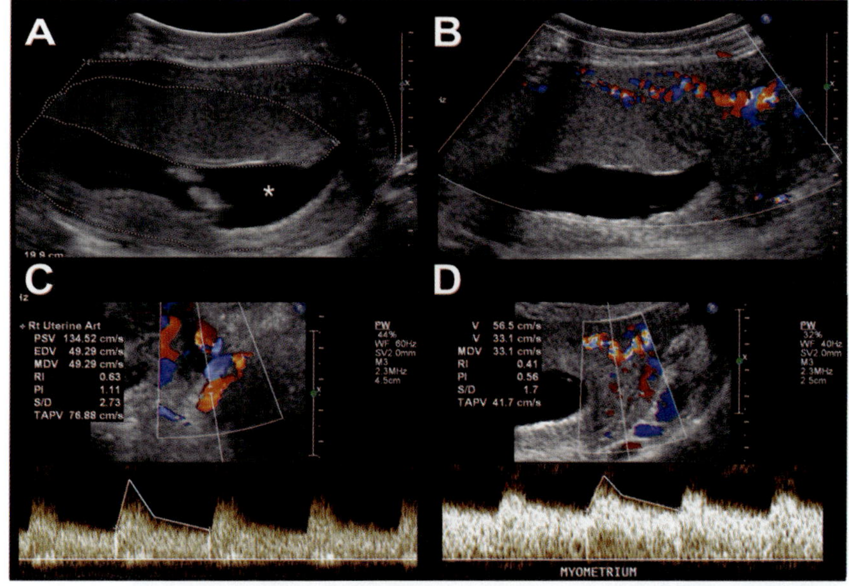

Fig. 23.1 Blood flow to the uterus and placenta at 12 weeks of gestation. (A) Real-time imaging in the transverse plane shows the uterus (outer line) and definitive placenta (inner line) with the intervening tissue being myometrium. *Denotes the amniotic fluid. (B) Corresponding image with color flow Doppler shows strong blood flow signals in the myometrium, but not inside the placenta. (C) Pulsed Doppler waveforms from the proximal left uterine artery in the same plane below the uterus – note high peak systolic velocity (134 cm/second) and low pulsatility index (PI) indicating a low-impedance circulation. (D) Corresponding pulsed Doppler recordings from the myometrial arteries showing similar low-impedance waveforms. No arterial signals are obtained inside the placenta.

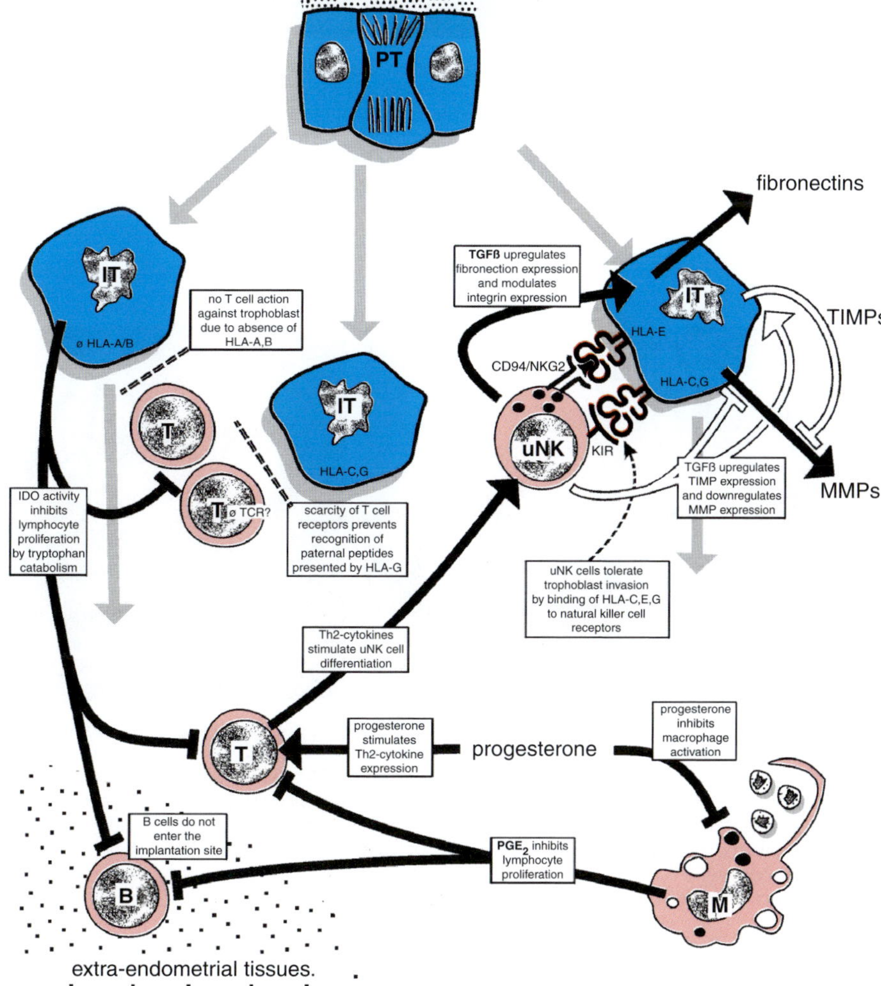

Fig. 23.3 Schematic overview of interaction of maternal immune cells with trophoblast cells in the implantation site and their effects on trophoblast invasion. Gray arrows: routes of trophoblast invasion; black arrows: interactions that are thought to exert a promoting net effect in trophoblast invasion. Blue: trophoblast cells; pink: maternal cells; PT, proliferative extravillous trophoblast; IT, invasive extravillous trophoblast; uNK, uterine natural killer cell; M, macrophage; T, T cell; B, B cell. Reproduced with permission from David *et al.* [96].

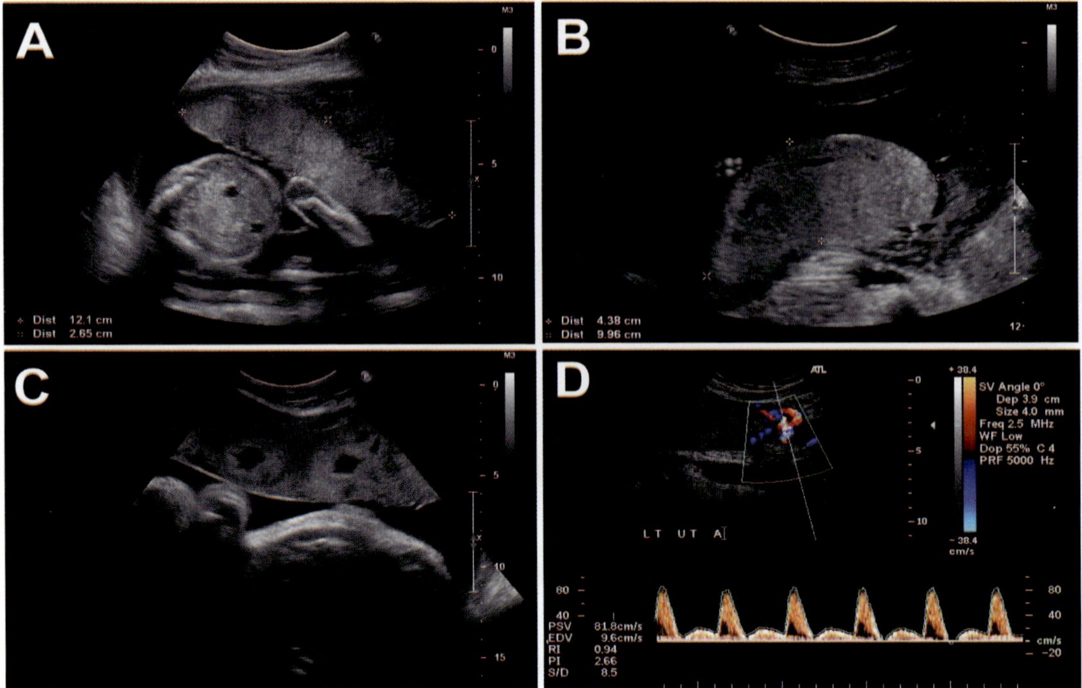

Fig. 23.4 Placental ultrasound and abnormal uterine artery Doppler at 19–22 weeks in women with low PAPP-A (< 0.3 MOM) values at 11–13 weeks. (A) The normal placenta is typically 12 cm long and 2.5 cm thick. Note the normal granular texture, created by the interdigitating villous trees anchored to the basal plate. (B) A small placental footprint increases the risk of stillbirth and severe IUGR in this study. In this situation, the umbilical cord insertion is usually at the edge, indicating 'chorion regression' at the end of the first trimester. The placental insufficiency initiated by a small footprint may then be compounded by subsequent injury to the placental tissue (C). (C) These echogenic cystic lesions (ECLs) are non-functioning tissue due to intervillous thrombosis and are a poor prognostic sign. (D) ECLs and wedge-shaped infarcts usually develop in the placentae of women with persistently abnormal uterine artery Doppler characterized by an elevated pulsatility index (PI) > 1.45, in this case 2.6.

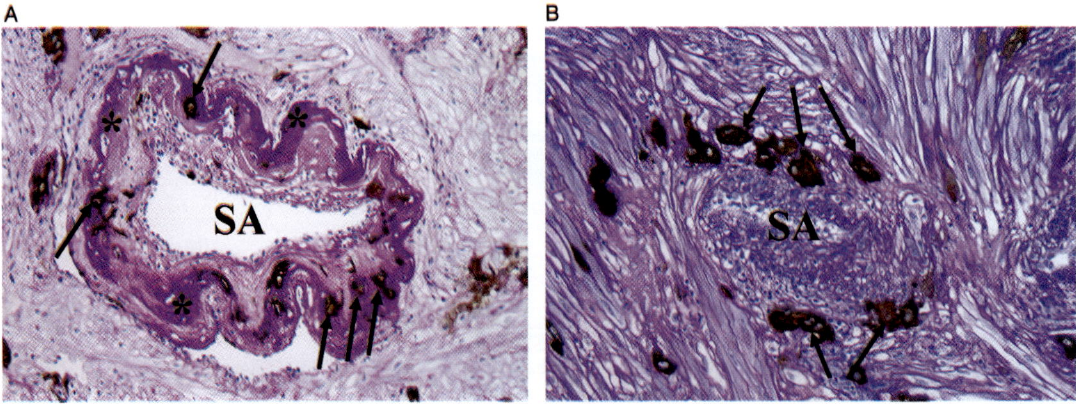

Fig. 24.1 (A) Physiological transformation of myometrial spiral artery in a placental bed biopsy specimen from a normal pregnant woman at 40 weeks of gestation (cytokeratin 7/PAS, ×200). The lumen of the spiral arteries (SA) is dilated. The fibrinoid material, which replaces the media of the 'physiologically transformed spiral arteries', is purple in color (PAS positive) and labeled with an asterisk (*). Trophoblastic cells, which are cytokeratin positive (brown and labeled with arrows), are infiltrating the wall of the spiral artery. (B) Failure of physiological transformation of myometrial spiral arteries in a placental bed biopsy specimen from a patient with preterm labor (without a small-for-gestational age fetus) at 31 weeks of gestation (cytokeratin 7/PAS, ×200). The lumen of the artery (SA) is not dilated. The medial layers of the spiral artery are intact. Fibrinoid material (PAS positive) is not present. Although plenty of interstitial trophoblasts surround the spiral arteries, which are cytokeratin positive (brown and labeled with arrows), trophoblasts have not invaded the vessel wall.

Section 8 Chapter 22

Translation to obstetrics

Periconceptual and early pregnancy approach

Gordon C. S. Smith

Department of Obstetrics and Gynaecology, University of Cambridge, Robinson Way, Cambridge, UK

Introduction

Even up to the nineteenth century, there was professional discussion of the possibility that congenital abnormalities might be caused by exposure of the mother to a related shock in late pregnancy, a belief known as maternal impression [1]. We now know that the vast majority of congenital structural malformations of the fetus are a consequence of dysfunctional embryogenesis in early pregnancy. However, when researchers address the causes of placental dysfunction resulting in growth restriction or pre-eclampsia, they might be accused of having a view that has parallels with the concept of maternal impression, in that they are studying a process in late pregnancy that was determined, at least in part, during the weeks immediately following conception. The biology of implantation and placentation are addressed in detail in other chapters of this book. The aim of the present chapter is to address the clinical evidence that complications in the second half of gestation are manifestations of dysfunctional formation of the placenta in early pregnancy. The following specific issues will be addressed in relation to early pregnancy markers of subsequent adverse outcome: (1) study design, (2) assessment of fetal growth, (3) ultrasonic assessment of placentation, (4) maternal circulating concentrations of placentally derived proteins, (5) combined ultrasonic and biochemical assessment of the placenta, and (6) clinical and epidemiological implications.

Study design in analyses of early pregnancy and periconceptual factors

Retrospective versus prospective studies

In general, there are many more studies of women who are known to have complications (retrospective analyses) than of women who are studied prior to the onset of some complication (prospective studies). In reality, in most obstetric populations, the majority of women have an uncomplicated pregnancy. Hence, the decision to study women prior to the onset of clinical manifestation of a given condition means that a large number of healthy women need to be recruited and studied. Hence, for a given amount of activity, the number of women studied who ultimately manifest an abnormality is lower if women are studied prospectively rather than retrospectively. However, the advantage of studying women prior to development of a complication is that any abnormalities observed are more likely to have a role in the development of the condition, as opposed to being epiphenomena. Moreover, associations determined from prospective studies may allow development of a predictive test. In general, the weakness of methods for prediction is a greater problem in obstetrics than the weakness of diagnostic methods. Therefore, when designing a study, these two conflicting interests have to be balanced.

Studies in the periconceptual period

The problems alluded to above are increased further if the aim is to study periconceptual factors. This requires recruitment of women prior to pregnancy. Hence, as well as the (relatively) wasted activity of obtaining data and samples from women who experience uncomplicated pregnancies, there is also the wasted activity of obtaining data and samples from women who do not ultimately have a pregnancy within the period of study. A large-scale cohort study in the south of England, the Southampton Women's Study, recruited women prior to pregnancy. The ratio of women recruited to women who were followed through to pregnancy was greater than 4:1 [2]. While there are clearly real strengths in a study design where prepregnancy data are available, this involves the expense of retrieving information from large numbers of women who do not have a pregnancy in the timescale of the study.

Studying selected populations

The proportion of women experiencing problems can be increased in prospective studies by recruiting high-risk women. However, many of these studies have the ultimate goal of developing a screening test. It is a very basic principle of screening that the performance of a screening test will tend to be overestimated if it is evaluated in a high-risk population. Another approach to improving the efficiency of such studies is to confine analysis to primiparous women. There are a number of reasons why this is an attractive option. First, primiparity is associated with increased risks of a number of adverse outcomes of pregnancy, including preterm birth, preeclampsia, stillbirth, and intrapartum cesarean section [3,4,5]. By focusing on primiparous women, a greater proportion of a cohort will experience an adverse event. Second, one of the best predictors of the outcome of pregnancy is the outcome of a woman's previous pregnancy. This information is clearly not available for primipara, hence, there is a particular need for tests to predict risk in this population. Third, any model derived from women of mixed parity would have to incorporate previous pregnancy outcome for those who were multiparous. In a cohort of mixed parity, this information will be variably present and hence complicate the process of modeling. Finally, in studies which are conducted in the same location over a prolonged period of time, it is likely that a subset of women will attend the hospital for consecutive pregnancies. This would mean that, within the cohort of pregnancies, some would be to the same women. Non-independence of observations is a further complicating factor for statistical analysis.

Selecting controls

One of the most important features of all scientific analyses is having an appropriate control group. Another major advantage of prospective studies is that the cohort provides a clear source of appropriate controls. Broadly, controls can be selected from within a cohort in three ways. First, all cases may be compared with all women who did not experience the event. This can be done where the given measurement is available in the whole population. However, in many biological studies, specific tests will be performed which can be expensive. Two other main approaches involve selection of controls, primarily to reduce the costs of a given comparison. In a case–cohort design, a random sample of the cohort (the subcohort) is selected as the control group at the start of the study. Measurements are made on the subcohort and on all cases and a common group of controls can be selected for all adverse outcomes [6]. The analysis for a given adverse event compares cases with the members of the subcohort who did not experience the given outcome. Typically, control for potential confounding factors (such as variation in body mass index or smoking status) is achieved by multivariate statistical analysis. However, this approach may be problematic where very expensive or labor-intensive methodologies are planned, such as proteomic analysis of serum or gene expression array analysis of placental RNA. Multivariate analysis is impractical using these methods, given that small numbers are employed. The second major approach to selecting controls can deal with this, namely, a nested case–control design. In this event controls are selected from the unaffected population and matched to cases on key maternal characteristics to address the potential for confounding. Subsequent analyses utilize paired statistical methods and paired comparison accounts for any confounding by the maternal characteristics used for matching [7].

Relationship between early embryonic and fetal growth and outcome

Estimating fetal growth in the first trimester

The major ultrasonic measure of fetal growth in early pregnancy is the crown–rump length (CRL), which is conceptually self-explanatory and technically described elsewhere [8]. Early fetal growth can be assessed by comparing the actual size of the embryo or fetus with the expected size on the basis of standard growth charts and the last menstrual period (LMP) [9]. Use of the LMP assumes ovulation occurs on day 14, where day 1 is the first day of the last menses. While this is true on average, the actual timing of ovulation will be scattered around this mode. Therefore, variation between the observed and expected size of the fetus will also in part reflect variation in the timing of ovulation. The expected size of the fetus will be systematically overestimated when the cycle length is longer than

28 days and systematically underestimated when the cycle length is shorter. Other factors which may undermine interpretation of estimated gestation based on LMP are recent use of hormonal contraception, bleeding since the presumed last menstrual period, or uncertain date of LMP. Quantification of the difference between the observed and expected size can also be attempted in other specialized situations. First, pregnancies conceived using assisted reproductive technology (ART) will often have well-defined dates of conception, either due to known timing of ovulation or through *in vitro* fertilization. Second, in twin pregnancies, comparison can be made between the crown–rump lengths and differences correlated with eventual differences in birth weight.

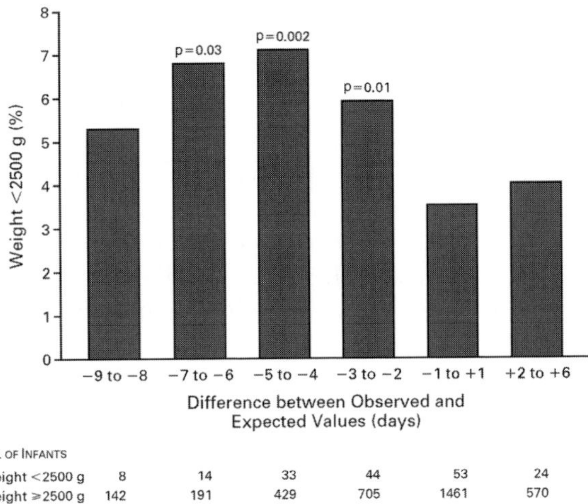

Fig. 22.1 Proportion of infants with birth weights of less than 2500 g according to the difference between observed and expected first trimester crown–rump lengths. p values are for the comparison with the group with normal crown–rump length (−1 to +1 day) by Fisher's exact test (two-tailed). The crown–rump length was expressed as deviation from the expected size on the basis of the LMP, quantified as equivalent days of growth. Reproduced with permission from Smith *et al.* [10].

Early growth and later outcome

The first large-scale study to address early fetal growth and eventual birth weight examined the relationship between the observed and expected first trimester crown–rump length in a cohort of over 4000 women [10]. The study group was derived from approximately 30 000 women attending for prenatal care at a single institution. The expected size of the fetus was accurately determined by confining the analysis to women who had not used oral contraception in the preceding 3 months and described a certain date of LMP and regular 28-day cycle. There was a clear relationship between a smaller than expected crown–rump length (within the range −6 to +6 days) and the risk of delivering a low birth weight baby (Fig. 22.1). A smaller than expected crown–rump length was also found to be associated with low birth weight at term, birth weight small for gestational age (< 5th percentile), and extreme preterm birth (defined as 24–32 weeks' gestation). Relative risks were in the region of 2–3. All associations were tested in multivariate analysis and were independent of maternal age, parity, previous abortions, vaginal bleeding, pregnancy-induced hypertension, elective delivery, fetal sex, and the timing of the ultrasound scanning.

Studies in ART and twin pregnancy

Some early studies of early growth following assisted reproductive technologies demonstrated possible associations between early fetal growth and birth weight [11, 12]. More recently, analysis of a large-scale prospective cohort study conducted in the USA confirmed that smaller than expected CRL was associated with variation in birth weight. Data were available from approximately 1000 women who conceived using ART with a known date of conception. Variation in the observed and expected CRL was associated both with the birth weight and the risk of being delivered small for gestational age (Fig. 22.2) [13]. A further analysis of the same cohort also demonstrated that male fetuses were slightly larger than female fetuses in the first trimester [14]. This indicated that genetic determinants of variation in growth were manifested in early pregnancy and that the phenomenon of sexual size dimorphism was apparent in the first trimester. A large-scale study of dichorionic twins also demonstrated a highly statistically significant correlation between discordance in the CRLs and the risk of significant birth weight discordance: a discrepancy equivalent to more than 3 days of growth was associated with a six-fold risk of birth weight discordance > 20% [15].

Fetal and placental volume ratios

In practice, the majority of pregnancies do not have good information on the likely timing of conception. Hence, while these studies demonstrate an interesting biological point in relation to early fetal growth, the

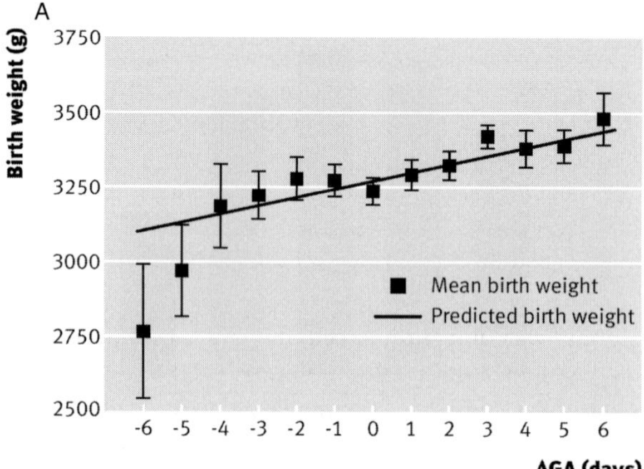

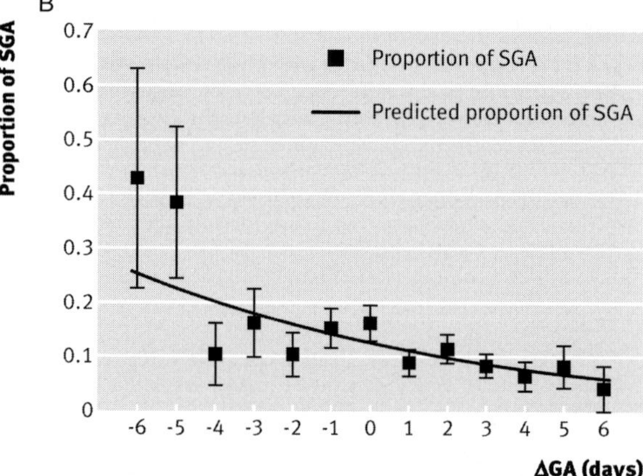

Fig. 22.2 Relationship between variation in observed and expected size of the fetus in the first trimester in 976 singleton ART conceptions. (A) Birth weight as a function of ΔGA (difference between observed and expected size of fetus in first trimester of pregnancy). Mean (±SE) birth weights and fitted values from multivariable linear regression are plotted for each day of ΔGA discrepancy. (B) Proportion of small-for-gestational age (SGA) neonates by size of ΔGA discrepancy (difference between observed and expected size of fetus in first trimester of pregnancy). Reproduced with permission from Bukowski *et al.* [13].

clinical utility of these associations is less evident. This has led some groups to compare the size of the CRL to the placental volume, presented as the placental quotient. A study of almost 2500 singleton pregnancies demonstrated that the first trimester placental quotient was reduced among women who went on to develop complicated preeclampsia or who ultimately delivered a small-for-gestational age infant. However, the association was too weak to be clinically useful [16]. Interestingly, a lower placental quotient at 11–13 weeks was associated with increased uterine artery mean PI and notching in the second trimester, indicating that pregnancies exhibiting the 'classic' markers of impaired trophoblast invasion in the middle of pregnancy are demonstrably abnormal even in the first trimester [17].

First trimester ultrasonic assessment of placentation

A number of studies have addressed ultrasonic assessment of the placenta in the first trimester and the two main approaches have been three-dimensional ultrasound to estimate placental volume and Doppler flow velocimetry to assess resistance in the uterine circulation. Serial assessment of placental volume in approximately 1200 singleton pregnancies, with measurements at 12, 16, and 22 weeks' gestation, demonstrated a complex pattern of associations. Among women who subsequently developed preeclampsia, the mean placental volume was greater at 12 and 16 weeks but exhibited a reduced rate of growth from 16 to 22 weeks. Among women who subsequently delivered a small-for-gestational age (SGA) infant, the mean placental volume was small compared with the average at 12 weeks but maintained a normal rate of growth (i.e. remained small but with the same proportional deviation from the mean). Among women who subsequently developed preeclampsia and delivered a SGA infant, the mean placental volume was persistently smaller in all three measurements [18].

A number of studies have addressed the relationship between first trimester uterine artery Doppler resistance indices and the risk of adverse outcome, which follows from the good predictive associations between second trimester Doppler and both preeclampsia [19] and stillbirth [20]. One of the earliest studies demonstrated that there was no association between measurements at 7–11 weeks and outcome, but being in the top quartile of pulsatility index (PI, a quantitative measure positively correlated with vascular resistance) at 12–13 weeks was associated with a four-fold risk of hypertensive disorders [21]. A study of over 3000 women assessed the screening properties of this measurement. A uterine artery mean PI at 11–14 weeks in the top 5% of the population was associated with an increased risk of both preeclampsia and delivery of an SGA infant. The sensitivity for the detection of all preeclampsia was 27% but the sensitivity for preeclampsia requiring delivery prior to 34 weeks was 50%. The equivalent figures for delivery of a small-for-gestational age infant were 12% and 24% [22].

Maternal circulating concentrations of placentally derived proteins and outcome

Pregnancy-associated plasma protein-A (PAPP-A)

First trimester maternal serum levels of PAPP-A have been widely studied in the assessment of Down's syndrome risk. However, the biology of the protein is such that associations might be anticipated for other complications of pregnancy. PAPP-A is part of the system controlling the insulin-like growth factors (IGF) in trophoblast, being a protease for insulin-like growth factor binding protein (IGFBP-)4 [23]. IGFBPs bind IGF-I and IGF-II, inhibiting their interaction with cell surface receptors and have, therefore, a key role in modulating IGF activity [24]. Since PAPP-A breaks down IGFBP [23], low levels of PAPP-A would be expected to be associated with high levels of IGFBP and, therefore, low levels of free IGF. Messenger RNA for PAPP-A has been identified in syncytiotrophoblast and mononuclear cells of possible extravillous trophoblast origin, and the protein has been localized to placental septae, anchoring villi, and chorionic villi [25]. The IGFs have a key role in regulating fetal growth [26], have also been shown to control uptake of glucose and amino acids in cultured trophoblast [27], and are thought to have an important role in the autocrine and paracrine control of trophoblast invasion of the decidua [28]. Finally, mice which were null mutant for the gene encoding PAPP-A exhibited severe, early onset intrauterine growth restriction [29]. An association between PAPP-A and later outcome was, therefore, biologically plausible.

Early studies relating first trimester measurement of PAPP-A to perinatal outcome reported inconsistent results. One study compared first trimester PAPP-A levels in 73 babies ultimately born weighing less than the 5th percentile for gestational age and 87 babies ultimately born preterm with matched controls. There was no statistically significant difference between the groups [30]. However, another study found a positive correlation between PAPP-A at 8–14 weeks and eventual birth weight [31] and an analysis of 60 *in vitro* fertilization pregnancies described lower concentrations of PAPP-A in the first trimester among eight women who eventually delivered preterm [32]. A further study of 5297 women demonstrated lower PAPP-A at 10–14 weeks' gestation among women who miscarried, delivered babies small for gestational age, and developed preeclampsia [33]. However, PAPP-A was used in these women to estimate the risk of the fetus having Down's syndrome which is a potential cause of confounding.

Two large-scale studies evaluated first PAPP-A measurement in a non-interventional way, i.e. data were ascertained but the management of the pregnancy was not influenced by the early pregnancy assessment. Both studies demonstrated that low levels of PAPP-A at 10–13 weeks were associated with an increased risk of delivery of an SGA infant, preterm delivery, preeclampsia, and stillbirth [34, 35]. The associations persisted in multivariate analysis. A further analysis of the earlier of the two cohorts assessed whether PAPP-A levels prior to 13 weeks' gestation were associated with fetal growth and the timing of labor among entirely uncomplicated pregnancies. A total of 4288 women who had PAPP-A assayed at 8–12 weeks of gestation (dated by ultrasound, equivalent to 6–10 weeks after conception) who ultimately had uncomplicated singleton pregnancies and delivered normal, live babies at full term were studied [36]. This demonstrated that both the eventual birth weight (stratified by gestational age) and the timing of labor at term were correlated with the early pregnancy levels of PAPP-A (Fig. 22.3).

Stillbirth, i.e. intrauterine fetal death at a birth weight or gestational age where the infant is viable, is one of the most common devastating complications of pregnancy. The majority of stillbirths are thought to be a consequence of some form of placental dysfunction, for example associated with preeclampsia, placental abruption, and intrauterine growth restriction [37]. Both of the large-scale cohort studies of early pregnancy PAPP-A demonstrated associations with stillbirth but lacked detailed information on the cause of stillbirth. In order to address this, data from the multicenter Scottish cohort study were linked to a national registry of perinatal deaths. Moreover, the number of participants in the cohort was sufficient to allow limitation of the analysis to women who were, by strict definition, in the first trimester (i.e. prior to 13 weeks gestational age). This analysis demonstrated that low first trimester levels of PAPP-A were very strongly associated with stillbirth due to placental causes (i.e. associated with growth restriction, placental abruption, or preeclampsia) but not stillbirths due to other causes (Fig. 22.4A) [38]. Women with PAPP-A

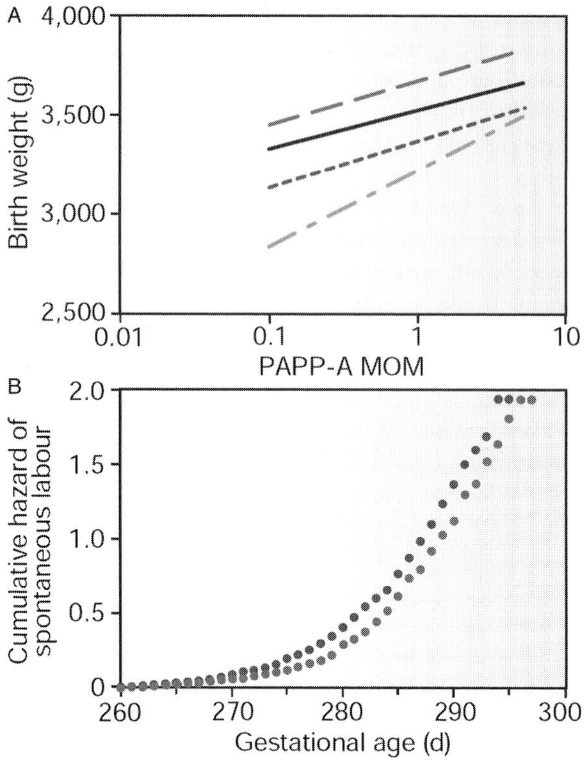

Fig. 22.3 Association between PAPP-A and birth weight at 38–41 weeks of gestation and timing of labor at term. (A) Predicted values of birth weight plotted against PAPP-A multiples of the median (MOM) (on $\log_{10}$ scale) from linear regression analysis. Coefficients (95% CI) for change in birth weight (in grams) associated with a one $\log_{10}$ unit change in PAPP-A MOM: 38 weeks 380 (209 to 552), 39 weeks 231 (113 to 349), 40 weeks 196 (104 to 289) and 41 weeks 221 (112 to 331). All $P < 0.0001$. Coefficients were virtually unchanged after adjusting for age, parity, body mass index, height, smoking status, and race. (B) Cumulative hazard of spontaneous labor at each day of gestation at term comparing lowest and highest quintiles of first trimester PAPP-A MOMs. Univariate comparison: $P = 0.0003$ (log rank test). Reproduced with permission from Smith *et al.* [36].

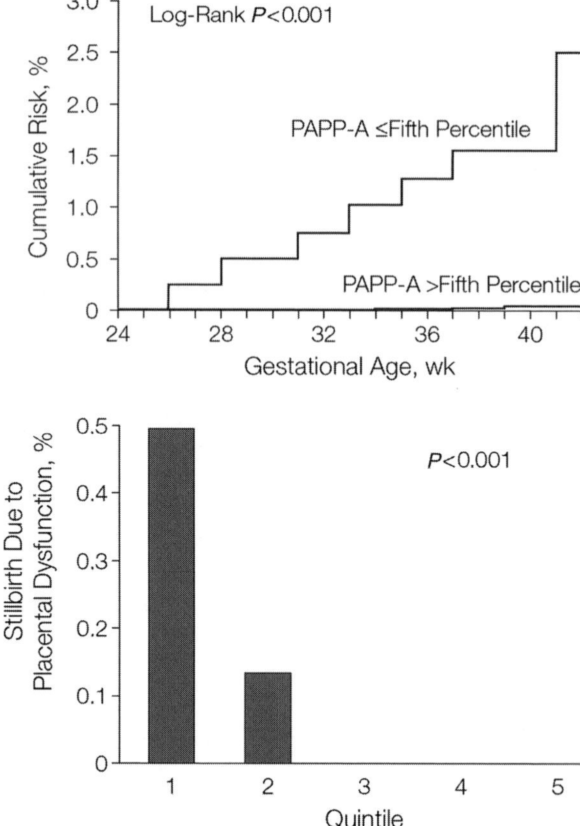

Fig. 22.4 Relationship between first trimester PAPP-A levels and the risk of stillbirth due to a placental cause (growth restriction, abruption or preeclampsia). (A) Cumulative risk of stillbirth due to a placental cause. Hazard ratio for PAPP-A < 5th percentile 46.0 (95% CI 11.9–178.0) $P < 0.001$). (B) Proportion of stillbirths due to placental dysfunction in relation to first trimester levels of PAPP-A, expressed as quintiles. *P* value from Fisher's exact test. Reproduced with permission from Smith *et al.* [38].

levels in the lowest 5% had a 40- to 50-fold risk of stillbirth compared with the rest of the population. Moreover, when analyzed by quintiles of PAPP-A, there were no placentally related stillbirths among women with maternal serum levels in the top 60% (Fig. 22.4B). When analyzed by gestational age, the increased risk of stillbirth was apparent across the whole range of gestation, indicating that these devastating events at term may be determined by placental function even prior to a woman's first visit for prenatal care. This observation raises the hope that effective clinical prediction of the most severe complications of late pregnancy may be possible in the first trimester. However, the positive predictive value of low PAPP-A on its own was too low to be clinically useful. The very high relative risk partly reflects the extreme rarity of the outcome in women with normal levels rather than a strong predictive association among women with low PAPP-A.

Other biochemical markers of first trimester placental function

First trimester Down's syndrome screening also involves measurement of the free beta subunit of human chorionic gonadotropin. However, serum levels of this substance are not independently associated with the outcomes discussed above [34, 38]. In the last 5 years, there has been considerable interest in placentally derived regulators of angiogenesis and the risk of preeclampsia. The main studies identifying these associations have focused on second and third trimester levels [39]. The key proteins identified thus far are soluble fms-like tyrosine kinase 1 (sFlt1) and placental growth factor (PlGF). sFlt1 is a soluble form of the membrane-bound vascular endothelial growth factor receptor 1 (VEGFR1), which is synthesized and released by endothelial cells and the placenta. It is produced by alternative splicing of VEGFR1 and binds VEGF-A and PlGF, preventing them from exerting their biological effects through their membrane-bound receptors. PlGF is a type of vascular endothelial growth factor expressed both in the placenta and normal endothelial cells which binds specifically to VEGFR1. The current model is that sFlt1 is released by the placenta, probably in response to placental hypoxia, and the increased levels of sFlt1 reduce the levels of PlGF and VEGF, which has an antiendothelial effect [40].

A nested case–control study conducted within the Scottish multicenter cohort study analyzed sFlt1 and PlGF at 10–14 weeks in relation to the ultimate outcome of the pregnancy. Low PlGF was associated with subsequent development of preeclampsia whereas there was no association with levels of sFlt1 [41]. The results were similar when confined to samples obtained prior to 13 weeks gestational age and when confined to women with severe preeclampsia. This suggests that PlGF is low independently of increased binding by sFlt1, at least in early pregnancy, and could reflect less release of PlGF from the placenta of women who ultimately will develop the condition. Low PlGF was also associated with an increased risk of delivering a small-for-gestational age infant, but there was no association with the risk of preterm birth [41]. These findings were very similar to a previous report of a smaller nested case–control study [42]. However, in contrast to the earlier study, analysis of the Scottish data demonstrated that higher levels of sFlt1 were associated with a reduced risk of delivering a small-for-gestational age infant, delivering preterm, and the risk of stillbirth. Moreover, the apparent protective effect of high levels of sFlt1 was greater among women with low or average levels of PlGF [41]. These findings point to a more complex model of the relationship between circulating angiogenic factors and outcome than originally proposed and further large-scale studies of high methodological quality are awaited.

A number of other studies have reported the relationship between maternal serum concentrations of other placentally derived proteins and adverse outcome. A nested case–control study of about 50 women who went on to develop preeclampsia with approximately 100 controls (matched on maternal characteristics) confirmed the association with low PAPP-A and PlGF, but also found associations with high inhibin A and activin A. In contrast, there were no associations with pregnancy-specific β1-glycoprotein, placental lactogen, leptin, interleukin 8, or C-reactive protein [43]. The associations with inhibin A and activin A have subsequently been confirmed. Moreover, the predictive ability of activin A was comparable to PAPP-A and that of inhibin A was somewhat stronger [44]. Another IGFBP protease has been studied (ADAM12, a protease for IGFBP3 and 5). The risk of preeclampsia was increased among women with low levels of ADAM12 in the first trimester whereas high levels in the second trimester were associated with an increased risk of the condition. In the first trimester, analysis of the protein added little to the prediction obtained from PAPP-A [45]. Finally, the placentally produced galectin, placental protein 13 (PP13), has been the focus of a number of studies for the first trimester prediction of preeclampsia. Low levels were very strongly predictive of early onset preeclampsia but less predictive of disease at term whether mild or severe [46].

Combined ultrasonic and biochemical assessment of the placenta

A number of studies have examined the interrelationships between the ultrasonic and biochemical measurements discussed above. Higher values of PAPP-A have been demonstrated where the placental quotient was higher in the first trimester [47]. Moreover, first trimester levels of PAPP-A are positively correlated with second trimester growth of femur length and abdominal circumference [48]. A study comparing first trimester assessment of uterine artery Doppler and maternal serum PP13 confirmed that both were associated with preeclampsia requiring delivery prior to 34 weeks but that there was no correlation between PP13 and uterine artery mean PI. The implication of the finding is that measurement of both parameters may be useful. A number of studies have directly compared the screening performance of combining ultrasonic and biochemical measurements. Two studies have demonstrated that adding PAPP-A to uterine artery Doppler had a minimal effect on the prediction of preeclampsia [49, 50]. However, adding PAPP-A to uterine artery Doppler has been shown to improve prediction of an SGA infant [49] and the same was found for maternal serum PlGF [51]. One study combined PAPP-A, PlGF, and uterine artery mean PI and found that, although PAPP-A was associated with preeclampsia and was more strongly predictive of severe disease, adding it to a model with uterine artery mean PI and PlGF had a minimal effect on the predictive ability obtained by the latter two parameters on their own [52]. Finally, a Chinese study used z-scores to quantify deviation of both PAPP-A and CRL from expected values. Although the z-scores for both parameters were associated with low birth weight, they did not perform well as a screening test [53]. Hence, a complex pattern of association exists between ultrasonic measures of growth and the risk of different adverse outcomes. Large-scale prospective cohort studies would help resolve the details of these interrelationships and would also yield screening performance indices from an unselected population.

Clinical and epidemiological implications of early pregnancy determination of risk

Clinical utility of first trimester assessment of risk

The studies described above clearly indicate that serious complications of pregnancy, such as growth restriction, preeclampsia and stillbirth, exhibit abnormalities in the first 10 weeks postconception. Although based on clinical observations, these findings are relevant to understanding the biology of normal pregnancy and the pathophysiology of complicated pregnancies. Aside from the biological significance of these observations, the primary clinical purpose of tests which discriminate women destined to have complications is that such tests may be used to screen the whole population. The necessity for such an approach is underlined by the fact that the majority of serious complications of pregnancy occur in women with no known risk factors. The exemplar of obstetric screening is the approach to detecting fetuses affected by Down's syndrome. Previously, the offer of an invasive diagnostic test (with its associated risk of inducing a loss) was conducted on the basis of specific clinical risk factors, principally advanced maternal age. However, this approach detected a small proportion of Down's cases (low sensitivity) and the personal risk of Down's in many of these women was low (low positive predictive value). In the last 20 years, a highly effective screening programme, based on ultrasonic and biochemical associations with Down's, has led to methods for screening which detect in the region of 90% of cases of Down's for a less than 5% rate of invasive testing [54].

When considering screening for other complications of pregnancy using early pregnancy markers there are two main considerations. First, how effectively do the measures discriminate between women who are going to have complicated or uncomplicated pregnancies? Second, if a woman is known to be at high risk, how might this information be used to inform management? In relation to the first question, the important point is that most serious complications of pregnancy are relatively rare. For example, among a population of nulliparous women in the west of Scotland who attended for biochemical screening for Down's syndrome, the risk of antepartum stillbirth occurring between 24 and 28 weeks' gestation was 1.25 per 1000 [55] and the risk of spontaneous preterm birth between 24 and 28 weeks' gestation was 2.4 per 1000 [56]. Hence, even if tests were capable of identifying women with a 10-fold risk of such an event, the vast majority of such women would still not have the specific complication.

Meta-analysis of randomized controlled trials of screening tests in later pregnancy demonstrated that the most promising method of fetal assessment to reduce perinatal mortality is the use of umbilical artery Doppler flow velocimetry in high-risk pregnancies [57]. However, there is only a trend toward a reduction in perinatal mortality and the analysis is also consistent with no effect on mortality. Meta-analyses of current methods of fetal monitoring do not indicate any methods of fetal assessment which reduce the risk of stillbirth when used as a screening tool in an unselected population [37]. Interpretation of the negative results is, however, problematic and the meta-analysis of umbilical artery Doppler in low-risk pregnancies is a good illustration of the problems of interpretation [58]. First, the trials in this meta-analysis were designed in the absence of reliable information on how the test performed as a predictor of stillbirth in a population of low-risk women. The adequate design of an interventional trial requires knowledge of how the test performs in identifying women at increased risk. In the case of stillbirth, this includes both the discriminative power of the test and the gestational age dependence [59]. Without this information, a trial cannot be adequately designed.

The second problem in interpreting these data is the failure to distinguish between the two major components of successful screening, namely, effective detection of women at increased risk and effective intervention in high-risk women. A trial of an effective prenatal screening tool may yield a negative result because the intervention is ineffective at preventing the outcome among high-risk women. Only one of the RCTs included in the Cochrane meta-analysis of umbilical artery Doppler had a protocol for the treatment of women who screened positive. It is impossible, therefore, to determine whether these trials yielded a negative result due to failure of the screening tool or failure of the intervention. The same issues will be encountered when evaluating early pregnancy screening tests. Future studies of population-based screening for stillbirth at all gestational ages need to be preceded by high quality, non-interventional prospective cohort studies characterizing the screening properties of novel methods of risk assessment in an unselected population. Such an approach should be feasible, as this has been achieved for the evaluation of novel methods of screening for Down's syndrome risk, [54] a condition which is less common than stillbirth. Having identified effective screening tools, candidate interventions could be evaluated in RCTs among women who screen positive.

Candidate medical interventions for women with abnormal early placentation

Understanding the pathophysiology and etiological factors for placentally related causes of complications of pregnancy has led to evaluation of a number of prophylactic medical treatments to try and prevent the onset of complications among high-risk women. There is a large body of work that indicates an important role for endothelial dysfunction in preeclampsia and other pregnancy complications. This led to the evaluation of antiplatelet agents, principally aspirin, as a means of preventing preeclampsia in a series of trials. A meta-analysis using individual patient data demonstrated modest benefits of antiplatelet treatment, specifically, 10% reductions in the risk of preeclampsia and preterm birth before 34 weeks [60]. The analysis did not demonstrate significant heterogeneity in the effect in subgroups, i.e. the different types of high-risk women. However, despite its size, the study lacked power to detect such heterogeneity. Moreover, none of the sub-groups included low-risk women who had screened positive with either biochemical or ultrasonic markers of preeclampsia.

A body of evidence indicates associations between inherited and acquired thrombophilia and the risk of placentally related complications of pregnancy [61]. This suggests that low-molecular-weight heparin or administration of high doses of folic acid (the latter to normalize homocysteine levels in women with the prothrombotic methylene-tetrahydrofolate reductase mutation, C677T) may reduce the risks of these complications. However, no high-quality data exist on the effects of these interventions and the current recommendations for pregnant women in the second half of pregnancy with a thrombophilia are that anticoagulant treatment should be for prevention of thromboembolic disease only [62]. In view of the association between fetal hypoxia and stillbirth, a number of studies have evaluated supplemental maternal oxygen therapy as a means of reducing perinatal death among women with a growth restricted infant. A meta-analysis of three studies involving 94 women demonstrated a 50% reduction in perinatal mortality [63]. However, only one of the studies was blinded. This intervention is not in routine use, would be impractical in many settings, and widespread application of this method would require confirmation of this finding in a large-scale high-quality randomized controlled trial. Recent trials of antioxidant vitamins have demonstrated no reduction in the risk of preeclampsia and, indeed, there is some evidence that the intervention increased rates of perinatal complications [64].

Birth weight and the risk of cardiovascular disease

As discussed above, impaired growth is associated with many complications of pregnancy, in particular antepartum stillbirth [65, 66]. However, fetal growth is also thought to be important as a determinant of later adult disease. There are many studies which demonstrate associations between low birth weight and an individual's risk of a range of diseases in later life. Diseases of the cardiovascular system have been a major focus, in particular ischemic heart disease (IHD). A meta-analysis of 18 eligible observational studies demonstrated that the finding was consistent and that the odds of ischemic heart disease decreased by 16% for every 1 kg increase in birth weight [67].

Statistical adjustment for available confounders had a minimal effect on the strength of the association. Barker has hypothesized that these associations reflect a causal association between maternal diet during pregnancy and key aspects of fetal physiology, stating 'that alterations in fetal nutrition and endocrine status result in developmental adaptations that permanently change structure, physiology, and metabolism, thereby predisposing individuals to cardiovascular, metabolic, and endocrine disease in adult life' [68]. Lifelong changes in physiology induced by the intrauterine environment are referred to as 'fetal programing'. The phenomenon of fetal programing is real and has been confirmed in multiple animal models under controlled conditions [69]. Hence, understanding the timing of onset of fetal growth disorders may be important in understanding the associations between intrauterine environment and later disease.

Birth weight and the mother's risk of cardiovascular disease

The data described in the preceding section indicate that a proportion of both preterm birth and intrauterine growth restriction (the determinants of birth weight) have their origin in very early pregnancy, before the conceptus makes significant calorific demands on the mother. These observations potentially undermine the proposal that maternal diet is the mechanism that leads to increased risk of diseases in later life in the offspring. Another possibility is that common factors determine pregnancy complications and some of these diseases in later life. These common factors could include genetic, socioeconomic, and environmental characteristics. Such characteristics tend to persist within families, a property known as familial aggregation [70]. One way to address whether this may explain, at least in part, the association between an individual's birth weight and their later risk of disease is to determine the relationship between birth weight and the disease experience of other family members. We [71] and others [72] have tested the specificity of the associations with birth weight by examining the association between the birth weight of the baby and the mother's risk of disease in later life. The relative risk of death due to ischemic heart disease (adjusted for maternal age, height, socioeconomic deprivation, and essential hypertension) for a woman giving birth to a baby weighing less than 2500 g in comparison to a woman giving birth to a baby of ≥ 3500 g was 11.3 [71]. In fact, this is much stronger than the association between birth weight and the personal risk of IHD.

This observation suggests that pregnancy complications may be a manifestation of characteristics which will also predispose a woman to cardiovascular disease in later life. Implantation of the embryo and early placentation involve complex adaptations of the mother's cardiovascular and microvascular systems. These early pregnancy events influence the risk of preterm birth and intrauterine growth restriction, the determinants of low birth weight. It is plausible that occult cardiovascular, microvascular, or hemostatic dysfunction is manifested in pregnancy complications during reproductive years and in overt cardiovascular disease in later life. Understanding the nature of the common determinants of pregnancy complications and cardiovascular disease may reveal insights into the pathophysiology and prevention of both.

References

1. Bynum W. Discarded diagnoses. *The Lancet* 2002; **359**: 898.
2. Southampton Woman's Survey. 2008. Available at http://www.mrc.soton.ac.uk/sws
3. Smith G C S. Life-table analysis of the risk of perinatal death at term and post term in singleton pregnancies. *Am J Obstet Gynecol* 2001; **184**(3): 489–96.
4. Patel R R, Peters T J, Murphy D J. Prenatal risk factors for Caesarean section: analyses of the ALSPAC cohort of 12,944 women in England. *Int J Epidemiol* 2005; **34**(2): 353–67.
5. Smith G C S, Shah I, Pell J P, Crossley J A, Dobbie R. Maternal obesity in early pregnancy and risk of spontaneous and elective preterm deliveries: a retrospective cohort study. *Am J Public Health* 2007; **97**(1): 157–62.
6. Rothman K J, Greenland S, Lash T L. Case-control studies. In: Rothman K J, Greenland S, Lash T L, eds. *Modern epidemiology*, 3rd ed. Philadelphia: Lippincott, Williams & Wilkins; 2008: pp. 111–27.
7. Pasupathy D, Dacey A, Cook E *et al.* Study protocol. A prospective cohort study of unselected primiparous women: the pregnancy outcome prediction study. *BMC Pregnancy Childbirth* 2008; **8**(1): 51.
8. Evans E, Farrant P, Gowland M, McNay M B, Richards B. *Clinical applications of ultrasonic fetal measurements.* London: British Medical Ultrasound Society/British Institute of Radiology; 1990.
9. Robinson H P, Fleming J E E. A critical evaluation of sonar "crown-rump length" measurements. *Br J Obstet Gynaecol* 1975; **82**(9): 702–10.

10. Smith G C S, Smith M F S, McNay M B, Fleming J E E. First-trimester growth and the risk of low birth weight. *N Engl J Med* 1998; **339**: 1817–22.

11. Dickey R P, Olar T T, Taylor S N *et al.* Incidence and significance of unequal gestational sac diameter or embryo crown-rump length in twin pregnancy. *Hum Reprod* 1992; **7**: 1170–2.

12. Sebire N J, D'Ercole C, Soares W, Nayar R, Nicolaides K H. Intertwin disparity in fetal size in monochorionic and dichorionic pregnancies. *Obstet Gynecol* 1998; **91** (1): 82–5.

13. Bukowski R, Smith G C S, Malone F D *et al.* Fetal growth in early pregnancy and risk of delivering low birth weight infant: prospective cohort study. *BMJ* 2007; **334** (7598): 836.

14. Bukowski R, Smith G C S, Malone F D *et al.* Human sexual size dimorphism in early pregnancy. *Am J Epidemiol* 2007; **165**(10): 1216–18.

15. Kalish R B, Chasen S T, Gupta M *et al.* First trimester prediction of growth discordance in twin gestations. *Am J Obstet Gynecol* 2003; **189**(3): 706–9.

16. Hafner E, Metzenbauer M, Hofinger D *et al.* Comparison between three-dimensional placental volume at 12 weeks and uterine artery impedance/ notching at 22 weeks in screening for pregnancy-induced hypertension, pre-eclampsia and fetal growth restriction in a low-risk population. *Ultrasound Obstet Gynecol* 2006; **27**(6): 652–7.

17. Hafner E, Metzenbauer M, Dillinger-Paller B *et al.* Correlation of first trimester placental volume and second trimester uterine artery Doppler flow. *Placenta* 2001; **22**(8–9): 729–34.

18. Hafner E, Metzenbauer M, Hofinger D *et al.* Placental growth from the first to the second trimester of pregnancy in SGA-foetuses and pre-eclamptic pregnancies compared to normal foetuses. *Placenta* 2003; **24**(4): 336–42.

19. Yu C K, Smith G C S, Papageorghiou A T *et al.* An integrated model for the prediction of preeclampsia using maternal factors and uterine artery Doppler velocimetry in unselected low-risk women. *Am J Obstet Gynecol* 2005; **193**(2): 429–36.

20. Smith G C S, Yu C K, Papageorghiou A T, Cacho A M, Nicolaides K H. Maternal uterine artery Doppler flow velocimetry and the risk of stillbirth. *Obstet Gynecol* 2007; **109**(1): 144–51.

21. van den Elzen H J, Cohen-Overbeek T E, Grobbee D E, Quartero R W, Wladimiroff J W. Early uterine artery Doppler velocimetry and the outcome of pregnancy in women aged 35 years and older. *Ultrasound Obstet Gynecol* 1995; **5**(5): 328–33.

22. Martin A M, Bindra R, Curcio P, Cicero S, Nicolaides K H. Screening for pre-eclampsia and fetal growth restriction by uterine artery Doppler at 11–14 weeks of gestation. *Ultrasound Obstet Gynecol* 2001; **18**(6): 583–86.

23. Lawrence J B, Oxvig C, Overgaard M T *et al.* The insulin-like growth factor (IGF)-dependent IGF binding protein-4 protease secreted by human fibroblasts is pregnancy-associated plasma protein-A. *Proc Natl Acad Sci U S A* 1999; **96**(6): 3149–53.

24. Clemmons D R. Role of insulin-like growth factor binding proteins in controlling IGF actions. *Mol Cell Endocrinol* 1998; **140**(1–2): 19–24.

25. Bonno M, Oxvig C, Kephart G M *et al.* Localization of pregnancy-associated plasma protein-A and colocalization of pregnancy-associated plasma protein-A messenger ribonucleic acid and eosinophil granule major basic protein messenger ribonucleic acid in placenta. *Lab Invest* 1994; **71**(4): 560–6.

26. van Kleffens M, Groffen C, Lindenbergh-Kortleve D J *et al.* The IGF system during fetal-placental development of the mouse. *Mol Cell Endocrinol* 1998; **140**(1–2): 129–35.

27. Kniss D A, Shubert P J, Zimmerman P D, Landon M B, Gabbe S G. Insulinlike growth factors: their regulation of glucose and amino acid transport in placental trophoblasts isolated from first-trimester chorionic villi. *J Reprod Med* 1994; **39**(4): 249–56.

28. Irwin J C, Suen L F, Martina N A, Mark S P, Giudice L C. Role of the IGF system in trophoblast invasion and pre-eclampsia. *Hum Reprod* 1999; **14** (Suppl 2): 90–6.

29. Conover C A, Bale L K, Overgaard M T *et al.* Metalloproteinase pregnancy-associated plasma protein A is a critical growth regulatory factor during fetal development. *Development* 2004; **131**(5): 1187–94.

30. Morssink L P, Kornman L H, Hallahan T W *et al.* Maternal serum levels of free beta-hCG and PAPP-A in the first trimester of pregnancy are not associated with subsequent fetal growth retardation or preterm delivery. *Prenat Diagn* 1998; **18**(2): 147–52.

31. Pedersen J F, Sorensen S, Ruge S. Human placental lactogen and pregnancy-associated plasma protein A in first trimester and subsequent fetal growth. *Acta Obstet Gynecol Scand* 1995; **74**(7): 505–8.

32. Johnson M R, Riddle A F, Grudzinskas J G *et al.* Reduced circulating placental protein concentrations during the first trimester are associated with preterm labour and low birth weight. *Hum Reprod* 1993; **8**: 1942–7.

33. Ong C Y, Liao A W, Spencer K, Munim S, Nicolaides K H. First trimester maternal serum free beta human chorionic gonadotrophin and pregnancy associated

plasma protein A as predictors of pregnancy complications. *BJOG* 2000; **107**(10): 1265–70.

34. Smith G C S, Stenhouse E J, Crossley J A *et al.* Early pregnancy levels of pregnancy-associated plasma protein A and the risk of intra-uterine growth restriction, premature birth, pre-eclampsia and stillbirth. *J Clin Endocrinol Metab* 2002; **87**: 1762–7.
35. Dugoff L, Hobbins J C, Malone F D *et al.* First-trimester maternal serum PAPP-A and free-beta subunit human chorionic gonadotropin concentrations and nuchal translucency are associated with obstetric complications: a population-based screening study (the FASTER Trial). *Am J Obstet Gynecol* 2004; **191**(4): 1446–51.
36. Smith G C S, Stenhouse E J, Crossley J A *et al.* Development early-pregnancy origins of low birth weight. *Nature* 2002; **417**: 916.
37. Smith G C S, Fretts R C. Stillbirth. *Lancet* 2007; **370** (9600): 1715–25.
38. Smith G C S, Crossley J A, Aitken D A *et al.* First-trimester placentation and the risk of antepartum stillbirth. *JAMA* 2004; **292**(18): 2249–54.
39. Levine R J, Maynard S E, Qian C *et al.* Circulating angiogenic factors and the risk of preeclampsia. *N Engl J Med* 2004; **350**(7): 672–83.
40. Maynard S, Epstein F H, Karumanchi S A. Preeclampsia and angiogenic imbalance. *Annu Rev Med* 2008; **59**: 61–78.
41. Smith G C S, Crossley J A, Aitken D A *et al.* Circulating angiogenic factors in early pregnancy and the risk of preeclampsia, intrauterine growth restriction, spontaneous preterm birth, and stillbirth. *Obstet Gynecol* 2007; **109**(6): 1316–24.
42. Thadhani R, Mutter W P, Wolf M *et al.* First trimester placental growth factor and soluble fms-like tyrosine kinase 1 and risk for preeclampsia. *J Clin Endocrinol Metab* 2004; **89**(2): 770–5.
43. Zwahlen M, Gerber S, Bersinger N A. First trimester markers for pre-eclampsia: placental vs. non-placental protein serum levels. *Gynecol Obstet Invest* 2007; **63**(1): 15–21.
44. Spencer K, Cowans N J, Nicolaides K H. Maternal serum inhibin-A and activin-A levels in the first trimester of pregnancies developing pre-eclampsia. *Ultrasound Obstet Gynecol* 2008; **32**(5): 622–6.
45. Spencer K, Cowans N J, Stamatopoulou A. ADAM12s in maternal serum as a potential marker of pre-eclampsia. *Prenat Diagn* 2008; **28**(3): 212–16.
46. Romero R, Kusanovic J P, Than N G *et al.* First-trimester maternal serum PP13 in the risk assessment for preeclampsia. *Am J Obstet Gynecol* 2008; **199**(2): 122.
47. Metzenbauer M, Hafner E, Hoefinger D *et al.* Three-dimensional ultrasound measurement of the placental volume in early pregnancy: method and correlation with biochemical placenta parameters 7. *Placenta* 2001; **22** (6): 602–5.
48. Leung T Y, Chan L W, Leung T N *et al.* First-trimester maternal serum levels of placental hormones are independent predictors of second-trimester fetal growth parameters. *Ultrasound Obstet Gynecol* 2006; **27**(2): 156–61.
49. Pilalis A, Souka A P, Antsaklis P *et al.* Screening for pre-eclampsia and fetal growth restriction by uterine artery Doppler and PAPP-A at 11–14 weeks' gestation. *Ultrasound Obstet Gynecol* 2007; **29**(2): 135–40.
50. Spencer K, Cowans N J, Chefetz I, Tal J, Meiri H. First-trimester maternal serum PP-13, PAPP-A and second-trimester uterine artery Doppler pulsatility index as markers of pre-eclampsia. *Ultrasound Obstet Gynecol* 2007; **29**(2): 128–34.
51. Poon L C, Zaragoza E, Akolekar R, Anagnostopoulos E, Nicolaides K H. Maternal serum placental growth factor (PlGF) in small for gestational age pregnancy at 11(+0) to 13(+6) weeks of gestation. *Prenat Diagn* 2008; **28**(12): 1110–5.
52. Akolekar R, Zaragoza E, Poon L C, Pepes S, Nicolaides K H. Maternal serum placental growth factor at 11 + 0 to 13 + 6 weeks of gestation in the prediction of pre-eclampsia. *Ultrasound Obstet Gynecol* 2008; **32**(6): 732–9.
53. Leung T Y, Sahota D S, Chan L W *et al.* Prediction of birth weight by fetal crown-rump length and maternal serum levels of pregnancy-associated plasma protein-A in the first trimester. *Ultrasound Obstet Gynecol* 2008; **31** (1): 10–14.
54. Malone F D, Canick J A, Ball R H *et al.* First-trimester or second-trimester screening, or both, for Down's syndrome. *N Engl J Med* 2005; **353**(19): 2001–11.
55. Smith G C S, Shah I, White I R *et al.* Maternal and biochemical predictors of antepartum stillbirth among nulliparous women in relation to gestational age of fetal death. *BJOG* 2007; **114**(6): 705–14.
56. Smith G C S, Shah I, White I R *et al.* Maternal and biochemical predictors of spontaneous preterm birth among nulliparous women: a systematic analysis in relation to the degree of prematurity. *Int J Epidemiol* 2006; **35**(5): 1169–77.
57. Neilson J P, Alfirevic Z. Doppler ultrasound for fetal assessment in high risk pregnancies. *Cochrane Database Syst Rev* 2000; (2): CD000073.
58. Bricker L, Neilson J P. Routine Doppler ultrasound in pregnancy. *Cochrane Database Syst Rev* 2000; (2): CD001450.

59. Smith G C S. Estimating risks of perinatal death. *Am J Obstet Gynecol* 2005; **192**(1): 17–22.

60. Askie L M, Duley L, Henderson-Smart D J, Stewart L A. Antiplatelet agents for prevention of pre-eclampsia: a meta-analysis of individual patient data. *Lancet* 2007; **369**(9575): 1791–8.

61. Wu O, Robertson L, Twaddle S *et al.* Screening for thrombophilia in high-risk situations: systematic review and cost-effectiveness analysis. The Thrombosis: Risk and Economic Assessment of Thrombophilia Screening (TREATS) study. *Health Technol Assess* 2006; **10**(11): 1–110.

62. Bates S M, Greer I A, Hirsh J, Ginsberg J S. Use of antithrombotic agents during pregnancy: the Seventh ACCP Conference on Antithrombotic and Thrombolytic Therapy. *Chest* 2004; **126**(Suppl 3): 627S–644S.

63. Say L, Gulmezoglu A M, Hofmeyr G J. Maternal oxygen administration for suspected impaired fetal growth. *Cochrane Database Syst Rev* 2003; (1): CD000137.

64. Rumbold A, Duley L, Crowther C A, Haslam R R. Antioxidants for preventing pre-eclampsia. *Cochrane Database Syst Rev* 2008; (1): CD004227.

65. Smith G C S. A population study of birthweight and the risk of cesarean section: Scotland 1980–1996. *BJOG* 2000; **107**(6): 740–4.

66. Smith G C S. Sex, birth weight and the risk of stillbirth in Scotland, 1980–1996. *Am J Epidemiol* 2000; **151**: 614–19.

67. Huxley R, Owen C G, Whincup P H *et al.* Is birth weight a risk factor for ischemic heart disease in later life? *Am J Clin Nutr* 2007; **85**(5): 1244–50.

68. Godfrey K M, Barker D J. Fetal nutrition and adult disease. *Am J Clin Nutr* 2000; **71**(Suppl 5): 1344S–1352S.

69. Gluckman P D, Hanson M A, Cooper C, Thornburg K L. Effect of in utero and early-life conditions on adult health and disease. *N Engl J Med* 2008; **359**(1): 61–73.

70. Susser E, Susser M. Familial aggregation studies: a note on their epidemiologic properties. *Am J Epidemiol* 1989; **129**(1): 23–30.

71. Smith G C S, Pell J P, Walsh D. Pregnancy complications and maternal risk of ischaemic heart disease: a retrospective cohort study of 129,290 births. *Lancet* 2001; **357**: 2002–6.

72. Davey S G, Hypponen E, Power C, Lawlor D A. Offspring birth weight and parental mortality: prospective observational study and meta-analysis. *Am J Epidemiol* 2007; **166**(2): 160–9.

New concepts and recommendations on clinical management and research

Caroline Dunk, Sascha Drewlo, Leslie Proctor, and John C. P. Kingdom

Centre for Women's and Infant's Health, Samuel Lunenfeld Research Institute and Department of Obstetrics & Gynecology, Mount Sinai Hospital, University of Toronto, Ontario, Canada

Introduction

Adverse pregnancy outcomes are associated with impaired placental perfusion which can be documented *in vivo* using color/pulsed Doppler ultrasound of the proximal uterine arteries. Persistent high-resistance waveforms in the uterine arteries (PI > 1.45 associated with a small placenta defined as uteroplacental vascular insufficiency, UPVI) were found in 85% of such cases at 22 weeks' gestation in the Placenta Clinic at Mount Sinai Hospital [1,2]. Deficient physiological transformation of the spiral arteries is observed in these pathological cases at the level of the decidual myometrial junction, accompanied by vascular lesions (atherosis and luminal thrombosis) [3,4,5,6], which can be collectively described as 'myometrial junctional zone vasculopathy'. Physiological transformation is thought to be mediated by the progressive invasion of two extravillous trophoblast populations, the interstitial trophoblast which target the spiral arteries leading to smooth muscle disruption and endothelial loss, and the eventual relining of the vessels by endovascular trophoblast [7]. The failed physiological transformation and vascular lesions in the pathological placental bed have been documented in a number of studies using placental bed biopsies, containing one or more myometrial spiral arteries and the more distal decidual arterioles, reviewed in Lyall [8]. Although placental bed biopsies can provide valuable insights into the events underlying vascular transformation they do have limitations dependent on sampling site within the context of the placental bed and the number collected for analysis. Studies of pregnant hysterectomy specimens have elegantly demonstrated a gradient in the number of spiral arteries targeted and the depth of trophoblast invasion with the highest density and depth in the center of the placental site decreasing to the periphery [7,9]. Furthermore, the more proximal (arcuate and radial) branches of the uterine circulation are not accessible, unless a cesarean hysterectomy is performed [10]. While it is established that these vessels are not directly invaded by trophoblast in either humans or mice both the uterine artery and the systemic and cardiovascular vasculature also undergo remodeling in order to accommodate the increase in blood volume [11,12,13]. It is important to acknowledge that our understanding of cellular and molecular mechanisms underlying the development of UPVI remains limited. Placental bed pathology is an important subject of study for two reasons. First, at an epidemiological level, women who deliver preterm as a result of placental complications of pregnancy have increased rates of long-term cardiovascular morbidity and mortality, suggesting that these vascular defects may be present in a more widespread, but subclinical fashion [14]. As an example, we recently correlated abnormal uterine artery Doppler studies in mid-pregnancy with increased maternal carotid artery intima-media thickness [15]. Second, at an individual patient level, whilst uterine artery Doppler is far from being a robust screening test in pregnancy, new research reveals its potential when combined with other modalities of placental or maternal vascular function [16,17]. Clearly the attainment of a high-flow low-resistance uteroplacental circulation has implications for both the mother and her developing fetus. In this chapter, we therefore pose a series of questions, designed to emphasize some of the more intriguing current concepts in clinical and basic placentology that remain poorly understood – yet are very relevant to researchers and clinicians whose day-to-day activities focus on the placenta.

Why is an exponential rise in pelvic blood flow important for normal pregnancy?

A key aspect of placental function is to promote maternal perfusion of the implantation site. Indeed, this is a central objective across many animal species, where extravillous cytotrophoblast invasion of maternal blood vessels directs blood into an intervillous space. Maternal blood thus bathes the placental villi, which in turn become specialized to enhance gaseous diffusion and mediate active nutrient transport to the developing fetus. The exponential nature of the rise in uterine artery blood flow during human pregnancy, from around 50 ml/minute to > 600 ml/minute, was initially documented by Konje *et al.* [18], and is self-evident to obstetricians especially when dealing with problems like placenta previa or placenta increta. The rise in blood flow is assumed to cater for the metabolic demands of the fetus, and assumes that this increase is mostly directed to the intervillous space of the placenta. This assumption is reinforced by the observation that the uterine artery Doppler waveforms become transformed to a high-flow low-resistance pattern [19] and that this Doppler transformation is associated with successful term pregnancy – however several pieces of information challenge this association.

First, most pregnancies with incidental isolated findings of abnormal uterine artery Doppler at 20–22 weeks' gestation progress to term, suggesting that physiological uterine artery blood flow (and Doppler) changes occur in excess of that required for fetal growth via perfusion of the intervillous space. Consequently, the low (20%) positive predictive value of this test in isolation for preterm delivery due to IUGR/preeclampsia means that uterine artery Doppler is not recommended as a screening test of uteroplacental function in unselected, or 'low-risk', pregnancies [20]. We suggest the alternate hypothesis that the exponential rise in blood flow may be designed to ensure adequate placental perfusion during labor, as opposed to the antenatal period, since uterine contractions obstruct blood flow. If so, persistent abnormal uterine artery Doppler in late gestation could be associated with the development of fetal distress in labor. Surprisingly this concept has not received much research attention because the focus of research has been the association with preterm delivery due to preeclampsia and/or IUGR. However, in one small study uterine artery Doppler studies were shown not to be predictive of fetal distress during oxytocin challenge tests (OCT) in 67 high-risk women [21], although an increase in umbilical artery resistance as was seen in fetuses displaying heart rate decelerations during OCT induced uterine contraction [22].

Second, color Doppler ultrasound imaging suggests a low-flow maternal circulation inside the placenta, whereas the surrounding myometrium is very vascular (Fig. 23.1). Doppler signals can be obtained from spiral arteries entering through the placental

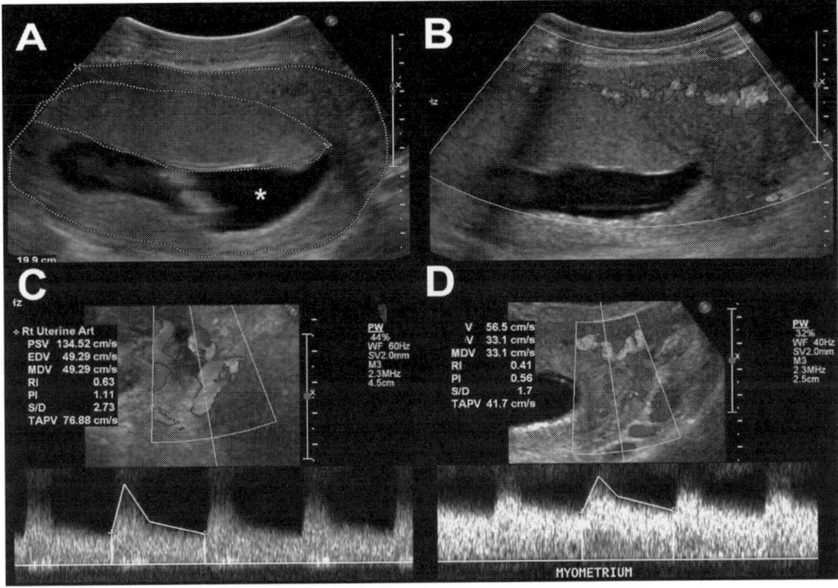

Fig. 23.1 Blood flow to the uterus and placenta at 12 weeks of gestation. (A) Real-time imaging in the transverse plane shows the uterus (outer line) and definitive placenta (inner line) with the intervening tissue being myometrium. *Denotes the amniotic fluid. (B) Corresponding image with color flow Doppler shows strong blood flow signals in the myometrium, but not inside the placenta. (C) Pulsed Doppler waveforms from the proximal left uterine artery in the same plane below the uterus – note high peak systolic velocity (134 cm/second) and low pulsatility index (PI) indicating a low-impedance circulation. (D) Corresponding pulsed Doppler recordings from the myometrial arteries showing similar low-impedance waveforms. No arterial signals are obtained inside the placenta. See plate section for color version.

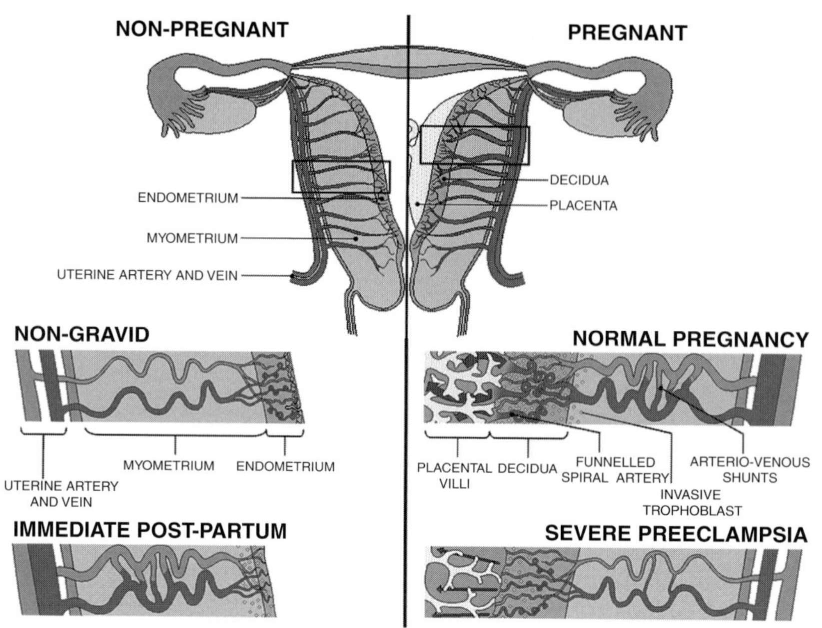

Fig. 23.2 Diagrammatic representation of uterine and placental vasculature (dark shading = arterial; light shading = venous) in the non-pregnant, pregnant, and immediate postpartum state. Normal pregnancy is characterized by the formation of large arteriovenous shunts that persist in the immediate postpartum period. By contrast pregnancies complicated by severe preeclampsia are characterized by minimal arteriovenous shunts and thus narrower uterine arteries. Extravillous cytotrophoblast invasion in normal pregnancy (diamonds) extends beyond the decidua into the inner myometrium resulting in the formation of funnels at the discharging tips of the spiral arteries. Contrast with severe preeclampsia. Reproduced with permission from Burton *et al.* [28].

basal plate [23] but intervillous blood flow velocity is below the detection limits of color Doppler (i.e. below 10 m/second) [24]. Third, the increased use of magnetic resonance imaging (MRI) in obstetrics, in particular with gadolinium definition of blood flow, suggests the possibility of arteriovenous shunts in the myometrium, allowing most maternal blood to bypass the spiral arteries and intervillous space [25,26]. A challenging viewpoint is therefore that uterine artery blood flow by mid-gestation is indeed greatly in excess of that needed to ensure fetal survival at term, but that these changes are actually not critical for fetal growth and survival to term. Why therefore, from an evolutionary perspective, does this phenomenon occur?

Our alternative view is that the formation of myometrial arteriovenous shunts provides the capability to accommodate the increase in maternal blood volume in order to protect against maternal death at delivery from hemorrhage. The maternal cardiovascular changes of normal pregnancy, namely a 40% increase in both blood volume and cardiac output, are achieved in the first half of pregnancy [27]. These changes would cause severe hypertension in a non-pregnant woman, yet blood pressure falls: this reconciliation is made possible by a profound reduction in systemic arterial vascular resistance and an increase in venous capacitance – the pooling of blood in veins. Normal pregnancy is thus characterized by warm skin, prominent veins, and a tendency to dizziness, termed orthostatic hypotension, when lying flat. By contrast the hypertensive complication of pregnancy termed severe preeclampsia is characterized by several abnormal aspects of cardiovascular function: hypertension due to increased systemic vascular resistance, contracted blood volume, hemo-concentration, and abnormal uterine artery Doppler. As such abnormal uterine artery Doppler may be viewed as part of a more generalized systemic vasculopathy, which can be imaged non-invasively during pregnancy and may mediate future cardiovascular risk [15]. These vascular differences between normal and severely preeclamptic pregnancies at the level of the uterus are summarized in Fig. 23.2 [28].

> The progressive increase in pelvic blood flow of pregnancy, accompanied by changes in uterine artery Doppler, may be a local expression of the systemic vascular adaptation to pregnancy, as opposed to meeting a local demand for the delivery of maternal blood to the placental villi.

Can EVT cells mediate maternal physiological changes of pregnancy?

Extravillous cytotrophoblast (EVT) cells proliferate, invade, and differentiate as they surround and transform the distal segments of the uteroplacental spiral arteries. In normal pregnancy, dilated transformed segments of these vessels contain perivascular aggregates of interstitial EVT that have fused together [29]. The nuclei in these multinucleated aggregates may be larger, indicating a degree of endo-duplication [30] as part of this process; mitosis is suppressed. These observations are similar in many ways to the observed differentiation of EVT in mice to form so-called 'giant cells'. The molecular control of trophoblast differentiation in mice is now well appreciated [31] and some of this knowledge is steadily being translated to our understanding of human trophoblast differentiation.

Placental development in both mice and humans is conditional upon a steady supply of trophoblast differentiating along both the EVT and villous/labyrinthine pathways. Trophoblast stem (TS) cells have been isolated in mice [32] and these cells supply progenitors for each trophoblast lineage [33]. Murine TS cells require FGF4/FGFR2 signaling for maintenance, and similarly a subset of first trimester villous cytotrophoblasts express FGFR2 and proliferate in response to FGF4/heparin, analogous to TS cell maintenance in mice [34]. Along the proximal EVT pathway, the expression of the transcription factor Mash2 in the murine spongiotrophoblast corresponds with expression of MASH2 (or HASH2) in cytotrophoblast columns [35,36,37]. In mice, another key transcription factor glial cell missing-1 (Gcm-1) is absolutely required for chorionic trophoblast differentiation into syncytiotrophoblast and thus morphogenesis of the labyrinth [38]. Whilst Gcm-1 expression has not been studied in murine giant cell formation, the human ortholog GCM1 is expressed in a subset of cytotrophoblast in placental villi, but also in postmitotic EVT [39]. We recently demonstrated that GCM1 is indeed required for differentiation of both the villous and extra-villous trophoblast lineages in the first trimester human placenta [40]. Gcm-1 is known to mediate the arrest of mitosis and stimulate the expression of the fusogenic proteins Syncytin 1 and 2 implicated in trophoblast cell fusion [41,42]. Our EVT data are further supported by the observation that distal EVT also focally express Syncytin as they form mature aggregates around transformed vessels [43]. Interestingly, we have recently shown that a 30–50% repression of GCM1, in both floating villous explants and in Matrigel-invading villous tip explants, recapitulates the observed defects found in placentas and placental bed biopsies of severely preeclamptic women, namely an increase in proliferating cells at the expense of differentiated trophoblast, either syncytiotrophoblast or invasive EVT [40]. Since GCM1 expression is similarly reduced in severely preeclamptic placentae at delivery [44], the evidence suggests that dysregulation of this transcription factor, expressed at the beginning of trophoblast differentiation, could be responsible for defects in both trophoblast differentiation pathways and thus impact the placental phenotype. Moreover, our most recent data show that GCM1 repression causes floating villous explants to release a 3.5-fold increase in the antiangiogenesis protein sFlt1 and a proportional suppression of VEGF secretion [45]. These findings provide a molecular link between the observed structural changes in trophoblast differentiation and the reversible vasculopathy that characterizes severe preeclampsia, especially the increased systemic vascular resistance and renal glomerular injury [46,47,48].

Another candidate gene recently suggested to contribute to a defect in EVT differentiation is the transcription factor storkhead box 1 (STOX1). Five missense mutations in STOX1 have been identified, identical in sequence between preeclampsia-affected sisters and segregating with the preeclamptic phenotype in the Dutch population [49]. Although other genetic studies have not confirmed this finding in other populations [50, 51] recent studies have defined a potential linkage mechanism for STOX1 action. STOX1 has been shown to transactivate the catenin-associated protein alpha 3 gene (CTNNA3) in an allele-dependent manner in SGHPL5 cells, with mutant STOX1 showing a much stronger induction of this gene than the wild-type STOX1. Moreover, silencing of STOX1 in villous explants leads to an increase in the invasive capability of the EVT [52]. This is of interest as the protein encoded by this gene, αT-catenin, is implicated in cell–cell adhesion, dysregulation of which would impact trophoblast invasion and differentiation, factors thought to contribute to the etiology of preeclampsia. Overexpression of STOX1 in choriocarcinoma cells also results in a gene expression profile that strongly correlates with transcriptome alterations in preeclamptic placentae [53]. STOX1 is intriguing, because haplotype frequency variations by ethnicity also correlate with ethnically derived risks for severe preeclampsia [54]. It is suggested that haplotype variations in STOX1 interacting with its partner (CTNNA3) may explain the recurrence of severe preeclampsia in Dutch families [52]. Such genetic data add weight to the hypothesis that severe placental phenotypes have a distinct genetic basis in the maternal EVT cell lineage.

Molecular defects that impact on progenitor trophoblast can impact both villous and extravillous trophoblast differentiation. In turn these may create the 'antiangiogenic' environment that is expressed maternally as severe preeclampsia.

The major emphasis thus far on EVT differentiation in the human has been upon the capacity of these cells to invade and physically transform the distal uterine spiral arteries. However in mice, EVT behave differently, enlarging to form giant cells that physically displace the decidua, and only a small degree of EVT invasion of the central spiral artery within the ectoplacental cone occurs, and is thus of questionable physiological relevance in this species [55]. This small degree of vascular invasion is not consistent across different species, as reviewed in Chapter 12. However, this observation has suggested that these giant cells and the analogous human interstitial EVT may mediate increased blood flow locally via paracrine signals that affect a much greater extent of this circulation than that part with which these cells are physically connected. For example, in the guinea-pig the spiral arteries become dilated in advance of EVT invasion [56] and in mice, changes in uterine artery Doppler and in the arcuate artery vasculature occur much more proximally than growth of the giant cells [13]. The potential list of paracrine candidates for EVT-mediated vasodilation includes several diffusible gases with limited (nitric oxide) [56] or more potent local vasodilator properties (carbon monoxide [57,58], hydrogen sulfide [59]).

More classic hormones may be responsible for mediating increased blood flow to the implantation site. In a recent study by Kanasaki *et al.* in 2008, reduced expression of catechol-*O*-methyl transferase (COMT), an enzyme promoting the conversion of estradiol to the vasodilator product 2-methoxyestradiol (2-ME), results in a preeclamptic phenotype in mice [60]. The same enzyme was shown to be reduced in preeclamptic placentae in the third trimester [60].

EVT cells populating the placental bed appear to do more than erode the distal uteroplacental arteries. EVT may exist in the uterine wall to function as a 'dispersed' endocrine organ, interacting with the systemic vasculature, much as B-cell islands in the pancreas regulate the metabolic state of the mother.

Is host-induced uteroplacental vascular insufficiency possible?

Abnormal uterine artery Doppler at 22 weeks' gestation confers a five-fold increased risk of all forms of preeclampsia, but a much greater risk of early-onset disease with associated IUGR. Placental bed biopsies from these subjects at delivery demonstrate a vasculopathy characterized by a failure of endovascular EVT invasion into the walls of myometrial spiral arteries and decreased levels of vascular smooth muscle disruption, despite the presence of interstitial EVT [8,10,61]. The nature of the block in the invasion of semi-allogenic EVT is presently unknown, but may be influenced by the maternal immune system.

Successful tissue engraftment of the placenta to the maternal host is challenged by human genetic diversity. This genetic conflict results in varying degrees of placental vascular pathology at an epidemiological level, from low rates in Asians through intermediate rates in Caucasians to much higher levels in African-American couples [62,63,64]. The risk may be transmitted by certain high-risk men or by primipaternity [65] and is higher in assisted conception pregnancies, especially with donor gametes [66]. The risk is reduced by intercourse prior to conception suggesting that 'graft tolerance' may be induced by vaginal paternal leukocyte exposure (for review [67]). Under optimal circumstances, maternal leukocyte lineages may be capable of promoting EVT invasion, whereas the same cell types may also be capable of attacking and killing these cells.

Normal pregnancy is characterized on the whole by a shift in the maternal immune system from a Th1 dominated system, into a Th2 immune response that is mediated by macrophage and dendritic cells; however, other key cellular players specialized to the decidua are also implicated as discussed below [68,69]. The trophoblast surrounding the conceptus comes into direct contact with maternal cells in the decidua, a unique tissue that develops from the late secretory endometrium via progesterone, human chorionic gonadotropin (hCG), and human placental lactogen (hPL) [70,71,72]. During the first trimester further spatial differentiation of the decidua occurs into the decidua basalis, underlying the implantation site, the adjacent decidua parietalis, and the more distant decidual secretory endometrium with corresponding changes in vascular density, vessel type, and maturity [73]. In the decidua basalis, vessel density is reduced in favor of larger vessels, where the expression of the angiogenic factors PlGF, its receptor Flt1, and angiopoetin-2 are increased [74], in preparation for vascular transformation. It is these vessels of decidua basalis and their associated myometrial portions that are targeted for transformation by the endovascular EVT.

Immune cells are a significant constituent of the normal cycling endometrium [75], and are a potent source of the growth factors and proteases believed to be important for endometrial angiogenesis. Menstrual cycle-dependent changes are apparent in leukocyte numbers and subtypes within the endometrial stroma, corresponding to distinct repair and remodeling events [76,77]; for review see Dunk *et al.* [78]. Following ovulation there is a marked increase in endometrial leukocyte numbers comprising 40% of endometrial cells in the mid–late secretory phase. They promote spiral artery angiogenesis and subsequent decidualization; they mediate maternal tolerance of the fetal allograft and regulate EVT invasion [79,80,81]. The main subpopulation (70%) are uterine natural killer (uNK) cells. The remainder comprises macrophages, dendritic cells and CD4+ T helper cells, a few CD8+ T-cytotoxic cells, T-regulatory cells, and NK T cells [82]. Vascular and decidual cells in the decidua express a range of chemokines with potential chemoattractant activity for uNK cells [83,84,85,86,87]. Thus the decidualized spiral arteries are intrinsically capable of honing uNK cells to the perivascular regions [84].

Uterine NK cells are distinct from peripheral blood NK (PBNK) cells in that they have a unique phenotype (CD3-, CD16- and $CD56_{bright}$) [88] and a markedly different gene expression profile [89]. Expression of mRNA for a range of angiogenic factors (VEGF-C, PlGF, Ang2) by uNK cells has been demonstrated both *in vitro* and *in vivo* [90,91], and isolated uNK cells from early pregnancies secrete Ang1, Ang2, VEGF-C, and TGFβ-1 [92]. These findings strongly support key roles for uNK immune cells in the process of decidualization including regulating vascular tone in spiral arteries. Macrophages form the second largest immune cell population and also express a range of cytokines with potent angiogenic activity, including IL-8 and VEGF [93,94,95] (Fig. 23.3). Recently, in sheep, selective upregulation of VEGF signaling via adenovirus transfection of the uterine artery was shown to increase local uterine artery blood flow [96].

The varied properties of uNK cells are mediated via a series of inhibitory or activating receptors whose ligands are the HLA class 1 molecules expressed on EVT; namely HLA-C, HLA-E, and HLA-G [82]. EVT may therefore inhibit uNK cytotoxicity when their HLA class 1 molecules bind to a variety of inhibitory receptors, ILT2, CD94/NKG2, and KIR, although when these class I ligands are blocked *in vitro*, trophoblast cells are not killed by uNK cells [97]. Although a highly complex process, data are now emerging that begin to explain how maternal leukocytes can mediate the risk of developing uteroplacental vascular pathology. Novel work by Hiby *et al.* begins to explain global ethnic differences in preeclampsia susceptibility via polymorphisms in a specific ligand–receptor pairing (HLA-C in EVT with maternal uNK KIR activating receptors). Mothers lacking KIR-activating uNK cells (AA genotype) when the fetally derived EVT expressed HLA-C2 were at high risk of preeclampsia [98]. These findings have recently been extended to the related pathology of recurrent unexplained miscarriages where a high frequency of HLA-C2 in both parents was found in combination with a high frequency of maternal KIR AA genotype [99].

Intriguingly it has recently been shown that there is a temporal change in the expression pattern of both activating and inhibitory KIR specific for HLA-C in isolated first trimester uNK cells, with a decline in both intensity of expression and frequency throughout the first trimester of pregnancy [100]. KIR expression by uNK cells is likely to be regulated by the decidual microenvironment around the activated spiral arterioles before EVT invasion. Interestingly, our collaborators have recently demonstrated an accumulation of uNK cells and macrophages in the arterial wall of first trimester decidual spiral arterioles prior to invasion of the vascular lumen by endovascular EVT [101]. These immune cells appear to contribute to the smooth muscle cell disruption through the secretion of MMP-9 and we suggest that this vascular interaction may modulate their subsequent behavior [101]. A similar phenomenon is also observed in our *in vitro* model of EVT-mediated decidual transformation but only in the presence of a placental explant suggesting that the placenta may provide the chemotactic stimulus for uNK cells and macrophage infiltration of the vessel wall [102]. This is a potentially powerful model that could, for example, be exploited to test the hypothesis that an initial uNK cell–trophoblast interaction can stimulate and amplify further EVT-mediated spiral artery transformation.

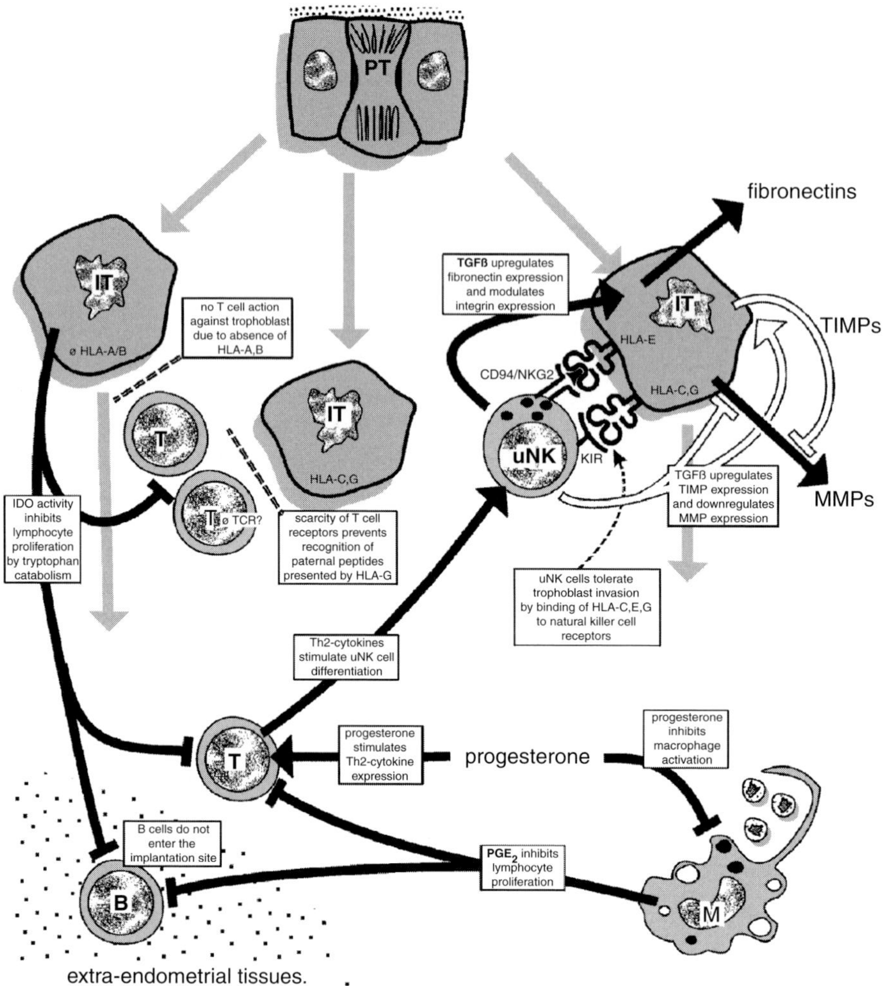

Fig. 23.3 Schematic overview of interaction of maternal immune cells with trophoblast cells in the implantation site and their effects on trophoblast invasion. Gray arrows: routes of trophoblast invasion; black arrows: interactions that are thought to exert a promoting net effect in trophoblast invasion. Blue: trophoblast cells; pink: maternal cells; PT, proliferative extravillous trophoblast; IT, invasive extravillous trophoblast; uNK, uterine natural killer cell; M, macrophage; T, T cell; B, B cell. Reproduced with permission from David *et al.* [96]. See plate section for color version.

These data consolidate the hypothesis that impaired decidualization represents failure to activate beneficial uNK cells that in turn encourage vascular transformation and endovascular EVT invasion. Chronic overexposure of uNK cells to activating ligands exhausts this beneficial uNK status, decreasing angiogenic capability at the expense of increased cytotoxic interferon-gamma (IFN-γ) production [79]. Women who suffer from recurrent miscarriages or preeclampsia display altered uNK cell profiles and persistent IFN-γ production in the secretory menstrual phase, and excessive Th1 response in the peripheral circulation [103,104,105,106]. The persistent IFN-γ expression by uNK cells may activate maternal macrophages and T cells to kill EVT. In support of this concept, hostile activated uNK cells and macrophages coincide with apoptotic EVT in non-transformed vessels in the preeclamptic placental bed [10,61,107]. Furthermore, IFN-γ activates macrophages to secrete the cytotoxin TNF-α and indole amine 2,3-dioxygenase (IDO) that induces trophoblast apoptosis via tryptophan starvation [61].

Finally, an extension of this process into later placentation is illustrated by the exclusion of maternal T cells from the placental villi in normal pregnancy. By contrast, the invasion of placental villi by maternal T cells is described by perinatal pathologists as 'villitis of unknown etiology' (VUE) [48]. This lesion is observed in a subset of severe IUGR and preeclamptic pregnancies

[108,109] suggesting activation of the maternal immune system against the placenta and fetus in these cases. VUE does not appear to have any direct detrimental effects during pregnancy, however this inappropriate invasion of the placental villous core, and thus fetus, by maternal immune cells could provide an explanation for certain autoimmune diseases including systemic lupus erythematosus (SLE) [110].

> Maternal uNK cells and macrophages play integral roles in decidual matrix destruction, angiogenesis, and vascular remodeling. All of these processes participate in EVT invasion. Polymorphic receptor–ligand interactions between uNK cells and trophoblast can have either beneficial or harmful effects, which can then determine the extent of trophoblast invasion.

Why erode the distal portions of the spiral arteries if the proximal segments are dilated by other mechanisms?

If the exponential increase in uterine artery blood flow in pregnancy is considered merely part of the generalized cardiovascular adaptation to normal pregnancy, what then is the residual role of distal transformation of the spiral arteries by invasive extravillous cytotrophoblast? In humans, studies of reconstructed histological sections from full-thickness myometrial specimens at cesarean hysterectomy suggest that only the myometrial segment of a spiral artery wall is invaded in normal pregnancy [10]. As stated in the section 'Why is an exponential rise in pelvic blood flow important for normal pregnancy?', several pieces of evidence suggest that maternal blood flow in the intervillous space is at a low velocity. This is important for two reasons. First, blood flow velocity around the placental villi needs to be reduced, to facilitate gaseous exchange, especially as the two circulations are not arranged in a formal countercurrent way [111]. Second, a significant fall in blood pressure must occur across the spiral arteries to keep intervillous pressure low; this is necessary because fetal perfusion of floating villi is at low pressure and thus transmission of arterial blood pressure to the intervillous space would collapse the floating villi, compressing the villous capillaries, and thereby prevent maternal–fetal diffusional exchange (discussed in detail in Burton *et al.* [28]). Finally, the anatomical changes induced in the distal portions of the anatomically transformed spiral arteries are predicted to create a Venturi effect so that the villi are sprayed gently with maternal blood (Figs 23.1 and 23.2).

How does 'uteroplacental vascular insufficiency' mediate serious fetal complications of pregnancy?

The above discussions imply that impaired uterine artery Doppler studies alone likely have minimal impact on fetal growth, because most blood entering the radial arteries traverses the uterus via arteriovenous shunts [25], and only a small proportion enters the intervillous space – at low pressure and velocity [28]. These physiological considerations therefore explain why recent systematic reviews show poor test characteristics of abnormal UTA Doppler alone at 20–22 weeks of gestation for the prediction of adverse outcomes (preeclampsia, small-for-gestational age [SGA] infant, stillbirth) attributed to 'placental insufficiency' – especially in low-risk women [20]. The association is stronger when these outcomes result in delivery before 34 weeks [112], though not to the extent that uterine artery Doppler is recommended as a screening test for either preeclampsia [113] or IUGR [114]. Since the placenta villous tree is responsible for maternal–fetal exchange, one solution to defining the role of uterine artery Doppler in clinical practice is to study the placenta at delivery in relation to Doppler test results. However, few studies of uterine artery Doppler include pathological examination of the placenta.

Several components of pathological examination are relevant to a diagnosis of placental insufficiency [2]. The first is simply placental weight for gestation. In our recent cohort study experience of 60 high-risk pregnancies with abnormal uterine artery Doppler, 74% of placentas were < 10th centile for weight [16]. A study combining placental pathology with placental bed biopsy in 47 IUGR pregnancies found normal placental bed biopsies in all 25 controls, and a 17% and 79% rate of abnormal placental bed pathology when IUGR pregnancies had normal or abnormal uterine artery Doppler [115]. The second component is injury to the remaining placental villous tissue. In the Toal series, abnormal uterine artery Doppler conferred a 30% risk of severe IUGR with abnormal umbilical artery Doppler. Both studies demonstrated high rates of placental villous infarction; in the Toal cohort, only 16% of placentas were normal at

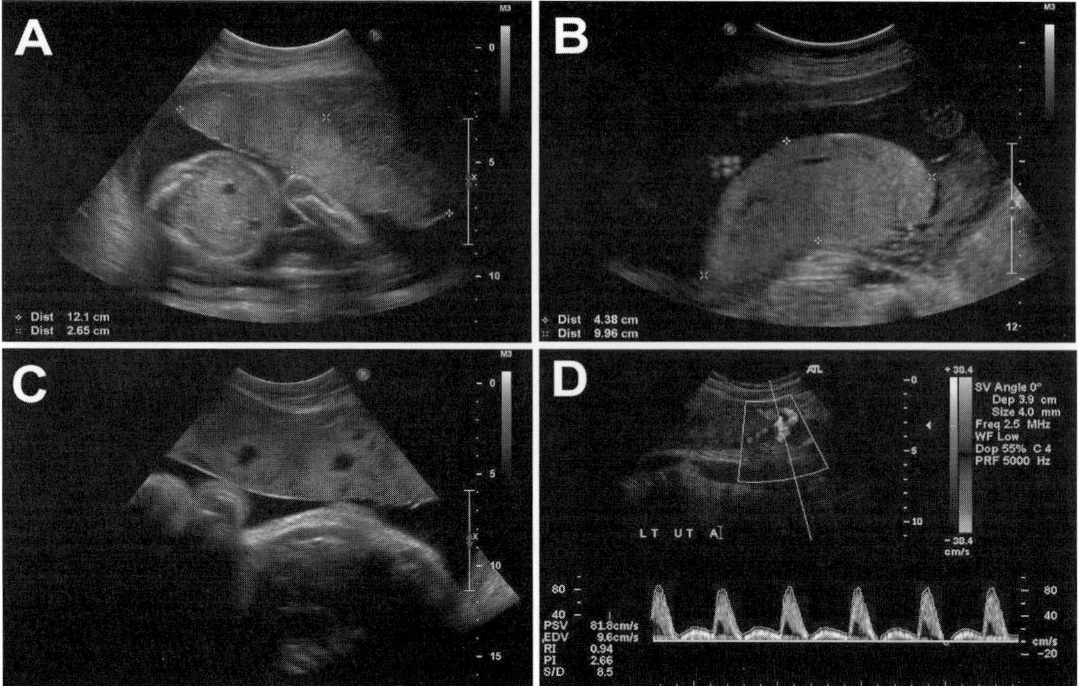

Fig. 23.4 Placental ultrasound and abnormal uterine artery Doppler at 19–22 weeks in women with low PAPP-A (< 0.3 MOM) values at 11–13weeks. (A) The normal placenta is typically 12 cm long and 2.5 cm thick. Note the normal granular texture, created by the interdigitating villous trees anchored to the basal plate. (B) A small placental footprint increases the risk of stillbirth and severe IUGR in this study. In this situation, the umbilical cord insertion is usually at the edge, indicating 'chorion regression' at the end of the first trimester. The placental insufficiency initiated by a small footprint may then be compounded by subsequent injury to the placental tissue (C). (C) These echogenic cystic lesions (ECLs) are non-functioning tissue due to intervillous thrombosis and are a poor prognostic sign. (D) ECLs and wedge-shaped infarcts usually develop in the placentae of women with persistently abnormal uterine artery Doppler characterized by an elevated pulsatility index (PI) > 1.45, in this case 2.6. See plate section for color version.

delivery [16]. The third component is basal plate pathology, mediated by various factors already discussed in this chapter. A simplistic view is that the pathological lesion decidual vasculopathy directly causes both regression of placental size and villous infarction. However, placental bed biopsy studies have occasionally demonstrated a high prevalence of vascular pathology in control pregnancies; for example, 40% amongst 27 controls in one study of preeclampsia [116] and similar numbers of partially transformed vessels seen in both normal, preeclamptic, and preterm pregnancies [6]. We would therefore suggest that decidual vasculopathy alone probably does not cause either regression of placental size or a tendency to multifocal placental infarction.

To shed light on the likely origins of clinically significant UPVI, we have studied placental ultrasound and uterine artery Doppler in over 70 women with very low (<0.3 multiples of median) maternal serum levels of the syncytiotrophoblast-derived pregnancy-associated plasma protein A (PAPP-A) [117] measured at 11–13 weeks of gestation to define the risk for trisomy 21 [118,119]. The rationale of the study is that low PAPP-A is associated with early severe preeclampsia [120] and stillbirth [121]. Severe IUGR and preterm stillbirth were common in this cohort and strongly associated with small placentae and eccentric cords. We term this phenomenon 'chorion regression' [122] (Fig. 23.4).

The pathological basis of multifocal placental infarction is important to appreciate, because it leads to acute fetal deterioration from IUGR and severe preeclampsia. Systematic review suggests at best only a weak association between IUGR and thrombophilia [123] in that, while women with thrombophilia are at increased risk of placental complications [124], the majority of IUGR pregnancies that have placental lesions do not have thrombophilia [1]. An alternative explanation is that the process of normal syncytiotrophoblast differentiation (to a pseudoendothelial phenotype) in turn promotes local inhibition of coagulation [125]. There are currently clinical trials underway investigating the use of anticoagulants such as unfractionated heparin (UFH) or low molecular weight heparin (LMWH) in pregnancies at risk of placental thrombosis. In a recent Canadian pilot randomized control trial (RCT) of 110 women with a complex past obstetrical history and a negative thrombophilia screen, the administration of subcutaneous LMWH significantly reduced the risk of a composite of adverse perinatal outcomes attributable to placental thrombosis, principally early-onset preeclampsia [126]. A deficiency of this study was the lack of antenatal evaluation of placental function (e.g. using second trimester uterine artery Doppler or reinterpretation of IPS tests) and of placental pathological evaluation.

The utility of uterine artery Doppler is improved when targeted to women with risk factors for placental dysfunction, especially women with abnormal first or second trimester screening results [2]. As a result of increasing publications, one guideline now suggests this test be offered to women in this setting [127]. In the second trimester, the combined elevation of hCG and inhibin, both derived from syncytiotrophoblast, is associated with adverse outcomes and is compounded by elevated AFP, since this fetally derived protein enters the maternal circulation via defects in the villous trophoblast [128]. Since, for example, hCG levels normally peak at 13 weeks, persistently elevated hCG at 16 weeks implies excessive villous trophoblast differentiation. This phenomenon can be recapitulated *in vitro* by upregulating GCM1 but is associated with depletion of underlying cytotrophoblasts [40], as is found at delivery in severe IUGR placentae [129].

Therefore the pregnancy with an 'at risk' placenta, based upon multiple test categories (abnormal IPS test results, small/thick placenta on ultrasound, abnormal uterine artery Doppler) has a much higher risk of serious adverse perinatal events; from the Toal study when two, or all three, of these test categories were abnormal, the positive predictive value for stillbirth or delivery before 32 weeks was over 30% [16]. These data form the rationale of the HEPRIN (HEparin to PRevent placental Insufficiency) (ISRCTN: 88675588) pilot RCT that randomizes women between 18 and 23 weeks to UFH 7500 units SC BD.

Though presently only IPS tests are used real-time with uterine artery Doppler for trial recruitment, other blood or urine assays may become integrated in the future, such as maternal serum expression of pro- and antiangiogenesis proteins [130].

> The concept of assessing placental function in clinical practice has entered the realm of clinical trials, but sequential testing is recommended (blood markers followed by uterine artery Doppler and ultrasound of placental shape and texture) to attain high positive predictive values for serious adverse perinatal outcomes causing stillbirth or iatrogenic preterm delivery.

Research questions

1. What are the molecular mechanisms linking control of trophoblast differentiation and the production of antiangiogenesis proteins?
2. How does the normal placenta prevent pathological coagulation in the intervillous space?
3. What is the genetic basis of the racial disparity in risk of severe preeclampsia?
4. What is the molecular basis of chorion regression in women with either low PAPP-A at 11–13 weeks or with persistently abnormal uterine artery Doppler at 20–22 weeks?

Practice points

1. Uterine artery Doppler alone is not a useful screening test in clinical practice, especially in low-risk women.
2. The combination of uterine artery Doppler with one or more factors (maternal clinical risk factors (hypertension, obesity), integrated prenatal serum (IPS) screening blood tests, placental shape) results in clinically useful positive predictive values for clinical practice and for trial recruitment.
3. Women identified as being high-risk for adverse clinical outcomes by use of such methods benefit from enhanced maternal–fetal surveillance, though to date no therapeutic randomized control trials have demonstrated any significant impact upon perinatal survival or handicap.
4. Prophylactic anticoagulation with subcutaneous heparin may reduce the risk of severe preeclampsia, but current trials (e.g. HEPRIN trial ISRCTN: 88675588) are designed to test the mechanism of potential benefit via pathological analysis of the placenta following delivery.
5. Careful postnatal evaluation of cardiovascular health and targeted programs of exercise, weight loss, and even lipid-lowering drugs, may have an

impact upon longer-term cardiovascular risks in formerly preeclamptic women. Women recovering from severe preeclampsia should therefore receive ongoing medical advice once their blood pressure has subsided.

References

1. Viero S, Chaddha V, Alkazaleh F *et al.* Prognostic value of placental ultrasound in pregnancies complicated by absent end-diastolic flow velocity in the umbilical arteries. *Placenta* 2004; **25**(8–9): 735–41.
2. Whittle W, Chaddha V, Wyatt P *et al.* Ultrasound detection of placental insufficiency in women with 'unexplained' abnormal maternal serum screening results. *Clin Genet* 2006; **69**(2): 97–104.
3. Brosens I A, Robertson W B, Dixon H G. The role of the spiral arteries in the pathogenesis of preeclampsia. *Obstet Gynecol Annu* 1972; **1**: 177–91.
4. Brosens I, Dixon H G, Robertson W B. Fetal growth retardation and the arteries of the placental bed. *Br J Obstet Gynaecol* 1977; **84**(9): 656–63.
5. Pijnenborg R, Anthony J, Davey D A *et al.* Placental bed spiral arteries in the hypertensive disorders of pregnancy. *Br J Obstet Gynaecol* 1991; **98**(7): 648–55.
6. Kim Y M, Chaiworapongsam T, Gomez R *et al.* Failure of physiologic transformation of the spiral arteries in the placental bed in preterm premature rupture of membranes. *Am J Obstet Gynecol* 2002; **187**(5): 1137–42.
7. Pijnenborg R, Bland J M, Robertson W B *et al.* Uteroplacental arterial changes related to interstitial trophoblast migration in early human pregnancy. *Placenta* 1983; **4**(4): 397–413.
8. Lyall F. The human placental bed revisited. *Placenta* 2002; **23**(8–9): 555–62.
9. Pijnenborg R, Bland J M, Robertson W B *et al.* The pattern of interstitial trophoblastic invasion of the myometrium in early human pregnancy. *Placenta* 1981; **2**(4): 303–16.
10. Kadyrov M, Kingdom J C, Huppertz B. Divergent trophoblast invasion and apoptosis in placental bed spiral arteries from pregnancies complicated by maternal anemia and early-onset preeclampsia/ intrauterine growth restriction. *Am J Obstet Gynecol* 2006; **194**(2): 557–63.
11. Palmer S K, Zamudio S, Coffin C *et al.* Quantitative estimation of human uterine artery blood flow and pelvic blood flow redistribution in pregnancy. *Obstet Gynecol* 1992; **80**(6): 1000–6.
12. Moll W. [Physiological cardiovascular adaptation in pregnancy – its significance for cardiac diseases.] *Z Kardiol* 2001; **90** (Suppl 4): 2–9.
13. Mu J, Adamson S L. Developmental changes in hemodynamics of uterine artery, utero- and umbilicoplacental, and vitelline circulations in mouse throughout gestation. *Am J Physiol Heart Circ Physiol* 2006; **291**(3): H1421–8.
14. Ray J G, Vermeulen M J, Schull M J *et al.* Cardiovascular health after maternal placental syndromes (CHAMPS): population-based retrospective cohort study. *Lancet* 2005; **366**(9499): 1797–803.
15. Lausman A, Kingdom J, Bradley T *et al.* Subclinical atherosclerosis in association with elevated placental vascular resistance in early pregnancy. *Artherosclerosis* 2009. doi.org/10.1016/j.atherosclerosis.2009.02.007.
16. Toal M, Keating S, Machin G *et al.* Determinants of adverse perinatal outcome in high-risk women with abnormal uterine artery Doppler images. *Am J Obstet Gynecol* 2008; **198**(3): 330 e1–7.
17. Costa S L, Proctor L, Dodd J M *et al.* Screening for placental insufficiency in high-risk pregnancies: is earlier better? *Placenta* 2008; **29**(12): 1034–40.
18. Konje J C, Kaufmann P, Bell S C *et al.* A longitudinal study of quantitative uterine blood flow with the use of color power angiography in appropriate for gestational age pregnancies. *Am J Obstet Gynecol* 2001; **185**(3): 608–13.
19. McCowan L M, Ritchie K, Mo L Y *et al.* Uterine artery flow velocity waveforms in normal and growth-retarded pregnancies. *Am J Obstet Gynecol* 1988; **158**(3 Pt 1): 499–504.
20. Cnossen J S, Morris R K, ter Riet G *et al.* Use of uterine artery Doppler ultrasonography to predict preeclampsia and intrauterine growth restriction: a systematic review and bivariable meta-analysis. *CMAJ* 2008; **178**(6): 701–11.
21. Li H, Gudmundsson S, Olofsson P. Clinical significance of uterine artery blood flow velocity waveforms during provoked uterine contractions in high-risk pregnancy. *Ultrasound Obstet Gynecol* 2004; **24**(4): 429–34.
22. Li H, Gudmundsson S, Olofsson P. Acute increase of umbilical artery vascular flow resistance in compromised fetuses provoked by uterine contractions. *Early Hum Dev* 2003; **74**(1): 47–56.
23. Matijevic R, Johnston T. In vivo assessment of failed trophoblastic invasion of the spiral arteries in pre-eclampsia. *Br J Obstet Gynaecol* 1999; **106**(1): 78–82.
24. Kurjak A, Kupesic S, Hafner T *et al.* Conflicting data on intervillous circulation in early pregnancy. *J Perinat Med* 1997; **25**(3): 225–36.
25. Schaaps J P, Tsatsaris V. [Uteroplacental vascularization.] *Gynecol Obstet Fertil* 2001; **29**(7–8): 509–11.
26. Schaaps JP, Tsatsaris V, Goffin F *et al.* Shunting the intervillous space: new concepts in human uteroplacental vascularization. *Am J Obstet Gynecol* 2005; **192**(1): 323–32.

27. Hunter S, Robson S C. Adaptation of the maternal heart in pregnancy. *Br Heart J* 1992; **68**(6): 540–3.
28. Burton G, Woods A, Kingdom J *et al.* Rheological and physiological consequences of conversion of the maternal spiral arteries for uteroplacental blood flow during human pregnancy. *Placenta* 2009; **30**: 473-82.
29. Pijnenborg R, Luyten C, Vercruysse L *et al.* Attachment and differentiation in vitro of trophoblast from normal and preeclamptic human placentas. *Am J Obstet Gynecol* 1996; **175**(1): 30–6.
30. Zybina T G, Frank H G, Biesterfeld S *et al.* Genome multiplication of extravillous trophoblast cells in human placenta in the course of differentiation and invasion into endometrium and myometrium. II. Mechanisms of polyploidization. *Tsitologiia* 2004; **46**(7): 640–8.
31. Cross J C. How to make a placenta: mechanisms of trophoblast cell differentiation in mice – a review. *Placenta* 2005; **26** (Suppl A): S3–9.
32. Tanaka S, Kunath T, Hadjantonakis A K *et al.* Promotion of trophoblast stem cell proliferation by FGF4. *Science* 1998; **282**(5396): 2072–5.
33. Uy G D, Downs K M, Gardner R L. Inhibition of trophoblast stem cell potential in chorionic ectoderm coincides with occlusion of the ectoplacental cavity in the mouse. *Development* 2002; **129**(16): 3913–24.
34. Baczyk D, Dunk C, Huppertz B *et al.* Bi-potential behaviour of cytotrophoblasts in first trimester chorionic villi. *Placenta* 2006; **27**(4–5): 367–74.
35. Guillemot F, Nagy A, Auerbach A *et al.* Essential role of Mash-2 in extraembryonic development. *Nature* 1994; **371**(6495): 333–6.
36. Alders M, Hodges M, Hadjantonakis A K *et al.* The human Achaete-Scute homologue 2 (ASCL2, HASH2) maps to chromosome 11p15.5, close to IGF2 and is expressed in extravillus trophoblasts. *Hum Mol Genet* 1997; **6**(6): 859–67.
37. Janatpour M J, Utset M F, Cross J C *et al.* A repertoire of differentially expressed transcription factors that offers insight into mechanisms of human cytotrophoblast differentiation. *Dev Genet* 1999; **25**(2): 146–57.
38. Anson-Cartwright L, Dawson K, Holmyard D *et al.* The glial cells missing-1 protein is essential for branching morphogenesis in the chorioallantoic placenta. *Nat Genet* 2000; **25**(3): 311–4.
39. Baczyk D, Satkunaratnam A, Nait-Oumesmar B *et al.* Complex patterns of GCM1 mRNA and protein in villous and extravillous trophoblast cells of the human placenta. *Placenta* 2004; **25**(6): 553–9.
40. Baczyk D, Drewlo S, Proctor L *et al.* Glial cell missing-1 transcription factor is required for the differentiation of the human trophoblast. *Cell Death Differ* 2009; **16**: 719-27.
41. Yu C, Shen K, Lin M *et al.* GCMa regulates the syncytin-mediated trophoblastic fusion. *J Biol Chem* 2002; **277**(51): 50062–8.
42. Lin C, Lin M, Chen H. Biochemical characterization of the human placental transcription factor GCMa/1. *Biochem Cell Biol* 2005; **83**(2): 188–95.
43. Malassine A, Handschuh K, Tsatsaris V *et al.* Expression of HERV-W Env glycoprotein (syncytin) in the extravillous trophoblast of first trimester human placenta. *Placenta* 2005; **26**(7): 556–62.
44. Chen C P, Chen C Y, Yang Y C *et al.* Decreased placental GCM1 (glial cells missing) gene expression in pre-eclampsia. *Placenta* 2004; **25**(5): 413–21.
45. Drewlo S B, Kingdom D J. GCM1 regulation of sflt-1 expression in first trimester placental villi: the missing link between disordered trophoblast differentiation and the development of severe early-onset preeclampsia. *J Reprod Invest* 2009; **16**(3 Suppl): 90A.
46. Sankaralingam S, Arenas I A, Lalu M M *et al.* Preeclampsia: current understanding of the molecular basis of vascular dysfunction. *Expert Rev Mol Med* 2006; **8**(3): 1–20.
47. Maynard S, Epstein F H, Karumanchi S A. Preeclampsia and angiogenic imbalance. *Annu Rev Med* 2008; **59**: 61–78.
48. Redline R W. Villitis of unknown etiology: noninfectious chronic villitis in the placenta. *Hum Pathol* 2007; **38**(10): 1439–46.
49. van Dijk M, Mulders J, Poutsma A *et al.* Maternal segregation of the Dutch preeclampsia locus at 10q22 with a new member of the winged helix gene family. *Nat Genet* 2005; **37**(5): 514–9.
50. Berends A L, Bertoli-Avella A M, de Groot C J *et al.* STOX1 gene in pre-eclampsia and intrauterine growth restriction. *BJOG* 2007; **114**(9): 1163–7.
51. Kivinen K, Peterson H, Hiltunen L *et al.* Evaluation of STOX1 as a preeclampsia candidate gene in a population-wide sample. *Eur J Hum Genet* 2007; **15**(4): 494–7.
52. van Djik M, Dunk C, Oudejans C B *et al.* Preeclampsia susceptibility gene STOX1 in migration and invasion of extravillous trophoblasts. *Placenta* 2008; **29**(8): A7.
53. Rigourd V, Chauvet C, Chelbi S T *et al.* STOX1 overexpression in choriocarcinoma cells mimics transcriptional alterations observed in preeclamptic placentas. *PLoS ONE* 2008; **3**(12): e3905.
54. Oudejans C B, van Dijk M, Oosterkamp M *et al.* Genetics of preeclampsia: paradigm shifts. *Hum Genet* 2007; **120**(5): 607–12.
55. Adamson S L, Lu Y, Whiteley K J *et al.* Interactions between trophoblast cells and the maternal and fetal

circulation in the mouse placenta. *Dev Biol* 2002; **250**(2): 358–73.

56. Nanaev A, Chwalisz K, Frank H G *et al.* Physiological dilation of uteroplacental arteries in the guinea pig depends on nitric oxide synthase activity of extravillous trophoblast. *Cell Tissue Res* 1995; **282**(3): 407–21.
57. Lyall F. Development of the utero-placental circulation: the role of carbon monoxide and nitric oxide in trophoblast invasion and spiral artery transformation. *Microsc Res Tech* 2003; **60**(4): 402–11.
58. Bainbridge S A, Smith G N. HO in pregnancy. *Free Radic Biol Med* 2005; **38**(8): 979–88.
59. Patel P, Vatish M, Heptinstall J *et al.* The endogenous production of hydrogen sulphide in intrauterine tissues. *Reprod Biol Endocrinol* 2009; **7**: 10.
60. Kanasaki K, Palmsten K, Sugimoto H *et al.* Deficiency in catechol-O-methyltransferase and 2-methoxyoestradiol is associated with pre-eclampsia. *Nature* 2008; **453**(7198): 1117–21.
61. Reister F, Frank H G, Kingdom J C *et al.* Macrophage-induced apoptosis limits endovascular trophoblast invasion in the uterine wall of preeclamptic women. *Lab Invest* 2001; **81**(8): 1143–52.
62. Williams K P, Baldwin V. The effect of ethnicity on the development of small for gestational age infants associated with hypertension in pregnancy. *Am J Perinatol* 1998; **15**(2): 125–8.
63. Samadi A R, Mayberry R M, Reed J W. Preeclampsia associated with chronic hypertension among African-American and White women. *Ethn Dis* 2001; **11**(2): 192–200.
64. Caughey A B, Stotland N E, Washington A E *et al.* Maternal ethnicity, paternal ethnicity, and parental ethnic discordance: predictors of preeclampsia. *Obstet Gynecol* 2005; **106**(1): 156–61.
65. Deen M E, Ruurda L G, Wang J *et al.* Risk factors for preeclampsia in multiparous women: primipaternity versus the birth interval hypothesis. *J Matern Fetal Neonatal Med* 2006; **19**(2): 79–84.
66. Chen X K, Wen S W, Bottomley J *et al.* In vitro fertilization is associated with an increased risk for preeclampsia. *Hypertens Pregnancy* 2009; **28**(1): 1–12.
67. Saito S, Sakai M, Sasaki Y *et al.* Inadequate tolerance induction may induce pre-eclampsia. *J Reprod Immunol* 2007; **76**(1–2): 30–9.
68. Chaouat G. The Th1/Th2 paradigm: still important in pregnancy? *Semin Immunopathol* 2007; **29**(2): 95–113.
69. Chaouat G. Innately moving away from the Th1/Th2 paradigm in pregnancy. *Clin Exp Immunol* 2003; **131**(3): 393–5.
70. Bonvissuto A C, Lala P K, Kennedy T G *et al.* Induction of transforming growth factor-alpha gene expression in rat decidua is independent of the conceptus. *Biol Reprod* 1992; **46**(4): 607–16.
71. Bell S C. Secretory endometrial and decidual proteins: studies and clinical significance of a maternally derived group of pregnancy-associated serum proteins. *Hum Reprod* 1986; **1**(3): 129–43.
72. Hochner-Celnikier D, Ron M, Eldor A *et al.* Growth characteristics of human first trimester decidual cells cultured in serum-free medium: production of prolactin, prostaglandins and fibronectin. *Biol Reprod* 1984; **31**(4): 827–36.
73. Vailhe B, Kapp M, Dietl J *et al.* Human first-trimester decidua vascular density: an immunohistochemical study using VE-cadherin and endoglin as endothelial cell markers. *Am J Reprod Immunol* 2000; **44**(1): 9–15.
74. Plaisier M, Rodrigues S, Willems F *et al.* Different degrees of vascularization and their relationship to the expression of vascular endothelial growth factor, placental growth factor, angiopoietins, and their receptors in first-trimester decidual tissues. *Fertil Steril* 2007; **88**(1): 176–87.
75. Klentzeris L D, Bulmer J N, Warren A *et al.* Endometrial lymphoid tissue in the timed endometrial biopsy: morphometric and immunohistochemical aspects. *Am J Obstet Gynecol* 1992; **167**(3): 667–74.
76. Salamonsen L A, Lathbury L J. Endometrial leukocytes and menstruation. *Hum Reprod Update* 2000; **6**(1): 16–27.
77. King A, Burrows T, Verma S *et al.* Human uterine lymphocytes. *Hum Reprod Update* 1998; **4**(5): 480–5.
78. Dunk C, Smith S, Hazan A *et al.* Promotion of angiogenesis by human endometrial lymphocytes. *Immunol Invest* 2008; **37**(5): 583–610.
79. Hanna J, Goldman-Wohl D, Hamani Y *et al.* Decidual NK cells regulate key developmental processes at the human fetal-maternal interface. *Nat Med* 2006; **12**: 1065-74.
80. Sargent I L, Borzychowski A M, Redman C W. NK cells and human pregnancy – an inflammatory view. *Trends Immunol* 2006; **27**(9): 399–404.
81. Riley J K, Yokoyama W M. NK cell tolerance and the maternal-fetal interface. *Am J Reprod Immunol* 2008; **59**(5): 371–87.
82. Tabiasco J, Rabot M, Aguerre-Girr M *et al.* Human decidual NK cells: unique phenotype and functional properties – a review. *Placenta* 2006; **27** (Suppl A): S34–9.
83. Wu X, Jin L P, Yuan M M *et al.* Human first-trimester trophoblast cells recruit CD56brightCD16- NK cells into

decidua by way of expressing and secreting of CXCL12/ stromal cell-derived factor 1. *J Immunol* 2005; **175**(1): 61–8.

84. Jones R L, Hannan N J, Kaitu'u T J *et al.* Identification of chemokines important for leukocyte recruitment to the human endometrium at the times of embryo implantation and menstruation. *J Clin Endocrinol Metab* 2004; **89**(12): 6155–67.

85. Hannan N J, Jones R L, Critchley H O *et al.* Coexpression of fractalkine and its receptor in normal human endometrium and in endometrium from users of progestin-only contraception supports a role for fractalkine in leukocyte recruitment and endometrial remodeling. *J Clin Endocrinol Metab* 2004; **89**(12): 6119–29.

86. Sentman C L, Meadows S K, Wira C R *et al.* Recruitment of uterine NK cells: induction of CXC chemokine ligands 10 and 11 in human endometrium by estradiol and progesterone. *J Immunol* 2004; **173**(11): 6760–6.

87. Engert S, Rieger L, Kapp M *et al.* Profiling chemokines, cytokines and growth factors in human early pregnancy decidua by protein array. *Am J Reprod Immunol* 2007; **58**(2): 129–37.

88. Moffett-King A. Natural killer cells and pregnancy. *Nat Rev Immunol* 2002; **2**(9): 656–63.

89. Koopman L A, Kopcow H D, Rybalov B *et al.* Human decidual natural killer cells are a unique NK cell subset with immunomodulatory potential. *J Exp Med* 2003; **198**(8): 1201–12.

90. Jokhi P P, King A, Sharkey A M *et al.* Screening for cytokine messenger ribonucleic acids in purified human decidual lymphocyte populations by the reverse-transcriptase polymerase chain reaction. *J Immunol* 1994; **153**(10): 4427–35.

91. Li X F, Charnock-Jones D S, Zhang E *et al.* Angiogenic growth factor messenger ribonucleic acids in uterine natural killer cells. *J Clin Endocrinol Metab* 2001; **86**(4): 1823–34.

92. Lash G E, Schiessl B, Kirkley M *et al.* Expression of angiogenic growth factors by uterine natural killer cells during early pregnancy. *J Leukoc Biol* 2006; **80**(3): 572–80.

93. Milne S A, Critchley H O, Drudy T A *et al.* Perivascular interleukin-8 messenger ribonucleic acid expression in human endometrium varies across the menstrual cycle and in early pregnancy decidua. *J Clin Endocrinol Metab* 1999; **84**(7): 2563–7.

94. Charnock-Jones D S, Macpherson A M, Archer D F *et al.* The effect of progestins on vascular endothelial growth factor, oestrogen receptor and progesterone receptor immunoreactivity and endothelial cell density in human endometrium. *Hum Reprod* 2000; **15** (Suppl 3): 85–95.

95. Milne S A, Henderson T A, Kelly R W *et al.* Leukocyte populations and steroid receptor expression in human first-trimester decidua; regulation by antiprogestin and prostaglandin E analog. *J Clin Endocrinol Metab* 2005; **90**(7): 4315–21.

96. David A L, Torondel B, Zachary I *et al.* Local delivery of VEGF adenovirus to the uterine artery increases vasorelaxation and uterine blood flow in the pregnant sheep. *Gene Ther* 2008; **15**(19): 1344–50.

97. Avril T, Jarousseau A C, Watier H *et al.* Trophoblast cell line resistance to NK lysis mainly involves an HLA class I-independent mechanism. *J Immunol* 1999; **162**(10): 5902–9.

98. Hiby S E, Walker J J, O'Shaughnessy M *et al.* Combinations of maternal KIR and fetal HLA-C genes influence the risk of preeclampsia and reproductive success. *J Exp Med* 2004; **200**(8): 957–65.

99. Hiby S E, Regan L, Lo W *et al.* Association of maternal killer-cell immunoglobulin-like receptors and parental HLA-C genotypes with recurrent miscarriage. *Hum Reprod* 2008; **23**(4): 972–6.

100. Sharkey A M, Gardner L, Hiby S *et al.* Killer Ig-like receptor expression in uterine NK cells is biased toward recognition of HLA-C and alters with gestational age. *J Immunol* 2008; **181**(1): 39–46.

101. Smith S, Dunk C, Aplin J *et al.* Evidence for immune cell involvement in decidual spiral arteriole remodeling in early human pregnancy. *Am J Pathol* 2009; **174**: 1959-71.

102. Dunk C, Jones R, Smith S, Lye S. Trophoblast leukocyte interactions mediate decidual vascular remodeling. *Placenta* 2007; **28**(8–9): A21.

103. Saito S, Umekage H, Sakamoto Y *et al.* Increased T-helper-1-type immunity and decreased T-helper-2-type immunity in patients with preeclampsia. *Am J Reprod Immunol* 1999; **41**(5): 297–306.

104. Lachapelle M H, Miron P, Hemmings R *et al.* Endometrial T, B, and NK cells in patients with recurrent spontaneous abortion: altered profile and pregnancy outcome. *J Immunol* 1996; **156**(10): 4027–34.

105. Aplin J D, Lacey H, Haigh T *et al.* Growth factor-extracellular matrix synergy in the control of trophoblast invasion. *Biochem Soc Trans* 2000; **28**(2): 199–202.

106. Raghupathy R, Makhseed M, Azizieh F *et al.* Cytokine production by maternal lymphocytes during normal human pregnancy and in unexplained recurrent spontaneous abortion. *Hum Reprod* 2000; **15**(3): 713–8.

107. Reister F, Frank H G, Heyl W *et al.* The distribution of macrophages in spiral arteries of the placental bed in

pre-eclampsia differs from that in healthy patients. *Placenta* 1999; **20**(2–3): 229–33.

108. Yusuf, K, Kliman H J. The fetus, not the mother, elicits maternal immunologic rejection: lessons from discordant dizygotic twin placentas. *J Perinat Med* 2008; **36**(4): 291–6.

109. Boog G. Chronic villitis of unknown etiology. *Eur J Obstet Gynecol Reprod Biol* 2008; **136**(1): 9–15.

110. Merbl Y, Zucker-Toledano M, Quintana F J *et al.* Newborn humans manifest autoantibodies to defined self molecules detected by antigen microarray informatics. *J Clin Invest* 2007; **117**(3): 712–8.

111. Benirschke K, Kaufman P, Baergen R. *Pathology of the human placenta*, 5th ed. New York: Springer; 2006.

112. Yu C K, Khouri O, Onwudiwe N *et al.* Prediction of pre-eclampsia by uterine artery Doppler imaging: relationship to gestational age at delivery and small-for-gestational age. *Ultrasound Obstet Gynecol* 2008; **31**(3): 310–3.

113. ACOG Practice Bulletin. Diagnosis and management of preeclampsia and eclampsia. Number 33, January 2002. *Obstet Gynecol* 2002; **99**(1): 159–67.

114. Chauhan S P, Gupta L M, Hendrix N W *et al.* Intrauterine growth restriction: comparison of American College of Obstetricians and Gynecologists practice bulletin with other national guidelines. *Am J Obstet Gynecol* 2009; **200**: e401–6.

115. Madazli R, Somunkiran A, Calay Z *et al.* Histomorphology of the placenta and the placental bed of growth restricted foetuses and correlation with the Doppler velocimetries of the uterine and umbilical arteries. *Placenta* 2003; **24**(5): 510– 6.

116. Aardema M W, Oosterhof H, Timmer A *et al.* Uterine artery Doppler flow and uteroplacental vascular pathology in normal pregnancies and pregnancies complicated by pre-eclampsia and small for gestational age fetuses. *Placenta* 2001; **22**(5): 405–11.

117. Guibourdenche J, Frendo J L, Pidoux G *et al.* Expression of pregnancy-associated plasma protein-A (PAPP-A) during human villous trophoblast differentiation in vitro. *Placenta* 2003; **24**(5): 532–9.

118. Nicolaides K H, Spencer K, Avgidou K *et al.* Multicenter study of first-trimester screening for trisomy 21 in 75 821 pregnancies: results and estimation of the potential impact of individual risk-orientated two-stage first-trimester screening. *Ultrasound Obstet Gynecol* 2005; **25**(3): 221–6.

119. Kagan K O, Wright D, Baker A *et al.* Screening for trisomy 21 by maternal age, fetal nuchal translucency thickness, free beta-human chorionic gonadotropin and pregnancy-associated plasma protein-A. *Ultrasound Obstet Gynecol* 2008; **31**(6): 618–24.

120. Smith G C, Stenhouse E J, Crossley J A *et al.* Early pregnancy levels of pregnancy-associated plasma protein a and the risk of intrauterine growth restriction, premature birth, preeclampsia, and stillbirth. *J Clin Endocrinol Metab* 2002; **87**(4): 1762–7.

121. Smith G C, Crossley J A, Aitken D A *et al.* First-trimester placentation and the risk of antepartum stillbirth. *JAMA* 2004; **292**(18): 2249–54.

122. Proctor L, Toil M, Keating S *et al.* Placental function testing predicts adverse perinatal outcomes in women with low PAPP-A at 11–13 weeks. *Am J Obstet Gynecol* 2008; **199**(6, Supplement 1): S125.

123. Howley H E, Walker M, Rodger M A. A systematic review of the association between factor V Leiden or prothrombin gene variant and intrauterine growth restriction. *Am J Obstet Gynecol* 2005; **192**(3): 694–708.

124. Rodger M A, Paidas M. Do thrombophilias cause placenta-mediated pregnancy complications? *Semin Thromb Hemost* 2007; **33**(6): 597–603.

125. Fan Z, Larson P J, Bognacki J *et al.* Tissue factor regulates plasminogen binding and activation. *Blood* 1998; **91**(6): 1987–98.

126. Rey E, Garneau P, David M *et al.* Dalteparin for the prevention of recurrence of placental-mediated complications of pregnancy in women without thrombophilia: a pilot randomized controlled trial. *J Thromb Haemost* 2009; **7**(1): 58–64.

127. Gagnon A, Wilson R D, Audibert F *et al.* Obstetrical complications associated with abnormal maternal serum markers analytes. *J Obstet Gynaecol Can* 2008; **30**(10): 918–49.

128. Dugoff L, Hobbins J C, Malone F D *et al.* Quad screen as a predictor of adverse pregnancy outcome. *Obstet Gynecol* 2005; **106**(2): 260–7.

129. Macara L, Kingdom J C, Kaufmann P *et al.* Structural analysis of placental terminal villi from growth-restricted pregnancies with abnormal umbilical artery Doppler waveforms. *Placenta* 1996; **17**(1): 37–48.

130. Diab A E, El-Behery M M, Ebrahiem M A *et al.* Angiogenic factors for the prediction of pre-eclampsia in women with abnormal midtrimester uterine artery Doppler velocimetry. *Int J Gynaecol Obstet* 2008; **102**(2): 146–51.

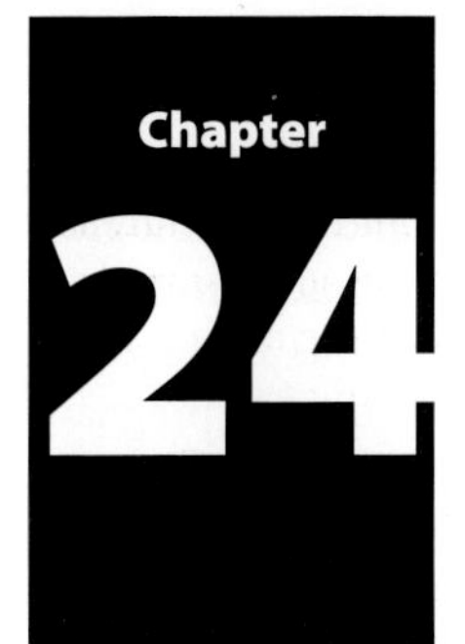

Placental bed disorders in the genesis of the great obstetrical syndromes

Roberto Romero[1,2], Juan Pedro Kusanovic[1,3], and Chong Jai Kim[1,4]

[1]Perinatology Research Branch, NICHD/NIH/DHHS, Bethesda, Maryland and Detroit, Michigan, USA
[2]Center for Molecular Medicine and Genetics, Wayne State University, Detroit, Michigan, USA
[3]Department of Obstetrics and Gynecology, Wayne State University/Hutzel Hospital, Detroit, Michigan, USA
[4]Department of Pathology, Wayne State University School of Medicine, Detroit, Michigan, USA

Recognition of the placental bed as a key interface in normal and abnormal human gestation

The recognition of the placental bed as a distinct anatomical site for the physiology and pathology of pregnancy began in 1958 after the pioneering studies of Dixon and Robertson [1] and the seminal contributions of Brosens [2] in 1964. The term 'placental bed' was purposely chosen to emphasize that the area of study was not the decidua basalis attached to the floor of the placenta, but rather the uterine tissues (endometrium and myometrium) underneath the placenta. This was important because the myometrium contains the origins of the spiral arteries. The investigators believed that these vessels were the target of lesions in preeclampsia on the basis that decreased utero-placental blood flow had been reported using a number of experimental techniques [3,4,5] coupled with the belief that the increased frequency of infarcts in the placenta of women with preeclampsia was due to interference with the maternal blood supply.

However, instead of finding the lesions associated with hypertension in target organs, Brosens discovered the lack of physiological transformation of the spiral arteries in the myometrium of women with preeclampsia [6,7,8]. These lesions were also found in pregnancies with intrauterine growth restriction [9] and subsequently, in patients with spontaneous abortion [10,11], placental abruption, [12], antiphospholipid syndrome [13], preterm labor with intact membranes leading to preterm delivery [14], and preterm premature rupture of membranes [15]. Therefore, research in the last 50 years has demonstrated that failure of physiological transformation of the myometrial segment of the spiral arteries can be present in a broad range of clinical disorders, and that it is not exclusive to preeclampsia or intrauterine growth restriction. These observations expand the importance of this developmental disorder in the pathology of abnormal pregnancies (for more details, the reader is referred to Chapters 1, 2, 3, and 11).

This chapter will review the evidence that failure of physiological transformation of the spiral arteries is observed in preterm labor, preterm premature rupture of membranes (PROM), and abruptio placentae. We will argue that this mechanism of disease is shared by many of the great obstetrical syndromes [16], and that the extent of the developmental failure and other features will determine the clinical phenotype.

Failure of physiological transformation in spontaneous abortion, fetal death, abruptio placentae, preterm labor, and preterm PROM

Spontaneous abortion

Spontaneous abortions in first trimester

The first study to examine the morphology of the placental bed in idiopathic, sporadic, and recurrent spontaneous abortion was reported by Khong *et al.* [10]. Twelve patients had spontaneous abortions. Four women composed the control group; three had elective terminations of pregnancy, and one had a late spontaneous abortion with a live fetus, due to cervical insufficiency. All patients in the control group had physiological transformation of the spiral arteries. In contrast, failure of physiological transformation of the decidual segments was seen in seven cases of spontaneous abortion. Only four of the twelve cases had myometrial segments of the spiral artery, and none had evidence of physiological transformation. It is important to note that this series included patients in the first trimester and midtrimester. Karyotyping of the products of conception was performed in six of the spontaneous abortions, and there was no relationship between the karyotype and the histology of the placental bed.

Michel *et al.* [11] examined placental bed biopsies from women with spontaneous abortions diagnosed with ultrasound (n = 6), those with a history of recurrent spontaneous abortion (n = 10), and patients undergoing elective terminations of pregnancy in the first trimester (n = 12). Physiological transformation was observed in 11 of the 12 patients who had an elective termination of pregnancy. These changes were demonstrated in the decidual segments of the spiral arteries. In contrast, five out of six women who had a spontaneous abortion (diagnosed as the presence of a gestational sac and the absence of fetal heart activity on two occasions) had inadequate development of most spiral arteries in the decidual bed with preservation of the musculoelastic tissue, and no evidence of invasion by extravillous trophoblasts of the decidual segment of the spiral artery. Finally, in the group of patients with recurrent spontaneous abortions (n = 10), four women had normal placental bed histology, and two others had findings which were nearly consistent with normal transformation, except for one area of abnormal vessels.

In the pathology specimens examined by Professor Khong, were assessed the number of cells with large granules (CLG). These cells probably correspond to large granular lymphocytes, which are now known to correspond to uterine natural killer (uNK) cells. The proportion of these cells was significantly higher in women undergoing elective terminations of pregnancy, rather than in those who had spontaneous abortions (either sporadic or recurrent).

Hustin *et al.* [17] evaluated the maternal–fetal interface in 184 specimens of complete spontaneous abortion (in which the gestational sac was expelled 'en bloc') as well as in a control group of 219 patients who underwent voluntary termination of pregnancy in the first trimester by uterine aspiration. There were three hysterectomy specimens with pregnancies *in situ* (before 10 weeks of gestation). The authors reported limited trophoblastic infiltration and physiological changes in 64% of those with embryonic demise and 77% of abnormal conceptuses, while this finding was observed in none of the patients with normal pregnancies. The authors concluded that most cases of spontaneous abortion are associated with defective trophoblast invasion into the decidua and spiral arteries (physiological changes were therefore limited or absent). Hustin *et al.* interpreted these findings as suggesting that untimely initiation of blood flow in the intervillous space may be associated with pregnancy failure and complete abortion, and noted that maternal blood could be observed with a higher frequency in the intervillous space in pathological cases than in normal pregnancy. This study is unique because it was based on the examination of the complete aborted material, rather than a biopsy of the placental bed [17].

In 2006, Gun *et al.* [18] reported a study in which the histology of the decidua was compared in women (n = 25) with spontaneous abortion (5–12 weeks) and the decidua of 40 women undergoing elective terminations of pregnancy (between 5 and 11 weeks). The authors found that transformation of the spiral arteries occurred in 90% of elective abortions, whereas lack of physiological transformation in the decidual segments was present in 48% of patients who had a spontaneous abortion ($p < 0.001$).

Ball *et al.* [19] have recently reported a large study in which placental bed biopsies obtained under ultrasound visualization were collected from 50 women who had a spontaneous abortion, and 78 women who underwent elective terminations of pregnancy. This study included only pregnancies dated with ultrasound who had spontaneous abortions at 12 weeks or less, and in which a karyotype was performed. Frozen sections were immunostained for cytokeratin, desmin, and von Willebrand factor (to detect trophoblasts, vascular and myometrial smooth muscle, and endothelium, respectively). Inclusion in the study required the presence of at least one spiral artery. In contrast to the previous studies reported above, trophoblast invasion of the decidua and spiral artery transformation did not differ between spontaneous abortion and elective terminations of pregnancy. Similarly, there were no differences in the histological features between patients with euploid and aneuploid conceptuses. This study did not include the trophoblastic shell or the very superficial placental bed, and therefore, no assessment of trophoblast shell thickness or plugging of the spiral arteries was possible.

The discrepancy among studies could be attributed to the nature of the specimens collected and the requirement for the presence of an embryo and gestational age. It seems that further investigation is required to elucidate the role of trophoblast plugging of the spiral arteries and physiological transformation of the decidual and myometrial segments in early spontaneous abortions. Since myometrial invasion of the spiral arteries does not occur until after 14 weeks of gestation, one may not expect that failure of transformation of this particular segment may be associated with spontaneous abortion. We also believe that systematic studies of the cell populations in the decidua are warranted. These efforts have been undertaken by some investigators, and the difficulties in interpreting whether the changes reported represent a causal shift in specific populations or an epiphenomenon resulting from pregnancy failure are acknowledged.

Spontaneous abortions in the second trimester

In addition to the study of Khong *et al.* [10] (described in the previous section) which supports a relationship between failure of physiological transformation of the spiral arteries and spontaneous abortion in the midtrimester, there is a recent study that provides support for this. Ball *et al.* [20] reported a study that included a large number of late sporadic miscarriages (n = 26; gestational age between 13 and 23.9 weeks) which underwent karyotyping, and gestational age matched ultrasound dated normal pregnancies undergoing elective termination. Frozen sections were subjected to the same treatment (reported in the previous paragraph) in early spontaneous abortions. Notably, a large number of spiral arteries were studied: 96 in cases of late spontaneous abortions, and 236 in the control group. Myometrial spiral arteries showed reduced endovascular (4% vs. 31%, p = 0.001), intramural trophoblasts (76% vs. 88%, p = 0.05), and less extensive fibrinoid change (4% vs. 18%, p = 0.01). In contrast, endovascular trophoblast in the decidual spiral arteries was higher in patients who had a spontaneous abortion than in the control group (66% vs. 40%, p = 0.04).

Collectively, the observations reported by Ball *et al.* [20] support the concept that failure of physiological transformation of the spiral arteries is a process with a broad spectrum of clinical presentation. The most severe forms would result in fetal death and would be clinically manifested as a midtrimester spontaneous abortion. Less severe defects would allow continuation of pregnancy and the development of other obstetrical syndromes such as intrauterine growth restriction, preeclampsia, preterm labor, and preterm PROM.

Preterm birth

Preterm birth is defined as delivery occurring before 37 weeks of gestation, and is the leading cause of perinatal morbidity and mortality worldwide [21]. Spontaneous preterm labor (with intact membranes or following preterm PROM) accounts for two-thirds of preterm births. The remaining third is due to maternal or fetal indications such as preeclampsia or intrauterine growth restriction.

Spontaneous preterm parturition is considered a syndrome [22] (whether it occurs with intact or ruptured membranes). The spectrum of the phenotype may range from cervical insufficiency, preterm labor with intact membranes, or preterm PROM. The causes of spontaneous preterm parturition have been proposed to include infection/inflammation [23,24,25,26,27,28,29,30,31,32,33,34,35], ischemia due to vascular disease [36,37], cervical disease [38,39,40], uterine overdistension [41], abnormal allograft reaction [42], allergy [43,44,45], and endocrine disorders [46,47,48,49]. Growing evidence suggests that vascular disorders may play a role in a subset of patients who have preterm labor with intact membranes or preterm PROM.

Spontaneous preterm labor leading to preterm delivery

Infection and inflammation are the most common lesions found in the placentae of patients with spontaneous preterm parturition, while vascular lesions are the second most common [36,37]. Vascular lesions in decidual vessels attached to the placenta have been reported by Arias *et al.* [36] in 34.1% of women with spontaneous preterm labor and intact membranes, while only in 11.8% of control women (term gestation without complications, p = 0.001). Vascular lesions in the decidual vessels of the placenta were more frequent in patients with preterm labor with intact membranes (odds ratio 3.8, 95% CI 1.3–11.1, p = 0.007). Moreover, abruptio placentae was more frequent in patients with preterm labor than in controls (9.5% vs. 0%, respectively; p = 0.001). Similarly, Germain *et al.* [50] reported a frequency of 25.4% of ischemic lesions in placentae from patients with preterm labor who delivered preterm, which is

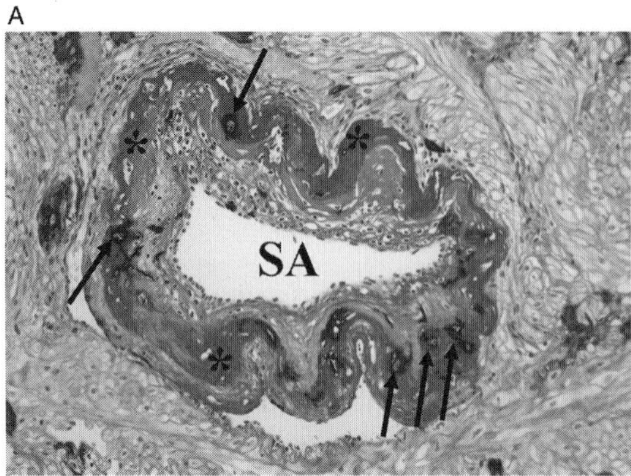

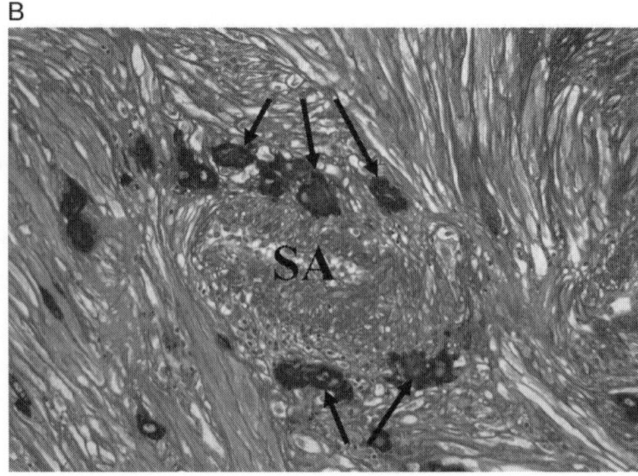

Fig. 24.1 (A) Physiological transformation of myometrial spiral artery in a placental bed biopsy specimen from a normal pregnant woman at 40 weeks of gestation (cytokeratin 7/PAS, × 200). The lumen of the spiral arteries (SA) is dilated. The fibrinoid material, which replaces the media of the 'physiologically transformed spiral arteries', is purple in color (PAS positive) and labeled with an asterisk (*). Trophoblastic cells, which are cytokeratin positive (brown and labeled with arrows), are infiltrating the wall of the spiral artery. (B) Failure of physiological transformation of myometrial spiral arteries in a placental bed biopsy specimen from a patient with preterm labor (without a small-for-gestational age fetus) at 31 weeks of gestation (cytokeratin 7/PAS, × 200). The lumen of the artery (SA) is not dilated. The medial layers of the spiral artery are intact. Fibrinoid material (PAS positive) is not present. Although plenty of interstitial trophoblasts surround the spiral arteries, which are cytokeratin positive (brown and labeled with arrows), trophoblasts have not invaded the vessel wall. See plate section for color version.

significantly higher than that of women with preterm labor who delivered at term (3.7%) and controls (0%, $p < 0.05$ for both comparisons).

The only systematic study of the placental bed of patients presenting with preterm labor who had a preterm delivery was reported by Kim *et al.* [14]. In this study, placental bed biopsies were obtained at the time of cesarean section under direct visualization. Specimens were immunostained for cytokeratin and counterstained with periodic acid Schiff (PAS) to detect trophoblasts and fibrinoid. The frequency of non-transformed spiral arteries was assessed in three groups of patients: (1) patients who had a cesarean section at term; (2) patients who had a spontaneous preterm labor/delivery with a cesarean section for obstetrical indications; and (3) patients with preeclampsia. The latter group was included as a positive control since patients with preeclampsia delivered at a median gestational age of 31 weeks.

The rate of failure of physiological transformation of the myometrial segment of the spiral arteries was significantly greater in patients with spontaneous preterm labor/delivery than in those who had a term delivery (30.9% vs. 13.6%, $p = 0.004$). The same was the case for the decidual segment in the basal plate of the placenta as well as in the placental bed. Figure 24.1 illustrates a typical lesion in a patient with preterm labor/delivery with failure of physiological transformation of the myometrial segment. Figure 24.2 describes the mean percentage of non-transformed spiral arteries in three different locations (myometrium, decidual segment of the placental bed, and decidua in the basal plate).

These observations indicate that patients with preterm labor and intact membranes who deliver a preterm neonate have a greater degree of failure of transformation of the spiral arteries in the myometrial and decidual segments than women who deliver at term. However, the extent of this defect was much greater in patients with preeclampsia than those in preterm labor with intact membranes. Of interest is that we could not document a difference in the frequency of lack of physiological transformation between patients with and without histological chorioamnionitis. The reasons why some women with failure of physiological transformation develop preterm labor, or other obstetrical syndromes, are presently unknown. Our view will be expressed at the end of this chapter. However, it is possible that the more extensive degree of vascular pathology in preeclampsia than in preterm labor may, in part, be responsible for the phenotype.

Preterm premature rupture of membranes

Preterm PROM accounts for one-third of all preterm births, and is often a leading cause of spontaneous preterm labor. Vascular lesions of the placental bed

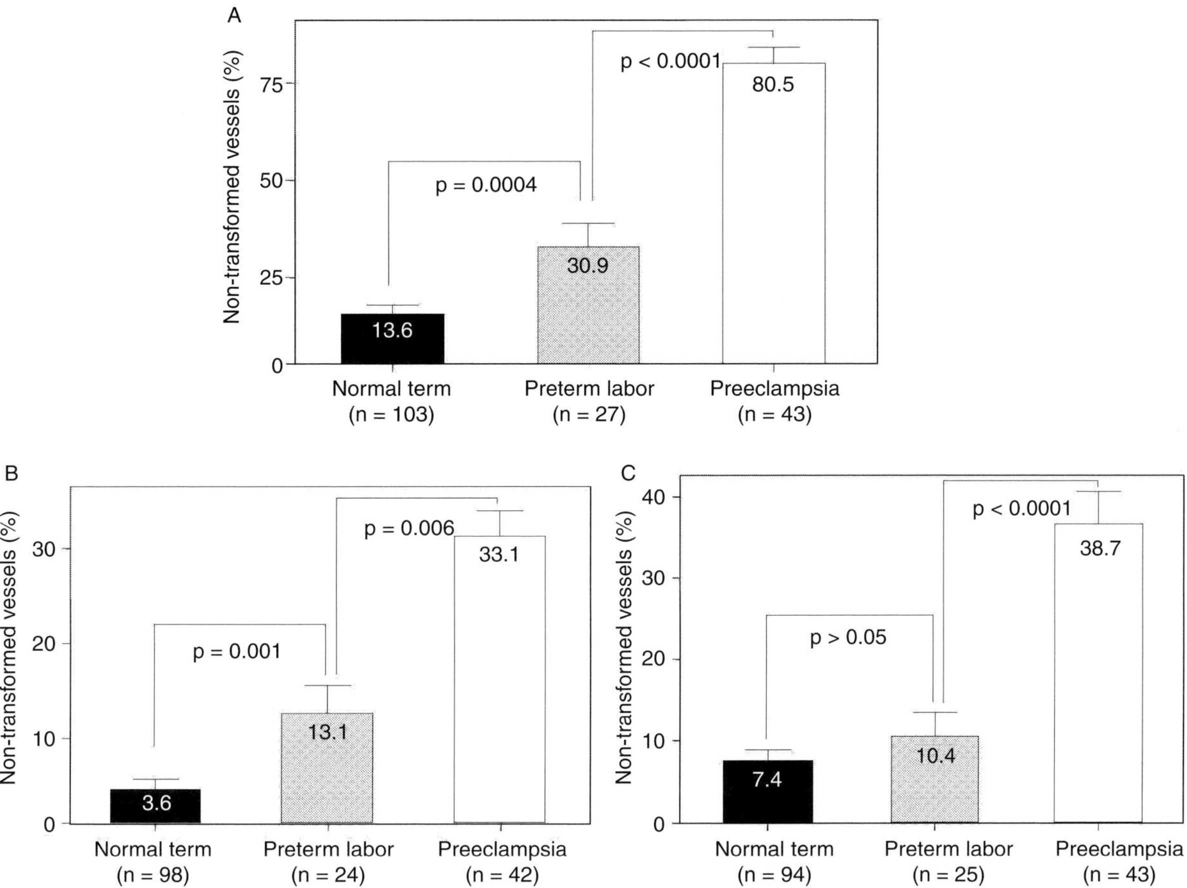

Fig. 24.2 Mean percentage of non-transformed spiral arteries weighted by the number of vessels. (A) The mean percentage of the spiral arteries that had failure of physiological transformation in the *myometrial segment* was significantly higher in patients with preterm labor and those with preeclampsia than in normal pregnant women at term (preterm labor; mean ± SEM 30.9% ± 5.8% vs. normal pregnant women; mean ± SEM 13.6% ± 2.1%; p = 0.0004 and preeclampsia; mean ± SEM 80.5% ± 3.8% vs. normal pregnant women; mean ± SEM 13.6% ± 2.1%; p < 0.0001). (B) Patients with preterm labor and intact membranes, as well as patients with preeclampsia, had a significantly higher mean percentage of the spiral arteries that had failure of physiological transformation in the *decidual segment of the placental bed* than normal pregnant women (preterm labor; mean ± SEM 13.1% ± 4.4% vs. normal pregnant women; mean ± SEM 3.6% ± 1.2%; p = 0.001 and preeclampsia; mean ± SEM 33.1% ± 4.5% vs. normal pregnant women; mean ± SEM 3.6% ± 1.2%; p < 0.0001). (C) The mean percentage of the spiral arteries that had failure of physiological transformation in *the decidual segments of the basal plate* was not significantly different between patients with preterm labor and normal pregnant women at term (preterm labor; mean ± SEM 10.4% ± 3.0% vs. normal pregnant women; mean ± SEM 7.4% ± 1.3%; p > 0.05). Patients with preeclampsia had a significantly higher mean percentage of the spiral arteries that had failure of physiological transformation in *the decidual segments of the basal plate* than patients with preterm labor and normal pregnant women (preeclampsia; mean ± SEM 38.7% ± 4.0% vs. preterm labor; mean ± SEM 10.4% ± 3.0%; p < 0.0001 and preeclampsia; mean ± SEM 38.7% ± 4.0% vs. normal pregnant women; mean ± SEM 7.4% ± 1.3%; p < 0.0001). Comparisons were performed with ANOVA, followed by student's t tests; p values > 0.017 became non-significant after adjusting for multiple comparisons.

have been described in patients with preterm PROM, including failure of physiological transformation of the decidual segment of the spiral arteries, thrombosis, and atherosis.

Only one study has examined the histology of the placental bed in patients with preterm PROM. Kim *et al.* [15] reported a blinded cross-sectional study to determine the frequency of non-transformed spiral arteries in placental bed biopsies obtained under direct visualization at the time of cesarean section in three groups of patients: (1) patients with normal pregnancies who delivered at term; (2) patients with preterm PROM that underwent cesarean section for obstetrical indications; and (3) patients with pre-eclampsia. Specimens were stained with cytokeratin and PAS. The study showed that the frequency of failure of physiological transformation of the myometrial segment of the spiral arteries was higher in

Table 24.1. The number (per cent) of patients who had failure of physiological transformation of the spiral arteries in normal pregnant women at term and patients with preeclampsia and preterm PROM

	Normal pregnancy at term	Preeclampsia	p value	Preterm PROM	p^a value	p^b value
Myometrial segment of the spiral arteries						
Total no. of patients	59	23		31		
Completely transformed in all vessels	31 (52.5%)	1 (4.3%)		9 (29%)		
Partially transformed or mixed transformed and non-transformed vessels	24 (40.7%)	10 (43.5%)		16 (51.6%)		
Non-transformed in all vessels	4 (6.8%)	12 (52.2%)	< 0.0001*	6 (19.4%)	0.016*	0.003*
Decidual segment of the spiral arteries in the basal plate						
Total no. of patients	52	22		30		
Completely transformed in all vessels	44 (84.6%)	8 (36.4%)		25 (83.3%)		
Partially transformed or mixed transformed and non-transformed vessels	8 (15.4%)	13 (59.1%)		5 (16.7%)		
Non-transformed in all vessels	0	1 (4.5%)	< 0.0001*	0	NS	0.001*

The p values for pairwise comparisons between diagnostic groups derived from the comparisons of shift in proportions of patients in each classification using Spearman rank correlation.
p, comparison between preeclampsia and normal pregnancy at term.
p^a, comparison between preterm PROM and normal pregnancy at term.
p^b, comparison between preeclampsia and preterm PROM.
*$p < 0.05$.
PROM, prelabor rupture of membranes; NS, not significant.

patients with preterm PROM than in patients who had a spontaneous delivery at term (completely transformed spiral arteries were observed in 59% of patients who delivered at term, 29% of those with preterm PROM, and 4.3% of patients with preeclampsia; Table 24.1). The lack of transformation of all vessels in the biopsy specimen was observed in only 6.8% of term deliveries, 52% of patients with preeclampsia, and in 19.4% of patients with preterm PROM. Notably, there was no difference in the rate of failure of physiological transformation in the decidual or myometrial segments of the spiral arteries in patients with and without histological chorioamnionitis (Table 24.2).

Vascular lesions in decidual vessels attached to the placenta also have been found in patients with preterm PROM. Arias *et al.* [36] reported maternal vascular lesions in 35.1% of patients with preterm PROM compared to 11.8% in patients with normal pregnancies ($p = 0.001$). An interesting observation was that the gestational age at delivery was greater in patients who had vascular lesions of the placenta than in those who had acute histological chorioamnionitis (30.1 weeks vs. 32.3 weeks, $p = 0.005$). This observation is consistent with the results of microbiological studies as well as those examining the frequency of intra-amniotic inflammation as a function of gestational age [32]. The importance of this is that there appear to be two major clusters of patients who delivered preterm: (1) patients with acute inflammatory lesions (acute chorioamnionitis); and (2) those who delivered preterm (but at a later gestational age) in whom the predominant lesions are vascular.

The same group of investigators evaluated the placental histology in 235 consecutive patients admitted with preterm PROM [37] and found the

Table 24.2. Comparison of number (count) of failure of physiological transformation of the spiral arteries between patients with preterm PROM with and without histological chorioamnionitis

	Preterm PROM		p value
	Without histological chorioamnionitis	With histological chorioamnionitis	
Myometrial segment of the spiral arteries			
Total no. of patients	11	20	
Non-transformed vessels (mean ± SE)	0.91 ± 0.37	0.90 ± 0.28	NS
Completely or partially transformed vessels (mean ± SE)	1.91 ± 0.79	2.75 ± 0.63	NS
Decidual segment of the spiral arteries in the basal plate			
Total no. of patients	11	19	
Non-transformed vessels (mean ± SE)	0.09 ± 0.09	0.32 ± 0.22	NS
Completely or partially transformed vessels (mean ± SE)	3.18 ± 0.69	3.37 ± 0.45	NS

NS, not significant.

presence of maternal or fetal vascular lesions was 20.4% (48/235). Acute histological chorioamnionitis was found in 43.4% of the cases. Maternal, rather than fetal, vascular lesions accounted for the majority (41/48) of these. Interestingly, most of the vascular lesions (77.1%) occurred in patients with preterm PROM after 30 weeks of gestation. It should be noted that the clusters were not pure, and there were some patients who had a mixed histological picture: acute chorioamnionitis as well as vascular lesions.

How can vascular lesions be linked to spontaneous onset of labor with intact or ruptured membranes?

Maternal vascular lesions could lead to preterm labor by causing uteroplacental ischemia. Compelling evidence supports a role for uteroplacental ischemia as a mechanism of disease leading to preterm labor: (1) experimental studies designed to generate a primate model for preeclampsia by causing uterine ischemia showed that a proportion of animals had spontaneous preterm labor and preterm birth [51]; (2) abruptio placentae, a lesion of vascular origin, is more frequent in women who deliver preterm with intact membranes [36,52] or rupture of membranes than in those who deliver at term [53,54,55]; (3) women presenting with preterm labor and intact membranes who have an abnormal uterine artery Doppler velocimetry are more likely to deliver preterm than those with normal Doppler velocimetry [56,57]. These results are similar to those reported by other investigators studying women before the onset of labor [58]; and (4) the frequency of small-for-gestational age infants is increased in women who delivered after preterm labor with intact membranes and preterm PROM [59,60,61,62,63,64,65]. Vascular lesions leading to compromise of the uterine supply line could account for both intrauterine growth restriction and preterm labor.

The precise mechanisms responsible for the onset of preterm parturition in women with uteroplacental ischemia have not been determined. A role for the renin–angiotensin system has been postulated as the fetal membranes are endowed with a functional renin–angiotensin system, [66] and uterine ischemia increases the production of uterine renin [67,68]. Angiotensin II can induce myometrial contractility directly [69] or through the release of prostaglandins [70]. When uteroplacental ischemia is severe enough to lead to decidual necrosis and hemorrhage, thrombin may activate the common pathway of parturition.

Evidence in support of this includes: (1) decidua is a rich source of tissue factor, the primary initiator of coagulation [71]; (2) intrauterine administration of whole blood to pregnant rats stimulates myometrial contractility [72], while heparinized blood does not (heparin blocks the generation of thrombin) [72]; (3) fresh whole blood stimulates myometrial contractility *in vitro*, and this effect is partially blunted by incubation with hirudin, a thrombin inhibitor [72]; (4) thrombin stimulates myometrial contractility in a dose-dependent manner [72]; (5) thrombin stimulates the production of matrix metalloproteinase-1 (MMP-1) [73], urokinase-type plasminogen activator (uPA), and tissue-type plasminogen activator (tPA) by endometrial stromal cells in culture [74]; matrix metalloproteinase-1 can digest collagen directly, while uPA and tPA catalyze the transformation of plasminogen into plasmin which, in turn, can degrade type III collagen and fibronectin [75], important components of the extracellular matrix in the chorioamniotic membranes [76]; (6) thrombin/antithrombin (TAT) complexes, markers of *in vivo* generation of thrombin, are increased in the plasma [77] and amniotic fluid [78] of women in preterm labor and with preterm PROM; (7) an elevation of plasma TAT complex concentration in the second trimester is associated with subsequent preterm PROM [79]; (8) the presence of retroplacental hematoma detected by ultrasound examination in the first trimester is associated with adverse pregnancy outcomes, including preterm birth and fetal growth restriction [80]; and (9) the presence of vaginal bleeding in the first or second trimester is associated with preterm birth and other adverse perinatal outcomes [81,82,83,84].

Placental abruption

Placental abruption occurs in 6.2/1000 pregnancies [85] and subclinical cases are more frequent than overt abruptio placentae, which is characterized by vaginal bleeding, abdominal pain, increased uterine contractility, increased uterine tone, and in extreme cases, fetal death and disseminated intravascular coagulation. It has been estimated that the histological diagnosis of placental abruption is ten times more frequent than the clinical diagnosis of this condition [86].

The initial event has been proposed to be an ischemic lesion of the decidua, leading to decidual necrosis, vascular disruption, and bleeding. As hemorrhage occurs, laceration and dissection along a decidual plane and placental separation takes place. The latter produces more vascular rhexis, arterial hemorrhage, and retroplacental accumulation of blood; this, in turn, furthers placental separation.

Dommisse and Tiltman [12] reported a study in which placental bed biopsies were obtained at the time of cesarean section in 18 women with the clinical diagnosis of placental abruption. Six biopsies did not include trophoblasts in the myometrium, and therefore were not considered to be representative of the placental bed. In this study, at least one spiral artery was seen in myometrium in each biopsy. Seven of the 12 specimens demonstrated an absence of physiological transformation of the spiral arteries. Hemorrhage was present in 83% (10/12) of these samples. Intimal or subintimal thickening was observed in five cases, and it was observed in non-transformed vessels. The authors indicated that the morphological changes were similar to those described by Brosens [6], who suggested that they may be the result of previous thrombosis. It is important to note that five of the patients included in this study had hypertension, and that four of them had an absence of physiological transformation.

Primary antiphospholipid syndrome

Primary antiphospholipid syndrome during pregnancy is associated with a higher rate of spontaneous abortion, intrauterine growth restriction, preeclampsia, preterm birth, and fetal death [87,88]. Studies of the placenta have demonstrated an excess of lesions associated with underperfusion; in particular, placental infarction, thrombosis, fibrinoid necrosis, and atherosis [89,90,91] as well as defective physiological transformation of the spiral arteries [90].

A study conducted by Stone *et al.* [13] systematically examined the characteristics of the placental bed in 12 patients with primary antiphospholipid syndrome and 16 controls. Placental bed biopsies were obtained from cases and controls at the time of cesarean section. The sections were stained with a panel of antibodies including vascular cell adhesion molecule-1 (VCAM-1) as a marker of endothelial cell activation, and also antibodies to CD68 for detection of macrophages. In addition, trophoblast was identified using cytokeratin, human alpha smooth muscle actin to identify smooth muscle, and PAS to detect fibrinoid. Orcein was used to detect the presence of elastin. The presence of extravillous trophoblasts was considered indicative that the sample was obtained from the placental bed, and decidua and myometrium were assessed individually for interstitial trophoblast distribution. Spiral arteries were assessed to determine the extent of vascular remodeling, which was described as the percentage of the muscular, elastic, and fibrinoid components in the vessel wall. Biopsies from seven of eleven women with antiphospholipid syndrome were confirmed to be from the placental bed because of the presence of extravillous trophoblasts, and one or more spiral arteries were present in six. Eleven of 16 biopsies from control patients were from the placental bed. Placental bed biopsies of patients with antiphospholipid antibodies had a higher density of inflammatory cells ($p = 0.0001$), and particularly macrophages ($p = 0.014$), than those of the control group. These inflammatory cells clustered around the blood vessels; however, there was no difference in the frequency of remodeled spiral arteries between cases and controls. Atherosis was not observed in any case. In three cases, the placental bed biopsies showed necrosis and hyperplastic vessels and one case had arterial thromboses.

This study is important because decidual vasculopathy of the basal plate of the placenta was described in cases with antiphospholipid antibodies and poor pregnancy outcome [89,90]. However, the decidual segments may not be representative of the events occurring in the myometrial segment of the spiral arteries. Perhaps the most striking observations in this study were the absence of impaired trophoblast invasion in women with antiphospholipid syndrome, the absence of endothelial cell activation (as determined by staining with VCAM-1), and the presence of an inflammatory reaction in the perivascular area. It should be noted that women with antiphospholipid syndrome were treated with 75 mg of aspirin from the preconception period and low-molecular-weight heparin after a positive pregnancy test if there was a history of thrombosis, previous late fetal loss, or recurrent miscarriages. An effect of these therapies on the placental bed findings cannot be excluded.

Recent observations in an animal model of antiphospholipid syndrome by Girardi *et al.* [92] have demonstrated C5a receptors and neutrophils as causal factors in the generation of the prothrombotic phenotype in this mouse model. In a second study, Girardi *et al.* reported that heparin prevented antiphospholipid antibody-induced fetal loss by inhibiting complement activation [93]. These two seminal studies suggest that inflammation plays a role in fetal death in this condition, and that heparin is acting not only by inhibiting thrombin, but also interfering with the local inflammatory process.

Sebire *et al.* [94] examined the products of conception obtained at 6–14 weeks of gestation from patients with a history of recurrent pregnancy loss classified by the following groups: (1) fetal chromosomal abnormality ($n = 34$); (2) primary antiphospholipid syndrome and normal karyotype ($n = 31$); and (3) normal karyotype without primary antiphospholipid syndrome ($n = 50$). Patients without a history of recurrent pregnancy loss and who underwent voluntary termination of pregnancy were included as controls ($n = 20$). Among patients with a normal karyotype, normal endovascular trophoblast invasion was identified only in 23% of patients with primary antiphospholipid syndrome, compared to 61% ($p = 0.02$) of those with a history of recurrent pregnancy loss but without primary antiphospholipid syndrome, and to 75% ($p < 0.01$) of those with a voluntary termination of pregnancy. The authors suggest that defective early trophoblast invasion, rather than placental thrombosis, may be the main cause of pregnancy failure in this condition [94]. It is important to realize that the observations derived from this study depend upon the examination of the products of conception rather than placental bed biopsies. It may be argued that this mode of sampling does not yield equivalent tissue to that obtained from a placental bed biopsy. Moreover, this study reports on the events in the first trimester of pregnancy rather than those observed at the end of pregnancy.

Vascular pathology as a mechanism of disease in obstetrics

Pregnancy requires vasculogenesis and angiogenesis in the fetal compartment and angiogenesis in the maternal compartment (for details, see Chapter 7). A monoallelic deletion of one of the many angiogenic factors, vascular endothelial growth factor (VEGF), causes embryo lethality due to the inability to form a vascular tree [95]. Similarly, deletion of several genes is incompatible with the development of a placenta. The maternal circulation must also undergo dramatic changes for a successful pregnancy. They include the development of the uteroplacental arteries from the spiral arteries to increase blood flow to the intervillous space. Although vasodilatation of the spiral arteries can occur before physiological transformation is completed, most investigators agree that remodeling and transformation of the spiral arteries is required to ensure adequate delivery of nutrients and oxygen to maintain pregnancy to term.

A unique feature of the biology of pregnancy (in contrast to that of other states such as angioinvasion in cancer) is that extravillous trophoblast invades the decidua and myometrium. This represents invasion of semi non-self cells into 'self' tissue. A counterpart of this phenomenon seems to be the microchimerism reported after successful transplantation of solid organs. Yet, extravillous invading trophoblast seems to play an important role in remodeling the maternal circulation, and probably in orchestrating the immunological dialogue that must occur in the maternal–fetal interface (for details, see Chapter 6). These processes are believed to be important, if not essential, to meet the requirements of the conceptus.

Inadequate angiogenesis, thrombosis, and/or inadequate physiological transformation of the spiral arteries can lead to ischemia of the placenta and the uterus. A catalogue of lesions in the human placenta has been considered the result of maternal underperfusion of the placenta. The focus of this book has not been the placenta, but rather the placental bed. This includes not only the uteroplacental or spiral arteries, but also the complex cellular and molecular network that operates in the decidua and myometrium to allow normal placentation.

What are the consequences of uteroplacental ischemia? Experimental evidence indicates that decreased blood supply can lead to fetal death, fetal growth restriction, maternal hypertension, and preterm labor. The specific clinical phenotype in response to ischemia is probably a function of the severity, timing, and duration of the ischemic insult. It is easy to understand that total occlusion of the uterine arteries will lead to sudden fetal death; this can be easily demonstrated in animal models. It could be argued that the closest human counterpart to this phenomenon can be a massive maternal floor infarction, in which extensive fibrin deposits in the intervillous space make impossible the exchange of gases and nutrients required for fetal survival. If the degree of ischemia is less severe, a different phenotype will result. Surgical removal of the caruncle in sheep is a well-established model for fetal growth restriction [96,97,98]. An inadequate supply of nutrients can be expected to decrease the rate of fetal growth. Deceleration of fetal growth can be considered to be adaptive if survival is the ultimate goal. In cases of a compromised supply line, fetal growth at a normal rate could lead to fetal death. The parallels between this and the necrosis observed in ischemic regions of tumors provide an understandable scenario of the consequences of mismatched growth (a mismatch between the availability of nutrients and the requirement of the growing fetus). If a reasonable compromise is reached between underperfusion and reduction of fetal growth, then the birth of a small-for-gestational age infant would be the expected result. On the other hand, if pregnancy continues and the delivery of nutrients is insufficient, nature has another mechanism to support the fetus: the induction of maternal hypertension to maintain or increase uterine blood flow. The phenotype would be gestational hypertension, and when this homeostatic response is driven to the pathological range, preeclampsia with maternal multiorgan damage. Thus, this adaptive mechanism is employed to support the fetus, but it occurs by placing the mother at risk. This situation is more likely to occur in preterm rather than in term gestations. When a fetus has undergone chronic underperfusion, reduction in fetal growth often results in accelerated maturation of multiple organ systems. Thus, when the fetus is close to maturity, the onset of preterm parturition (with intact or ruptured membranes) would solve the conundrum of both hosts. We propose that the different phenotypes are the result of adaptive mechanisms that, in general, have survival value. In early pregnancy, a severe antiangiogenic state is likely to lead to fetal death. Why continue to invest maternal resources when there is not enough of an angiogenic drive to maintain the placenta and fetus? In milder cases of uteroplacental ischemia, SGA, SGA plus hypertension, or late preterm labor could provide a solution.

The nature of obstetrical disease: The Great Obstetrical Syndromes

The current taxonomy of disease in obstetrics is based on the clinical presentation of the mother and/or fetus, and not on the mechanism of disease responsible for the clinical manifestations. For example, the term 'preterm labor' does not indicate whether this condition is caused by an infection, a vascular insult, uterine overdistension, abnormal allogeneic recognition, stress, or other pathological processes. The same applies to preeclampsia, small for gestational age, preterm PROM, fetal death, placental abruption, nausea and vomiting during pregnancy, miscarriage, and failure to progress in labor, in which the diagnoses simply describe the clinical manifestations without consideration of the specific etiology.

The established paradigm that pregnancy complications simply represent a collection of signs and symptoms with little reference to the underlying mechanisms of disease may be responsible for the expectation that one diagnostic test and treatment will detect and cure each of these conditions. The possibility that mechanisms of disease not yet discovered may be responsible for pregnancy complications must be considered given the unique biology of pregnancy which requires the pacific coexistence of two hosts. Therefore, the challenges presented by this intimate relationship could create conditions in which novel mechanisms of disease may emerge. The placental bed is strategically placed anatomically and functionally to be a site for the development of pathological processes. Although much of this book has focused on the important contribution of physiological transformation of the spiral arteries and lack thereof, chapters have been included about the immune cells in the placental bed (for details, see Chapter 6). It is likely that with the application of modern molecular pathology techniques and a deeper understanding of the immunobiology of the maternal–fetal interface, disorders in the stroma of the placental bed will be discovered.

We have proposed that the term 'syndrome' is more appropriate to refer to the previously mentioned obstetrical disorders. Syndrome is defined as 'a combination of symptoms and/or signs that form a distinct clinical picture indicative of a particular disorder'. The implicit meaning in this definition is that a syndrome can be caused by more than one mechanism of disease or etiology. We have argued that obstetrical disorders responsible for maternal death and perinatal morbidity and mortality are syndromes; hence, the designation of the 'Great Obstetrical Syndromes' [16]. Key features of these syndromes are: (1) multiple etiologies; (2) long preclinical stage; (3) frequent fetal involvement; (4) predisposition to a particular syndrome influenced by gene–environment interaction and/or complex gene–gene interactions involving maternal and/or fetal genotypes; and (5) clinical manifestations, which are often adaptive in nature [16].

A good example can be made with the preterm parturition syndrome: (1) '*Multiple etiologies*' have been implicated in the pathophysiology of this syndrome, such as intrauterine infection/inflammation [23,24,25,26,27,28,29,30,31,32,33,34,35], uterine ischemia [36,37], uterine overdistension [41], cervical disease [38,39,40], endocrine disorders [46,47,48,49], abnormal allogeneic recognition [42], and allergy-like reaction [43,44,45]. (2) Patients with a short cervix in the midtrimester of pregnancy or with increased concentrations of fetal fibronectin in the vaginal fluid are at increased risk for preterm labor or preterm delivery [39,99,100,101,102,103,104,105,106,107,108], suggesting that the pathological condition leading to these disorders is '*chronic*' in nature. For example, microbial invasion of the amniotic cavity can be detected at the time of routine midtrimester amniocentesis for genetic indications and become clinically evident weeks later with either spontaneous preterm labor or preterm PROM [109,110,111,112,113]. (3) '*Fetal involvement*' has been demonstrated in patients with microbial invasion of the amniotic cavity. Indeed, fetal bacteremia has been reported in 30% of cases of preterm PROM with a positive amniotic fluid for microorganisms [114]. Similarly, neonates born after spontaneous preterm labor or preterm PROM are more likely to be small-for-gestational age, suggesting a preexisting problem with the supply line [59,60,61,62,63,64,65]. (4) The inclination to use a mechanism of host defense may be determined by '*gene–environmental interaction*' as in other complex disorders, such as atherosclerosis, diabetes, etc. However, complexity is added during pregnancy by the presence, and even perhaps the conflicting interest, of two genomes (maternal and fetal) (for details, see Chapter 16). (5) The '*adaptive nature*' of the clinical manifestation has been proposed in the context of preterm labor with microbial invasion of the amniotic cavity, in which the onset of preterm labor and delivery can be considered as a mechanism of defense against intrauterine infection that allows the mother to eliminate an infected tissue by allowing the fetus to exit from a hostile environment. It is possible that other mechanisms of disease in preterm labor may also threaten the maternal/fetal pair, such as defects of the supply line, and so a key question to answer would be why some patients resort to fetal growth restriction, others to preeclampsia, and yet another group to the onset of preterm labor.

The same evidence outlined in the previous paragraph is available for preeclampsia. This condition has a characteristic phenotype: hypertension and proteinuria and also a common pathophysiological pathway responsible for the phenotype (poor placentation, oxidative-stressed placenta followed by a systemic inflammatory response including the endothelium). Preeclampsia has: (1) Multiple etiologies – it can occur with hydatidiform mole [115], 'Mirror syndrome' [116,117], or in the context of the first pregnancy of women at risk (e.g. women with metabolic syndrome). (2) A long preclinical phase has been known since 1973 when Gant *et al.* [118,119] reported that women destined to develop preeclampsia had an abnormal angiotensin II response at 22 weeks of gestation. Similarly, patients with a bilateral uterine artery notch in the Doppler waveform velocity are known to be at risk as early as the 24th week of gestation [120,121,122,123,124,125,126,127,128,129,130,131,132, 133] and, recently, changes in the Doppler waveform in the early second trimester have also been found to increase the risk for the development of the disease [134] (for details, see Chapter 22). The same can be said for change in the concentrations of antiangiogenic factors and angiogenic factors [135,136,137,138, 139,140,141,142,143,144,145,146,147,148,149,150,151, 152,153,154,155,156,157] (see Chapter 21 for details), as well as PP13 which can be uncovered as early as the first trimester [158,159,160,161,162]. (3) Fetal involvement can be demonstrated in preeclampsia because fetal growth restriction is present before the development of the disease in many cases [163]. (4) The adaptive nature of maternal hypertension was originally demonstrated by the classical experiments of Page *et al.* [164], in which ischemia of the pregnant uterus caused systemic maternal hypertension and a hysterectomy restored blood pressure to normal values indicating that the hypertension was the consequence of ischemia and not the cause (as many have believed). (5) Finally, genetic and environmental factors play a role in determining the risk of preeclampsia. For example, there is a rich literature documenting that preeclampsia clusters in families [165,166,167,168,169,170], linkage analysis [171,172,173,174,175,176,177,178] has identified chromosomal regions probably containing the genes conferring risk, and candidate genes have been identified [179]. Whole genome association studies are now in progress. Of interest is that DNA variants of both mothers and fetuses may confer risk. Moreover, such a risk is expressed not only by the mere carriage of a particular polymorphism but also the interaction between the fetal and maternal DNA variants and also 'maternal–fetal incompatibility' [180]. These would constitute examples of gene–gene interaction or epistasis. Examples of environmental factors that may modify the underlying genetic risk include the presence of obesity [181,182,183,184,185] or exposure to microbial products during early pregnancy which may increase the baseline risk [186,187,188]. The same arguments can be made for SGA, fetal death, and other great obstetrical syndromes (for more details, the reader is referred to Chapter 17).

We propose that pathology of the placental bed, primarily through ischemia, but perhaps through other mechanisms (e.g. immune related), may give rise to preeclampsia, small-for-gestational age, preterm labor with intact or ruptured membranes, abruptio placentae, and fetal death. Why a similar insult would result in a different clinical phenotype is dependent upon genetic and environmental factors, as well as the time of onset, duration, and extent of the ischemic insult. Evolutionary pressures derived from the potential conflictual relationship between the fetus and mother are likely to play a role.

Acknowledgment

This work was supported by the Perinatology Research Branch, Division of Intramural Research, *Eunice Kennedy Shriver* National Institute of Child Health and Human Development, NIH, DHHS.

References

1. Dixon H G, Robertson W B. A study of the vessels of the placental bed in normotensive and hypertensive women. *J Obstet Gynaecol Br Emp* 1958; **65**: 803–09.
2. Brosens I. A Study of the spiral arteries of the decidua basalis in normotensive and hypertensive pregnancies. *J Obstet Gynaecol Br Commonw* 1964; **71**: 222–30.
3. Browne J C, Veall N. The maternal placental blood flow in normotensive and hypertensive women. *J Obstet Gynaecol Br Emp* 1953; **60**: 141–7.
4. Meschia G. Techniques for the study of the uteroplacental circulation. In: Rosenfeld C R, ed. *The uterine circulation.* Ithaca, NY: Perinatology Press; 1989: pp. 35–51.
5. Clavero-Nunez J A. Uteroplacental blood flow in pregnant women: its measurement by radioisotope techniques. In: Moawad A H, Lindheimer M D, eds. *Uterine and placental blood flow.* New York: Masson Publishing USA, Inc.; 1982: pp. 53–9.
6. Brosens I, Robertson W B, Dixon H G. The physiological response of the vessels of the placental bed to normal pregnancy. *J Pathol Bacteriol* 1967; **93**: 569–79.

7. Brosens I A, Robertson W B, Dixon H G. The role of the spiral arteries in the pathogenesis of preeclampsia. *Obstet Gynecol Annu* 1972; **1**: 177–91.

8. Brosens I A. The uteroplacental vessels at term – the distribution and extent of physiological changes. *Trophoblast Res* 1988; **3**: 61–7.

9. Khong T Y, De Wolf F, Robertson W B, Brosens I. Inadequate maternal vascular response to placentation in pregnancies complicated by pre-eclampsia and by small-for-gestational age infants. *Br J Obstet Gynaecol* 1986; **93**: 1049–59.

10. Khong T Y, Liddell H S, Robertson W B. Defective haemochorial placentation as a cause of miscarriage: a preliminary study. *Br J Obstet Gynaecol* 1987; **94**: 649–55.

11. Michel M Z, Khong T Y, Clark D A, Beard R W. A morphological and immunological study of human placental bed biopsies in miscarriage. *Br J Obstet Gynaecol* 1990; **97**: 984–88.

12. Dommisse J, Tiltman A J. Placental bed biopsies in placental abruption. *Br J Obstet Gynaecol* 1992; **99**: 651–54.

13. Stone S, Pijnenborg R, Vercruysse L *et al.* The placental bed in pregnancies complicated by primary antiphospholipid syndrome. *Placenta* 2006; **27**: 457–67.

14. Kim Y M, Bujold E, Chaiworapongsa T *et al.* Failure of physiologic transformation of the spiral arteries in patients with preterm labor and intact membranes. *Am J Obstet Gynecol* 2003; **189**: 1063–69.

15. Kim Y M, Chaiworapongsa T, Gomez R *et al.* Failure of physiologic transformation of the spiral arteries in the placental bed in preterm premature rupture of membranes. *Am J Obstet Gynecol* 2002; **187**: 1137–42.

16. Romero R. Prenatal medicine: the child is the father of the man. *J Mat Fet Neonat Med*, in press.

17. Hustin J, Jauniaux E, Schaaps J P. Histological study of the materno-embryonic interface in spontaneous abortion. *Placenta* 1990; **11**: 477–86.

18. Gun B D, Numanoglu G, Ozdamar S O. The comparison of vessels in elective and spontaneous abortion decidua in first trimester pregnancies: importance of vascular changes in early pregnancy losses. *Acta Obstet Gynecol Scand* 2006; **85**: 402–6.

19. Ball E, Robson S C, Ayis S, Lyall F, Bulmer J N. Early embryonic demise: no evidence of abnormal spiral artery transformation or trophoblast invasion. *J Pathol* 2006; **208**: 528–34.

20. Ball E, Bulmer J N, Ayis S, Lyall F, Robson S C. Late sporadic miscarriage is associated with abnormalities in spiral artery transformation and trophoblast invasion. *J Pathol* 2006; **208**: 535–42.

21. Goldenberg R L, Culhane J F, Iams J D, Romero R. Epidemiology and causes of preterm birth. *Lancet* 2008; **371**: 75–84.

22. Romero R, Espinoza J, Kusanovic J P *et al.* The preterm parturition syndrome. *BJOG* 2006; **113** (Suppl 3): 17–42.

23. Naeye R L, Ross S M. Amniotic fluid infection syndrome. *Clin Obstet Gynaecol* 1982; **9**: 593–607.

24. Minkoff H. Prematurity: infection as an etiologic factor. *Obstet Gynecol* 1983; **62**: 137–44.

25. Romero R, Mazor M, Wu Y K *et al.* Infection in the pathogenesis of preterm labor. *Semin Perinatol* 1988; **12**: 262–79.

26. Romero R, Mazor M. Infection and preterm labor. *Clin Obstet Gynecol* 1988; **31**: 553–84.

27. Romero R, Sirtori M, Oyarzun E *et al.* Infection and labor. V. Prevalence, microbiology, and clinical significance of intraamniotic infection in women with preterm labor and intact membranes. *Am J Obstet Gynecol* 1989; **161**: 817–24.

28. Gibbs R S, Romero R, Hillier S L *et al.* A review of premature birth and subclinical infection. *Am J Obstet Gynecol* 1992; **166**: 1515–28.

29. Goldenberg R L, Hauth J C, Andrews W W. Intrauterine infection and preterm delivery. *N Engl J Med* 2000; **342**: 1500–7.

30. Yoon B H, Romero R, Moon J B *et al.* Clinical significance of intra-amniotic inflammation in patients with preterm labor and intact membranes. *Am J Obstet Gynecol* 2001; **185**: 1130–36.

31. Goncalves L F, Chaiworapongsa T, Romero R. Intrauterine infection and prematurity. *Ment Retard Dev Disabil Res Rev* 2002; **8**: 3–13.

32. Shim S S, Romero R, Hong J S *et al.* Clinical significance of intra-amniotic inflammation in patients with preterm premature rupture of membranes. *Am J Obstet Gynecol* 2004; **191**: 1339–45.

33. Kusanovic J P, Espinoza J, Romero R *et al.* Clinical significance of the presence of amniotic fluid 'sludge' in asymptomatic patients at high risk for spontaneous preterm delivery. *Ultrasound Obstet Gynecol* 2007; **30**: 706–14.

34. Romero R, Kusanovic J P, Espinoza J *et al.* What is amniotic fluid 'sludge'? *Ultrasound Obstet Gynecol* 2007; **30**: 793–98.

35. Romero R, Schaudinn C, Kusanovic J P *et al.* Detection of a microbial biofilm in intraamniotic infection. *Am J Obstet Gynecol* 2008; **198**: 135.

36. Arias F, Rodriquez L, Rayne S C, Kraus F T. Maternal placental vasculopathy and infection: two distinct subgroups among patients with preterm labor and

preterm ruptured membranes. *Am J Obstet Gynecol* 1993; **168**: 585–91.

37. Arias F, Victoria A, Cho K, Kraus F. Placental histology and clinical characteristics of patients with preterm premature rupture of membranes. *Obstet Gynecol* 1997; **89**: 265–71.
38. Iams J D, Johnson F F, Sonek J *et al.* Cervical competence as a continuum: a study of ultrasonographic cervical length and obstetric performance. *Am J Obstet Gynecol* 1995; **172**: 1097–103.
39. Hassan S S, Romero R, Berry S M *et al.* Patients with an ultrasonographic cervical length < or = 15 mm have nearly a 50% risk of early spontaneous preterm delivery. *Am J Obstet Gynecol* 2000; **182**: 1458–67.
40. Romero R, Espinoza J, Erez O, Hassan S. The role of cervical cerclage in obstetric practice: can the patient who could benefit from this procedure be identified? *Am J Obstet Gynecol* 2006; **194**: 1–9.
41. Phelan J P, Park Y W, Ahn M O, Rutherford S E. Polyhydramnios and perinatal outcome. *J Perinatol* 1990; **10**: 347–50.
42. Romero R, Sepulveda W, Baumann P *et al.* The preterm labor syndrome: biochemical, cytologic, immunologic, pathologic, microbiologic, and clinical evidence that preterm labor is a heterogeneous disease. *Am J Obstet Gynecol* 1993; **168**(1 part 2): 287.
43. Romero R, Mazor M, Avila C, Quintero R, Munoz H. Uterine "allergy": a novel mechanism for preterm labor. *Am J Obstet Gynecol* 1991; **164**(1 part 2): 375.
44. Garfield R E, Bytautiene E, Vedernikov Y P, Marshall J S, Romero R. Modulation of rat uterine contractility by mast cells and their mediators. *Am J Obstet Gynecol* 2000; **183**: 118–25.
45. Bytautiene E, Romero R, Vedernikov Y P *et al.* Induction of premature labor and delivery by allergic reaction and prevention by histamine H1 receptor antagonist. *Am J Obstet Gynecol* 2004; **191**: 1356–61.
46. Csapo A I, Pohanka O, Kaihola H L. Progesterone deficiency and premature labour. *Br Med J* 1974; **1**: 137–40.
47. Check J H, Lee G, Epstein R, Vetter B. Increased rate of preterm deliveries in untreated women with luteal phase deficiencies: preliminary report. *Gynecol Obstet Invest* 1992; **33**: 183–84.
48. Mazor M, Hershkovitz R, Chaim W *et al.* Human preterm birth is associated with systemic and local changes in progesterone/17 beta-estradiol ratios. *Am J Obstet Gynecol* 1994; **171**: 231–36.
49. Fidel P I Jr, Romero R, Maymon E, Hertelendy F. Bacteria-induced or bacterial product-induced preterm parturition in mice and rabbits is preceded by a significant fall in serum progesterone concentrations. *J Matern Fetal Med* 1998; **7**: 222–26.
50. Germain A M, Carvajal J, Sanchez M *et al.* Preterm labor: placental pathology and clinical correlation. *Obstet Gynecol* 1999; **94**: 284–89.
51. Combs C A, Katz M A, Kitzmiller J L, Brescia R J. Experimental preeclampsia produced by chronic constriction of the lower aorta: validation with longitudinal blood pressure measurements in conscious rhesus monkeys. *Am J Obstet Gynecol* 1993; **169**: 215–23.
52. Arias F. Placental insufficiency: an important cause of preterm labor and preterm premature ruptured membranes. *Society of Perinatal Obstetricians (10th Annual Meeting)* 1990; **158**.
53. Vintzileos A M, Campbell W A, Nochimson D J, Weinbaum P J. Preterm premature rupture of the membranes: a risk factor for the development of abruptio placentae. *Am J Obstet Gynecol* 1987; **156**: 1235–38.
54. Moretti M, Sibai B M. Maternal and perinatal outcome of expectant management of premature rupture of membranes in the midtrimester. *Am J Obstet Gynecol* 1988; **159**: 390–96.
55. Major C, Nageotte M, Lewis D. Preterm premature rupture of membranes and placental abruption: is there an association between these pregnancy complications? *Am J Obstet Gynecol* 1991; **164**: 381.
56. Brar H S, Medearis A L, DeVore G R, Platt L D. Maternal and fetal blood flow velocity waveforms in patients with preterm labor: prediction of successful tocolysis. *Am J Obstet Gynecol* 1988; **159**: 947–50.
57. Brar H S, Medearis A L, De Vore G R, Platt L D. Maternal and fetal blood flow velocity waveforms in patients with preterm labor: relationship to outcome. *Am J Obstet Gynecol* 1989; **161**: 1519–22.
58. Strigini F A, Lencioni G, De Luca G *et al.* Uterine artery velocimetry and spontaneous preterm delivery. *Obstet Gynecol* 1995; **85**: 374–77.
59. Weiner C P, Sabbagha R E, Vaisrub N, Depp R. A hypothetical model suggesting suboptimal intrauterine growth in infants delivered preterm. *Obstet Gynecol* 1985; **65**: 323–26.
60. MacGregor S N, Sabbagha R E, Tamura R K, Pielet B W, Feigenbaum S L. Differing fetal growth patterns in pregnancies complicated by preterm labor. *Obstet Gynecol* 1988; **72**: 834–37.
61. Ott W J. Intrauterine growth retardation and preterm delivery. *Am J Obstet Gynecol* 1993; **168**: 1710–15.
62. Zeitlin J, Ancel P Y, Saurel-Cubizolles M J, Papiernik E. The relationship between intrauterine growth restriction and preterm delivery: an empirical approach using data

from a European case-control study. *BJOG* 2000; **107**: 750–58.

63. Bukowski R, Gahn D, Denning J, Saade G. Impairment of growth in fetuses destined to deliver preterm. *Am J Obstet Gynecol* 2001; **185**: 463–67.

64. Morken N H, Kallen K, Jacobsson B. Fetal growth and onset of delivery: a nationwide population-based study of preterm infants. *Am J Obstet Gynecol* 2006; **195**: 154–61.

65. Espinoza J, Kusanovic J P, Kim C J *et al.* An episode of preterm labor is a risk factor for the birth of a small-for-gestational-age neonate. *Am J Obstet Gynecol* 2007; **196**: 574–75.

66. Poisner A M. The human placental renin-angiotensin system. *Front Neuroendocrinol* 1998; **19**: 232–52.

67. Katz M, Shapiro W B, Porush J G, Chou S Y, Israel V. Uterine and renal renin release after ligation of the uterine arteries in the pregnant rabbit. *Am J Obstet Gynecol* 1980; **136**: 676–78.

68. Woods L L, Brooks V L. Role of the renin-angiotensin system in hypertension during reduced uteroplacental perfusion pressure. *Am J Physiol* 1989; **257**: R204–R209.

69. Lalanne C, Mironneau C, Mironneau J, Savineau J P. Contractions of rat uterine smooth muscle induced by acetylcholine and angiotensin II in Ca^{2+}-free medium. *Br J Pharmacol* 1984; **81**: 317–26.

70. Campos G A, Guerra F A, Israel E J. Angiotensin II induced release of prostaglandins from rat uterus. *Arch Biol Med Exp (Santiago)* 1983; **16**: 43–9.

71. Lockwood C J, Krikun G, Papp C *et al.* The role of progestationally regulated stromal cell tissue factor and type-1 plasminogen activator inhibitor (PAI-1) in endometrial hemostasis and menstruation. *Ann N Y Acad Sci* 1994; **734**: 57–79.

72. Elovitz M A, Saunders T, Ascher-Landsberg J, Phillippe M. Effects of thrombin on myometrial contractions in vitro and in vivo. *Am J Obstet Gynecol* 2000; **183**: 799–804.

73. Rosen T, Schatz F, Kuczynski E *et al.* Thrombin-enhanced matrix metalloproteinase-1 expression: a mechanism linking placental abruption with premature rupture of the membranes. *J Matern Fetal Neonatal Med* 2002; **11**: 11–17.

74. Lockwood C J, Krikun G, Aigner S, Schatz F. Effects of thrombin on steroid-modulated cultured endometrial stromal cell fibrinolytic potential. *J Clin Endocrinol Metab* 1996; **81**: 107–12.

75. Lijnen H R. Matrix metalloproteinases and cellular fibrinolytic activity. *Biochemistry (Mos.)* 2002; **67**: 92–8.

76. Aplin J D, Campbell S, Allen T D. The extracellular matrix of human amniotic epithelium: ultrastructure, composition and deposition. *J Cell Sci* 1985; **79**: 119–36.

77. Chaiworapongsa T, Espinoza J, Yoshimatsu J *et al.* Activation of coagulation system in preterm labor and preterm premature rupture of membranes. *J Matern Fetal Neonatal Med* 2002; **11**: 368–73.

78. Gomez R, Athayde N, Pacora P *et al.* Increased thrombin in intrauterine inflammation. *Am J Obstet Gynecol* 1998; **178**: S62.

79. Rosen T, Kuczynski E, O'Neill L M, Funai E F, Lockwood C J. Plasma levels of thrombin-antithrombin complexes predict preterm premature rupture of the fetal membranes. *J Matern Fetal Med* 2001; **10**: 297–300.

80. Nagy S, Bush M, Stone J, Lapinski R H, Gardo S. Clinical significance of subchorionic and retroplacental hematomas detected in the first trimester of pregnancy. *Obstet Gynecol* 2003; **102**: 94–100.

81. Funderburk S J, Guthrie D, Meldrum D. Outcome of pregnancies complicated by early vaginal bleeding. *Br J Obstet Gynaecol* 1980; **87**: 100–5.

82. Williams M A, Mittendorf R, Lieberman E, Monson R R. Adverse infant outcomes associated with first-trimester vaginal bleeding. *Obstet Gynecol* 1991; **78**: 14–18.

83. Signore C C, Sood A K, Richards D S. Second-trimester vaginal bleeding: correlation of ultrasonographic findings with perinatal outcome. *Am J Obstet Gynecol* 1998; **178**: 336–40.

84. Gomez R, Romero R, Nien J K *et al.* Idiopathic vaginal bleeding during pregnancy as the only clinical manifestation of intrauterine infection. *J Matern Fetal Neonatal Med* 2005; **18**: 31–7.

85. Ananth C V, Wilcox A J. Placental abruption and perinatal mortality in the United States. *Am J Epidemiol* 2001; **153**: 332–37.

86. Mooney E E, al Shunnar A, O'Regan M, Gillan J E. Chorionic villous haemorrhage is associated with retroplacental haemorrhage. *Br J Obstet Gynaecol* 1994; **101**: 965–69.

87. Branch D W, Dudley D J, Scott J R, Silver R M. Antiphospholipid antibodies and fetal loss. *N Engl J Med* 1992; **326**: 952–54.

88. Stone S, Hunt B J, Seed P T *et al.* Longitudinal evaluation of markers of endothelial cell dysfunction and hemostasis in treated antiphospholipid syndrome and in healthy pregnancy. *Am J Obstet Gynecol* 2003; **188**: 454–60.

89. Abramowsky C R, Vegas M E, Swinehart G, Gyves M T. Decidual vasculopathy of the placenta in lupus erythematosus. *N Engl J Med* 1980; **303**: 668–72.

90. De Wolf F, Carreras L O, Moerman P *et al.* Decidual vasculopathy and extensive placental infarction in a patient with repeated thromboembolic accidents,

recurrent fetal loss, and a lupus anticoagulant. *Am J Obstet Gynecol* 1982; **142**: 829–34.

91. Out H J, Kooijman C D, Bruinse H W, Derksen R H. Histopathological findings in placentae from patients with intra-uterine fetal death and anti-phospholipid antibodies. *Eur J Obstet Gynecol Reprod Biol* 1991; **41**: 179–86.
92. Girardi G, Berman J, Redecha P *et al.* Complement C5a receptors and neutrophils mediate fetal injury in the antiphospholipid syndrome. *J Clin Invest* 2003; **112**: 1644–54.
93. Girardi G, Redecha P, Salmon J E. Heparin prevents antiphospholipid antibody-induced fetal loss by inhibiting complement activation. *Nat Med* 2004; **10**: 1222–26.
94. Sebire N J, Fox H, Backos M *et al.* Defective endovascular trophoblast invasion in primary antiphospholipid antibody syndrome-associated early pregnancy failure. *Hum Reprod* 2002; **17**: 1067–71.
95. Ferrara N, Carver-Moore K, Chen H *et al.* Heterozygous embryonic lethality induced by targeted inactivation of the VEGF gene. *Nature* 1996; **380**: 439–42.
96. Robinson J S, Kingston E J, Jones C T, Thorburn G D. Studies on experimental growth retardation in sheep: the effect of removal of endometrial caruncles on fetal size and metabolism. *J Dev Physiol* 1979; **1**: 379–98.
97. Robinson J S, Hart I C, Kingston E J, Jones C T, Thorburn G D. Studies on the growth of the fetal sheep. The effects of reduction of placental size on hormone concentration in fetal plasma. *J Dev Physiol* 1980; **2**: 239–48.
98. Falconer J, Owens J A, Allotta E, Robinson J S. Effect of restriction of placental growth on the concentrations of insulin, glucose and placental lactogen in the plasma of sheep. *J Endocrinol* 1985; **106**: 7–11.
99. Lockwood C J, Wein R, Lapinski R *et al.* The presence of cervical and vaginal fetal fibronectin predicts preterm delivery in an inner-city obstetric population. *Am J Obstet Gynecol* 1993; **169**: 798–804.
100. Iams J D, Goldenberg R L, Meis P J *et al.* The length of the cervix and the risk of spontaneous premature delivery: National Institute of Child Health and Human Development Maternal Fetal Medicine Unit Network. *N Eng J Med* 1996; **334**: 567–72.
101. Goldenberg R L, Mercer B M, Iams J D *et al.* The preterm prediction study: patterns of cervicovaginal fetal fibronectin as predictors of spontaneous preterm delivery: National Institute of Child Health and Human Development Maternal-Fetal Medicine Units Network. *Am J Obstet Gynecol* 1997; **177**: 8–12.
102. Taipale P, Hiilesmaa V. Sonographic measurement of uterine cervix at 18–22 weeks' gestation and the risk of preterm delivery. *Obstet Gynecol* 1998; **92**: 902–07.
103. Andrews W W, Copper R, Hauth J C *et al.* Second-trimester cervical ultrasound: associations with increased risk for recurrent early spontaneous delivery. *Obstet Gynecol* 2000; **95**: 222–26.
104. Goldenberg R L, Iams J D, Das A *et al.* The Preterm Prediction Study: sequential cervical length and fetal fibronectin testing for the prediction of spontaneous preterm birth: National Institute of Child Health and Human Development Maternal-Fetal Medicine Units Network. *Am J Obstet Gynecol* 2000; **182**: 636–43.
105. Heath V C, Daskalakis G, Zagaliki A, Carvalho M, Nicolaides K H. Cervicovaginal fibronectin and cervical length at 23 weeks of gestation: relative risk of early preterm delivery. *BJOG* 2000; **107**: 1276–81.
106. To M S, Skentou C, Liao A W, Cacho A, Nicolaides K H. Cervical length and funneling at 23 weeks of gestation in the prediction of spontaneous early preterm delivery. *Ultrasound Obstet Gynecol* 2001; **18**: 200–3.
107. Shennan A, Jones G, Hawken J *et al.* Fetal fibronectin test predicts delivery before 30 weeks of gestation in high risk women, but increases anxiety. *BJOG* 2005; **112**: 293–98.
108. Hassan S, Romero R, Hendler I *et al.* A sonographic short cervix as the only clinical manifestation of intra-amniotic infection. *J Perinat Med* 2006; **34**: 13–19.
109. Cassell G H, Davis R O, Waites K B *et al.* Isolation of Mycoplasma hominis and Ureaplasma urealyticum from amniotic fluid at 16–20 weeks of gestation: potential effect on outcome of pregnancy. *Sex Transm Dis* 1983; **10**: 294–302.
110. Gray D J, Robinson H B, Malone J, Thomson R B Jr. Adverse outcome in pregnancy following amniotic fluid isolation of Ureaplasma urealyticum. *Prenat Diagn* 1992; **12**: 111–17.
111. Horowitz S, Mazor M, Romero R, Horowitz J, Glezerman M. Infection of the amniotic cavity with Ureaplasma urealyticum in the midtrimester of pregnancy. *J Reprod Med* 1995; **40**: 375–79.
112. Gerber S, Vial Y, Hohlfeld P, Witkin S S. Detection of Ureaplasma urealyticum in second-trimester amniotic fluid by polymerase chain reaction correlates with subsequent preterm labor and delivery. *J Infect Dis* 2003; **187**: 518–21.
113. Nguyen D P, Gerber S, Hohlfeld P, Sandrine G, Witkin S S. Mycoplasma hominis in mid-trimester amniotic fluid: relation to pregnancy outcome. *J Perinat Med* 2004; **32**: 323–26.

114. Carroll S G, Papaioannou S, Ntumazah I L, Philpott-Howard J, Nicolaides K H. Lower genital tract swabs in the prediction of intrauterine infection in preterm prelabour rupture of the membranes. *Br J Obstet Gynaecol* 1996; **103**: 54–9.

115. Stepan H, Faber R. Cytomegalovirus-induced mirror syndrome associated with elevated levels of angiogenic factors. *Obstet Gynecol* 2007; **109**: 1205–6.

116. Espinoza J, Romero R, Nien J K *et al.* A role of the anti-angiogenic factor sVEGFR-1 in the 'mirror syndrome' (Ballantyne's syndrome). *J Matern Fetal Neonatal Med* 2006; **19**: 607–13.

117. Rana S, Venkatesha S, DePaepe M *et al.* Cytomegalovirus-induced mirror syndrome associated with elevated levels of circulating antiangiogenic factors. *Obstet Gynecol* 2007; **109**: 549–52.

118. Gant N F, Daley G L, Chand S, Whalley P J, MacDonald P C. A study of angiotensin II pressor response throughout primigravid pregnancy. *J Clin Invest* 1973; **52**: 2682–89.

119. Gant N F, Chand S, Whalley P J, MacDonald P C. The nature of pressor responsiveness to angiotensin II in human pregnancy. *Obstet Gynecol* 1974; **43**: 854.

120. Harrington K F, Campbell S, Bewley S, Bower S. Doppler velocimetry studies of the uterine artery in the early prediction of pre-eclampsia and intra-uterine growth retardation. *Eur J Obstet Gynecol Reprod Biol* 1991; **42** (Suppl): S14–S20.

121. Bower S, Bewley S, Campbell S. Improved prediction of preeclampsia by two-stage screening of uterine arteries using the early diastolic notch and color Doppler imaging. *Obstet Gynecol* 1993; **82**: 78–83.

122. Harrington K, Cooper D, Lees C, Hecher K, Campbell S. Doppler ultrasound of the uterine arteries: the importance of bilateral notching in the prediction of pre-eclampsia, placental abruption or delivery of a small-for-gestational-age baby. *Ultrasound Obstet Gynecol* 1996; **7**: 182–88.

123. Irion O, Masse J, Forest J C, Moutquin J M. Prediction of pre-eclampsia, low birthweight for gestation and prematurity by uterine artery blood flow velocity waveforms analysis in low risk nulliparous women. *Br J Obstet Gynaecol* 1998; **105**: 422–29.

124. Aardema M W, De Wolf B T, Saro M C *et al.* Quantification of the diastolic notch in Doppler ultrasound screening of uterine arteries. *Ultrasound Obstet Gynecol* 2000; **16**: 630–34.

125. Albaiges G, Missfelder-Lobos H, Lees C, Parra M, Nicolaides K H. One-stage screening for pregnancy complications by color Doppler assessment of the uterine arteries at 23 weeks' gestation. *Obstet Gynecol* 2000; **96**: 559–64.

126. Chien P F, Arnott N, Gordon A, Owen P, Khan K S. How useful is uterine artery Doppler flow velocimetry in the prediction of pre-eclampsia, intrauterine growth retardation and perinatal death? An overview. *BJOG* 2000; **107**: 196–208.

127. Lees C, Parra M, Missfelder-Lobos H *et al.* Individualized risk assessment for adverse pregnancy outcome by uterine artery Doppler at 23 weeks. *Obstet Gynecol* 2001; **98**: 369–73.

128. Papageorghiou A T, Yu C K, Bindra R, Pandis G, Nicolaides K H. Multicenter screening for pre-eclampsia and fetal growth restriction by transvaginal uterine artery Doppler at 23 weeks of gestation. *Ultrasound Obstet Gynecol* 2001; **18**: 441–49.

129. Papageorghiou A T, Yu C K, Cicero S, Bower S, Nicolaides K H. Second-trimester uterine artery Doppler screening in unselected populations: a review. *J Matern Fetal Neonatal Med* 2002; **12**: 78–88.

130. Yu C K, Papageorghiou A T, Boli A, Cacho A M, Nicolaides K H. Screening for pre-eclampsia and fetal growth restriction in twin pregnancies at 23 weeks of gestation by transvaginal uterine artery Doppler. *Ultrasound Obstet Gynecol* 2002; **20**: 535–40.

131. Papageorghiou A T, Yu C K, Erasmus I E, Cuckle H S, Nicolaides K H. Assessment of risk for the development of pre-eclampsia by maternal characteristics and uterine artery Doppler. *BJOG* 2005; **112**: 703–9.

132. Yu C K, Smith G C, Papageorghiou A T, Cacho A M, Nicolaides K H. An integrated model for the prediction of preeclampsia using maternal factors and uterine artery Doppler velocimetry in unselected low-risk women. *Am J Obstet Gynecol* 2005; **193**: 429–36.

133. Espinoza J, Romero R, Nien J K *et al.* Identification of patients at risk for early onset and/or severe preeclampsia with the use of uterine artery Doppler velocimetry and placental growth factor. *Am J Obstet Gynecol* 2007; **196**: 326.e1–326.e13.

134. Plasencia W, Maiz N, Poon L, Yu C, Nicolaides K H. Uterine artery Doppler at 11 + 0 to 13 + 6 weeks and 21 + 0 to 24 + 6 weeks in the prediction of pre-eclampsia. *Ultrasound Obstet Gynecol* 2008; **32**: 138–46.

135. Livingston J C, Haddad B, Gorski L A *et al.* Placenta growth factor is not an early marker for the development of severe preeclampsia. *Am J Obstet Gynecol* 2001; **184**: 1218–20.

136. Su Y N, Lee C N, Cheng W F *et al.* Decreased maternal serum placenta growth factor in early second trimester and preeclampsia. *Obstet Gynecol* 2001; **97**: 898–904.

137. Tidwell S C, Ho H N, Chiu W H, Torry R J, Torry D S. Low maternal serum levels of placenta growth factor as an antecedent of clinical preeclampsia. *Am J Obstet Gynecol* 2001; **184**: 1267–72.

138. Tjoa M L, van Vugt J M, Mulders M A *et al.* Plasma placenta growth factor levels in midtrimester pregnancies. *Obstet Gynecol* 2001; **98**: 600–7.

139. Chappell L C, Seed P T, Briley A *et al.* A longitudinal study of biochemical variables in women at risk of preeclampsia. *Am J Obstet Gynecol* 2002; **187**: 127–36.

140. Taylor R N, Grimwood J, Taylor R S *et al.* Longitudinal serum concentrations of placental growth factor: evidence for abnormal placental angiogenesis in pathologic pregnancies. *Am J Obstet Gynecol* 2003; **188**: 177–82.

141. Krauss T, Pauer H U, Augustin H G. Prospective analysis of placenta growth factor (PlGF) concentrations in the plasma of women with normal pregnancy and pregnancies complicated by preeclampsia. *Hypertens Pregnancy* 2004; **23**: 101–11.

142. Levine R J, Maynard S E, Qian C *et al.* Circulating angiogenic factors and the risk of preeclampsia. *N Engl J Med* 2004; **350**: 672–83.

143. Thadhani R, Mutter W P, Wolf M *et al.* First trimester placental growth factor and soluble fms-like tyrosine kinase 1 and risk for preeclampsia. *J Clin Endocrinol Metab* 2004; **89**: 770–75.

144. Chaiworapongsa T, Romero R, Kim Y M *et al.* Plasma soluble vascular endothelial growth factor receptor-1 concentration is elevated prior to the clinical diagnosis of pre-eclampsia. *J Matern Fetal Neonatal Med* 2005; **17**: 3–18.

145. Parra M, Rodrigo R, Barja P *et al.* Screening test for preeclampsia through assessment of uteroplacental blood flow and biochemical markers of oxidative stress and endothelial dysfunction. *Am J Obstet Gynecol* 2005; **193**: 1486–91.

146. Levine R J, Lam C, Qian C *et al.* Soluble endoglin and other circulating antiangiogenic factors in preeclampsia. *N Engl J Med* 2006; **355**: 992–1005.

147. Moore Simas T A, Crawford S L, Solitro M J *et al.* Angiogenic factors for the prediction of preeclampsia in high-risk women. *Am J Obstet Gynecol* 2007; **197**: 244–48.

148. Ohkuchi A, Hirashima C, Matsubara S *et al.* Alterations in placental growth factor levels before and after the onset of preeclampsia are more pronounced in women with early onset severe preeclampsia. *Hypertens Res* 2007; **30**: 151–59.

149. Robinson C J, Johnson D D. Soluble endoglin as a second-trimester marker for preeclampsia. *Am J Obstet Gynecol* 2007; **197**: 174–75.

150. Stepan H, Unversucht A, Wessel N, Faber R. Predictive value of maternal angiogenic factors in second trimester pregnancies with abnormal uterine perfusion. *Hypertension* 2007; **49**: 818–24.

151. Unal E R, Robinson C J, Johnson D D, Chang E Y. Second-trimester angiogenic factors as biomarkers for future-onset preeclampsia. *Am J Obstet Gynecol* 2007; **197**: 211–14.

152. Akolekar R, Zaragoza E, Poon L C, Pepes S, Nicolaides K H. Maternal serum placental growth factor at 11 + 0 to 13 + 6 weeks of gestation in the prediction of pre-eclampsia. *Ultrasound Obstet Gynecol* 2008; **32**: 732–39.

153. Baumann M U, Bersinger N A, Mohaupt M G *et al.* First-trimester serum levels of soluble endoglin and soluble fms-like tyrosine kinase-1 as first-trimester markers for late-onset preeclampsia. *Am J Obstet Gynecol* 2008; **199**: 266.

154. Crispi F, Llurba E, Dominguez C *et al.* Predictive value of angiogenic factors and uterine artery Doppler for early- versus late-onset pre-eclampsia and intrauterine growth restriction. *Ultrasound Obstet Gynecol* 2008; **31**: 303–9.

155. Erez O, Romero R, Espinoza J *et al.* The change in concentrations of angiogenic and anti-angiogenic factors in maternal plasma between the first and second trimesters in risk assessment for the subsequent development of preeclampsia and small-for-gestational age. *J Matern Fetal Neonatal Med* 2008; **21**: 279–87.

156. Lim J H, Kim S Y, Park S Y *et al.* Effective prediction of preeclampsia by a combined ratio of angiogenesis-related factors. *Obstet Gynecol* 2008; **111**: 1403–9.

157. Stepan H, Geipel A, Schwarz F *et al.* Circulatory soluble endoglin and its predictive value for preeclampsia in second-trimester pregnancies with abnormal uterine perfusion. *Am J Obstet Gynecol* 2008; **198**: 175–76.

158. Nicolaides K H, Bindra R, Turan O M *et al.* A novel approach to first-trimester screening for early pre-eclampsia combining serum PP-13 and Doppler ultrasound. *Ultrasound Obstet Gynecol* 2006; **27**: 13–17.

159. Chafetz I, Kuhnreich I, Sammar M *et al.* First-trimester placental protein 13 screening for preeclampsia and intrauterine growth restriction. *Am J Obstet Gynecol* 2007; **197**: 35–7.

160. Gonen R, Shahar R, Grimpel Y I *et al.* Placental protein 13 as an early marker for pre-eclampsia: a prospective longitudinal study. *BJOG* 2008; **115**: 1465–72.

161. Romero R, Kusanovic J P, Than N G *et al.* First-trimester maternal serum PP13 in the risk assessment for preeclampsia. *Am J Obstet Gynecol* 2008; **199**: 122.

162. Khalil A, Cowans N J, Spencer K *et al.* First trimester maternal serum placental protein 13 for the prediction of pre-eclampsia in women with a priori high risk. *Prenat Diagn*, in press.

163. McCowan L M, North R A, Harding J E. Abnormal uterine artery Doppler in small-for-gestational-age

pregnancies is associated with later hypertension. *Aust N Z J Obstet Gynaecol* 2001; **41**: 56–60.

164. Page E W. On the pathogenesis of pre-eclampsia and eclampsia. *J Obstet Gynaecol Br Commonw* 1972; **79**: 883–94.

165. Adams E M, Finlayson A. Familial aspects of pre-eclampsia and hypertension in pregnancy. *Lancet* 1961; **2**: 1375–78.

166. Chesley L C, Annitto J E, Cosgrove R A. The familial factor in toxemia of pregnancy. *Obstet Gynecol* 1968; **32**: 303–11.

167. Cooper D W, Liston W A. Genetic control of severe pre-eclampsia. *J Med Genet* 1979; **16**: 409–16.

168. Sutherland A, Cooper D W, Howie P W, Liston W A, MacGillivray I. The indicence of severe pre-eclampsia amongst mothers and mothers-in-law of pre-eclamptics and controls. *BJOG* 1981; **88**: 785–91.

169. Arngrimsson R, Bjornsson S, Geirsson R T *et al.* Genetic and familial predisposition to eclampsia and pre-eclampsia in a defined population. *BJOG* 1990; **97**: 762–69.

170. Alexander B T. Prenatal influences and endothelial dysfunction: a link between reduced placental perfusion and preeclampsia. *Hypertension* 2007; **49**: 775–76.

171. Harrison G A, Humphrey K E, Jones N *et al.* A genomewide linkage study of preeclampsia/eclampsia reveals evidence for a candidate region on 4q. *Am J Hum Genet* 1997; **60**: 1158–67.

172. Arngrimsson R, Sigurard T S, Frigge M L *et al.* A genome-wide scan reveals a maternal susceptibility locus for pre-eclampsia on chromosome 2p13. *Hum Mol Genet* 1999; **8**: 1799–805.

173. Moses E K, Lade J A, Guo G *et al.* A genome scan in families from Australia and New Zealand confirms the presence of a maternal susceptibility locus for pre-eclampsia, on chromosome 2. *Am J Hum Genet* 2000; **67**: 1581–85.

174. Lachmeijer A M, Arngrimsson R, Bastiaans E J *et al.* A genome-wide scan for preeclampsia in the Netherlands. *Eur J Hum Genet.* 2001; **9**: 758–64.

175. Laivuori H, Lahermo P, Ollikainen V *et al.* Susceptibility loci for preeclampsia on chromosomes 2p25 and 9p13 in Finnish families. *Am J Hum Genet.* 2003; **72**: 168–77.

176. Kalmyrzaev B, Aldashev A, Khalmatov M *et al.* Genome-wide scan for premature hypertension supports linkage to chromosome 2 in a large Kyrgyz family. *Hypertension* 2006; **48**: 908–13.

177. Moses E K, Fitzpatrick E, Freed K A *et al.* Objective prioritization of positional candidate genes at a quantitative trait locus for pre-eclampsia on 2q22. *Mol Hum Reprod* 2006; **12**: 505–12.

178. Johnson M P, Fitzpatrick E, Dyer T D *et al.* Identification of two novel quantitative trait loci for pre-eclampsia susceptibility on chromosomes 5q and 13q using a variance components-based linkage approach. *Mol Hum Reprod* 2007; **13**: 61–67.

179. Goddard K A, Tromp G, Romero R *et al.* Candidate-gene association study of mothers with pre-eclampsia, and their infants, analyzing 775 SNPs in 190 genes. *Hum Hered* 2007; **63**: 1–16.

180. Parimi N, Tromp G, Kuivaniemi H *et al.* Analytical approaches to detect maternal/fetal genotype incompatibilities that increase risk of pre-eclampsia. *BMC Med Genet* 2008; **9**: 60.

181. Stone J L, Lockwood C J, Berkowitz G S *et al.* Risk factors for severe preeclampsia. *Obstet Gynecol* 1994; **83**: 357–61.

182. Sibai B M, Gordon T, Thom E *et al.* Risk factors for preeclampsia in healthy nulliparous women: a prospective multicenter study. The National Institute of Child Health and Human Development Network of Maternal-Fetal Medicine Units. *Am J Obstet Gynecol* 1995; **172**: 642–48.

183. O'Brien T E, Ray J G, Chan W S. Maternal body mass index and the risk of preeclampsia: a systematic overview. *Epidemiology* 2003; **14**: 368–74.

184. Bodnar L M, Ness R B, Markovic N, Roberts J M. The risk of preeclampsia rises with increasing prepregnancy body mass index. *Ann Epidemiol* 2005; **15**: 475–82.

185. Bodnar L M, Catov J M, Klebanoff M A, Ness R B, Roberts J M. Prepregnancy body mass index and the occurrence of severe hypertensive disorders of pregnancy. *Epidemiology* 2007; **18**: 234–39.

186. Faas M M, Schuiling G A, Baller J F, Visscher C A, Bakker W W. A new animal model for human preeclampsia: ultra-low-dose endotoxin infusion in pregnant rats. *Am J Obstet Gynecol* 1994; **171**: 158–64.

187. Faas M M, Schuiling G A, Linton E A, Sargent I L, Redman C W. Activation of peripheral leukocytes in rat pregnancy and experimental preeclampsia. *Am J Obstet Gynecol* 2000; **182**: 351–57.

188. Conde-Agudelo A, Villar J, Lindheimer M. Maternal infection and risk of preeclampsia: systematic review and metaanalysis. *Am J Obstet Gynecol* 2008; **198**: 7–22.

Index

Note: Page numbers in *italics* refer to figures and tables.